DIFFERENTIAL DIAGNOSIS *of*

ORAL *and* MAXILLOFACIAL LESIONS

FIFTH EDITION

DIFFERENTIAL DIAGNOSIS *of*
ORAL *and*
MAXILLOFACIAL
LESIONS

NORMAN K. WOOD, D.D.S., M.S., Ph.D.
Professor of Oral Health Sciences,
Faculty of Medicine and Oral Health Sciences,
University of Alberta,
Edmonton, Alberta, Canada

PAUL W. GOAZ, B.S., D.D.S., S.M. (deceased)
Professor, Department of Oral Diagnosis and Oral Radiology,
Baylor Dental College,
Dallas, Texas

with 1343 illustrations and 120 color plates

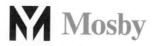

St. Louis Baltimore Boston Carlsbad Chicago Naples New York Philadelphia Portland
London Madrid Mexico City Singapore Sydney Tokyo Toronto Wiesbaden

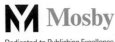

Mosby

Dedicated to Publishing Excellence

A Times Mirror Company

Publisher: Don Ladig
Executive Editor: Linda L. Duncan
Developmental Editor: Melba Steube
Project Manager: Carol Sullivan Weis
Production Editor: Rick Dudley
Designer: Sheilah Barrett
Manufacturing Manager: Dave Graybill

FIFTH EDITION

Copyright © 1997 by Mosby-Year Book, Inc.

Previous editions copyrighted 1975, 1980, 1985, 1991

Printed in the United States of America
Composition by TSI Graphics
Lithography/color film by Color Dot Graphics, Inc.
Printing/binding by The Maple-Vail Book Manufacturing Group

Mosby-Year Book, Inc.
11830 Westline Industrial Drive
St. Louis, Missouri 63146

Library of Congress Cataloging in Publication Data
Wood, Norman K. (Norman Kenyon), 1935-
    Differential diagnosis of oral and maxillofacial lesions / Norman
K. Wood, Paul W. Goaz. --5th ed.
      p. cm.
    Rev. ed. of: Differential diagnosis of oral lesions / Norman K.
Wood, Paul W. Goaz. 4th ed. c1991.
    Includes bibliographical references and index.
    ISBN 0-8151-9432-3
     1. Mouth—Diseases—Diagnosis.   2. Face—Diseases—Diagnosis.
3. Maxilla—Diseases—Diagnosis.   4. Diagnosis, Differential.
I. Goaz, Paul W., 1922-1995.   II. Wood, Norman K. (Norman Kenyon),
1935-   Differential diagnosis of oral lesions.   III. Title.
    [DNLM: 1. Mouth Diseases—diagnosis.   2. Diagnosis, Differential.
3. Maxillary Diseases—diagnosis.   WU 140 W877d 1996]
RC815.W66   1996
616.3' 1075--dc20
DNLM/DLC
for Library of Congress   96-7855
                                 CIP

97 98 99 00 / 9 8 7 6 5 4 3 2

Contributors

CHARLES B. BAKER, D.M.D., M.Sc.D., F.R.C.D.(C)
Professor and Head,
Division of Radiology,
Faculty of Medicine and Oral Health Sciences,
University of Alberta,
Edmonton, Alberta, Canada

BRUCE F. BARKER, D.D.S.
Professor of Oral Pathology,
Department of Oral Pathology,
University of Missouri, Kansas City,
School of Dentistry,
Kansas City, Missouri

RONALD J. BARR, M.D.
Professor, Departments of Dermatology and Pathology;
Director, Section of Dermal Pathology,
University of California,
Irvine, California

ROLLEY C. BATEMAN, D.D.S.
Professor Emeritus,
Department of Radiology,
Loyola University of Chicago,
School of Dentistry,
Maywood, Illinois

GEORGE G. BLOZIS, D.D.S., M.S.
Professor Emeritus,
Section of Diagnostic Services,
The Ohio State University,
College of Dentistry,
Columbus, Ohio

HENRY M. CHERRICK, D.D.S., M.S.D.
Professor of Dentistry,
School of Dentistry,
University of California at Los Angeles,
Center for Health Sciences,
Los Angeles, California

HENRY M. DICK, D.D.S., M.Sc., F.R.C.D.(C)
Professor Emeritus,
Faculty of Medicine and Oral Health Sciences,
University of Alberta,
Edmonton, Alberta, Canada

THOMAS E. EMMERING, D.D.S., F.I.C.D.
Formerly Professor,
Department of Dental Radiology,
Loyola University of Chicago,
School of Dentistry,
Maywood, Illinois

STUART L. FISCHMAN, D.M.D.
Professor of Oral Medicine,
School of Dental Medicine,
State University of New York at Buffalo;
Director of Dentistry,
Erie County Medical Center,
Buffalo, New York

RONALD E. GIER, D.M.D., M.S.D.
Professor, Department of Oral Diagnosis and Oral Radiology,
University of Missouri, Kansas City,
School of Dentistry,
Kansas City, Missouri

MARIE C. JACOBS, D.D.S.
Formerly Professor,
Department of Oral Diagnosis, Pathology, and Radiology,
Loyola University of Chicago,
School of Dentistry,
Maywood, Illinois

JERALD L. JENSEN, D.D.S., M.S.
Oral Pathologist, Laboratory Service,
Veterans Administration Medical Center,
Long Beach, California;
Associate Clinical Professor of Pathology,
University of California,
Irvine, California

ROGER H. KALLAL, D.D.S., M.S.
Professor, Clinical Orthodontics,
Department of Orthodontics,
Northwestern University Dental School;
Attending Oral and Maxillofacial Surgeon,
Northwestern Memorial Hospital;
Private Practice of Oral Surgery and Maxillofacial Surgery,
Chicago, Illinois

IRIS M. KUC, D.D.S., Ph.D.
Associate Professor of Oral Health Sciences,
Faculty of Medicine and Oral Health Sciences,
University of Alberta,
Edmonton, Alberta, Canada

JAMES F. LENNERT, D.D.S.
Formerly Associate Professor,
Department of Oral Diagnosis, Pathology, and Radiology;
Director, Division of Oral Diagnosis,
Loyola University of Chicago,
School of Dentistry,
Maywood, Illinois;
Attending, Foster McGaw Hospital,
Maywood, Illinois

THOMAS M. LUND, D.D.S., M.S.
Professor Emeritus,
Northwestern University Dental School,
Chicago, Illinois

RUSSELL J. NISENGARD, D.D.S., Ph.D.
Professor of Periodontology and Microbiology,
State University of New York at Buffalo,
Schools of Dental Medicine and Medicine,
Buffalo, New York

DANIEL J. PEHOWICH, B.Sc., Ph.D.
Associate Professor of Physiology,
Faculty of Medical and Oral Health Sciences,
University of Alberta,
Edmonton, Alberta, Canada

EDWARD PETERS, D.D.S., Ph.D.
Professor of Pathology,
Faculty of Medicine and Oral Health Sciences,
University of Alberta,
Edmonton, Alberta, Canada

DANNY R. SAWYER, D.D.S., Ph.D.
Professor and Chairman,
Department of Oral Diagnosis and Radiology,
School of Dentistry;
Professor of Pathology,
School of Medicine,
Case Western Reserve University,
Cleveland, Ohio

ORION H. STUTEVILLE, D.D.S., M.D.S., M.D.†
Professor Emeritus of Surgery and Former Chief,
Section of Plastic Surgery,
Loyola University of Chicago,
School of Medicine,
Maywood, Illinois

RAYMOND L. WARPEHA, D.D.S., M.D., Ph.D.
Professor and Chairman,
Division of Plastic Surgery,
Loyola University of Chicago,
School of Medicine,
Maywood, Illinois

†Deceased.

Preface

The purposes of this book remain the same: (1) to serve as an interface textbook between oral pathology/oral medicine/oral radiology and clinical practice, (2) to simplify the classification of lesions by clinical or radiographic appearances, and (3) to help the practitioner arrive at a working (clinical) diagnosis through the differential diagnosis process.

The expanded title of this edition to include *maxillofacial* lesions gives a truer indication of the regions covered. Lesions of the face, neck, lips, and jawbones are covered, as well as lesions of the oral soft tissues. This also follows the trend set in recent years by oral pathology, oral surgery, and oral radiology academies and some journals.

The present edition represents a major overhaul. This is due in part to the author's other responsibilities during the preparation of the previous edition, which precluded heavy revision. Much new information has appeared during the last 5 years as well. The following housekeeping chores have been rigorously attended to: (1) redundancy has been significantly reduced; (2) more crispness of expression, simpler sentence structure, and clarity of wording has been accomplished for improved readability and understanding; (3) up-to-the-minute references have been introduced and selected older ones retained; (4) the reference style has been changed from author names to numbers for both conciseness and unhindered thought; and (5) pictures have been cropped judiciously so that the lesion is shown with just enough anatomic landmarks to identify location. This makes the lesion itself larger, clearer, and more prominent.

The following changes have been made in content. In Chapter 2, discussion of the patient history section and a detailed treatment of radiologic views have been deleted or condensed because more thorough works are available from other sources. This leaves room for deeper discussion of material more pertinent to our book. Some ranking of lesions according to frequency has been changed because of new literature and quiet reflection. Some fairly common lesions left out of former editions have been included in this edition. More rarities gathered from the monthly journals have been included in their proper place, often with references.

Chapters 35 (Oral Cancer), 36 (AIDS), and 37 (Viral Hepatitis) have been added. A variety of pulpoperiapical lesions that produce various radiographic changes in the bony and soft tissue floor of the maxillary sinus have been added to Chapter 16 (Periapical Radiolucencies). Both candidiasis and oral cancer are discussed in much greater detail and current methods of management dealt with at length.

All illustrations have been carefully reviewed. Many black and white pictures have been replaced with more characteristic examples or better quality pictures. Judicious cropping has helped also. The color plates have been much improved in quality and the numbers more than doubled. New Plates E through H are devoted to the many appearances and types of oral cancer. These are arguably among the best collections of colored pictures of oral cancer available today. Recent shifts in philosophy and specific information that appeared in literature during the past 6 years have been included throughout. A new index more suitable to the differential style of the textbook has been developed.

As in past editions, the author is indebted to many confreres who have helped with the preparation of the fifth edition. Authors and coauthors are listed at the head of chapters. Numerous colleagues have supplied excellent slides from their personal collections, and others have given permission to use previously published information, charts, tables, or pictures. In this regard, I mention the material borrowed from an article by Dr. L. Gold, et al, on the uniform use of surgical procedure terms, which we have included in the introduction to the Bony Lesions section. We have endeavored to use correct surgical procedure terms throughout discussions of the management of bony lesions. Global usage of a uniform system would make the surgical literature more meaningful and enrich assessment of various procedures.

I am indebted to Ms. Colleen Murdock, who kindly gave much assistance in printing a number of black and white glossies. I especially express my deepest gratitude to my wife Carole, who typed the manuscripts of new chapters and altered other chapters using the material provided on diskettes by the publisher.

NORMAN K. WOOD

Contents

1 Introduction, 1

PART I

GENERAL PRINCIPLES OF DIFFERENTIAL DIAGNOSIS

2 History and Examination of the Patient, 5
Norman K. Wood and Paul W. Goaz

3 Correlation of Gross Structure and Microstructure with Clinical Features, 14
Norman K. Wood and Paul W. Goaz

4 The Diagnostic Sequence, 39
Norman K. Wood

PART II

SOFT TISSUE LESIONS

5 Solitary Red Lesions, 49
Norman K. Wood, Edward Peters, and George G. Blozis

6 Generalized Red Conditions and Multiple Ulcerations, 71
Stuart L. Fischman, Russell J. Nisengard, and George G. Blozis

7 Red Conditions of the Tongue, 90
Norman K. Wood and George G. Blozis

8 White Lesions of the Oral Mucosa, 96
Norman K. Wood and Paul W. Goaz

9 Red and White Lesions, 127
Norman K. Wood and Henry M. Dick

10 Peripheral Oral Exophytic Lesions, 130
Norman K. Wood and Paul W. Goaz

11 Solitary Oral Ulcers and Fissures, 162
Norman K. Wood and Paul W. Goaz

12 Intraoral Brownish, Bluish, or Black Conditions, 182
Norman K. Wood, Paul W. Goaz, and Danny R. Sawyer

13 Pits, Fistulae, and Draining Lesions, 209
Henry M. Cherrick and Norman K. Wood

14 Yellow Conditions of the Oral Mucosa, 225
Ronald E. Gier

PART III

BONY LESIONS

Section A   Radiolucencies of the Jaws

15 Anatomic Radiolucencies, 238
Norman K. Wood and Paul W. Goaz

16 Periapical Radiolucencies, 252
Norman K. Wood, Paul W. Goaz, and Marie C. Jacobs

17 Pericoronal Radiolucencies, 279
Norman K. Wood and Iris M. Kuc

18 Interradicular Radiolucencies, 296
Norman K. Wood and Charles G. Baker

19 Solitary Cystlike Radiolucencies Not Necessarily Contacting Teeth, 309
Norman K. Wood and Paul W. Goaz

20 Multilocular Radiolucencies, 333
Norman K. Wood, Paul W. Goaz, and Roger H. Kallal

21 Solitary Radiolucencies with Ragged and Poorly Defined Borders, 356
Norman K. Wood, Paul W. Goaz, and Orion H. Stuteville

22 Multiple Separate, Well-Defined Radiolucencies, 380
Norman K. Wood, Paul W. Goaz, and Marie C. Jacobs

23 Generalized Rarefactions of the Jawbones, 392
Norman K. Wood, Daniel J. Pehowich, and Rolley C. Bateman

Section B   Radiolucent Lesions with Radiopaque Foci or Mixed Radiolucent-Radiopaque Lesions

24 Mixed Radiolucent-Radiopaque Lesions Associated with Teeth, 415
Norman K. Wood, Paul W. Goaz, and James F. Lehnert

25 Mixed Radiolucent-Radiopaque Lesions Not Necessarily Contacting Teeth, 433
Norman K. Wood and Paul W. Goaz

Section C   Radiopacities of the Jawbones

26 Anatomic Radiopacities of the Jaws, 449
Thomas M. Lund and Norman K. Wood

xi

27 Periapical Radiopacities, 457
Norman K. Wood, Paul W. Goaz, and James F. Lehnert

28 Solitary Radiopacities Not Necessarily Contacting Teeth, 477
Norman K. Wood and Paul W. Goaz

29 Multiple Separate Radiopacities, 500
Norman K. Wood and Paul W. Goaz

30 Generalizcd Radiopacities, 509
Thomas E. Emmering and Norman K. Wood

PART IV

LESIONS BY REGION

31 Masses in the Neck, 521
Raymond L. Warpeha

32 Lesions of the Facial Skin, 540
Jerald L. Jensen and Ronald J. Barr

33 Lesions of the Lips, 561
Bruce F. Barker

34 Intraoral Lesions by Anatomic Region, 580
Danny R. Sawyer and Norman K. Wood

PART V

ADDITIONAL SUBJECTS

35 Oral Cancer, 587
Norman K. Wood and Danny R. Sawyer

36 Acquired Immunodeficiency Syndrome, 596
Norman K. Wood and Danny R. Sawyer

37 Viral IIepatitis, 611
James F. Lehnert and Norman K. Wood

APPENDIX A Lesions of Bone That May Have Two or More Major Radiographic Appearances, 620

APPENDIX B Normal Values for Laboratory Tests, 621

COLOR PLATES A-D, 82-83
E-I, 466-467

Differential Diagnosis *of*

Oral *and* Maxillofacial Lesions

CHAPTER 1

Introduction

The objective of this text is to present a systematic discussion of the differential diagnosis of oral lesions based on a classification of lesions, which are grouped according to their similar clinical or radiographic appearances.

Part I consists of three *preparatory chapters.* Chapter 2 is devoted to a review of pertinent steps and modalities to follow in the examination of the patient. Chapter 3 explains on a functional and histologic basis the clinical and radiographic features of lesions discovered during the clinical examination. Chapter 4 outlines the diagnostic sequence we prefer, commencing with the detection of the lesion and progressing through intermediate steps until a final diagnosis is established.

Parts II and III make up the *differential diagnosis section* of the text, which deals with the specific disease entities. Part II is devoted primarily to the soft tissue lesions (Chapters 5 to 14), and Part III deals with lesions that originate in bone (Chapters 15 to 30). In each part the individual entities are classified into groups consisting of similar-appearing lesions, and each group forms the subject of a chapter.

Part IV is devoted to the presentation and discussion of lesions according to specific anatomic location. Thus Chapters 31 to 34 deal with masses in the neck, lesions of the facial skin, lesions of the lips, and intraoral lesions by anatomic region.

Part V deals with additional subjects. Thus Chapters 35 to 37 present oral cancer, acquired immunodeficiency syndrome (AIDS), and viral hepatitis.

Although our text is primarily for the clinician, the microscopic picture is also discussed, but this aspect is stressed only when it contributes to the recognition and comprehension of the clinical or radiologic features. This approach evolved from our observation of dental students entering the clinic and encountering great difficulty as they attempted to relate their knowledge of histopathology to the clinical features of lesions. Apparently, students experience this difficulty because, first, they are not adequately instructed in the simple but meaningful correlations between the histologic and clinical pictures. Second, they

lack experience in the grouping of lesions according to clinical and radiographic appearances, which is necessary before a usable differential diagnosis can be developed.

Of course, there are several excellent textbooks of oral pathology that complement the clinical study of oral lesions, but these books classify and discuss lesions according to etiology, tissue of origin, microscopic nature, or areas of occurrence. Although such an approach has proved to be effective for presenting a course in pathology, our experience has shown it to be cumbersome. In an attempt to alleviate this problem, we group and discuss lesions according to their clinical or radiographic appearance. Regardless of etiology or area of occurrence, *all similar-appearing lesions are grouped together* and discussed in the same chapter.

Although some experts may object to our particular ranking of lesions, no inerrant authority is claimed. We have attempted to rank the entities in each category according to *frequency of occurrence*—with the discussion of the most common being first. The very rare lesions are simply listed. This particular arrangement was borne out of our personal experience, as well as from our assessment of other authors' statistics.* It is not intended to be an authoritative statement but merely an aid to the clinician in the development of a differential diagnosis.

Our ranking of lesions must be taken in the general context of this book, since different frequency rates occur in different age groups and are modified by socioeconomics, as well as by cultural and geographic factors. Also, new journal articles may modify these rankings from time to time, but we doubt that these changes will detract significantly from the usefulness of the arrangement presented here.

Pathoses of the dental hard tissues, gingivitis, temporomandibular joint problems, and facial and oral pain

---

*We are particularly indebted to Drs. Charles Halstead and Dwight Weathers[1] of Emory University, who have graciously made available to us statistical rankings from their extensive computerized study on the differential diagnosis of oral lesions.

have been excluded because they are adequately discussed elsewhere. In some cases, entire books have been devoted to these difficult and sometimes unresolvable diagnostic problems.

It is important to recognize that discussions of entities included in this text are not intended to be exhaustive descriptions of any disease but only to present pertinent points that will minimize confusion and contribute to the development of a differential diagnosis. Specifically, we have avoided controversial issues concerning etiology and tissue of origin that are unresolved, since they have been exhaustively discussed in other sources and contribute little that is clinically useful to the dental practitioner.

Also, the discussions of the features of particular lesions have not been specifically subdivided on the basis of clinical, radiographic, and histologic characteristics. On the contrary, these have been blended in an attempt to illustrate how the three disciplines interrelate and to aid in the explanation of the features found in each.

Again the primary aim of this book is to provide the clinician with the pertinent features of relatively common oral diseases that we consider necessary to the differentiation of similar-appearing lesions.

The diagnoses that appear in the descriptions of the reproduction of the clinical pictures and radiographs have been determined by microscopic examination in the vast majority of cases.

REFERENCE

1. Halstead CL, Weathers DR: *Differential diagnosis of oral soft tissue pathoses: site unit(s)-3379: instructional materials for health professional education,* National Library of Medicine/National Medical Audiovisual Center, Washington, DC, 1977, US Department of Health, Education, and Welfare.

PART I

GENERAL PRINCIPLES
OF DIFFERENTIAL DIAGNOSIS

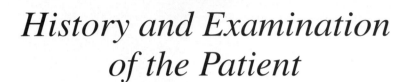

CHAPTER 2

History and Examination of the Patient

NORMAN K. WOOD

PAUL W. GOAZ

Collecting the information necessary to determine the cause of a patient's complaint is accomplished by determining the patient's medical and dental history and performing a physical examination. Properly performed, the history and physical examination are frequently the most definitive of the diagnostic procedures. Without the information provided by the history and physical examination, the diagnostic process is reduced to hazardous speculation. These diagnostic procedures include the following:

RECORDING THE IDENTIFYING DATA
HISTORY AND PHYSICAL
    EXAMINATION
CHIEF COMPLAINT
PRESENT ILLNESS
PAST MEDICAL HISTORY
    Family history
    Social history
    Occupational history
    Dental history
REVIEW OF SYMPTOMS BY SYSTEM

PHYSICAL EXAMINATION
    Radiologic examination
DIFFERENTIAL DIAGNOSIS
WORKING DIAGNOSIS
    Medical laboratory studies
    Dental laboratory studies
    Biopsy
      Incisional
      Excisional
      Fine-needle aspiration
    Exfoliative cytology

    Toluidine blue staining
    Consultation
FINAL DIAGNOSIS
TREATMENT PLAN

HISTORY AND PHYSICAL EXAMINATION

The reader is referred to other books[1-4] for information on history and physical examination because space does not permit an adequate description of these aspects. Oral chief complaints are detailed in Chapter 4, and physical characteristics of lesions and masses are covered in Chapter 3.

Radiologic Examination

The use of diagnostic radiology is not routinely prescribed. After completion of the history and physical examination, the examiner may order pertinent views that will most likely contribute to the further description and diagnosis of the lesion. Radiographs should never be accepted as the sole criterion for the diagnosis or selection of treatment.

Most routine examinations may require one or more of the following traditional radiographic projections whose images are produced on film:

I. Intraoral radiographic examinations; periapical, interproximal (bitewing), and occlusal projections[5]

II. Extraoral radiographic examinations of oral and perioral areas

    A. Panoramic projection

B. Lateral oblique projection
1. Mandibular (anterior or posterior) body projection
2. Mandibular ramus projection
C. Skull projections
1. Posteroanterior (anteroposterior) projection
2. Lateral skull (cephalometric) projection
D. Facial projections
1. Waters' projection
2. Submentovertex projection
3. Reverse Towne's projection
E. Temporomandibular joint projection
1. Transpharyngeal (infracranial) projection
2. Transorbital (Zimmer) projection
3. Facial projections
F. Conventional tomography

For a description of the structures that these technical procedures demonstrate and how they are performed, see Goaz and White.[6]

Panoramic radiography. The mechanics and images of panoramic radiography have been described adequately elsewhere.[6-8] The finer detail obtained by intraoral radiation source machines has been described by Jensen.[9]

Conventional tomography (laminography) Often, images produced by the previously described techniques are obscured because of superimposition of details of the complete thickness of the anatomic region radiographed. Tomography eliminates this superimposition by selectively imaging a layer or "slice" of an object so that it may be clearly seen, while overlying and underlying structures are blurred or not imaged at all. For a description of the technology, the reader is referred elsewhere.[6,10]

The basic principle applied in conventional tomography is also used in computed tomography (CT), sonography, single-photon emission tomography, positron emission tomography, and magnetic resonance imaging (MRI).

In general, motion tomography finds its major application in imaging fine-detail, high-contrast objects. In dentistry, tomography is frequently used for the demonstration of the temporomandibular joint (Fig. 2-1) and for the identification and location of facial fractures. Tomograms in straight anteroposterior and lateral views assess more accurately than plain films the extent of both soft tissue disease and bony destruction of the paranasal sinuses.[11]

Computer-Assisted Imaging

Developments and refinements in imaging technology have appeared with the advent of scanning and digital computer techniques to supplement the information gained by traditional radiology. These developments permit discrimination between small differences in physical densities and tend to eliminate the confusion caused by superimposition. In addition, these new imaging technologies have provided access to lesions in such areas as the pharyngeal space and the pterygopalatine fossa that were not easily evaluated by conventional x-ray imaging. Some

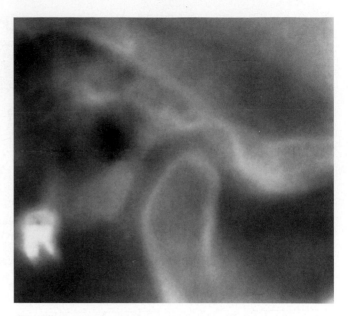

Fig. 2-1. Lateral tomography of right temporomandibular joint.

of the modern imaging procedures such as digital radiography, subtraction radiography, CT, radionuclide scanning, MRI, and ultrasound imaging are introduced here. More detailed information may be found elsewhere.[6]

Digital radiography Digital radiography (digital x-ray imaging) is a technique that is fundamental to CT, MRI, diagnostic ultrasound, nuclear medicine, and even film radiography. The remnant beam of x-rays is directed onto a phosphor screen instead of a film. The screen is scanned by a television type of camera whose output is directed into a data acquisition system (digital computer). The computer digitizes the image, that is, divides the image into small areas, or pixels, and assigns a number to each pixel proportional to the intensity of the light at that pixel. These numbers can be stored in the computer and used to reconstruct the original image on a TV monitor by converting the numbers to light of appropriate intensity. The computer or digital processor performs a variety of functions, including: (1) image acquisition control, (2) image reconstruction, (3) image storage and retrieval, (4) image processing, and (5) image analysis. Unlike the other techniques described here, the digital imaging equipment does not provide a cross-sectional image.

The image from a conventional radiograph can also be digitized, improved, and stored for future viewing. To improve the quality of an image, the operator manipulates its pixel numbers, thereby changing the density and contrast of selected areas or of the entire image (Fig. 2-2).

Subtraction radiography. Subtraction radiography is an extension of digital radiography. To subtract images, the computer digitizes two radiographs of the same area and electronically subtracts the numbers representing the intensity of light at each pixel of the second radiograph from the numbers in analogous locations on the first radi-

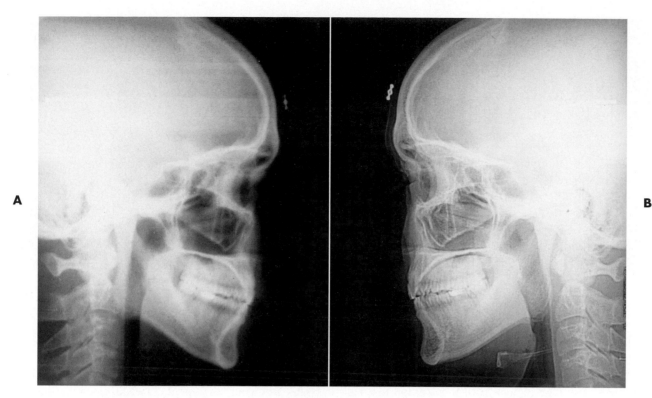

Fig. 2-2. Comparison of **A,** a conventional lateral cephalometric projection with **B,** a view of the video conversion of its digitized image, illustrating the increase in detail achieved by contrast modification. (Courtesy Peter H. Buschang, Dallas.)

ograph. If the two films are made one before and one after an event such as bone loss in an area, the area of change will be the only image that is clearly apparent (without superimpositions) on the subtracted image.

The greatest use of subtraction techniques in dentistry are being applied to the detection of changes in alveolar bone.[12] Currently it is best described as a subject for research rather than a routine methodology for the evaluation of changes in the periodontal apparatus.

Computed tomography CT, originally termed *computerized axial tomography* or *computer-assisted tomography,* has since been referred to as computerized reconstruction tomography, computed tomographic scanning, axial tomography, and computerized transaxial tomography. The acronym "CAT," or "CAT scan," appears in the literature. However, CT is now the preferred abbreviation in the diagnostic radiographic literature.[13]

In CT, a fan-shaped x-ray beam is rotated around the patient, along with a ring of detector elements that detect the remnant radiation. The detectors convert the radiation to electric impulses that are in turn fed into a digital computer, which then constructs an image of the "slice" through the regional tissues. This image may be projected onto a TV display, stored on magnetic tape, or converted to a hard copy (Fig. 2-3). The primary advantage of this system is that it eliminates superimposition of structures.

CT scanning can also distinguish between tissues that differ in physical density by less than 1%, in contrast to the 10% difference required by conventional radiology.[14,15] Although computer scanning of the oral cavity is not practical because of the artifacts caused by dental restorations (Fig. 2-4), it is frequently useful in determining how far a lesion may have extended from the oral cavity into the base of the skull, cervical spine, or paranasal sinuses.[16] A more detailed image of the paranasal sinuses, the nasopharynx, or the base of the skull and surrounding area is possible with CT than with conventional tomography.[17] CT has been described by some as the method of choice for evaluating salivary masses.[18] It is also more reliable for the evaluation of tumor extent, but it does not image in the sagittal plane, nor does it readily distinguish between tumor and inflammatory change in the sinuses.[19] For a detailed description of the physical principles of CT, as well as how to interpret the CT image, see Sprawls[20] and Valvassori et al.[21]

Radionuclide imaging Radionuclide imaging takes advantage of the propensity of particular substances to concentrate selectively in certain "target" tissues and organs. These substances can be chemically tagged with radionuclides, and in some cases the ionic form of a nuclide selectively concentrates at the "target." The radionuclides used for this procedure are γ-ray producers with relatively

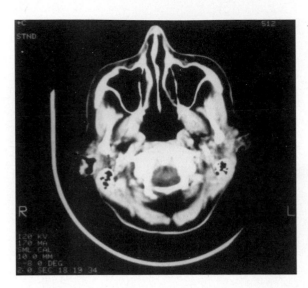

Fig. 2-3. Computed tomography scan. Such features as the nasal cavity and septum, nasopharynx, maxillary sinus, zygoma, mandibular ramus, lateral pterygoid muscles, mastoid processes, and air cells can be seen.

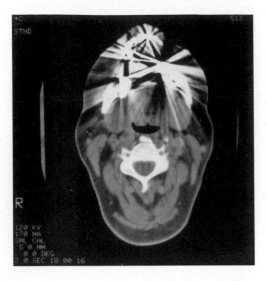

Fig. 2-4. Computed tomography scan illustrating artifacts produced by metal dental restorations.

short half-lives (a few hours to a day). These agents are injected or ingested. The γ-rays from the isotope that has concentrated at a particular area in the body are then detected by a gamma camera that converts the energy to electric impulses that are used by a computer to form an image on a cathode ray tube, transfer it to a film (Polaroid or x-ray), or store it for future viewing.[13]

The radionuclide imaging techniques delineate areas of increased or decreased metabolism (Fig. 2-5). To determine the cause of the altered function, the clinician must qualify this information with other diagnostic tests and clinical deductions. This technique demonstrates abnormalities in tissue and the extent of these changes even before they are demonstrable on routine radiographs.[22,23]

Bone resorption and formation such as bony metastases, primary bone tumors, infections, metabolic bone diseases, and stress fractures may be detected with this technique.[24] Scintigraphy is a "part of the standard diagnostic program in planning the therapy of malignant tumors of the oral cavity."[25] The technique has been used as an indication of the rate of alveolar crest bone loss, and the results are verifiable by sequential radiographic examinations. This examination delivers a radiation dose of less than 0.5 rem to the individual.[26]

A variation of this nuclear imaging is *positron emission tomography,* in which the radiopharmaceuticals are labeled with positron-emitting isotopes ($^{11}C, ^{18}F, ^{13}N, ^{15}O$) and the gamma camera is moved around the patient. The information from the camera is analyzed by a computer, which constructs sectional images using the same mathematical models used in computed tomography.[27]

Magnetic resonance imaging Chemical elements with nuclei that have an odd number of nucleons have a magnetic moment and a characteristic resonant frequency (in the FM radio range) when placed in a magnetic field. This frequency is unique to each element (nuclei) and varies with the strength of the magnetic field. If such elements are subjected to electromagnetic radiation (EMR) when they are in a magnetic field, they absorb energy and radiate it when the EMR is terminated. Since hydrogen represents at least 60% of the atoms in the body and hydrogen has the strongest MRI signal, most MRI systems are tuned to the resonant frequency of hydrogen.[28] These radio signals from hydrogen are detected by an antenna (field coil[s]), and a computer constructs the MR image, which is displayed on a TV screen that is similar to that used by the CT scanner. It may also be recorded on film or magnetic tape for later interpretation.

MRI is being adapted for use in the diagnosis of almost all body organs and systems. MRI images of normal and abnormal tissues have better contrast and resolution than CT (Fig. 2-6). Because of these improved image characteristics, tumor margins in the nasopharynx, oropharynx, and base of the skull are more sharply represented. MRI has proved useful for demonstrating the oral cavity, temporomandibular joint, and salivary glands. It can also differentiate between muscles, tonsils, mucosa, and lymph nodes. In contrast to CT, there is an absence of artifact generation by dental restorations. In CT, these artifacts frequently obscure regions of the oropharynx. Also, major blood vessels can be visualized in MRI without contrast medium, and images of transverse, coronal, and sagittal sections can be produced without repositioning the patient as is necessary with CT.

A disadvantage of MRI is its poor visualization of air spaces, subtle osseous abnormalities, and bone in general. The low concentration of magnetic nuclei in air and the rigid fixation of hydrogen in the bony matrix (pre-

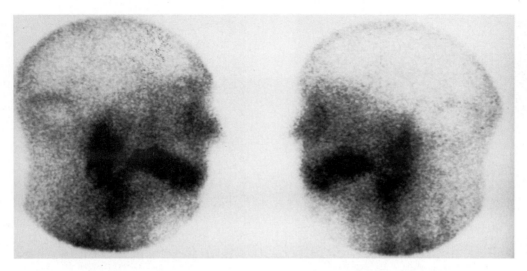

Fig. 2-5. Right and left radionuclide image of head showing more intense uptake in right parotid caused by chronic parotitis with accompanying abscess formation in this gland. The accumulation of activity in oral cavity is due to gingival inflammation and the appearance of the isotope in the saliva. (Courtesy Byron W. Benson, Dallas.)

cluding resonance) cause MRI to produce weak signals and poor images. However, with improved soft tissue contrast and the capacity to image exact tumor borders (Fig. 2-7), this disadvantage is minimal.

For a detailed description of the physical principles of MRI, and for interpreting the MR image, see Sprawls[20] and Mills et al.[29]

Sonography Ultrasonic examination does not use any form of electromagnetic radiation. Instead high-frequency sound pulses (approximately 1×10^{-6}/sec) are directed into the body (500 pulses/sec) from a handheld transducer in contact with the skin. The sound is reflected by tissue interfaces, and the resulting echoes are detected by the same transducer, which then converts them to electrical signals that are fed into a computer. Small and more superficially located organs and structures lend themselves to this procedure.[30] The images can be recorded like a moving picture and stored, or they can be viewed in real time on a TV monitor (Fig. 2-8).

Air and bone and other heavily calcified materials absorb almost all of the sound and are less echogenic than soft tissue. Fluid transmits sound so well that it is echo free, but it transmits echoes from underlying structures. Consequently, ultrasound can be used to determine whether a structure is solid or cystic. The walls of a cyst produce good echoes, but the cystic fluid does not. A cyst can also act as an acoustic enhancer, causing an amplification of the echoes from the tissues behind it. On the other hand, a stone causes a great reduction of echoes from the tissues behind it, producing a definitive acoustic shadow. Ultrasound has proved useful for examining salivary glands[31] and cysts and for similar processes in the soft tissue of the cervicofacial region.[32] Diagnostic sonography only images structure, so assessments of physiology or pathologic changes are possible only when architecture is affected. The reliability of an examination depends on the examiner's experience. Piette et al found that results are more reliable when the maxillofacial surgeon performs the sonography.[33]

To date, no harmful effects of this relatively inexpensive ultrasound examination have been documented. For a detailed description of the physical principles of sonography, as well as how to interpret the ultrasound image, see Sprawls[20] and Yoshida et al.[34]

DIFFERENTIAL DIAGNOSIS

This process is discussed in Chapter 4.

Working Diagnosis

This process is discussed in Chapter 4.

Medical Laboratory Studies

Certain pertinent laboratory tests may give helpful diagnostic information on clinical conditions whose identities remain obscure after the patient's history and physical examination. Such tests are useful, however, only if the clinician is aware of what tests to order and how to interpret the results. For a description of the bewildering array of laboratory procedures available, their technical aspects, the circumstances in which they are appropriate, and the possibilities of both error and false reports, and for lists of substances that interfere with certain laboratory tests and the clinical application of test results, see Ravel.[35]

Dental Laboratory Studies

The fabrication and analysis of articulated models of the dental arches and the attendant records are an integral

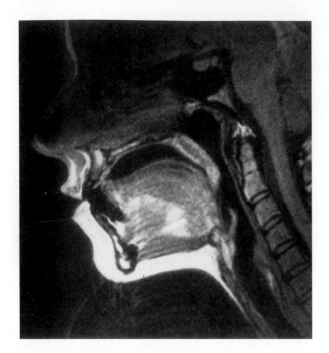

Fig. 2-6. Sagittal magnetic resonance scan through tongue and surrounding structures showing the mandible, hyoid bone, geniohyoid and genioglossus muscles, epiglottis, oropharynx, hard and soft palate, nasal turbinate, sphenoid sinus, pons, and medulla oblongata. (Courtesy Dan Waite, Dallas.)

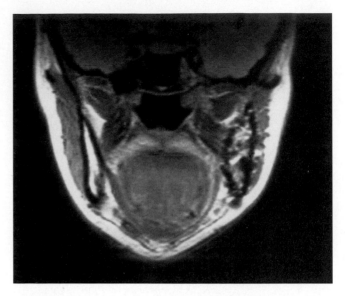

Fig. 2-7. Magnetic resonance image in coronal plane demonstrating a mass (desmoplastic fibroma) in the left ramus and angle of the mandible. (Courtesy Dan Waite, Dallas.)

part of the examination of many patients. Metabolic diseases, neoplasms, odontogenic diseases, congenital deformities, developmental malformations, and acquired maladies affecting the configurations of the oral cavity are often well visualized in properly prepared models.

Biopsy

Biopsy is the term used to describe the process of surgically removing tissue from a patient for histopathologic examination. The procedure is undertaken as the most accurate means of establishing a definitive diagnosis (confirming the working diagnosis) usually before the initiation of therapy. Biopsy should be pursued in the case of oral ulcers that persist for 2 to 3 weeks beyond the elimination of their suspected cause, persistent red and white lesions on the oral mucosa, suspected neoplasms, or any unidentified tissue mass or any pathologic mass that has been removed. Artifacts can develop in the excised tissue if handled improperly. These can be caused by crushing the tissue with forceps, fulguration, injection, improper fixation, freezing, and curling of the specimen.[36]

There are at least three types of biopsy: excisional biopsy, incisional biopsy, and fine-needle aspiration. It is important that the tissue be sent to a specialist, such as a certified oral pathologist, trained in microscopic examination of disease from the oral cavity and maxillofacial region.[37,38]

The tissue specimen should be placed in a solution of 5% to 10% formalin and fixed immediately. If there are two or more samples, each should be placed in a separate container. Each container should then be identified with the patient's name, the clinician's name, and the specimen's measurements and location of the lesion from which the sample came. An adequate patient history should also be included with the specimen.

Excisional biopsy An excisional biopsy is a therapeutic and diagnostic procedure performed when the lesion is no larger than 1 cm or so in diameter and when its removal does not necessitate a major surgical procedure. Excisional biopsy has the advantage of only requiring one surgical encounter. In addition, it does not transect tumor tissue as in incisional biopsy.

Incisional biopsy An incisional biopsy is indicated if the lesion is too large for an excisional procedure. However, multiple tissue samples may be required (i.e., serial biopsy). The sample, taken from the most suspect area, should be relatively large and deep and should include the junction with surrounding normal tissue. Necrotic areas generally should be avoided because they will not be diagnostic. The sample should be handled gently, and electrosurgery should not be used to remove it.

Punch biopsies are a type of incisional biopsy that may be used on surface oral lesions.[39] Wedge-shaped biopsies may be used for vesiculoerosive disease and to minimize postsurgical discomfort.[40]

For more detailed discussions of the indications for a biopsy and the mechanics of the techniques, see Bernstein[41] and Sabes.[42]

Fine-needle aspiration In fine-needle aspiration (FNA, fine-needle biopsy, aspiration biopsy) a fine-needle (21-gauge to 23-gauge) is inserted into a tissue or suspected lesion. The needle may be guided with a fluoroscope or with ultrasound to ensure that an exact area of tissue is

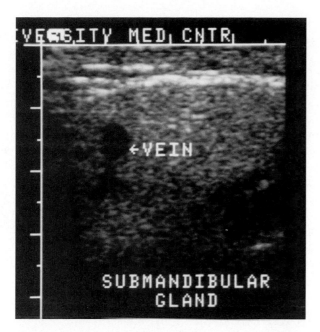

Fig. 2-8. Ultrasound image of a portion of normal submandibular gland. Note lack of internal echoes from the vein. The bright line at the top of the illustration is from fat on the surface of gland, which is more reflective than the salivary parenchyma. (Courtesy Robert Burpo, Dallas.)

sampled.[35] A minute piece of tissue is sucked into the needle tip, expressed onto a glass slide, dried, and rapidly stained.[43] The cytomorphology of the aspirated tissue is then studied. The main advantages of FNA are simplicity of technique (it can be easily performed on an outpatient basis using a local anesthetic), greater patient acceptance and less risk of delayed wound healing and infection than with incisional or excisional biopsy, rapid diagnosis, and economy (it eliminates the need for hospitalization and tissue processing and saves operating room time). Another advantage is that different areas within a mass can easily be sampled to ensure that representative material has been obtained.[44] The risk of seeding the needle track with cancer cells that accompanies the use of a large needle is unlikely with FNA.[45] A 90% to 100% accuracy range for the technique has been reported in lymph node aspiration (for metastatic carcinoma and melanoma, Hodgkin's and non-Hodgkin's lymphoma), salivary glands and the head and neck region (oral cavity, maxillary antrum, oropharynx, and nasopharynx), and other neck swelling.[46-51] The positive predictive value of FNA for malignancy in the head and neck is considered to be 100% for patients with or without a prior history of malignancy. It is considered the definitive diagnostic technique and allows the clinician to begin treatment. A negative, unsatisfactory, or suspect FNA diagnosis should be considered an indication for open biopsy to confirm the nature of the lesion. FNA is a safe, reliable method of diagnosing suspect lesions in the head and neck area and greatly aids and speeds the implementation of appropriate treatment.

Exfoliative Cytology

The technique for the cytologic examination of exfoliated cells scraped from suspect oral lesions is similar to that used for the detection of uterine cervix cancer. However, it has not provided the same level of reliability in the diagnosis of oropharyngeal malignancy. The lesion is scraped with a moistened tongue blade or a cement spatula, and the cells obtained are smeared evenly over a glass slide, fixed, stained, and examined under the microscope for the presence of viral or fungal disease or malignant-appearing cells.[52,53] The oral exfoliative technique has a tendency to produce a false-negative result an average of 37% of the time.[45] Most of the false-negative results stem from unappreciated limitations of this modality. Exfoliative cytology is unsuitable for the following lesions: homogeneous leukoplakias, smooth-surfaced exophytic lesions, submucosal lesions, unulcerated pigmented lesions, verruca vulgaris, papilloma, condyloma acuminata, etc. On the other hand, exfoliative cytology can give useful information for erythroplakia, the "erythro" patch of erythroleukoplakia, ulcers, erosions, and fungal and viral infections such as oral herpes simplex.[52,53] Bernstein and Miller discussed in detail the indications and contraindications of oral cytology.[53] Oral exfoliative cytology is recommended as an adjunct to open biopsy, for prebiopsy assessment, for the examination of broad surface lesions, and for the evaluation of patients after definitive treatment.

Toluidine Blue Staining

Most epithelial surfaces stain blue after the application of a 1% toluidine blue solution, but the stain is lost after application of a 1% acetic acid solution to a normal epithelial surface or to benign erythematous lesions on oral mucosa. In contrast, premalignant and malignant erythematous lesions are not decolorized by the acetic acid. Toluidine blue is not a specific stain for cancer cells but is an acidophilic, metachromatic nuclear dye that selectively stains acid tissue components, particularly nucleic acids such as deoxyribonucleic acid (DNA) and ribonucleic acid (RNA). It is believed to have greater affinity for nucleic DNA than for cytoplasmic RNA,[54] and dysplastic and anaplastic cells contain more DNA than normal cells.

Although toluidine blue staining has shown to be ineffective when applied to hamster cheek pouch carcinomas,[55] in humans it has been shown effective in demonstrating dysplastic (premalignant) and early malignant lesions not otherwise clinically recognizable on most of the mucous membrane surfaces and linings of the body, including the oral cavity.[56] The technique may be useful for differentiating the small dysplastic erythroplakia that requires biopsy from small erythematous lesions caused by infection, inflammation, or trauma. Also, benign ulcerations usually have a well-defined uptake of dye at the margins, whereas a diffuse marginal pattern is characteristic of the dysplastic or malignant lesion.[57]

Nearly all false-positive staining (e.g., persistent blue color, no carcinoma) occurs (in 8% to 10% of cases) in keratotic lesions and at the regenerating edges of erosions and ulcerations. It follows that if all keratotic and erosive lesions are excluded, the test is highly sensitive and specific for dysplastic mucosal epithelium.[58] False-negative results (no persistent blue staining, carcinoma present in 6% to 7% of cases) may occur in dysplasia with significant keratosis, which prevents penetration of the stain so the dye does not reach submucosal extensions of a tumor.[59]

Although some contend that preoperative toluidine blue staining more reliably indicates the border of a lesion and serves as a guide for its surgical excision than does clinical examination alone,[60] the technique cannot show tumor that is present under normal epithelium.[61] A good general rule is that if positive staining occurs, biopsy is in order.[62] In screening studies, sensitivity ranged from 93.5% to 97.8% and specificity from 73.3% to 92.9%.[63] The use of toluidine blue and Lugol's iodine in combination has produced better specificity than toluidine alone.[63] These authors do not recommend the routine use of toluidine blue and Lugol's iodine for screening all patients, but they recommend this technique as an additional aid "in assessing high risk patients and suspicious oral lesions."[63]

It would seem that the routine use of toluidine blue oral rinse would make apparent some small or unnoticed red lesions that practitioners might miss clinically (NKW).

Toxic effects of toluidine blue have been described but are not associated with the minute doses incurred during vital staining of mucosal surfaces.[64] Toluidine blue has been shown not to be carcinogenic in hamsters.[65]

Consultation

Before considering a consultation, the clinician should be satisfied that he or she, by taking a reliable history and conducting a thorough physical examination, has made an effort to solve the problem. Reasonable consideration should also be given to the identity of an appropriate consultant. There should be a written form of the request for consultation, which includes a brief summary of the patient's history and physical examination, a description of the problem, and an indication of the nature of the request: advice, treatment of the patient, or transfer of the patient. Finally, when the report from the consultant is received, it should always be placed in the patient's record along with the consultant's name and address.

FINAL DIAGNOSIS

The final diagnosis is a statement that a precise diagnosis has been made on the basis of all required observations: the identification of definitive symptoms, the pathologist's report, and the patient's response to therapy.

TREATMENT

Treatment of specific lesions is discussed throughout this text.

REFERENCES

1. Rose LF, Kaye D: *Internal medicine for dentistry,* ed 2, St Louis, 1990.
2. Bates B: *A guide to physical examination and history taking,* ed 4, New York, 1987, JB Lippincott.
3. Seidel HM, Ball JW, Dains JE, et al: *Mosby's guide to physical examination,* St Louis, 1987, Mosby.
4. Bricker SL, Langlais RP, Miller CS: *Oral diagnosis, oral medicine and treatment planning,* ed 2, Philadelphia, 1994, Lea & Febiger.
5. Tai CE, Miller PA, Packota GV, Wood RE: The occlusal radiograph revisited, *Oral Health* 84:47-53, 1994.
6. Goaz PW, White SC: *Oral radiology principles and interpretation,* ed 3, St Louis, 1994, Mosby.
7. Gratt BM: Panoramic radiography. In Goaz PW, White SC, editors: *Oral radiology principles and interpretation,* ed 3, St Louis, 1994, Mosby.
8. Langland OE, Langlis RP, McDavid WD, DelBalso AM: *Panoramic radiology,* ed 2, Philadelphia, 1989, Lea & Febiger.
9. Jensen TW: Fine-detail panoramic radiography by free-focus radiography: a clinical demonstration of diagnostic radiographs, *Oral Surg* 70:502-515, 1990.
10. Barrett HH, Swindell W: *Radiological imaging: the theory of image formation, detection, and processing, vols 1 and 2,* New York, 1981, Academic Press.
11. Som PM: The paranasal sinuses. In Bergeron RT, Osborn AG, Som PM, editors: *Head and neck imaging,* St Louis, 1984, Mosby.
12. Hausmann E, Dunford R, Christersson L, et al: Crestal alveolar bone changes in patients with periodontitis as observed by subtraction radiography: an overview, *Adv Dent Res* 2:378-381, 1988.
13. Grossman LD, Chew FS, Ellis DA, Brigham SC: *The clinician's guide to diagnostic imaging: cost effective pathways,* ed 2, New York, 1987, Raven Press.
14. Redington RW, Beninger WH: Medical imaging systems, *Physics Today* 34:36-44, 1981.
15. Thawley SE, Gado H, Fuller TR: Computerized tomography of head and neck lesions, *Laryngoscope* 88:451-459, 1978.
16. Nakagawa H, Wolf B: Delineation of lesions of the base of the skull by computed tomography, *Radiology* 124:75-180, 1977.
17. Carter BL, Bankoff MS: Facial trauma: computed versus conventional tomography. In Littleton JS, Durizch ML, editors: *Sectional imaging methods: a comparison,* Baltimore, 1983, University Park Press.
18. Rabinov K: CT of salivary glands, *Radiol Clin North Am* 22:145-149, 1984.
19. Lee Y, Van Tassel P: Craniofacial chondrosarcomas: imaging findings in 15 untreated cases, *AJNR* 10:165-170, 1989.
20. Sprawls P: *Physical principles of medical imaging,* Rockville, Md, 1987, Aspen Publishers.
21. Valvassori GE, Buckingham RA, Carter BL, et al: *Head and neck imaging,* New York, 1988, Thieme Medical Publishers.
22. Beirne OR, Leake DL: Technetium 99m pyrophosphate uptake in a case of unilateral condylar hyperplasia, *Oral Surg* 38:385-386, 1980.
23. Epstein JB, Hatcher DC, Graham M: Bone scintigraphy of fibro-osseous lesions of the jaw, *Oral Surg* 51:346-350, 1981.
24. Mettler FA, Guiberteau, MJ: *Essentials of nuclear medicine imaging,* New York, 1983, Grune & Stratton.
25. Fischer-Brandies E, Seifert C: Bone scintigraphy: an aid in deciding on the extent of bone resection in malignant oral tumors, *J Oral Maxillofac Surg,* 53:768-770, 1995.
26. Jeffcoat MK, Williams RC, Kaplan ML, Goldhaber P: Nuclear medicine techniques for the detection of active alveolar bone loss, *Adv Dent Res* 1:80-84, 1987.

27. Phelps ME, Mazziotta JC: Cerebral positron computed tomography. In Newton TH, Potts DG, editors: *Advanced imaging techniques,* San Anselmo, Calif, 1983, Clavadel Press.

28. Bushong SC: *Radiologic science for technologists,* ed 4, St Louis, 1988, Mosby.

29. Mills CM, de Groot J, Posin JP: *Magnetic resonance imaging: atlas of the head, neck, and spine,* Philadelphia, 1988, Lea & Febiger.

30. Wilson IR, Crocker EF, McKellar G, Rengaswamy V: An evaluation of the clinical applications of diagnostic ultrasonography in oral surgery, *Oral Surg* 67:242-248, 1989.

31. DeClerk LS, Corthouts R, Francx L, et al: Ultrasonography and computer tomography of the salivary glands in the evaluation of Sjögren's syndrome: comparison with parotid sialography, *J Rheumatol* 15:1777-1781, 1988.

32. Hell B: B-scan sonography in maxillofacial surgery, *J Craniomaxillofac Surg* 17:39-45, 1989.

33. Piette EJ, Lendoir L, Reychler H: The diagnostic limitations of ultrasonography in maxillofacial surgery, *J Craniomaxillofac Surg* 15:297-305, 1987.

34. Yoshida H, Akizuki H, Michi K: Intraoral ultrasonic scanning as a diagnostic aid, *J Craniomaxillofac Surg* 15:306-311, 1987.

35. Ravel R: *Clinical laboratory medicine: clinical application of laboratory data,* St Louis, 1989, Mosby.

36. Moenning JE, Tomich CE: A technique for fixation of oral mucosal lesions, *J Oral Maxillofac Surg* 50:1345, 1992.

37. Brannon RB, Kratochvil FJ, Warnock GR: Utilization of an oral pathology service: A professional responsibility, *Mil. Med* 157:31-32, 1992.

38. Allen CM: Patients requiring removal of impacted third molars should be referred to general surgeons: a modest proposal, *Oral Surg* 79:403, 1995 (editorial).

39. Lynch DP, Morris LF: The oral mucosal punch biopsy: indications and technique, *J Am Dent Assoc* 121:145-149, 1990.

40. Siegel MA: Intraoral biopsy technique for direct immunofluorescence studies, *Oral Surg* 72:681-684, 1991.

41. Bernstein ML: Biopsy techniques: the pathological considerations, *J Am Dent Assoc* 96:438-443, 1978.

42. Sabes WR: *The dentist and clinical laboratory procedures,* St Louis, 1979, Mosby.

43. Boccato P: Rapid staining techniques employed in fine-needle aspiration, *Acta Cytol* 27:82, 1983.

44. Raju G, Kakar PK, Das DK, et al: Role of fine-needle aspiration biopsy in head and neck tumors, *J Laryngol Otol* 102:248-251, 1988.

45. Scher RL, Oostingh PE, Levine PA, et al: Role of fine-needle aspiration in the diagnosis of lesions of the oral cavity, oropharynx and nasopharynx, *Cancer* 62:2602-2606, 1988.

46. Feldman PS, Kaplan MJ, Johns ME, et al: Fine-needle aspiration in squamous cell carcinoma of the head and neck, *Arch Otolaryngol Head Neck Surg* 109:735-742, 1983.

47. Frable MAS, Frable WJ: Fine-needle aspiration biopsy revisited, *Laryngoscope* 92:1414-1418, 1982.

48. Southam JC, Bradley PF, Musgrove BT: Fine-needle cutting biopsy of lesions of the head and neck, *Br J Oral Maxillofac Surg* 29:219-222, 1991.

49. Barnard NA, Paterson AW, Irvine GH, et al: Fine-needle aspiration cytology in maxillofacial surgery—experience in a district general hospital, *Br J Oral Maxillofac Surg* 31:223-226, 1993.

50. Platt JC, Davidson D, Nelson CL, Weisberger E: Fine-needle aspiration biopsy: an analysis of 89 head and neck cases, *J Oral Maxillofac Surg* 48:702-706, 1991.

51. Jayaram G, Verma AK, Sood N, Khurana N: Fine-needle aspiration cytology of salivary gland lesions, *J Oral Pathol Med* 23:256-261, 1994.

52. Barrett AP, Greenberg ML, Earl MJ, et al: The value of exfoliative cytology in the diagnosis of oral herpes simplex infection in immunosuppressed patients, *Oral Surg* 62:175-178, 1986.

53. Bernstein ML, Miller RL: Oral exfoliative cytology, *J Am Dent Assoc* 96:625-629, 1978.

54. Herlin P, Marnay J, Jacob JH, et al: A study of the mechanism of the toluidine blue dye test, *Endoscopy* 15:4-7, 1983.

55. Miller RL, Simms BW, Gould AR: Toluidine blue staining for detection of oral premalignant lesions and carcinomas, *J Oral Pathol Med* 17:73-78, 1988.

56. Hix WR, Wilson WR: Toluidine blue staining of the esophagus, *Arch Otolaryngol Head Neck Surg* 113:864-865, 1987.

57. Silverman S, Migliorati C, Barbosa J: Toluidine blue staining in the detection of oral precancerous and malignant lesions, *Oral Surg* 57:379-382, 1984.

58. Mashberg A: Reevaluation of toluidine blue application as a diagnostic adjunct in the detection of asymptomatic oral squamous carcinoma: a continuing prospective study of oral cancer, III, *Cancer* 46:758-763, 1980.

59. Mashberg A: Tolonium (toluidine blue) rinse—a screening method for recognition of squamous carcinoma: continuing study of oral cancer, IV, *JAMA* 245:2408-2410, 1981.

60. Eliezri YD: The toluidine blue test: an aid in the diagnosis and treatment of early squamous cell carcinomas of mucous membranes, *J Am Acad Dermatol* 18:1339-1349, 1988.

61. Bengel W, Veltman G, Loevy HT, et al: *Differential diagnosis of diseases of the oral mucosa,* Chicago, 1988, Quintessence Publishing Co.

62. Lundgren J, Olofasson J, Hellquist H: Toluidine blue: an aid in the microlaryngoscopic diagnosis of glottic lesions? *Arch Otolaryngol Head Neck Surg* 105:169-174, 1979.

63. Epstein JB, Scully C, Spinelli JJ: Toluidine blue and Lugol's iodine application in the assessment of oral malignant disease and lesions at risk of malignancy, *J Oral Pathol Med* 21:160-163, 1992.

64. *Registry of toxic effects of chemical substances,* Pub No 76-191, Rockville, Md, June 1975, National Institute for Occupational Safety and Health.

65. Redman RS, Krasnow SH, Sniffen RA: Evaluation of the carcinogenic potential of toluidine blue O in the hamster cheek pouch, *Oral Surg* 74:473-480, 1992.

CHAPTER 3

Correlation of Gross Structure and Microstructure with Clinical Features

NORMAN K. WOOD

PAUL W. GOAZ

IMPORTANCE OF NORMAL ANATOMY AND HISTOLOGY TO THE DIAGNOSTICIAN

The diagnosis of oral lesions is fundamentally an exercise in clinical pathology, which, in turn, is a study of changes. Usually such changes are precipitated by pathogenic or disease-producing agents. If the clinician is going to recognize and describe these changes, he or she must have a reference to contrast with the suspected area of pathology.

For the clinical oral diagnostician, this reference state is the state of oral health. Therefore a thorough and basic knowledge of the normal oral cavity and surrounding regions is fundamental to the detection of oral disease.

In addition, it is quite difficult to appreciate the physical characteristics of a tissue without an awareness of the tissue's microstructure because the microanatomy of the tissue establishes the clinical features on which diagnosticians base their judgments. Even the low-magnification photomicrograph of a tissue is very helpful.

Oral and Perioral Systems

The mucous membrane that lines the oral cavity consists of a layer of stratified squamous epithelium and a subepithelial layer, the lamina propria, which consists of a fibrous connective tissue and contains capillaries, nerves, and the minor salivary glands (Fig. 3-1).

The skin, like the mucous membrane, also possesses two layers—the epidermis and the underlying corium with its associated appendages, the sweat and sebaceous glands and the hair follicles (Fig. 3-2).

The remaining glandular systems of the perioral region of direct concern to the clinician are the major salivary glands and the thyroid and parathyroid glands. Either these glands are directly identified by the examiner or the effects of their pathologic involvement come to his or her attention when an adequate examination of the head and neck is completed.

When the examiner reviews radiographs of the region, knowledge of bone morphology and relationships of bones to each other is necessary to be able to anticipate and interpret the various forms their shadows may assume on the radiograph. The bones of the region include the maxilla, the mandible, the zygoma and vomer, the palatine, sphenoid, hyoid, and temporal bones, and the cervical vertebrae.

The oral examiner must be competent in appearances produced by the other systems, such as teeth, larynx, trachea, esophagus, and blood and lymphatic systems. Aberrations of these systems are also in the examiner's area of responsibility and must be recognized.

The muscle systems with which the oral diagnostician must be familiar are those of facial expression, mastication, and swallowing, as well as those involved in movements of the head. These muscles, along with the bony and cartilaginous structures and vessels, provide landmarks that facilitate an effective examination. They also with the fascial planes tend to mechanically obstruct or guide invading and spreading disease processes such as infections and neoplasms. Consequently, the examiner must be aware of the exact location and plane of each muscle and the extent of its normal movements during function.

Oral and Perioral Tissues

The epithelial tissues of the oral and perioral region include the following:

1. Stratified squamous epithelial lining
2. Mucous, serous, and sebaceous glandular units
3. Enamel

The connective tissues, located beneath the surface epithelium, include the following:

1. Fibrous, adipose, and loose connective tissue
2. Muscle (skeletal and smooth) and nerves
3. Cartilage and bone
4. Dentin, cementum, and dental pulp

A well-defined layer of loose connective tissue is usually present beneath the skin or mucous membrane and permits these superficial layers to move over the deeper, firmer tissues such as muscle and bone. If this loose connective tissue layer is absent, the superficial layer is bound to the deep layer, and it cannot be moved separately from the underlying structures. Such a situation is normally found on the anterior hard palate and on the attached gingivae. Loose connective tissue contains blood and lymphatic vessels, nerves, adipose tissue, myxomatous tissue, sparse fibrous tissue, reticular fibers (that is, precollagen fibers), elastic fibers, undifferentiated mesenchymal cells, and blast cells of many varieties.

Only through a thorough understanding of these tissues, their specific natures, their physical relationships to each other, how they support or fail to support each other when subjected to the deforming pressures of the examiner's fingers, and even the characteristic sensations the examiner can feel when palpating them will a full appreciation of the precepts of a physical examination be obtained.

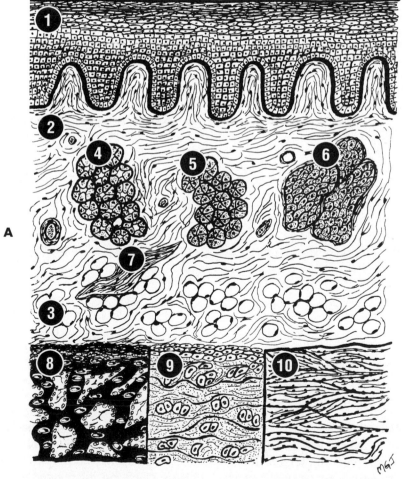

Fig. 3-1. A, Diagram of the oral tissues, illustrating the component tissues and their relative positions: *1,* stratified squamous epithelium; *2,* lamina propria; *3,* loose connective tissue; *4,* mucous glands; *5,* serous glands (occasionally); *6,* sebaceous glands (Fordyce's granules); *7,* nerve; *8,* bone; *9,* cartilage; *10,* skeletal muscle. Fortunately, a firm platform of muscle, bone, or cartilage is present beneath the superficial tissues. This facilitates examination and palpation of oral lesions.

Continued

Fig. 3-1, cont'd. B, Composite photomicrographs of tissue components diagrammed in **A.**

EXPLANATION OF CLINICAL FEATURES IN TERMS OF NORMAL AND ALTERED TISSUE STRUCTURE AND FUNCTION

Features Obtained by Inspection

The examiner can only visualize the surface tissue and its topography, including contours, color, and texture. For a more critical evaluation of irregularities, he or she must rely on other procedures.

Contours The diagnostician must be familiar with the normal tissue contours in and around the oral cavity to be able to detect any disorder that might alter the usual configuration of the area. Changes in contour, however, are not in themselves specifically diagnostic, since so many vastly different types of pathoses can produce similar alterations in contour.

Color The examiner must be familiar with the normal characteristic color of each region in the oral cavity and the normal variations in color and shadings these tissues can assume, and be able to recognize abnormal color changes in a specific region.

Pink. The normal color of the oral mucosa in whites is pink because healthy stratified squamous epithelium is semitransparent. Therefore the red of the blood in the extensive capillary bed beneath shows through. However the oral mucosa is *not* uniformly pink throughout but has

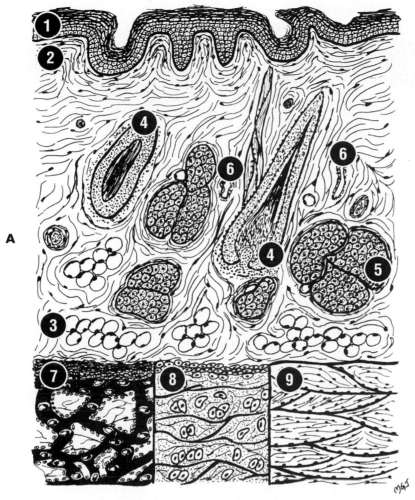

Fig. 3-2. A, Diagram of the skin and deeper tissues, illustrating the component tissues and their relative positions: *1,* keratinizing stratified squamous epithelium; *2,* corium; *3,* loose connective tissue; *4,* hair follicle; *5,* sebaceous glands; *6,* sweat glands; *7,* bone; *8,* cartilage; *9,* skeletal muscle. The firm platform below the oral tissues is also present beneath these dermal structures.

Continued

a deeper shade in some regions and a lighter shade in others. This is illustrated by the contrast between the darker red vestibular mucosa and the lighter pink gingiva.

Certain normal variations in the tissue that are related to function are known to influence this spectrum of pink and so shift the color toward the red or, in the opposite direction, toward a lighter pink. One of the two main factors that induce a transition to a whiter appearance is an increase in the thickness of the epithelial layer. This makes the epithelium more opaque and is normally the result of an increased retention of keratin (Fig. 3-3). The other modification responsible for a more blanched appearance of the mucosa is a less generous vascularity of the subepithelial tissues concomitant with a denser collagen component. These two modifications are often found simultaneously (Fig. 3-3), and the effective clinician must be able to correlate them with observed variations in microstructure and be able to interpret them as alterations caused by function, variations in function, or trauma.

For example, regions in the oral cavity that receive the greatest mechanical stimulation from mastication (the *masticatory mucosa*) react by developing a thicker layer of keratin for protection and a denser, less vascular lamina propria and so appear a light pink in color. These regions are the hard palate, the dorsal surface of the tongue, and the attached gingivae. On the other hand, regions such as the buccal mucosa, vestibule, floor of the mouth, and ventral surface of the tongue are not normally subjected to vigorous masticatory stimulation, so they require only a thin layer of stratified squamous epithelium, which retains little keratin and consequently permits the very vascular submucosa to show through and impart the redder color (Fig. 3-4). These areas are said to be covered with *lining mucosa.*

White. Because of the many white lesions that may occur in the oral cavity, not only must the clinician inspect the color of the soft tissues carefully, but he or she must also become intimately familiar with the normal color variations from region to region. These pathologic white lesions are discussed in detail in Chapter 8.

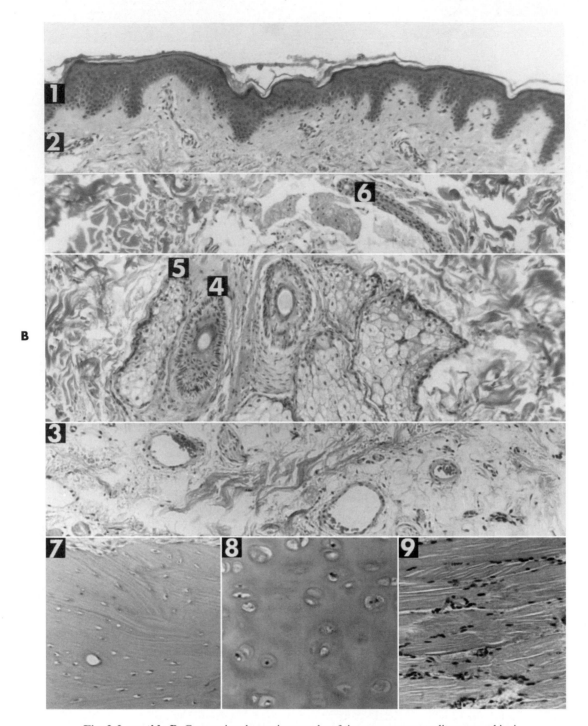

Fig. 3-2, cont'd. B, Composite photomicrographs of tissue components diagrammed in **A.**

For example, although a chronic mild irritation may act as a stimulus and induce the changes necessary to cause the mucosa to take on a lighter pink color, a more acute intense irritation will produce a thinning of the stratified squamous epithelium and a consequent inflammation of the subepithelial tissues. Thus such an involved area of the mucosa changes from pink to red because of (1) a thinning of the epithelial covering combined with (2) an increased vascularity and (3) a dissolution of part of the collagen content of the subepithelial tissue.

Yellow. The soft palate in many persons appears quite yellow. A moderate distribution of adipose tissue just beneath the basement membrane produces this color. Fordyce's granules, occurring in the buccal mucosa of most adults, are yellow, colored directly by the sebaceous material within the glandular units just beneath the epithelium.

Brownish, bluish, or black. Lesions of these colors are discussed in Chapter 12. The basis for the apparent clinical color of these lesions is frequently well demonstrated by

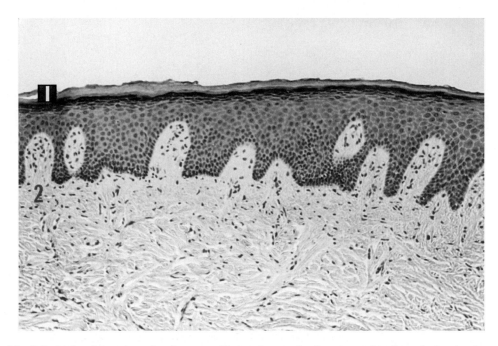

Fig. 3-3. Light pink region of oral mucosa. Photomicrograph of mucosa taken from the hard palate. The generous keratin layer *(1)* is combined with the dense fibrous and quite avascular lamina propria *(2)*. This combination accounts for the lighter coloration seen clinically on the hard palate and attached gingivae.

histologic study whether the color is induced by melanin, hemosiderin, heavy metals, or pools of clear fluid.

Surfaces Normal mucosa is smooth and glistening except for the area of the rugae and the attached gingiva, which frequently demonstrates stippling and pebbling.

The surface of a pathologic mass may be smooth, papillomatous, ulcerated, eroded, keratinized, necrotic, or bosselated.

Masses that arise in tissues *beneath* the stratified squamous lining are, almost without exception, smooth surfaced. They may originate from mesenchyme, the salivary glands, an abscess, or an embryonic rest. As the nest of cells enlarges below and presses against the stratified squamous epithelium, the epithelium responds by a combination of stretching and minimal mitotic activity. Therefore, as the mass becomes larger and bulges into the oral cavity, it is covered with a smooth epithelial surface. Examples of such masses are fibromas, osteomas, chondromas, hemangiomas, intradermal and compound nevi, many of the minor salivary gland tumors, cysts, retention phenomena, lipomas, myomas, schwannomas, neurofibromas, space abscesses, subepithelial bullae of erythema multiforme, bullous lichen planus, and bullous pemphigoid (Fig. 3-5).

Even the malignant counterparts of such tumors often have smooth surfaces, especially in their early phases, but when these bulging lesions are situated in a region subjected to repeated trauma, their smooth surfaces become ulcerated and necrotic.

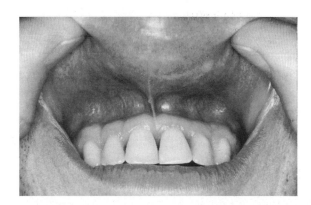

Fig. 3-4. This clinical picture illustrates the darker color of vestibular mucosa as contrasted with the lighter color of the attached gingivae. The histologic difference between the two regions explains these color differences.

Some exceptions to this rule are the intraepithelial vesicles and blebs seen in herpetic lesions and pemphigus. They are smooth despite the fact that they originate in the surface epithelium.

As a rule, however, masses that originate *in* the stratified squamous epithelium almost invariably have corrugated or papillomatous surfaces. Examples of these are papillomas, verrucae vulgari (warts), seborrheic keratoses, keratoacanthomas, verrucous carcinomas, and exophytic and ulcerative squamous cell carcinomas (Fig. 3-6). Exceptions would be the less than rough but pebbly surfaces

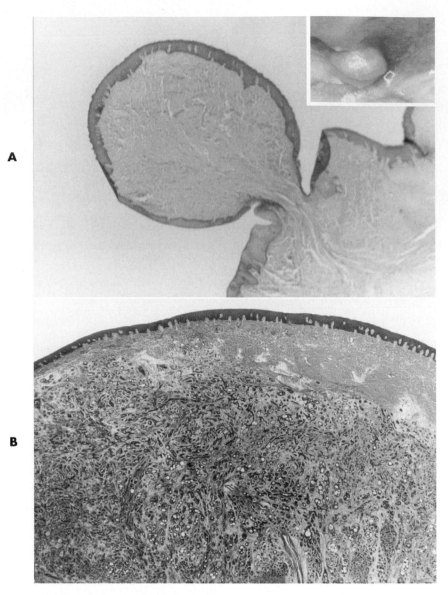

Fig. 3-5. Smooth-surfaced masses usually arise in tissues beneath the surface epithelium. **A,** Fibroma. **B,** Adenoid cystic carcinoma.

sometimes seen overlying a granular cell myoblastoma and a lymphangioma. The granular cell myoblastoma often induces a pseudoepitheliomatous hyperplasia in the overlying epithelium, and this sometimes is severe enough to produce a pebbly surface (Fig. 3-7). The superficial lymphangioma frequently has dilated lymphatic spaces that extend right to the basement membrane, and these produce folds in the surface epithelium (Fig. 3-8).

The smooth-surfaced and rough-surfaced masses are categorized in Table 3-1.

Flat and raised entities. A macule is the result of a localized color change produced by the deposition of pigments or slight alterations in the local vasculature or other minimal local changes. This is a flat lesion, since there is usually no significant increase in the number (hyperplasia) or size (hypertrophy) of the cells. Significant hyperplasia and hypertrophy always result in an eleva-

tion, which may take the shape of a papule, a nodule, a polypoid mass, or a papillomatous mass (see Chapter 10).

For example, an ephelis or freckle is a brownish macule that on histologic examination represents only an increased production of melanin by the normal number of melanocytes. On the other hand, an intradermal or intramucosal nevus shows a significantly increased number of nevus cells producing melanin and an increased amount of collagen in the subepithelial area. Therefore both hypertrophy and hyperplasia are present, and the lesion appears clinically to be pigmented and elevated (Fig. 3-9).

Aspiration The primary value of aspiration is to investigate the fluid contents of soft, cheesy, or rubbery masses whose characteristics suggest that they may contain fluid. An awareness therefore of the nature of the material contained in a mass will contribute significantly to the formulation of the appropriate differential diagnosis.

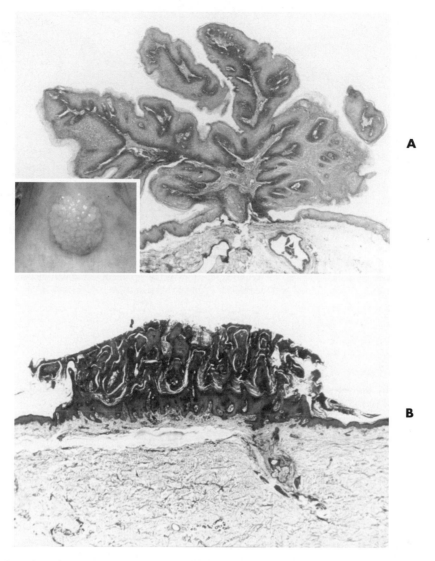

Fig. 3-6. Rough-surfaced masses usually arise within the surface epithelium. **A,** Papilloma. **B,** Seborrheic keratosis.

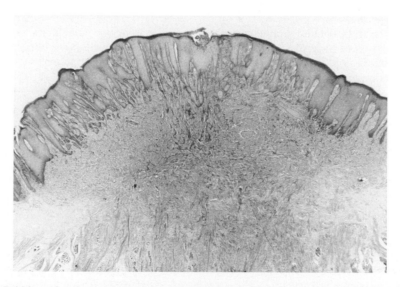

Fig. 3-7. Pebbly surfaced mass (granular cell myoblastoma). Note the presence of the pseudoepitheliomatous hyperplasia, which is often severe enough in these lesions to produce a pebbled surface.

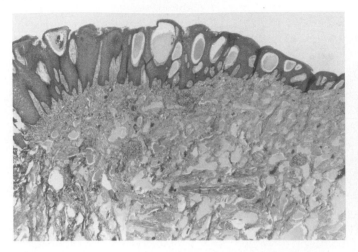

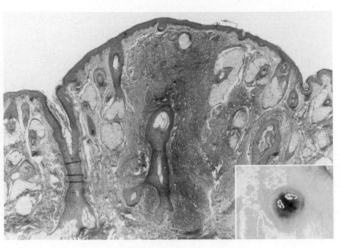

Fig. 3-8. Pebbly surfaced mass (lymphangioma). Note the numerous lymphatic channels throughout the tissue and especially those extending into the surface epithelium. A roughened surface frequently results from such extensions.

Fig. 3-9. Raised lesion (intradermal nevus). The large numbers of nevus cells present in the dermis produce the elevation of the lesion above the surface.

Table 3-1 Smooth-surfaced and rough-surfaced masses

Lesions	Exceptions
Smooth surface*	
Benign and malignant mesenchymal tumors	Highly malignant varieties
	Late stages of less malignant varieties
	Traumatized lesions
	Superficial lymphangiomas
Embryonal rests	Draining cysts with sinuses
Cysts and nevi	Some raised nevi with roughened surfaces
Space abscesses	Draining abscesses and parulides
Subepithelial bullae	
Erythema multiforme, bullous lichen planus, bullous pemphigoid, and epidermolysis bullosa	Ruptured bullae
Inflammatory hyperplasias	
Hormonal tumors, epulides fissurata, epulides granulomatosa, papillary hyperplasias, and fibrous hyperplasias	Pyogenic granulomas Epulides fissurata occasionally
Benign minor salivary gland tumors	Traumatized lesions
Early malignant salivary gland tumors	
Retention phenomena	Traumatized lesions
Mucoceles and ranulas	
Rough surface†	
Papillomas	None
Verrucae vulgares	None
Seborrheic keratoses	None
Keratoacanthomas	None
Verrucous carcinomas	None
Exophytic carcinomas	None
Ulcerative carcinomas	None
Condylomata latum	None

*All smooth-surfaced lesions, with the exception of intraepithelial bullae, originate *beneath* the surface epithelium.
†All rough-surfaced lesions, with the exception of those that were smooth surfaced and became roughened because of trauma, infection, or malignancy, originate *in* the surface epithelium.

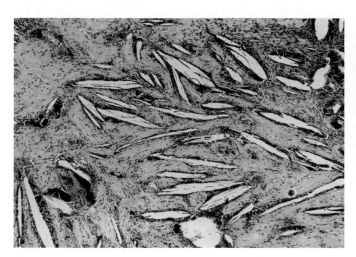

Fig. 3-10. Cholesterol clefts. The cholesterol crystals that occupy these clefts migrate to the luminal surface, are suspended in the cyst fluid, and may be subsequently discovered in the aspirate.

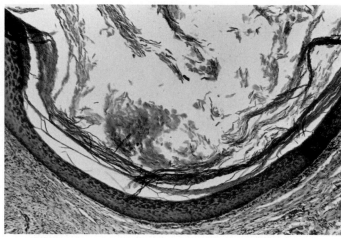

Fig. 3-11. Thick yellowish-white cyst aspirate. Note the large quantity of keratin that occupies the lumen of this epidermoid cyst and produces a viscous yellowish cystic fluid that would require a large-gauge needle for aspiration.

To aspirate masses indiscriminately is generally considered unwise. Most clinicians recommend that a mass not be subjected to aspiration until just before surgery because of the danger of introducing bacteria from the surface flora and thus secondarily infecting the mass. If the mass contains fluid, the fluid may be an excellent medium for the growth of bacteria. If the mass becomes subsequently infected, it may delay surgery until the infection has resolved. Even then the tissue in the immediate area that was infected will prove difficult to dissect because of poor texture and postinflammatory fibrosis. If the mass is aspirated immediately before surgery, the introduction of organisms will not pose such a problem, since the mass will have been enucleated before the potential bacterial infection could attain clinical significance.

The preoperative aspiration of a fluid-filled mass is a worthwhile precautionary procedure, and when carried out properly, it eliminates the unpleasant surprise of opening an innocuous-appearing lesion that proves to be a dangerous vascular tumor.

Aspirate. Examination of the fluid withdrawn at aspiration is essential. A straw-colored aspirate may be obtained from odontogenic and some fissural cysts and occasionally from cystic ameloblastomas. These generally have cholesterol crystals in their walls that are frequently shed into the lumen of the cyst and may be seen as small shiny particles when the syringe containing the aspirated fluid is transilluminated (Fig. 3-10). The crystals, which have a characteristic needlelike shape, may be studied in more detail under the microscope by placing a few drops of fluid on a slide under a coverslip.

Other types of cysts, such as epidermoid, sebaceous, and dermoid, which feel firmer on palpation than odontogenic cysts, yield more viscous aspirates and require at least a 15-gauge needle for successful aspiration.
1. The lumina of the epidermoid cyst and the keratocyst are filled with exfoliated keratin, and the aspirate is a

thick, yellowish-white, granular fluid (Fig. 3-11).
2. The sebaceous cyst yields sebum, which is *thick, homogeneous,* and *yellowish to gray.*
3. The walls of the dermoid cyst may contain most of the dermal appendages, including stratified, squamous, keratinizing epithelium with sebaceous and sweat glands and hair follicles. As a result the aspirate from this cyst is the *thickest of all, a yellowish, cheesy substance that can be aspirated only with difficulty* because it consists of keratin, sebum, sweat, and exfoliated squamous cells.

A dark, amber-colored fluid on aspiration may indicate a thyroglossal duct cyst (Fig. 3-12).

Lymph fluid may be aspirated from cystic hygromas and lymphangiomas. It is colorless, has a high lipid content, and so appears cloudy and somewhat frothy.

Bluish blood is aspirated from early hematomas, hemangiomas, and varicosities, whereas the blood from an aneurysm or an arteriovenous shunt is brighter red, reflecting the higher ratio of oxygenated to reduced hemoglobin of arterial blood (Fig. 3-13).

When a vascular lesion is suspected, care must be taken to use a needle of as small a gauge as possible to minimize postaspiration hemorrhage.

The aspiration of painful, warm, fluctuant swellings usually yields pus. The pus usually is yellow or yellowish white if the abscess is odontogenic. A superinfection with *Pseudomonas aeruginosa* produces greenish-blue pus.

Usually, aspirating a streptococcal infection such as Ludwig's angina is futile because streptococcal organisms causing this condition are usually not pyogenic and do not localize. Instead they produce spreading factors (e.g., the enzymes hyaluronidase, streptokinase, streptodornase, and coagulase), which facilitate their rapid dispersal through the tissues. Streptococcal organisms produce a red serosanguineous fluid, but usually not in large enough quantities to pool or be aspirated or to demonstrate fluctuance. Also, in contrast to staphylococcal infections, the streptococcal variety is more often associated with painful regional lymphadenitis.

Actinomycosis in its early stage is indicated by firm red swellings. Later, pus pools under the surface and produce fluctuance. At this intermediate stage, aspiration often yields a yellowish-white pus with a few firm yellow granules in it. These are the "sulfur granules," thought to be

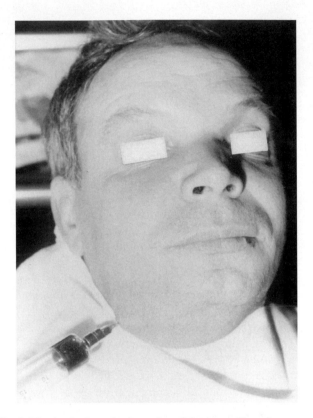

Fig. 3-12. Aspiration of a thyroglossal duct cyst. Note the unusual displacement of this particular cyst to the right of the midline.

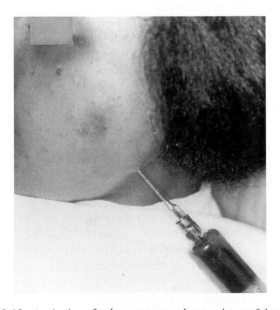

Fig. 3-13. Aspiration of a deep cavernous hemangioma of the face.

composed of mycelia and material produced as a by-product of the natural defenses of the host. Any aspirate from an infection should be sent to the laboratory for routine bacterial culture and sensitivity tests. If actinomycosis is suspected, special anaerobic cultures should be requested.

A sticky, clear, viscous fluid is obtained on aspiration of retention phenomena (mucoceles and cysts of the glands of Blandin and Nuhn and of the sublingual gland [ranula]) and sometimes from tumors of the minor salivary glands. This pooled liquid is a concentrated mucous secretion from which water is resorbed by the cells lining the cyst. Occasionally a low-grade mucoepidermoid tumor produces enough mucus to clinically resemble a mucocele and yields mucus on aspiration.

The papillary cystic adenoma and papillary cystadenoma lymphomatosum are often fluctuant and contain a thin, straw-colored liquid that can be aspirated.

Subcutaneous emphysemas and laryngoceles are soft masses that are filled with air, as are the rare pockets of carbon dioxide and hydrogen produced by *Clostridium perfringens* in gas gangrene. The former two entities can be completely deflated by aspiration.

Needle biopsy Needle biopsies can be performed with a special biopsy needle; this procedure can be advantageous in the biopsy of deeper structures such as the lymph nodes. The needle biopsy technique has the disadvantage of yielding a small-sized sample, and there is the added danger of lacerating some large blood vessels in the area (see Chapter 2, p. 10).

Features Obtained by Palpation

Knowledgeable examiners are able to distinguish the various tissues encountered in and around the oral cavity by palpation because, first, they are familiar with the normal gross anatomy of the structures and know where these tissues and organs are situated, their extent, in which plane they lie, and their anatomic relationship to each other. Second, examiners can visualize the microscopic structures of these tissues, which correlate so well with the tactile sensations elicited by the palpation of these structures and tissues.

Palpation is actually a "third eye"—the most informative method of clinically examining the tissues lying beneath the surface. Fortunately for the examiner, the soft tissues of the body lie over bones, cartilages, or skeletal muscles; therefore the superficial tissues can be palpated against a sturdy base.

Surface temperature Before attempting to make a judgment relative to the level of the surface temperature of a region or part, the examiner should first establish the patient's systemic temperature as indicated on an oral thermometer. A rise in surface temperature of the skin is simple to detect. The examiner places the fingers of one hand on the skin in the area of concern and the fingers of the other hand on the skin on the contralateral spot of the body. Relatively subtle differences in temperature may be rapidly and comfortably detected and can frequently contribute significantly to arriving at the diagnosis.

The skin generally has an increased temperature when it is inflamed or when it overlies an inflamed or infected region. The increased metabolic rate of the inflamed tissue, together with the increased vascularity of the area, is responsible for the increased local temperature of the part. The surface temperature of the skin overlying superficial aneurysms, arteriovenous shunts, and relatively large recent hematomas may also be elevated, since the higher deep body temperature is carried by the blood to the skin overlying these areas. The estimation of normal surface temperature is a useful test on the skin, but trying to transfer such a reference to the oral cavity is of little value, since the oral mucosa has a higher normal temperature than the skin.

Anatomic regions and planes involved Since many of the structures in the head and neck region can be at least partly palpated through the skin or oral mucosa or both, it becomes imperative that normal structures be anticipated and recognized.

For example, if the diagnostician locates a firm mass high in the submandibular space, he or she must be aware that the submaxillary gland is peculiar to that area and must then establish whether the mass is discrete from the salivary gland. If the mass is separate from the gland, pathoses of this gland will be deemphasized in the differential diagnosis. If this cannot be determined, the diagnostician must consider salivary gland pathoses as a probable diagnosis.

It is also essential that the examiner be able to detect, identify, and evaluate the condition of the regional tissues by manual examination. The acquisition of such a capability requires not only the basic anatomic knowledge but also considerable experience examining the area.

Sometimes the information gained by palpation is limited, and the palpation itself may be difficult—especially if the area is swollen because the swelling will tend to obscure the definition of structures. Furthermore, the patient will seldom permit a thorough palpation of painful tissue. In such a case a complete palpation may not be possible until the patient is anesthetized.

Initially the examiner must determine whether a mass in question is located superficially or deep. Then it is very helpful to identify the actual tissue involved because this may give a valuable clue to tissue of origin and to the clinical diagnosis.

Mobility Once the examiner has defined a mass in terms of its location in an anatomic plane and the tissue and organ involved, he or she will determine whether the mass is mobile or fixed with regard to its neighboring tissues. By palpation the examiner can establish whether the mass is freely movable in all directions. If it is freely movable, it is most likely a benign, possibly encapsulated, process originating in the loose subcutaneous or submucosal tissue (such as epidermoid or dermoid cyst or lymph node) (Fig. 3-14).

The mobility can be illustrated by fixing the mass with the fingers of one hand while moving the skin or mucosa over the mass with the other hand. Next, an attempt is made to move the mass independent of its underlying tissue. This demonstrates whether it is freely movable in all directions. If the mass is fixed to the skin but not to the underlying tissue, this is an important clue and limits the differential diagnosis list. For instance, epidermoid and dermoid cysts would be regarded as unlikely alternatives because they are freely movable in all directions, unless fibrosis has resulted from a previous infection. On the other hand, sebaceous cysts would be high on the list of possibilities, since they are freely movable over underlying tissues but are bound to the skin. This diagnosis is logical considering that sebaceous cysts form when sebaceous units of the skin become blocked but retain their continuity with the cystic glandular elements and the skin (Fig. 3-15).

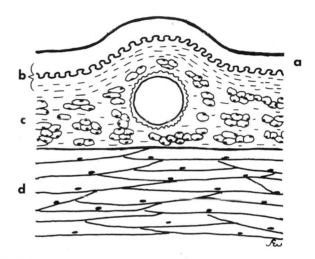

Fig. 3-14. Diagram of a freely movable mass. An example of this type of mass is the epidermoid cyst, which can be moved freely in all directions by digital pressure. *a*, Stratified squamous epithelium; *b*, mucosa or skin; *c*, loose connective tissue layer; *d*, skeletal muscle.

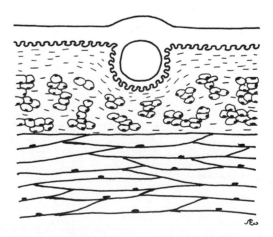

Fig. 3-15. Diagram of a mass attached to the skin. An example of this type of mass is the sebaceous cyst, which cannot be moved independent of the skin but is not attached to the deeper structures. This type of cyst thus can be moved as a unit with the skin.

The mass that is independent of the skin but attached to the deeper structures presents different possibilities. It could be attached to muscle, bone, cartilage, fat, salivary gland, or thyroid gland. The tissue or organ to which the mass is most intimately attached will most often prove to be the tissue of origin (Fig. 3-16). For example, if the mass is located in or bound to the parotid gland, the most likely possibility is that it is of parotid origin.

If the mass is bound to the skin or mucosa and to the underlying structures, however, there are only four possibilities:

1. Fibrosis after a previous inflammatory episode
2. An infiltrating malignant tumor that originated in the skin or mucous membrane and has invaded the deep structures (Fig. 3-17)
3. A malignancy that originated in a deep structure and has invaded the subcutaneous or submucosal tissue and the skin or mucosa
4. A malignancy that originated in the loose connective tissue and has invaded both the superficial and the deep layers

When examining the oral cavity, the diagnostician should remember that under normal conditions the mucosa covering the hard palate and the gingivae is bound tightly to the underlying bone. In addition, the loose submucosal layer under the papillated, keratinized, stratified squamous epithelium of the dorsal surface of the tongue is very thin and frequently nonexistent. Therefore the mucosa of the dorsal surface cannot normally be moved independent of the deeper muscular part. The remainder is lining mucosa and has a substantial loose submucosal layer, which in the absence of disease permits the surface epithelial layer to be moved independent of the deeper tissues and structures.

The palpation of a mass during function frequently reveals whether the mass is fixed to deeper structures—and if so, which ones. For example, if a fluctuant mass in the anterior midline of the neck moves up and down as the patient swallows, it may be diagnosed as part of, or at-

tached to, the hyoid bone, larynx, trachea, thyroid or parathyroid gland, or intervening muscles. If it elevates when the patient protrudes the tongue, the examiner may suspect that it is a thyroglossal cyst and that a persistent epithelial or fibrous cord or a fistula is leading to the tongue. (These are not always present in patients with thyroglossal cysts; however, if a mass does not elevate on protrusion of the tongue, a thyroglossal duct cyst is not necessarily ruled out.)

In some cases a mass may encroach on adjacent moving structures and impair or limit movement. For example, a chondroma or hyperplasia of the condyle may produce deviation and limitation of jaw movements.

Extent   The determination of the foregoing characteristics by palpation is important not only for masses located below the surface but also for visible superficial lesions.

Clinicians must always bear in mind that what is visible may represent just the tip of the iceberg. Consequently, it is important that the tissue surrounding and underlying the bases of these apparent surface lesions be carefully palpated to determine the maximum extension of the lesion into adjacent tissues. Positive identification of small cellular areas of penetration into the surrounding tissue can be made only by microscopic examination, but the surgeon must grossly estimate the extent of penetration in the surrounding tissue by palpation before surgery.

Whether a mass will have poorly defined, moderately defined, or well-defined borders, as determined by palpation, will depend on four factors:

1. Border characteristics of the mass
2. Relative consistency of the surrounding tissues
3. Thickness and nature of the overlying tissue
4. Sturdiness of the underlying tissue

Borders of the mass.   Malignancies usually have ill-defined borders that are extremely difficult to delineate

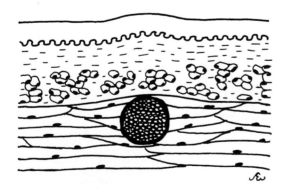

Fig. 3-16. Diagram of a mass attached to muscle. A rhabdomyoma is an example of this type of mass, which cannot be moved independent of the involved muscle but is not fixed to the skin or mucous membrane.

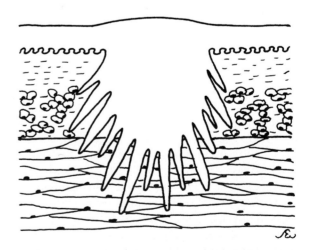

Fig. 3-17. Diagram of an epithelial mass—fixed to all layers of tissue. An invasive squamous cell carcinoma at this stage fixes the skin or mucous membrane to the deeper tissues.

by palpation. This observation is readily evident if we consider two features characteristic of these disorders:

1. Malignant tumors often infiltrate adjacent tissue by extending many *processes of tumor* into the surrounding normal tissue.
2. Malignant tumors produce a *scirrhous reaction* in the infiltrated tissue.

The processes of the tumor are irregular in size, shape, and distribution. The result is an irregular and vague outline. These extensions anchor the neoplasm to neighboring tissue and preclude the possibility that the tumor may be moved manually independent of its surroundings.

The tumor, with its extensions, elicits an inflammatory reaction in the adjacent tissue that is somewhat similar to an allergic or foreign body reaction. This inflammatory reaction results in the sequela of fibrosis. The fibrosis develops in the irregular and diffuse areas that are inflamed and results in a more tenacious binding of the tumor to the adjacent tissues by an ill-defined fibrous attachment whose limits are impossible to perceive by manipulation of the mass.

One exception involves some of the slow-growing malignancies that develop definable fibrous borders. The borders are composed of (1) connective tissue from the stroma of the dislodged normal tissue and (2) fibrous tissue newly formed in response to the tumor. These masses have borders that may be detected and delineated by palpation.

Inflammation occurs much more frequently as a response to other insults than as a response to malignant tumors, and it usually has poorly defined borders regardless of etiology.

Inflammation in a nonencapsulated organ or tissue seldom develops a smooth, well-defined border; the subsequent scarring in the areas of resolved inflammation will duplicate the limits of the inflammatory process, which is vague and irregular. On the contrary, if the inflammation of an encapsulated organ or tissue is confined within the capsule, the margins of the affected tissue will possess the well-defined characteristics of the encapsulated organ.

Also, the resolution of the inflammation and reparative scarring within the capsule (e.g., a lymph node, the parotid gland) will result in a mass with a well-defined detectable border. This of course is a consequence of the enclosing and restricting action of the capsule. If the inflammation breaks through the capsule and involves the surrounding tissue, however, the resultant extracapsular fibrosis will render the mass fixed to the surrounding tissue and the borders may then be ill defined. The postinflammatory fixed lymph node would be an example of such a process.

The limits of a pathologic process can be well defined by palpation depending on the shape of the lesion and the nature of its borders. The exact extent of a thin lesion or any lesion with a flattened, feather-edged border is difficult to determine. On the other hand, the limits of a plump lesion (e.g., spherical mixed tumor) are relatively easy to detect.

Consistency of surrounding tissue The consistency or the degree of firmness of a lesion, in contrast to that of its surrounding tissue, will affect the ease with which the lesion itself or its borders may be identified by palpation.

For example, the borders of a firm dermoid cyst occurring in loose subcutaneous tissue can be readily determined, whereas to ascertain the borders of a relatively soft lipoma when it occurs in the same type of loose connective tissue is difficult, if not impossible.

The same relative situation often pertains in the case of a firm mass occurring on or around the borders of a muscle. If the surrounding normal tissue is of the same consistency as the pathologic mass, the borders cannot be determined. Regardless of the physical circumstance attending the palpation of a lesion in or over bone, determining the extent of bony involvement without a radiograph is impossible.

When a radiograph indicates some degree of bone loss, identifying the site of origin as being soft tissue or bone itself without a biopsy may be difficult and often impossible. Even when the microscopic diagnosis is fibrosarcoma, the clinician still cannot be certain of the origin of the mass. If an adequate radiographic examination does not reveal a radiolucency in the bone, the clinician can proceed on the assumption that the lesion in question most likely has originated in the soft tissue.

Thickness of overlying tissue Clearly, the physical characteristics of a superficial mass are much easier to determine than in the case of a deep mass. Also, overlying dense fibrous tissue or tensed muscle tissue will obscure and may even obliterate the characteristic features of a lesion.

As an example, the borders of a branchial cleft cyst lying superficial to the sternocleidomastoid muscle may be readily delineated, and the mass is soft and fluctuant. In contrast, if the cyst lies beneath the sternocleidomastoid muscle, its borders may not be defined by palpation and the cystic mass feels firm and nonfluctuant. A covering of bone or cartilage precludes the palpation of an underlying mass, although if the mass has expanded the bone or cartilage, its presence may be suspected.

Sturdiness of underlying tissue Firm tissue situated beneath the mass promotes a more productive palpation of the mass. Soft issue platforms, on the other hand, frustrate the examiner. Fortunately, firm platforms for palpation are present in most regions of the body.

Size and shape The size and shape of a protuberant lesion may be determined by inspecting it and measuring it with a millimeter rule. In addition, a careful history frequently indicates the duration of the growth; on the basis of the present size, the growth rate can be approximated. Likewise, the history helps to establish whether a lesion is increasing in size at a steady rate, whether it is paroxysmal and predictable (like a retention phenomenon of the parotid gland, which enlarges just before eating), or whether it drains intermittently (like a rupturing abscess, which periodically decreases in size).

When masses are located within a tissue, however, palpation is necessary to determine their approximate size and shape. Round or ovoid masses are generally cysts, early benign tumors, or enlarged lymph nodes. Primary malignant tumors of lymph nodes and early metastatic tumors of lymph nodes are usually round or ovoid with a smooth border. As indicated, irregularly shaped masses are most likely to be inflammatory-fibrotic conditions or malignant tumors.

Consistency Consistency provides one of the most important clues to identification. Since the examiner must be as familiar with the texture and compressibility of normal tissue as with those of abnormal tissue, a description of the normal is given in Table 3-2.

The following terms are commonly used to define the consistency of tissue: soft, cheesy, rubbery, firm, and bony hard. The term *soft* is associated with easily compressible tissue such as a lipoma or a mucocele. Cysts filled with thin fluid are generally soft, but if they are under tension, they are rubbery. *Cheesy* indicates a somewhat firmer tissue that gives a more granular sensation but little or no rebound. *Rubbery* describes a tissue that is firm but can be compressed slightly and rebounds to its normal contour as soon as the pressure is withdrawn, such as skin. *Firm* identifies a tissue, such as fibrous tissue, that cannot be readily compressed. *Bony hard* is self-explanatory.

There are examples in each category that are borderline and appear to overlap adjacent categories, so it may not always be possible to explicitly describe a consistency with one of these terms. However, they are universally employed and connote a similar meaning to most individuals.

At least three different factors can modify the consistency of a tissue or mass as perceived by palpation:

1. The depth in the tissue will alter the consistency sensed by palpation; that is, a soft mass will seem firmer if it is deeper in the tissue than it would feel if it were situated more superficially.
2. A thick layer of overlying tissue, especially muscle or fibrous tissue, will appreciably modify or mask the true nature of a mass.
3. Soft glandular tissue surrounded by a dense connective capsule will be perceived as firmer than it is.

The examiner should be familiar with microstructure of tissue because it correlates so well with its consistency determined during palpation. The histologies of examples from each group of consistencies are shown together in Fig. 3-18 for comparison.

Once the examiner has become familiar with the location and consistency of normal tissues and organs, he or she will be quite capable of differentiating between normal and abnormal tissue when a consistency is detected that contrasts with the expected consistency of the tissue being palpated.

The consistency of abnormal tissue can be described with the same terms as those used for characterizing nor-

mal tissue: soft, cheesy, rubbery, firm, and bony hard. Representative segments of pathologic masses have been selected and categorized according to consistency in Table 3-3. Again, in an effort to underscore the correlation between microstructure and physical consistency, photomicrographs of pathologic tissues with similar consistencies have been grouped together in Fig. 3-19 on pp. 32-33.

Fluctuance and emptiability All soft, cheesy, or rubbery lesions or masses over 1 cm in diameter should be tested for fluctuance. This is done by placing the sensing fingers of one hand on one side of the mass and gently pressing on the mass with the probing fingers of the other hand. If the sensing fingers can detect a wave or force passing through the lesion, the mass is said to be fluctuant (Fig. 3-20 on p. 34). The following four factors determine whether fluctuance can be perceived in a soft, cheesy, or rubbery lesion (Table 3-4 on p. 34):

1. *The mass must contain liquid or gas in a relatively enclosed cavity* (Fig. 3-20). Examples of such fluctuant masses are cysts, mucoceles, ranulas, pyogenic space abscesses, early hematomas, subcutaneous emphysemas, varicosities, Warthin's tumors, papillary cyst adenomas, lipomas, and plexiform neurofibromas (Fig. 3-21 on p. 35). Although a lipoma and a plexiform neurofibroma do not

Table 3-2	**Consistency of normal tissues and organs***
Consistency	**Tissues or organs**
Soft	Adipose tissue
	Fasciae
	Veins
	Loose connective tissue
	Glandular tissue, minor salivary glands, and sublingual salivary gland
Cheesy	Brain tissue
Rubbery	Skin
	Relaxed muscle
	Glandular tissue with capsule
	Arteries and arterioles
	Liver
Firm	Fibrous tissue
	Tensed muscle
	Large nerves
	Cartilage†
Bony hard	Bone
	Enamel
	Dentin
	Cementum
	Cartilage†

*Many normal tissues and organs (e.g., dental pulp, thyroid and parathyroid glands, lymph nodes, and lymphatic vessels) usually cannot be palpated under normal conditions, so they have not been categorized here.

†Cartilage is difficult to classify; it seems to fall into an intermediate category, being too firm to be included in the firm group and not firm enough to be placed in the bony hard group.

have a true lumen containing a fluid, the high liquid content of the cells and interstitial tissue is apparently sufficient to produce fluctuance in these tumors.

2. *The mass must be located in a superficial plane.* If the mass is covered by a thick layer of relatively inflexible tissue or a structure such as a muscle, it cannot be palpated in a manner that might demonstrate fluctuance (Fig. 3-22 on p. 35).

3. *The mass must be in a fluctuant stage.* Some clinical lesions represent a fluctuant stage in a multiphasic disease process. For example, an odontogenic infection that has broken through the cortical plates and commenced to involve the adjacent soft tissue is tender, red, and firm. As the process continues, pus produced by the typical odontogenic space infection results in a soft, fluctuant, painful, nonemptiable mass. As the abscess resolves, regardless of the treatment, the fluctuant stage gives way to a firm stage and the firm stage may either disappear completely or leave a small area of fibrosis. Actinomycosis often demonstrates the same cycle, as do infected cysts to some extent.

4. *Developing fibrosis around the mass may obscure the fluctuance.* Chronically infected cysts that flare up

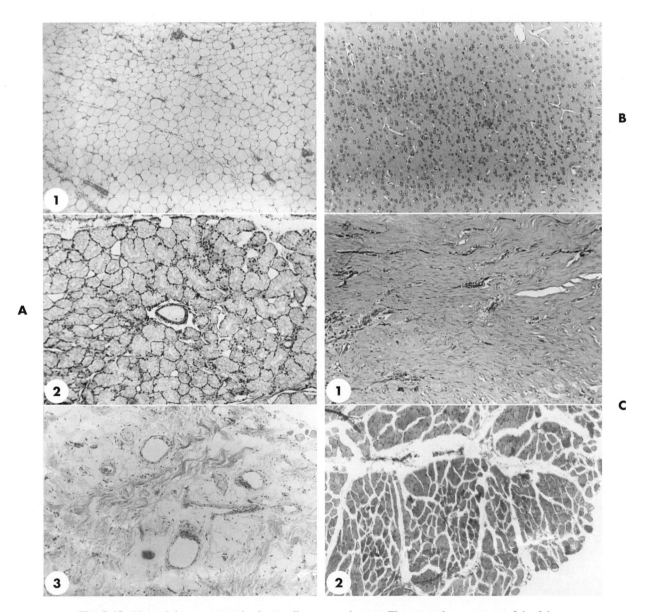

Fig. 3-18. Normal tissues categorized according to consistency. The general appearance of the following normal tissues at low magnification reflects the consistency of the tissue to palpation. **A,** Tissues with soft consistency: *1,* adipose tissue; *2,* unencapsulated mucous glands; *3,* loose connective tissue; note the presence of thin-walled vessels. **B,** Tissue with cheesy consistency: brain tissue. **C,** Tissues with firm consistency: *1,* fibrous tissue; *2,* skeletal muscle; tensed muscle feels firm, whereas relaxed muscle feels rubbery.   *Continued*

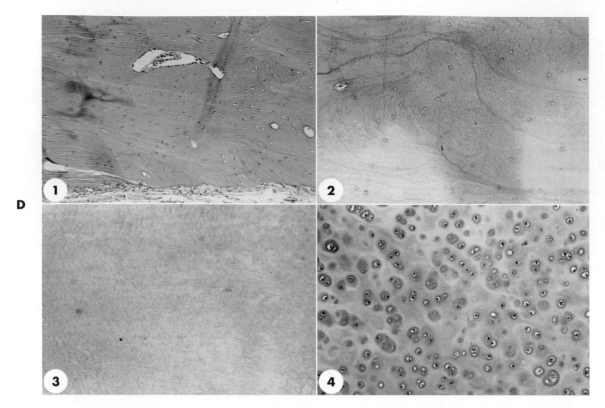

Fig. 3-18, cont'd. D, Tissues with bony hard consistency: *1,* bone; *2,* cementum; *3,* dentin; *4,* cartilage.

Table 3-3   Consistency of pathologic masses

Lesions	Exceptions
Soft	
Cysts	Cysts under tension—rubbery
	Infected and fibrosed cysts—firm
	Sebaceous cysts, keratocysts, and dermoid cysts—cheesy
Warthin's tumors and papillary cystic adenomas	Occasionally sclerosed types firm in some areas
Vascular tumors and phenomena	Sclerosing types—firm
Hemangiomas, lymphangiomas, varicosities, and cystic hygromas	Hemangioendotheliomas—firm
	Hemangiosarcomas—firm
Fatty tumors	Sclerosing types of liposarcoma—firm
Lipomas, hibernomas, xanthomas, and liposarcomas	
Myxomas	None
Plexiform neurofibromas	None
Inflammatory hyperplasias (granulomatous stage)	Fibrosed types—firm
Emphysemas	None
Laryngoceles	None
Retention phenomena	If high tension, rubbery
Mucoceles and ranulas	If fibrosed, firm
Cheesy	
Cysts	Infected and fibrosed types—firm or alternate areas of
Sebaceous, dermoid, and epidermoid	cheesiness and firmness
Tuberculous nodes	Early or late tuberculosis nodes—firm

Table 3-3   Consistency of pathologic masses—cont'd

Lesions	Exceptions
Rubbery	
Cysts with contents under tension	None
Lymphomas	None
Myomas	None
Myoblastomas	Those with severe pseudoepitheliomatous hyperplasia—firm
Aneurysms	None
Pyogenic space infection	Early stages—firm
Edematous tissue	None
Early hematomas	If not much tension, soft
Firm	
Infection	None
Streptococcus, early staphylococcus, early actinomycosis, and histoplasmosis	
Benign tumors of soft tissue	Fatty tumors, plexiform neurofibromas, myxomas, and hemangiomas
Fibromas, neurofibromas, schwannomas, and amputation neuromas	
Malignancies of soft tissues	None
Squamous cell carcinomas, melanomas, fibrosarcomas, and sclerosing liposarcomas	
Osteosarcomas	Occasionally bony hard
Chondrosarcomas	Occasionally bony hard
Metastatic carcinomas	Occasionally (osteoblastic, metastatic, and prostatic carcinomas) bony hard
Benign and malignant salivary gland tumors	Warthin's tumors and papillary cyst adenomas—soft
	Occasionally mucoepidermoid tumors with alternate soft and firm areas
Inflammation and infection of parotid and submaxillary salivary glands	None
Inflammation and infection of lymph nodes	Caseous or liquefied nodes—soft and cheesy
Bony hard	
Osteomas	None
Exostoses	None
Osteogenic sarcomas	Undifferentiated—firm
Pleomorphic adenomas occasionally	Usually firm
Chondromas	Occasionally firm
Chondrosarcomas	Occasionally firm
Osteoblastic, metastatic, and prostatic carcinomas, occasionally	Usually firm

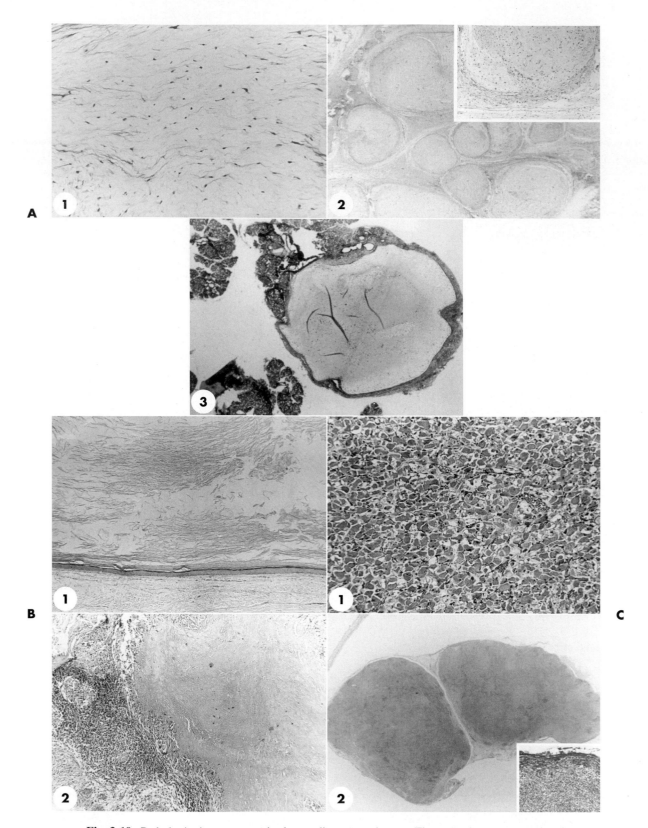

Fig. 3-19. Pathologic tissues categorized according to consistency. The general appearance of each of the following pathologic tissues at low magnification reflects the consistency of the tissue to palpation. **A,** Soft consistency: *1,* myxoma; *2,* plexiform neurofibroma (low and high magnifications); *3,* ranula. **B,** Cheesy consistency: *1,* epidermoid cyst; note that the lumen is filled with keratin, which imparts the cheesy consistency; *2,* tuberculous node; the large amorphous area is caseation necrosis, which imparts the cheesy consistency. **C,** Rubbery consistency: *1,* rhabdomyoma; *2,* lymphoma; the lymph node capsule helps to impart the rubbery consistency to this entity.

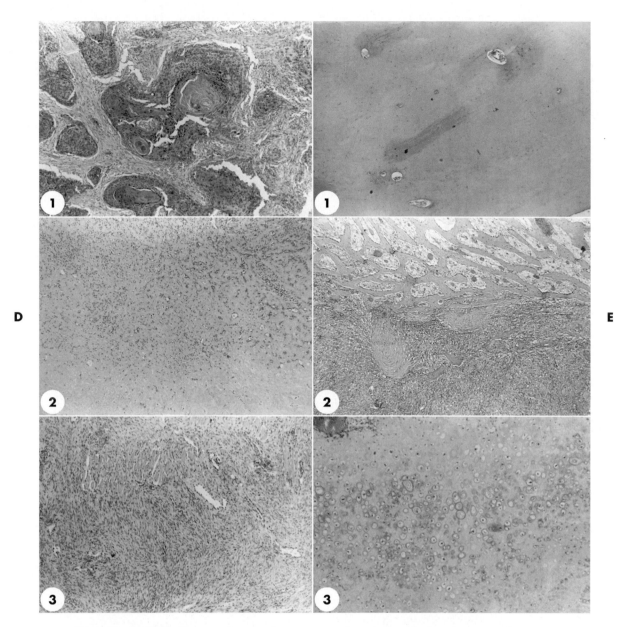

Fig. 3-19, cont'd. D, Firm consistency: *1,* squamous cell carcinoma; the keratin nests and surrounding fibrous tissue contribute to the firmness of this lesion; *2,* pleomorphic adenoma; the generous amount of hyaline in this tissue is responsible for the firmness; occasionally, cartilage and bone are present in this type of tumor and impart a bony hardness to some areas; *3,* fibrosarcoma; the amount of dense fibrous tissue imparts the firmness to this lesion. **E,** Bony hard consistency: *1,* torus; *2,* osteogenic sarcoma; frequently new bone formation and the production of fibrous tissue contribute to the consistency of this tumor; *3,* chondrosarcoma.

from time to time often lose their fluctuance and become hard and tender. This is an example in which inflammation and the resulting fibrosis around a fluid-filled cavity can mask fluctuance. Occasionally the epithelial lining and the lumen are destroyed, so the basic requirement for fluctuance, a fluid-filled cavity, is lost.

Lesions demonstrating variable fluctuance. Some examples of soft, cheesy, and rubbery lesions demonstrate fluctuance, whereas others of the same variety do not. This is usually related to the degree of emptiability

that a particular lesion has. All soft, cheesy, or rubbery lesions can be classified according to emptiability.

1. Some cannot be emptied at all by digital pressure (Fig. 3-23).
2. Others, such as hemangiomas, cystic hygromas, lymphangiomas, and laryngoceles, may show fluctuance or emptiability, depending on the individual structural characteristics of the specific lesion.
3. Still others, including aneurysms, most cavernous hemangiomas, draining cysts, and draining space

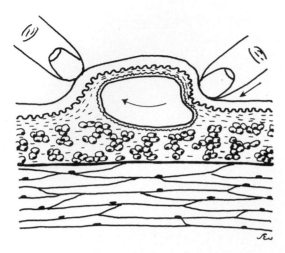

Fig. 3-20. Diagram illustrating fluctuance in a cystlike lesion.

Table 3-4 Characteristics of soft, cheesy, or rubbery masses		
Lesions	Fluctuant	Emptiable
Cysts	Yes	No
Abscesses	Yes	No
Mucoceles	Yes	No
Ranulas	Yes	No
Early hematomas	Yes	No
Subcutaneous emphysemas	Yes	No
Lipomas	Yes	No
Plexiform neurofibromas	Yes	No
Myxomas	Yes	No
Papillary cystic adenomas	Yes	No
Warthin's tumors	Yes	No
Varicosities	Variable	Variable
Cystic hygromas	Variable	Variable
Laryngoceles	Variable	Variable
Capillary hemangiomas*	Variable	Variable
Lymphangiomas	Usually	Usually not
Cavernous hemangiomas	Usually not	Usually
Aneurysms	No	Yes
Draining cysts	No	Yes
Draining abscesses	No	Yes
Inflammatory hyperplasias	No	No

*Capillary hemangiomas are often less than 1 cm in diameter and are usually too small for fluctuance to be accurately detected.

abscesses, are usually nonfluctuant and completely emptiable with ease. They rarely develop an architecture that results in fluctuance.

A number of factors influences the emptiability of a mass: course, number, diameter, and position of exit vessels or channels. Also, the width of the base of a lesion relates to the ease with which the lesion can be emptied.

Fig. 3-24 shows a diagram of an aneurysm. Note that the aneurysm could be readily emptied by digital pressure. The usual cavernous hemangioma is similar in this respect. The cavernous spaces are large but few, the exit channels large, and the base of the lesion sessile. Such a hemangioma would not demonstrate fluctuance, since it has all the features that permit rapid emptying.

Fig. 3-25, by contrast, is a diagram representing a capillary hemangioma with many blood sinuses connected by small vessels. Note that the exit vessels are few and small and the base is somewhat pedunculated. A hemangioma of this type would probably not be readily emptied by digital pressure, since the slight pressure that would empty the lesion would also tend to occlude the small exit vessels. Thus the lesion could consequently be partially fluctuant and partially emptiable.

Fig. 3-26 is an illustration of a capillary hemangioma that probably could not be emptied at all. The laryngocele, a developmental pouch projecting from the larynx, is inflated with air when the patient coughs. Frequently the connecting channel to the larynx is small and easily occluded, and although the laryngocele usually shows fluctuance, it can be slowly emptied by careful digital pressure. A cyst also would be fluctuant but not emptiable, since a channel for the egress of the fluid is not a usual feature of this lesion.

Position or location of the examiner's finger or fingers is important in determining whether a lesion can be emptied or not. In Fig. 3-27 the examiner's finger at point *X* would block the efferent channel and mask the fact that the lesion is really emptiable. This lesion would empty readily, however, with digital pressure if the finger were positioned at point *Y.*

The reason for the emptiability of a draining cyst or abscess is obvious and is illustrated in Fig. 3-28 on p. 38. Such a lesion generally is not fluctuant unless the opening is quite small.

Painless, tender, or painful During the digital examination it becomes apparent whether a mass is painless, tender, or painful. This information aids greatly in arranging a suitable list of diagnostic possibilities. In the development of a working diagnosis, it is helpful if the painful mass is evaluated on the basis of the following possible causes (Table 3-5):

1. *Pain because of inflammation.* The painful effect of an increase in the fluid content of a tissue by a pathologic agent is intensified when the tissue is confined within rigid or semirigid walls (dental pulp, lymph node, submaxillary or parotid salivary glands). The increased internal pressure that results from the interstitial accumulation of fluid is intensified by the external pressure of the examiner's fingers and is registered as pain or an increase in pain.

The most frequently encountered example is an inflammatory process resulting from mechanical trauma or

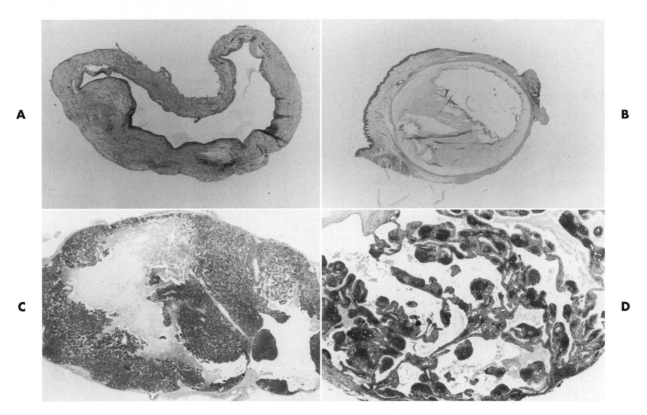

Fig. 3-21. Fluctuant pathologic masses. **A,** Radicular cyst. **B,** Mucocele. **C,** Papillary cyst adenoma. **D,** Warthin's tumor (papillary cystadenoma lymphomatosum).

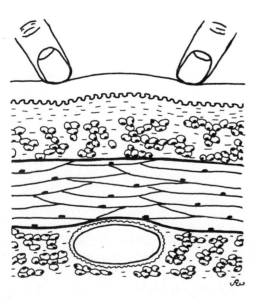

Fig. 3-22. Diagram of muscle overlying a cyst and masking its characteristics.

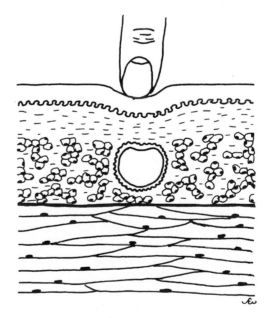

Fig. 3-23. Diagram illustrating a nonemptiable cystlike lesion.

Table 3-5   Painless, tender, and painful masses

Lesions	Exceptions
Painless	
Benign and malignant tumors	Amputation neuromas
	Adenoid cystic carcinomas
	Chondrosarcomas within bone occasionally
	Infected tumors
	Traumatized tumors
	Tumors pressing nerves
Cysts	Traumatized lesions
Benign hyperplasias	Traumatized lesions
Vascular phenomena, aneurysms, etc.	Traumatized lesions
Laryngoceles	Traumatized lesions
Late hematomas	Traumatized lesions
Sarcoidosis and tuberculosis	Traumatized lesions
Retention phenomena in nonencapsulated glands	Traumatized lesions
Tender	
Low-grade inflammations or infections	None
Mild physical trauma	None
Retention phenomena in encapsulated glands	Acute—painful
Bacterial, viral, fungal, and rickettsial infections	Acute mumps—painful
Mononucleosis	Occasionally nontender
Early hematomas	Occasionally nontender
Subcutaneous emphysemas	Occasionally nontender
Mikulicz's disease	Occasionally nontender
Sjögren's syndrome	Occasionally nontender
Painful	
Acutely inflamed tissue	None
Severe physical trauma and acute infections	None
Infected cysts	Those with draining sinuses
Infected tumors	None
Tumors	
Amputation neuromas	Early stage
Adenoid cystic carcinomas	Early stage
Chondrosarcomas	Peripheral

infection. Occasionally a tumor, especially of the malignant variety, indirectly causes pain by infiltrating a major duct of a major salivary gland—thereby inducing a retention phenomenon and an enlarged salivary gland that is tender or painful because of the markedly increased internal pressure. Also, a tumor located in adjacent normal tissue may become secondarily infected and thus change from a painless to an inflamed and painful lesion.

2. *Painful tumors.* Some neural tumors (e.g., the amputation neuroma, which actually is not a true neoplasm but represents an overexuberant misdirected repair process in a severed nerve) are commonly painful to palpation. As a rule, however, benign and malignant tumors are painless masses unless they are traumatized or secondarily infected.

3. *Pain because of sensory nerve encroachment.* Masses otherwise painless but located near relatively large sensory nerves may elicit pain when they rapidly enlarge and encroach on the nerve space. This most frequently happens when the nerve pathway is bone as opposed to soft tissue; in soft tissue, especially when the process is slow growing, the nerve is pushed ahead of the mass and pain is not elicited until an unyielding tissue is encountered. Occasionally a rapidly growing malignant tumor, such as an osteosarcoma growing within the bone, will cause pain because it expands more rapidly than the bone can be resorbed. Therefore the pressure on the surrounding bone and nerve tissue evokes pain.

Usually the pain produced by the encroachment of a malignant tumor on a sensory nerve is of short duration, since the rapidly growing tumor causes its early destruction. An exception is the adenoid cystic carcinoma, which frequently spreads through the perineural space.

Tenderness in a mass usually indicates the presence of a low-grade inflammation and internal pressure, which in

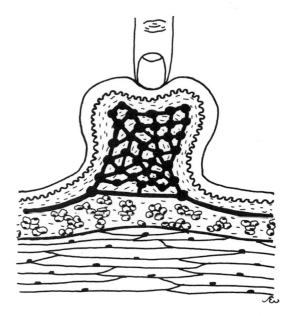

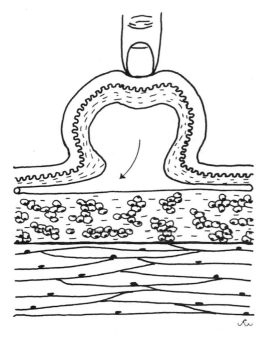

Fig. 3-24. Diagram illustrating complete emptiability in an aneurysm-like lesion.

Fig. 3-25. Diagram illustrating the difficulty encountered in attempting to completely empty a capillary hemangioma, which has many small channels and few exit vessels.

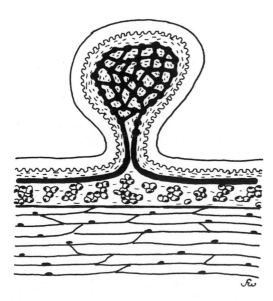

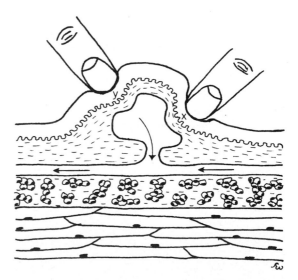

Fig. 3-26. Diagram illustrating a pedunculated capillary hemangioma, which would be nonemptiable by digital pressure.

Fig. 3-27. Diagram illustrating the importance of finger position when attempting to empty a lesion with this configuration. Careful pressure applied at point *Y* would readily empty the lesion, whereas rapid pressure applied at point *X* would tend to occlude the exit channel and render the lesion nonemptiable.

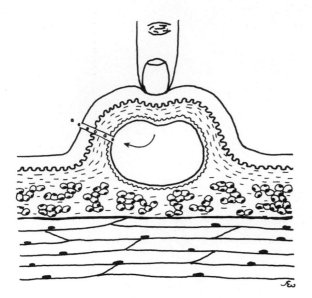

Fig. 3-28. Diagram illustrating the presence of a sinus draining a cyst or abscess. This causes a usually fluctuant lesion to become nonfluctuant and emptiable

practice are frequently induced by the repeated manipulation of a painless mass by a series of examiners. Frequently, however, a tender mass indicates the presence of a chronic infection.

The degree of pain that a mass produces often varies, depending on the stage of development of the mass or the type of infection that may have caused the pain. For example, a retention phenomenon of major glands may be tender in the early stages but become exquisitely painful as the situation worsens. Untreated bacterial infections are typically tender in the early stage, painful in the acute phase, and tender during resolution. Nevertheless, a low-grade bacterial infection occasionally may be tender throughout its course. Fungal, spirochetal, tuberculous, rickettsial, and viral infections, on the other hand, are more typically chronic in their nature and are tender throughout their development and resolution.

Unilateral or bilateral When a clinician encounters pathosis, he or she should investigate the contralateral region of the body to determine whether the condition is bilateral. As a rule, if similar masses are present bilaterally and in the same locations, they are most likely normal anatomic structures. The carotid bulb in the bifurcation of the artery, the mastoid process, the lateral processes of the cervical vertebrae, and the wings of the hyoid bone are such bilaterally occurring anatomic structures that are frequently mistaken for pathologic masses. Bilateral palpation coupled with a knowledge of anatomy is obligatory if these normal structures are to be differentiated from pathologic masses.

Solitary or multiple A solitary lesion nearly always indicates a local benign condition or an early malignancy. Multiple lesions, on the other hand, must alert the examiner to the following possibilities:

- Systemic diseases
- Disseminated disease
- Syndromes

Features Obtained by Percussion

Percussion is the act of tapping a part of the body to evaluate the quality of the echo produced. The physician routinely percusses the chest to determine the outline of the heart and to evaluate the lung fields. The dentist frequently percusses teeth to determine whether they have adequate bone support and to determine whether they are sensitive. Percussion is not particularly useful, however, for the examination of the lesions discussed in this text.

Features Obtained by Auscultation

Auscultation is the act of listening with or without the aid of a stethoscope to sounds produced inside the body. The physician routinely auscultates the chest to evaluate heart and lung sounds. The dentist may auscultate the temporomandibular joint to detect crepitus. Auscultation of pathologic masses is to be encouraged because this method detects the presence of bruits, which are a characteristic of aneurysms and arteriovenous shunts.

CHAPTER 4

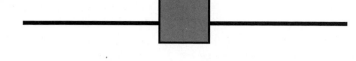

The Diagnostic Sequence

NORMAN K. WOOD

It is of paramount importance that the clinician follows a precisely formulated diagnostic sequence when a lesion is detected. Such an established approach will accomplish the following:
- *Time will be used effectively and efficiently.*
- *All the pertinent features will be identified.*
- *A high success rate in diagnosis will be achieved.*

Some authorities argue that the experienced diagnostician does not rely on such a cumbersome and formal procedure, since he or she is apparently able to diagnose a lesion after only a brief inspection. However, the expert diagnostician has seen many lesions on numerous occasions and is able to run through the diagnostic sequence very quickly in his or her mind and still maintain an excellent "batting average."

We have found the following diagnostic sequence to be both effective and practical:

DETECTION AND EXAMINATION OF THE PATIENT'S LESION
EXAMINATION OF THE PATIENT
   Chief complaint(s)
   Onset and course
REEXAMINATION OF THE LESION
CLASSIFICATION OF THE LESION

LISTING THE POSSIBLE DIAGNOSES
DEVELOPING THE DIFFERENTIAL
   DIAGNOSIS
DEVELOPING THE WORKING
   DIAGNOSIS (OPERATIONAL
   DIAGNOSIS, TENTATIVE DIAGNOSIS,
   CLINICAL IMPRESSION)

FORMULATING THE FINAL DIAGNOSIS
   (PROVED BY BIOPSY, CULTURE,
   AND/OR RESPONSE TO TREATMENT)

DETECTION AND EXAMINATION OF THE PATIENT'S LESION

Most lesions are discovered during routine examination, but in some cases, the patients are aware of their lesions and have come for help. This is especially so when pain or discomfort are the symptoms.

Once the clinician has recognized or at least suspects that an abnormal change is at hand, he or she proceeds to examine it using the modalities described in Chapters 2 and 3. These include visual examination in combination with palpation, percussion, and auscultation. The findings are noted and mentally evaluated. As a matter of personal preference, the clinician may elect to perform either a cur-

sory or a thorough examination of the lesion at this time, although the situation may dictate a thorough examination immediately. The importance of first examining the lesion is that the clinician can gain information that will alert him or her to look especially for possible related findings in the remainder of the patient examination.

EXAMINATION OF THE PATIENT

Patient examination has been discussed in depth in Chapters 2 and 3. In this chapter, we have chosen to enlarge on the sections of the interview dealing with the patient's chief complaint(s) and the onset and course of the present problem because information from these are so often pivotal.

Chief Complaint(s)

Common chief complaints related to oral diseases include sores, burning sensation, bleeding, loose teeth, recent occlusal problems, delayed tooth eruption, dry mouth, too much saliva, a swelling, bad taste, halitosis, paresthesia, and anesthesia.

Pain The patient should be encouraged to describe the main characteristics of the pain; its nature (sharp or dull), severity, duration, and location; and the precipitating circumstances.

The following entities may produce oral and facial pain:

1. Teeth
   a. Pulpal disease
   b. Pulpoperiapical disease
   c. Gingival and periodontal disease
2. Mucous membrane disease
3. Tongue conditions
4. Salivary gland inflammations and/or infection
5. Lesions of the jaw bones
6. Lymph node inflammations and infections
7. Temporomandibular joint diseases
8. Myofascial pain syndrome
9. Maxillary sinus disease
10. Ear diseases
11. Psychoses
12. Angina pectoris
13. Tonsillar disease
14. Pretender (e.g., drug addict)
15. Central nervous system diseases
16. Neuralgias
17. Neuritis
18. Vasculitis
19. Berry aneurysms
20. Diaphragmatic hernia
21. Esophageal diverticulum
22. Eagle's syndrome (calcification of stylohyoid ligament)
23. Trotter's syndrome (pain caused by carcinoma of pharynx)
24. Self-mutilation
25. Iatrogenic

Sores When a patient uses the term "sore" or "a sore" to describe a complaint, this may indicate the presence of mucosal inflammations or ulcers from any cause except early ulcerative malignancies (which are usually painless).

Burning sensation A burning sensation is usually felt in the tongue and is often caused by a thinning or erosion of the surface epithelium. The following disease states may produce a burning sensation:

1. Burning mouth syndrome
2. Psychosis
3. Neurosis
4. Viral infection
5. Fungal infection
6. Chronic bacterial infection
7. Geographic tongue
8. Fissured tongue
9. Generalized oral mucositis diseases
10. Xerostomic conditions
11. Anemia
12. Achlorhydria
13. Multiple sclerosis
14. Vitamin deficiencies

A generalized burning sensation in the mouth is also frequently found to be associated with an increased interalveolar space.

Bleeding Intraoral bleeding may be caused by these disturbances:

1. Gingivitis and periodontal disease
2. Traumatic incidents, including surgery
3. Inflammatory hyperplasias
4. Allergies
5. Tumors (traumatized tumors and tumors that are very vascular, e.g., hemangiomas)
6. Diseases that cause or are associated with deficiencies in hemostasis

Loose teeth Loss of supporting bone or the resorption of roots may result in loose teeth and may indicate the presence of any of the following:

1. Periodontal disease
2. Trauma
3. Normal resorption of deciduous teeth
4. Pulpoperiapical lesions
5. Malignant tumors
6. Benign tumors that may induce root resorption (chondromas, myxomas, hemangiomas)
7. Histiocytosis X
8. Hypophosphatasia
9. Familial hypophosphatemia
10. Papillon-Lefèvre syndrome
11. Acquired immunodeficiency syndrome (AIDS)

Recent occlusal problem When a patient complains that "recently the teeth don't bite right" or "recently some teeth are out of line," the clinician must consider overcontoured restorations or the following:

1. Periodontal disease
2. Traumatic injury (fracture of bone or tooth root)
3. Pericementitis or periapical abscess
4. Cysts or tumors of tooth-bearing regions of the jaws
5. Fibrous dysplasia

Delayed tooth eruption Delayed eruption of a tooth may be related to any of the following:

1. Malposed or impacted teeth
2. Cysts
3. Odontomas
4. Sclerosed bone
5. Tumors
6. Maldevelopment

If there is a generalized delay, the clinician should consider the possibilities of anodontia, cleidocranial dysplasia, or hypothyroidism.

Dry mouth (xerostomia) A dry mouth may result from the following disorders:

1. Local inflammation
2. Infection and fibrosis of major salivary glands
3. Dehydration states
4. Drug therapy
   a. Tranquilizers
   b. Antihistamines
   c. Anticholinergics
5. Autoimmune diseases
   a. Mikulicz's disease
   b. Sjögren's syndrome
6. Chemotherapy
7. Postradiation changes
8. Psychosis
9. Alcoholism

Too much saliva The complaint of excessive saliva may be related to psychosomatic problems. It may be associated with the insertion of new dentures; if it continues, it may indicate a decreased or an increased vertical dimension.

Swelling When a patient's chief complaint is a swelling, all the following entities must be considered as a probable cause:

1. Inflammations and infections
2. Cysts
3. Retention phenomena
4. Inflammatory hyperplasias
5. Benign and/or malignant tumors

Bad taste A complaint of bad taste may result from any of the following:

1. Aging changes
2. Heavy smoking
3. Poor oral hygiene
4. Dental caries
5. Periodontal disease
6. Acute necrotizing ulcerative gingivitis (ANUG)
7. Diabetes
8. Hypertension
9. Medication
10. Psychoses
11. Neurologic disorders
12. Decreased salivary flow
13. Uremia
14. Intraoral malignancies

Halitosis Although this is more frequently classified as an objective symptom, we have included it here because of its close relationship to bad taste.

1. Poor oral hygiene
2. Periodontal disease
3. Third molar opercula
4. Decayed teeth
5. ANUG
6. Oral cancer
7. Spicy food
8. Tobacco use
9. Nasal infection
10. Sinus infection
11. Tonsillitis
12. Pharyngeal infections or tumors
13. Gastric problems
14. Diabetes
15. Uremia

Paresthesia and anesthesia Such changes in sensation may be caused by any of the following:

1. Injury to regional nerves
   a. Anesthesia needles
   b. Jaw bone fractures
   c. Surgical procedures
2. Malignancies
3. Medications
   a. Sedatives
   b. Tranquilizers
   c. Hypnotics
4. Diabetes
5. Pernicious anemia
6. Multiple sclerosis
7. Acute infection of the jaw bone (unusual cause)
8. Psychoses

Onset and Course

The following classification of onsets and courses related to the growth rate of specific masses has proved helpful to us:

1. Masses that increase in size just before eating
   a. Salivary retention phenomena
2. Slow-growing masses (duration of months to years)
   a. Reactive hyperplasias
   b. Chronic infections
   c. Cysts
   d. Benign tumors
3. Moderately rapid-growing masses (weeks to about 2 months)
   a. Chronic infections
   b. Cysts
   c. Malignant tumors
4. Rapidly growing masses (hours to days)
   a. Abscesses (painful)
   b. Infected cysts (painful)
   c. Aneurysms (painless)
   d. Salivary retention phenomena (painless?)
   e. Hematomas (painless but sting on pressure)
5. Masses with accompanying fever
   a. Infections
   b. Lymphomas

REEXAMINATION OF THE LESION

At this point in the examination, unanswered questions frequently occur to the clinician, who may want to reexamine the lesion to reevaluate the original findings or to complete more detailed observations. For example, if the lesion is found to be soft, he or she may wish to determine whether it (1) is fluctuant, (2) can be emptied, (3) blanches on pressure, (4) pulsates, or (5) produces a gas or liquid on aspiration and what the nature of the aspirate is. On the other hand, if the lesion is firm, the clinician may want to determine its extent, whether it is freely movable, whether it is fixed to the mucosa or the underlying tissue, and so on.

CLASSIFICATION OF THE LESION

By the time the clinician has reached this point in the diagnostic sequence, he or she should be able to classify the lesion according to whether it has originated in soft tissue or bone. Having arrived at a conclusion, he or she must next describe the lesion in terms of its clinical or radiographic appearance.

For example, the soft tissue lesions will be subclassified as white, exophytic, ulcerative, and so on, whereas the bony lesions may be categorized as periapical radiolucencies, cystlike radiolucencies, multiple radiopacities, and so on. If the examiner is unsure of the correct classification, it will be helpful to refer to the diagram for soft tissue classification on p. 47 and for bony lesions on p. 234.

LIST OF THE POSSIBLE DIAGNOSES

When the lesion has been correctly classified, a list of all the lesions that may produce a similar clinical or radiographic picture should be compiled. It will be helpful to refer directly to the corresponding chapter and the list of lesions at the beginning. Initially the order of the list is not important, since the primary objective of this step is merely to include every entity that is clinically and/or radiographically similar to the condition under study.

DEVELOPMENT OF THE DIFFERENTIAL DIAGNOSIS

The process of developing a differential diagnosis may be defined briefly as the rearranging of the list of possible diagnoses, with the most probable lesion ranked at the top and the least likely at the bottom.

The actual process of ranking the lesions may become complicated as the clinician attempts to match the features of the lesion being examined with the usual (or characteristic) features of the specific lesions in his or her list. To become competent in the art of differential diagnosis, therefore, not only must the clinician be familiar with the signs and symptoms produced by many diseases, but he or she must also possess some statistical knowledge relative to the incidence of each disease entity. It is particularly important that the clinician be aware of the relative incidences of individual lesions because in the completed differential diagnosis the most commonly occurring lesion will usually be ranked above the least commonly occurring unless other features prompt a modification of this ranking. Halstead and Weathers,[1] Bouquot,[2] Goltry and Ayer,[3] and Weir et al,[4] have reported extensively on the frequency of lesions.

Consequently, we strongly recommend that in developing the differential diagnosis, the clinician first ranks the lesions in order of their *relative frequency of occurrence,* as they are in the list at the beginning of each chapter. This order by frequency will then need to be modified by consideration of age, gender, race, country of origin, and anatomic location.

Age

The age of a patient may greatly modify the rankings. For example, an ulcer occurring in the floor of a 50-year-old man's mouth indicates a reasonable probability of squamous cell carcinoma, but such a diagnosis would be unlikely if an ulcer occurred in a 10-year-old boy's mouth. The boxes on p. 43 and p. 44 group the soft tissue and bony lesions that tend to occur in patients within particular age spans. Hand and Whitehill[5] discussed the prevalence of oral mucosal lesions in elderly patients.

Gender

The fact that certain lesions occur more frequently in men or in women also contributes to the ranking of the lesions in the differential diagnosis. For example, squamous cell carcinoma affects men two to four times more often than women. On the other hand, about 80% of periapical cemental dysplasia occurs in women over 30 years of age. The boxes on p. 45 group the soft tissue and bony lesions that show a predilection for occurring in female or male patients.

Race

The importance of racial (and hereditary) influences on the incidence of some diseases is illustrated by the well-known fact that a preponderance of patients with sickle cell anemia is black. Also, florid cementoosseus dysplasia occurs predominantly in black women over 30 years of age.

Country of Origin

Information concerning the country of origin or residence may be an important clue for identification of the disease. Burkitt's lymphoma seldom affects people of non-African origin. Also, the greater use of chewing tobacco and snuff in the southeastern section of the United States is related to the increased incidence of intraoral verrucous carcinoma observed in that region.

Anatomic Location

The extent to which the anatomic location of the lesion may affect the lesion's ranking in the differential diagnosis is illustrated by the following examples:

1. Although the lower lip is a common site for the development of a mucocele but a rare location for a minor salivary gland tumor, both of these lesions may be in the same list of possible diagnoses.
2. The posterior region of the posterolateral hard palate is a characteristic location for a minor sali-

vary gland tumor but is an uncommon location for a mucocele.

3. Although the posterior hard palate is a characteristic site for a salivary gland tumor, this lesion is almost never found in the anterior hard palate and gingivae.

The box on p. 46 groups the various bony lesions that show a preference for either the maxilla or mandible and also for specific sites within these bones. Chapter 34 deals with intraoral lesions by anatomic region. Parapharyngeal masses are not discussed in this book. However, Pedlar and Ravindranathan[6] discussed the differential diagnosis of these lesions. Frommer[7] discussed differential diagnosis of lesions seen on panoramic radiographs.

The preceding pertinent facts are just a few examples from a large body of general information concerning the natural behavior of lesions that the clinician acquires from clinical experience in addition to the knowledge provided by formally structured sources.

After the ranking has been adjusted for incidence, the next step is to compare pertinent information, signs, symptoms, or other findings gained from examination of the patient with the usual features of the lesions in the list. The lesion showing the most correlation with the present findings should be ranked highest, and the lesion showing the least correlation should be ranked lowest. Halstead and Weathers[1] did an extensive differential diagnosis of soft tissue lesions.

PREDILECTION OF SOFT TISSUE LESIONS FOR SPECIAL AGE-GROUPS

Infants

Candidiasis*
Eruption cyst
Hemangioma (85% by 1 year of age)
Lingual thyroid
Lymphangioma
Neuroectodermal tumor (before 6 months of age)
White sponge nevus

Children

Albright's disease (ages 6-10)
Childhood infectious diseases
Eruption cyst
Herpes simplex
Infectious mononucleosis
Juvenile melanoma
Pulp polyps
White sponge nevus

Persons Under Age 40

Albright's disease (ages 6-10)
ANUG (ages 15-35; rare below age 12)
Benign salivary gland tumor (ages 30-39)
Branchial cyst
Candidiasis
Childhood infectious diseases
Cystic hygroma
Dermoid or epidermoid cyst
Eruption cyst
Erythema multiforme
Hemangioma (85% by 1 year of age)
Herpes simplex
Hodgkin's disease (ages 20-40)
Infectious mononucleosis
Juvenile melanoma
Lingual thyroid

Lymphangioma (88% before age 3)
Mucocele (65% before age 30)
Neuroectodermal tumor (before 6 months)
Palatal tori (peak before age 30)
Papilloma
Peripheral giant cell granuloma (over age 30)
Peripheral fibroma with calcification (peak at age 25)
Plasma cell gingivitis
Pulp polyps
Pyogenic granuloma (60%)
Recurrent aphthous ulcer
Thyroglossal cyst
White sponge nevus

Persons Over Age 40

Benign mucous membrane pemphigoid
Candidiasis†
Denture stomatitis
Desquamative gingivitis
Epulis fissuratum
Hemochromatosis
Inflammatory papillary hyperplasia
Keratoacanthoma
Leukoedema
Leukoplakia (90%)
Lichen planus
Lipoma
Lymphoma
Malignant salivary gland tumors (ages 40-60)
Melanoma
Metastatic carcinoma
Metastatic carcinoma to cervical nodes
Pemphigus (seldom under age 30)
Radiation mucositis
Squamous cell carcinoma
Verrucous carcinoma (ages 60-80)

*Also common in persons over age 40.
†Also common in infants.

PREDISPOSITION OF BONY OR CALCIFIED LESIONS FOR SPECIAL AGE-GROUPS

Infants

Caffey's disease (birth to 2 years of age)
Letterer-Siwe disease (ages 1-3)
Lingual mandibular bone defect?
Osteopetrosis (malignant)
Rickets
Thalassemia major

Children

Acute leukemia
Basal cell nevus syndrome (ages 5-30)
Burkitt's tumor (ages 2-14)
Central hemangioma (ages 10-20)
Cherubism
Dentigerous cyst (ages 10-20)
Fibrous dysplasia (ages 10-20)
Hand-Schüller-Christian disease (ages 1-10)
Lingual mandibular bone defect
Multilocular cyst (over age 15)
Osteoid osteoma
Osteopetrosis (malignant)
Proliferative periostitis (ages 5-12)
Rickets
Thalassemia major

Persons Under Age 30

Acute leukemia
Adenomatoid odontogenic tumor (peak at age 16)
Ameloblastic fibroma (peak at age 16)
Aneurysmal bone cyst (under age 20)
Basal cell nevus syndrome (ages 5-30)
Burkitt's tumor (ages 2-14)
Caffey's disease (birth to 2 years of age)
Cancer
    Ewing's sarcoma (peak at ages 14-18)
    Osteogenic sarcoma of jaws (ages 10-40, peak at age 27)
    Reticulum cell sarcoma of bone (70% under age 40)
Cementifying and ossifying fibroma (young adults)
Cementoblastoma (under age 25)
Central giant cell granuloma (60% under age 20)
Central hemangioma (ages 10-20)
Cherubism
Dentigerous cyst (ages 10-20)
Developing tooth crypt (under age 20)
Eosinophilic granuloma
Fibrous dysplasia (ages 10-20)

Hand-Schüller-Christian disease (ages 1-10)
Letterer-Siwe disease (ages 1-3)
Lingual mandibular bone defect
Multilocular cyst (over age 15)
Mural ameloblastoma (ages 18-30)
Odontogenic fibroma (under age 25)
Odontogenic keratocyst (ages 10-20)
Odontoma in developing stages (under age 20)
Osteoblastoma (75% under age 20)
Osteoid osteoma
Osteopetrosis (malignant)
Parulis
Primordial cyst (ages 10-30)
Proliferative periostitis (under age 25)
Rickets
Sickle cell anemia
Thalassemia major
Thalassemia minor
Traumatic bone cyst (under age 25)

Persons Over Age 30

Ameloblastoma (ages 20-50, peak at age 40)
Chondrosarcoma (ages 20-60, peak in 50s)
Osteopetrosis (benign)
Pindborg tumor (ages 28-48)
Primary hyperparathyroidism (ages 30-60)
Residual cyst (peak at age 52)
Florid cementoosseous dysplasia

Persons Over Age 40

Artery calcification
Calcified node
Cancer
    Chondrosarcoma (ages 20-60; peak in 50s)
    Metastatic carcinoma
    Minor salivary tumor
    Multiple myeloma (ages 40-70)
    Squamous cell carcinoma (peripheral)
Osteomalacia
Osteomyelitis
Paget's disease
Periapical cemental dysplasia
Postextraction sockets
Secondary hyperparathyroidism (ages 50-80)
Sialolith

TWO OR MORE LESIONS PRESENT

From time to time, clinicians examine patients with various combinations of lesions. Perhaps one patient will present with two lesions in the oral cavity. Another patient may have a lesion in the oral cavity and another in the neck. In still another patient the examination may reveal a lesion in the oral cavity and another in a more distant site, for example, the lung. After some thought, it becomes obvious that it is necessary to develop the differential diagnosis along distinctly contrasting lines in each of these cases.

Basically, when two or more lesions are present, seven possibilities or propositions must be considered (modified from Mitton et al[8]):

    1. Lesions are related
        a. Lesion A and lesion B are identical (two aphthous ulcers)

GENDER PREDILECTION OF SOFT TISSUE LESIONS (RATIOS OR PERCENTS ARE GIVEN IN PARENTHESES)

Male

Cancer (except minor salivary gland tumors and metastatic carcinoma from distant sites)
  Lymphoma (2:1)
  Melanoma (2:1)
  Metastatic carcinoma to cervical nodes
  Squamous cell carcinoma (3:1 to 2:1)
    Buccal (10:1)
    Floor (93%)
    Lip (98%)
    Tongue (75%)
  Verrucous carcinoma (3:1)
Erythema multiforme
Hemochromatosis
Keratoacanthoma (2:1)
Leukoplakia
Lymphoepithelial cyst (3:1)
Median rhomboid glossitis
Mucocele
Radiation mucositis

Female

Benign mucous membrane pemphigoid (2:1)
Desquamative gingivitis
Geographic tongue (2:1)
Hemangioma
Lichen planus (2:1)
Lipoma (7:1 or equal)
Palatal tori (2:1)
Peripheral giant cell granuloma (2:1)
Peripheral fibroma with calcification
Plasma cell gingivitis
Pyogenic granuloma (3:1)
Ranula
Recurrent aphthous ulcers
Salivary gland tumors (2:1)

GENDER PREDISPOSITION OF BONY LESIONS

Male

Cancer
  Chondrosarcoma
  Ewing's sarcoma (2:1)
  Lymphoma (2:1)
  Melanoma (2:1)
  Multiple myeloma (2:1)
  Osteogenic sarcoma
  Squamous cell carcinoma
    Central (2:1)
    Peripheral (3:1 to 2:1)
Cherubism
Eosinophilic granuloma (2:1)
Hand-Schüller-Christian disease (2:1)
Incisive canal cyst (3:1)
Lingual mandibular bone cavity
Osteoblastoma
Osteoid osteoma (2:1)
Osteomyelitis (5:1)
Residual cyst (2:1)
Traumatic bone cyst

Female

Cancer
  Metastatic carcinoma
  Minor salivary gland tumors
Central giant cell granuloma (2:1)
Central hemangioma (2:1)
Osteoporosis
Periapical cemental dysplasia
Primary hyperparathyroidism (7:1)
Florid cementoosseous dysplasia
Secondary hyperparathyroidism (2:1)

  b. Lesion B is secondary to lesion A (metastatic tumor and primary tumor)
  c. Lesion A is secondary to lesion B (metastatic tumor and primary tumor)
  d. Lesion A and lesion B are both secondary to a third lesion, which may be occult (metastatic tumors and primary tumor)
  e. Lesion A and lesion B are manifestations of systemic disease (infections, histiocytosis X, disseminated malignancy)
  f. Lesion A and lesion B form part of a syndrome (café-au-lait spots and multiple neurofibromas in von Recklinghausen's disease)
2. Lesions are completely unrelated to each other and occur together only as a matter of chance

DEVELOPING THE WORKING DIAGNOSIS (OPERATIONAL DIAGNOSIS, TENTATIVE DIAGNOSIS, CLINICAL IMPRESSION)

Although the clinician has completed a differential diagnosis, he or she is not yet completely prepared to treat the lesion. He or she must now recheck the *credibility* of these top choices. This is done by further examination of the lesion, by asking the patient more definitive questions to expand the history, by perhaps ordering additional tests, and finally by reevaluating all the assembled pertinent data. Once their validity has been supported, the top choices will be referred to as the working diagnosis or clinical impression. The clinician may in some cases be so confident of the first-ranked entity that he or she excludes all the others from the working diagnosis.

The *working diagnosis* will dictate the proper management, especially if the management is to include surgery,

---

JAWBONE AND REGIONAL PREDILECTION OF BONY LESIONS

Mandible and Predominant Region

Ameloblastic fibroma (molar, premolar)
Ameloblastoma (80%; posterior, 70%)
Aneurysmal bone cyst (much more common in molar)
Benign nonodontogenic tumors (molar, ramus)
Caffey's disease
Calcifying odontogenic cyst (70%)
Cancer
    Acute leukemia (molar)
    Ewing's sarcoma
    Metastatic carcinoma (95%; molar, premolar)
    Osteogenic sarcoma (body)
    Reticulum cell sarcoma (molar, angle, ramus)
    Squamous cell carcinoma
        Peripheral (3:1, molar)
        Central (2:1)
Cementifying and/or ossifying fibroma (molar, premolar)
Cementoblastoma (first molar, premolar)
Cementoma (90%; incisor)
Central giant cell granuloma (65%; two thirds are anterior to molar)
Central hemangioma (65%; ramus, premolar)
Cherubism (ramus, third molar)
Complex odontoma
Condensing osteitis
Eosinophilic granuloma
Follicular cyst

Garré's osteomyelitis
Odontogenic fibroma
Odontogenic keratocyst (65%)
Odontogenic myxoma (molar, premolar)
Osteomyelitis (7:1; body)
Pindborg tumor (2:1; molar, premolar)
Postextraction sockets
Primordial cyst (third molar)
Proliferative periostitis
Sclerosing cemental masses

Maxilla and Predominant Region

Adenomatoid odontogenic tumor (canine)
Chondrosarcoma (2:1)
Compound odontoma
Fibrous dysplasia (4:3)
Paget's disease (20:3)
Residual cyst (65%)

Rare in Maxilla

Caffey's disease
Cementifying and/or ossifying fibroma
Ewing's sarcoma
Osteomyelitis
Proliferative periostitis
Reticulum cell sarcoma
Traumatic bone cyst

---

because it will aid the surgeon in planning any operation—how long to reserve the operating room, what instrument setups to have prepared, whether to do an incisional or an excisional biopsy or a frozen section, whether to have blood available, and, if so, how much and what type.

Before the surgery commences, the surgeon may choose to do one last test, such as aspiration of the lesion. This is an excellent precaution in certain instances and will rule out or identify vascular tumors, thereby avoiding the dangerous surprise that awaits the unsuspecting surgeon who encounters an unrecognized vascular tumor at surgery.

FORMULATING THE FINAL DIAGNOSIS

The final diagnosis in most cases of oral pathoses is provided by the oral pathologist who evaluates a biopsy in light of all the available clinical data. In some instances the microscopic picture is quite diagnostic. In other cases, however, the microscopic picture may be so equivocal that the pathologist must depend heavily on the accompanying clinical symptoms in establishing the final diagnosis. In still other cases (e.g., an empty traumatic bone cyst) the clinician must establish the final diagnosis at the time of the surgery, since there may not be a specimen available for microscopic examination.

REFERENCES

1. Halstead CL, Weathers DR: *Differential diagnosis of oral soft tissue pathoses: site unit(s)-3379: instructional materials for health professional education,* National Library of Medicine/National Medical Audiovisual Center, Washington, DC, 1977, US Department of Health, Education, and Welfare.
2. Bouquot JE: Common oral lesions found during a mass screening examination, *J Am Dent Assoc* 112:50-57, 1986.
3. Goltry RR, Ayer WA: Head, neck, and oral abnormalities in dentists participating in the health assessment program, *J Am Dent Assoc* 112:338-341, 1986.
4. Weir JC, Davenport WD, Skinner RL: A diagnostic and epidemiologic survey of 15,783 oral lesions, *J Am Dent Assoc* 115:439-442, 1987.
5. Hand JA, Whitehall JM: The prevalence of oral mucosal lesions in an elderly population, *J Am Dent Assoc* 112:73-76, 1987.
6. Pedlar J, Ravindranathan N: Differential diagnosis and surgical management of parapharyngeal masses: review and an unusual illustrative case, *Oral Surg* 63:412-416, 1987.
7. Frommer HH: Differential diagnosis from pantomograms, *Dent Radiogr Photogr* 55:25-36, 1982.
8. Mitton VA, Eversole LR, Kramer HS, Stern M: Clinical-Pathological Conference: case 16, part 1 and part 2. Stafne's bone cyst of the mandible and concurrent pulmonary coccidioidomycosis, *J Oral Surg* 34:616-617, 715-716, 1976.

PART II

SOFT TISSUE LESIONS

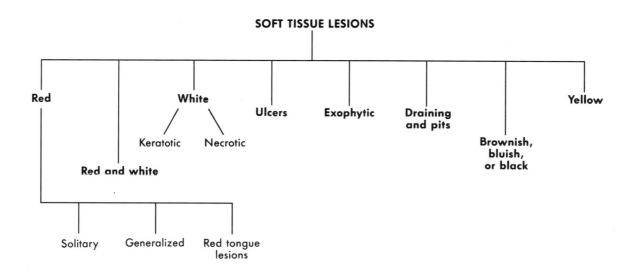

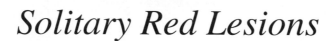

CHAPTER 5

Solitary Red Lesions

NORMAN K. WOOD

EDWARD PETERS

GEORGE G. BLOZIS

This chapter deals primarily with pathologic conditions appearing as single red lesions or else diffuse lesions that affect only one mucosal surface. These are listed as follows:

PATHOLOGIC RED LESIONS
TRAUMATIC ERYTHEMATOUS MACULES AND EROSIONS
PURPURIC MACULES (EARLY STAGE)
INFLAMMATORY HYPERPLASIA LESIONS
REDDISH ULCERS OR ULCERS WITH RED HALOS
NONPYOGENIC SOFT TISSUE ODONTOGENIC INFECTION (CELLULITIS)
CHEMICAL OR THERMAL ERYTHEMATOUS MACULE
NICOTINE STOMATITIS
ERYTHROPLAKIA, CARCINOMA IN SITU, AND RED MACULAR SQUAMOUS CELL CARCINOMA
EXOPHYTIC, RED SQUAMOUS CELL CARCINOMA
CANDIDIASIS
 Atrophic/erythematous candidiasis
 Denture stomatitis
 Angular cheilitis

MACULAR HEMANGIOMA AND TELANGIECTASIA
ALLERGIC MACULES
HERALD LESION OF GENERALIZED STOMATITIS OR VESICULOBULLOUS DISEASE
METASTATIC TUMORS TO SOFT TISSUE
KAPOSI'S SARCOMA (AIDS)
RARITIES
 Actinomycosis
 Anemia (solitary red patch)
 Amyloidosis
 Angiosarcoma
 Blastomycosis
 Candidiasis endocrinopathy syndrome
 Crohn's disease
 Coccidioidomycosis
 Dermatitis herpetiformis
 Erysipelas
 Exfoliative cheilitis
 Gonococcal infection
 Graft-versus-host disease (GVHD)

Herpangina
Histoplasmosis
Hyperemic oral tonsils
Larva migrans
Lichen planus
Lupus erythematosus
Ludwig's angina
Lymphonodular pharyngitis (Coxsackie A)
Multinucleate cell angiohistiocytoma
Mycosis fungoides
Non-Hodgkin's lymphoma
Peripheral ameloblastoma
Plasma cell gingivitis
Psoriasis, oral
Sarcoidosis
Secondary syphilis
Self-mutilation
Subacute necrotizing sialadenitis
Tuberculosis
Tumoral calcinosis

NORMAL VARIATION IN ORAL MUCOSA

Masticatory and Lining Mucosa

The normal oral mucosa demonstrates a wide spectrum of pink colors, varying from a dark pink (reddish) to a very pale pink (almost white).

The healthy masticatory mucosa (over the hard palate, the gingiva, and dorsal surface of the tongue) is light pink (Fig. 5-1). These surfaces are exposed to forces and pres-

sure of mastication and have adapted by producing (1) a protective layer of keratin and (2) a subepithelial connective tissue that is densely fibrous, relatively avascular, and firmly attached to bone or muscle.

In contrast, the lining mucosa (the oral mucosa over the vestibule, cheeks, lips, floor of the mouth, and ventral surface of the tongue) is protected from such intense mechanical and chemical stimulations, so similar tissue

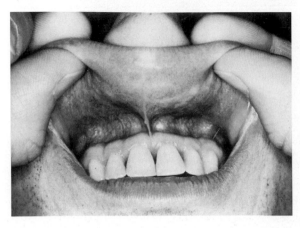

Fig. 5-1. Clinical view showing the paler pink of the attached gingiva (masticatory mucosa) in contrast to the deeper pink of the vestibular mucosa (lining mucosa).

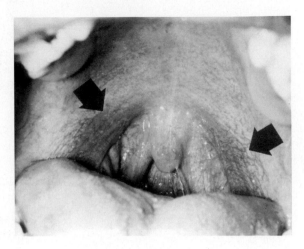

Fig. 5-2. Note the red appearance of the palatoglossal arch *(arrows)* in this healthy asymptomatic patient.

modification does not occur in these areas. Therefore the color from the underlying vasculature is transmitted through the more transparent overlying tissue and imparts a more reddish color to the surface in comparison with the light pinkish hue of the masticatory mucosa.

Individual variations in the color of the oral mucosa will be apparent and are probably an expression of one or more genetically controlled factors; that is, some people readily form keratin as a result of minor stimuli, whereas others require a strong stimulus to produce minimal keratinization. Also, a patient's hemoglobin concentration will affect the shade of pink. For example, the patient with polycythemia will have a redder mucosa than will the patient with anemia.

Palatoglossal Arch Region

In a significant number of individuals, areas of apparently normal mucosa covering the palatoglossal arch region are a deep dusky red in contrast to the light red color of the surrounding tissues (Fig. 5-2 and Plate A, 1).

These entirely painless red macular bands are usually present bilaterally and, although the size and shape of the areas in the same individual may not be uniform, persist unchanged. In some cases, bands are also found on the mucosa lining the tonsillar fossa, particularly in individuals who have had tonsillectomies some years before. These regions have a richer blood supply than the surrounding tissues and may be associated with Waldeyer's ring. Although this entity must be considered an individual normal variation, it is important that the clinician be familiar with the condition because it is often misdiagnosed as "sore throat."

PATHOLOGIC RED LESIONS

The basic tissue changes or causes that produce abnormal red conditions are as follows:

I. Vascular dilatation from:
  A. Inflammation (erythema)
    1. Mechanical trauma (e.g., cheek biting, ill-fitting denture)
    2. Thermal trauma (e.g., hot food)
    3. Chemical trauma (strong mouthwashes, iatrogenic spills)
    4. Infection (cellulitis, Ludwig's angina)
    5. Allergy or autoimmune disease (e.g., Sjögren's syndrome)
    6. Ulcer with inflamed rim (e.g., recurrent herpetic lesion)
  B. Congenital defects (e.g., hemangioma)
II. Extravasation of blood (e.g., trauma or hemostatic disease or both)
III. Atrophy or erosion of mucosa (e.g., atrophic candidiasis [inflammatory component usually present also])
IV. Marked increase in hemoglobin concentration of circulating blood (polycythemia)

White keratin areas and sloughing white patches, representing necrotic tissue and fibrinous exudate, may appear in areas where the mucosa is erythematous (see Chapter 9).

TRAUMATIC ERYTHEMATOUS MACULES AND EROSIONS

Mechanical trauma to the oral mucosa can produce a variety of clinical lesions depending on the nature and circumstances of the insult, as well as factors that govern reactions in the host. Some of the clinical lesions are listed in the box on p. 51.

The erythematous macule and erosion, the purpuric macule, and the granulomatous stage of the inflammatory hyperplastic lesion are essentially red and are discussed in this chapter.

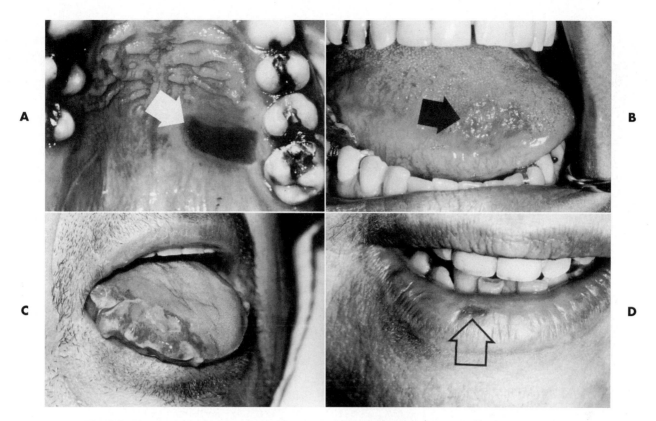

Fig. 5-3. Traumatic erythematous macules. These red patches all blanched on digital pressure. **A,** Palatal lesion caused by ill-fitting palatal connector of a partial denture. **B,** Red lesion at anterolateral border of tongue caused by a carious tooth with a sharp edge. **C,** Red and white traumatic lesion of the tongue caused by the patient chewing his tongue while it was anesthetized. The darker areas (red) are erythematous, and the white areas are necrotic. **D,** Small red macule on lip of middle-aged woman who repeatedly touched this spot with the incisal edge of her maxillary incisor.

RESPONSE TO TRAUMA

- Keratotic lesion (increased retention of keratin)
- Necrotic white lesion (necrosis of the epithelium and possibly the subepithelial tissue to some extent)
- Reddish erythematous macule (an area of inflammation)
- Purpuric macule (subepithelial hemorrhage within the tissue spaces)
- Bleb (a pooling of tissue fluid in the tissue)
- Erosion
- Ulcer
- Exophytic lesion (inflammatory hyperplasia)

Traumatic erythematous macules are produced by a low-grade, usually chronic physical insult. A more intense degree of brief trauma would be expected to produce a purpuric macule, an erosion, or a frank ulcer, in order of increasing severity. Common causes include sharp margins of teeth or restorations and ill-fitting prostheses. Self-inflicted trauma such as cheek biting or other habits also may produce traumatic erythematous macules.

Features

The usual sites for erythematous macules are on the anterior and lateral borders of the tongue, the floor of the mouth, the posterior palate, buccal mucosa, and mucosal surfaces of the lips. The macule may show considerable variation in the intensity of its red color. The size of the red zone corresponds closely to the size of the traumatic agent. Consequently, size and shape may vary considerably. The margins of macular lesions are not usually sharply defined but may be in some instances (Fig. 5-3 and Plate A, 2). Symptoms may vary from mild tenderness to considerable pain. The causative agent is usually easily identified through either the history or the clinical examination. The lesion generally regresses quickly after the cause is removed; however, if the lesion is located on the tongue, it may persist for several weeks and heal as a bald pink area devoid of papillae.

Microscopic changes include an inflamed lamina propria covered perhaps with a slightly thinned or eroded stratified squamous epithelium that is nonkeratinized. It may blanch when digital pressure is applied because this lesion is basically inflammatory.

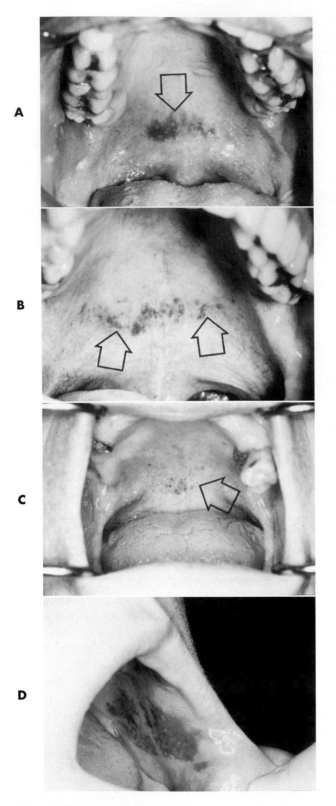

Fig. 5-4. Red purpuric macules. These lesions either blanched minimally or did not blanch at all to digital pressure. **A,** Palatal ecchymosis caused by fellatio. **B,** Palatal petechiae apparently caused by violent coughing, although a history of fellatio was not satisfactorily ruled out. **C,** Palatal petechiae in a patient with hemophilia. **D,** Reddish ecchymotic patch of the buccal mucosa after an oral surgical procedure.

Differential Diagnosis

For a discussion of the differential diagnosis of traumatic erythematous macules and erosions, refer to the differential diagnosis section under Purpuric Macules.

Management

The mechanical irritant should be identified and eliminated and the lesion kept under surveillance until it disappears. Healing noticeably occurs in 3 or 4 days. If the lesion does not disappear soon, additional workup should be done. If the suspicion index is high, a biopsy should be performed to rule out more serious conditions such as erythroplakia, squamous cell carcinoma, and fungal diseases such as candidiasis and histoplasmosis.

PURPURIC MACULES (EARLY STAGE)

The purpuric macule is produced by a blunt traumatic insult to the mucosa or skin of sufficient force to cause the extravasation of blood into the superficial tissues. If the patient is examined soon after the traumatic incident has occurred, petechial (small pinpoint) or ecchymotic (larger) areas that are quite red are observed. If sufficient time has lapsed for the reduction of oxyhemoglobin, the bruise will appear blue and later green and yellow as the hemoglobin pigment breaks down.

Features

The size of the purpuric macule varies according to the size and force of the physical agent inflicting the damage. Usually, the borders are poorly demarcated, blending almost imperceptibly with the surrounding normal tissue (Fig. 5-4). Blanching on pressure does not usually occur because the red blood cells are within the tissues rather than in vessels. Nevertheless, purpuric macules may also have an accompanying inflammatory component, and in such cases the clinician may observe some blanching on palpation. Virtually any of the oral surfaces may be involved, but the palate, buccal mucosa, and floor of the mouth are the most common sites.

Frequently, reddish elliptic purpuric macules occurring on the palatal mucosa near the junction of the hard and soft palate may result from oral sexual practices[1] and are caused by the repeated bumping of the male organ on the soft tissue in this region (Fig. 5-4). In such a case the lesion disappears within 2 or 3 days only to return again when the act is repeated.[2] A judicious history taken in a confidential setting frequently reveals the true identity of such a lesion.

Differential Diagnosis

When transient reddish macules are observed near the junction of the hard and soft palates, the following entities should be considered: traumatic erythematous macule, purpuric macule of oral sex, palatal bruising because of severe coughing or severe vomiting, macular hemangioma, atrophic candidiasis, mononucleosis, and herpangina. The first four lesions are usually painless, and a careful history establishes the occurrence of a traumatic incident. Hemangiomas seldom occur on the posterior palate, and both the erythematous macule and the hemangioma blanch somewhat on pressure. In contrast to the purpuric macule and the erythematous macule, the hemangioma is not transient.

Management

Once the diagnosis of purpuric macule has been established, the patient should be advised of its nature. Follow-up examinations are necessary to ensure that the lesion has disappeared.

If several purpuric areas are present, the patient should be asked if he or she has always bruised excessively and how extensive the trauma was. If the correlation is unsatisfactory, the patient should be tested for the presence of a bleeding disorder.

INFLAMMATORY HYPERPLASIA LESIONS

Inflammatory hyperplasia (IH) lesions are discussed in considerable detail in Chapter 10. Etiology is similar to the traumatic erythematous macule and the purpuric macule except that the precipitating insults are invariably chronic irritants such as calculus, ragged margins of cavities, overhanging restorations, overextended denture flanges, sharp spicules of bone, or chronic biting of the cheek or lip. Such prolonged chronic insults stimulate the production of granulation tissue. A list of IH lesions includes pyogenic granuloma, hormonal tumor, traumatic hemangioma, epulis fissuratum, epulis granulomatosum, papillary hyperplasia, peripheral giant cell granuloma, parulis, and the peripheral fibroma with calcification.

In the life cycle of one of these lesions the entity initially develops as a mass of inflamed granulation tissue and clinically appears soft and very red. Later, when fibrous tissue is laid down, the lesion becomes firmer and less red. If the irritant is eliminated at this stage, the remainder of the inflammation disappears and the lesion shrinks noticeably, becomes firm, and takes on a pale hue. This endpoint lesion is an inflammatory fibrous hyperplasia.

Features

Features of IH lesions are discussed in detail in Chapter 10. In the stage being considered here, the lesions are quite red, moderately soft, polypoid or nodular masses (Fig. 5-5 and Plates A, 4 to A, 6).

Microscopy of the early IH lesions reveals granulomatous tissue covered with an intact layer of stratified squamous epithelium that is nonkeratinized. If the surface becomes traumatized, a white necrotic area usually develops in the region of the injury and the lesion becomes a pyogenic granuloma.

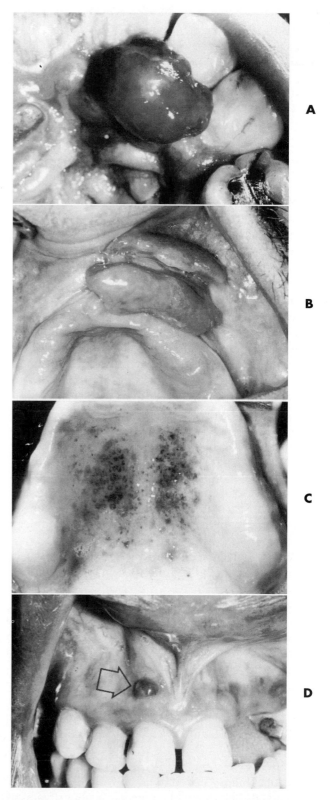

Fig. 5-5. Reddish IH lesions. All of these lesions contained a large inflammatory component. **A,** Red pyogenic granuloma of the lingual gingiva caused by the sharp edges of a large carious lesion on the lateral incisor. **B,** Large red epulis fissuratum. **C,** Red papillary hyperplasia in its earliest stages, caused by an ill-fitting upper denture. **D,** Red parulis on the labial mucosa in an early stage of development. Parulis at the opening of a sinus that was draining the infected periapical region of the maxillary right central incisor. (**A** courtesy E. Seklecki, Tucson, Ariz.)

DIFFERENTIAL DIAGNOSIS OF RED IH LESIONS

- Hemangioma
- Metastatic tumor
- Primary malignant tumor
- Kaposi's sarcoma (Chapters 12, 36)
- Papilloma/condyloma/verruca

Differential Diagnosis

The early IH lesion must be differentiated from other raised lesions listed in the box above. In the case of most IH lesions in their early stages of development, a precipitating irritant is usually identifiable. This strengthens the impression and supports a working diagnosis of IH.

However, if an irritant is not apparent, the possibility the lesion is either a primary (probably not squamous cell carcinoma [SCC]) or secondary malignant tumor beginning beneath a normal surface epithelium is given more consideration in the differential diagnosis. In turn, a history of treatment or symptoms of a primary tumor elsewhere prompts the ordering of these possibilities in favor of a metastatic tumor (see Fig. 5-21). Excluding SCC and salivary gland tumors, primary malignant tumors of the oral soft tissue are quite uncommon. It is rare for a squamous cell carcinoma to appear as a small exophytic red lesion with a smooth nonulcerated surface.

In the case of gingival IH lesions adjacent to alveolar bony changes, malignant tumors must be given a high ranking except in the case of obvious chronic infection of the bone.

A congenital *hemangioma* is present from birth, whereas a traumatic (acquired) hemangioma is really a type of IH lesion.

Papillomas, *condylomas*, *verrucae*, and *verrucous* and *squamous cell carcinomas* are included for the sake of completeness. However, since the IH lesions have a basically smooth, evenly contoured surface, they should be readily differentiated from these epithelial growths that have rough pebbly to a cauliflower-like surface. The pyogenic granuloma may have an area on its otherwise smooth surface that is white, but this is necrotic material and can be easily removed, leaving a raw bleeding surface.

Management

Excisional biopsy in combination with elimination of the irritant is the treatment of choice for lesions of substantial size when the suspicion index is moderate to high. When the suspicion index is low, elimination of the irritant will result in significant reduction of the inflammatory component, making surgery easier. Small red lesions may shrink to a size that precludes treatment when the irritant is eliminated.

REDDISH ULCERS OR ULCERS WITH RED HALOS

Ulcers are discussed at length in Chapter 11. They are included here for completeness because ulcerative conditions frequently are first manifested as erythematous macules, for example, the recurrent herpetic lesion and the recurrent aphthous ulcer. Furthermore, in these conditions, when the reddish area ultimately ulcerates, the defect frequently has a reddish border (Fig. 5-6 and Plate B, 4). Such an observation might prompt the clinician to classify the entity as a red lesion; however, experience has demonstrated that for the purpose of a differential diagnosis it is more beneficial to classify these lesions as ulcers.

Differential Diagnosis

The differential diagnosis of the various oral ulcers is covered in Chapter 11.

NONPYOGENIC SOFT TISSUE ODONTOGENIC INFECTION (CELLULITIS)

This section includes a discussion of soft tissue odontogenic infections that either are caused by nonpyogenic bacteria or represent prepyogenic or postpyogenic stages of infections; that is, the causative bacteria may be nonpyogenic, or the infection has not reached the pus-forming or pus-pooling stage. Odontogenic infection may originate in three sites: the canals and periapex of pulpless teeth, the gingiva or bony pockets in periodontal disease, and the gingival operculum over an erupting tooth.

Features

In most of these cases a suitable history and clinical and radiographic examinations coupled with pulp testing usually clearly indicate the diagnosis of dental infection (Fig. 5-7).

The alveolar mucosa and gingiva are the most frequent sites of dental infection, but if the infection is permitted to spread, a number of the oral mucosal surfaces and the overlying skin may become involved. Various degrees of swelling show a hot, red, tender to painful surface. However, pus that has formed and pooled near the surface of the swollen tissue imparts a yellowish-white color to the central region of the swelling and renders the swelling rubbery and fluctuant to the touch (see Chapter 3).

Ludwig's angina is an unusual example of a reddish soft tissue infection that is produced by a mixed infection of nonspecific microorganisms, but a nonpyogenic strain of streptococcus is almost invariably present. This condition causes a sudden swelling of the floor of the mouth and also of the submental and submaxillary spaces, often of such a magnitude that obstruction of the airway is threatened. In most cases a very red, moderately firm, painful swelling of the floor of the mouth produces an elevation of the tongue. The skin of the neck overlying the

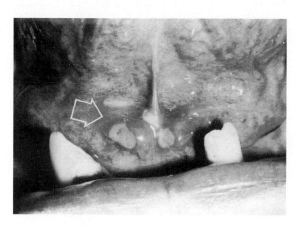

Fig. 5-6. Reddened mucosa surrounding three recurrent aphthous ulcers in the floor of the mouth.

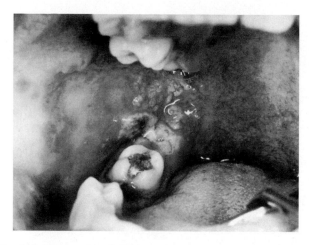

Fig. 5-7. Nonpurulent infection of retromolar region originating from a pericoronitis involving the erupting third molar tooth. The white necrotic material represents a localized ANUG. (Courtesy G. Blozis, Columbus, Ohio.)

swollen submental and submaxillary spaces is usually red and feels hot on palpation (Fig. 5-8 and Plate B, 3).

Cervical or intraoral actinomycosis is a specific infection that frequently occurs as a tender, reddish swelling (Fig. 5-8).

Differential Diagnosis

When a patient has a reddish painful swelling of the oral soft tissues with an accompanying tender cervical lymphadenitis, the diagnosis of infection is reasonably certain. An extremely high percentage of these infections are odontogenic in origin and therefore bacterial. However, the clinician should at least consider the less likely possibilities of actinomycosis, tuberculosis, and various fungal infections such as histoplasmosis, coccidioidomycosis, and blastomycosis.

Management

When a diagnosis of odontogenic infection has been established, the associated dental problem should be eliminated by root canal therapy, extraction, curettage, excision, or incision and drainage. In addition, in acute cases, concomitant oral administration of amoxicillin[3-7] is recommended.

Patients with infections that are or may become a threat to their airway should be hospitalized so that any respiratory complication can be managed promptly and properly.

CHEMICAL OR THERMAL ERYTHEMATOUS MACULE

The cause of a chemical or thermal erythematous macule is usually a caustic drug or hot foods or beverages. Obviously the severity of the tissue damage varies with the intensity and duration of the insult, so several different clin-

ical appearances may be produced. Caustic or hot agents may produce a coagulation necrosis of the superficial tissue that appears whitish and can be scraped off. Fig. 8-43 illustrates such a change precipitated by aspirin/acetaminophen. More intense or prolonged insults may still result in ulceration and possibly stripping of the mucosa. Milder agents or briefer applications of strong agents produce the mildest clinically detectable reaction, an *erythema* of the superficial tissues, which explains why this condition is included in this chapter (Fig. 5-9). Sometimes a mixed reaction is produced, so the clinical lesion may appear as necrotic white dots or patches on an erythematous base (Fig. 5-9).

Features

The red area is tender to painful, may blanch somewhat on pressure, and may bleed on the slightest manipulation. The size and shape corresponds to the area of contact with the caustic agent. The buccal and palatal mucosa are the sites most commonly affected. Mild aspirin burns are good examples, as are mild palatal burns from hot food. A careful history identifies the causative agent in almost all cases.

Differential Diagnosis

Many of the lesions discussed in this chapter should be considered in the differential diagnosis: erythema from mechanical trauma, purpuric macule, cellulitis (nonpyogenic odontogenic infection), allergic manifestations, erythroplakia, atrophic candidiasis (formerly known as atrophic candidosis), herald spot of disseminated red conditions, and fungal infections. A recent history of chemical or thermal injury along with uncomplicated resolution of the lesion in question eliminates these possibilities and establishes the correct diagnosis.

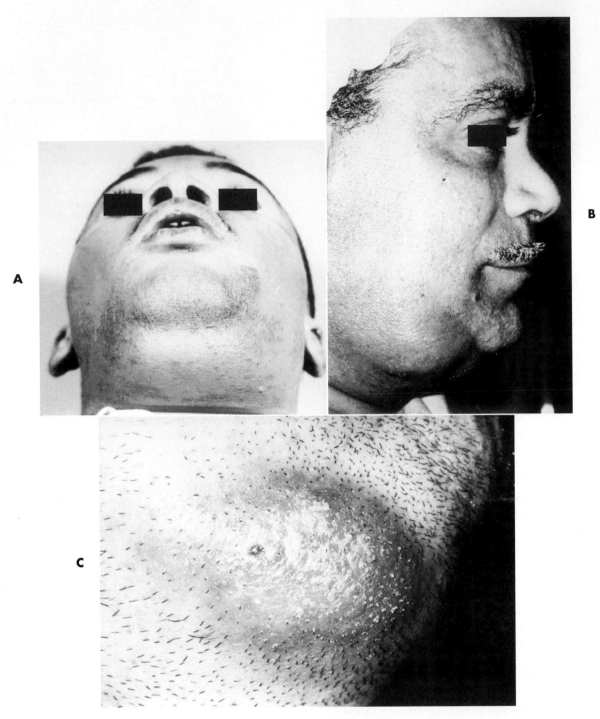

Fig. 5-8. Red infectious lesions. **A,** Ludwig's angina. Note the swelling of the submental and submandibular spaces. Unfortunately, the redness of the overlying skin does not show in this black-and-white photo. The patient also had a red painful sublingual swelling. **B** and **C,** A case of actinomycosis in the submandibular space of a 56-year-old man. **C** shows the redness of the lesion. (**B** and **C** courtesy E. Seklecki, Tucson, Ariz.)

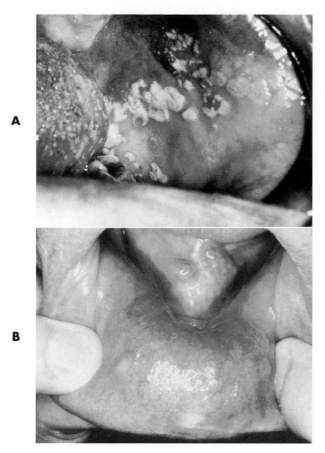

Fig. 5-9. Reddish lesions caused by chemical burns. **A,** Red and white acetaminophen burn. **B,** Reddish area on mucosa of lower lip represents a stage in healing of lesion caused by the overzealous use of Listerine mouthwash. (**B** from Bernstein ML: Oral mucosal white lesions associated with excessive use of Listerine mouthwash. Report of two cases, *Oral Surg* 46:781-785, 1978.)

Management

The majority of these cases are mild and relatively painless. Systemic analgesics and topical applications of corticosteroid in an emollient base can be used when pain is a problem. When diagnosis is uncertain or the injury appears to be superimposed on a serious lesion, surveillance is required. A biopsy should be performed if the lesion in question does not resolve promptly.

NICOTINE STOMATITIS

Nicotine stomatitis is discussed at length as a white lesion of the palate in Chapter 8. This lesion is included in the present chapter because it may be a red lesion in its earliest stage, before keratosis has been produced.[8] Also, in the later keratotic stage the inflamed minor salivary duct openings appear as small red dots in the center of low flat nodules of hyperplastic tissue. This mixed red-and-white appearance accounts for the inclusion of the lesion in Chapter 9. Nicotine stomatitis is seen primarily on the palate of pipe smokers.

Differential Diagnosis

The following conditions particularly have to be considered as somewhat similar clinical pictures when early-stage nicotine stomatitis is suspected: multiple papillomatosis, denture stomatitis, atrophic candidiasis, or atrophic/erythematous candiasis alone. Multiple papillomatosis and denture stomatitis can be quickly excluded if the condition is on the hard palate because nicotine stomatitis does not occur under a denture as do the former two entities. A smear quickly identifies atrophic candidiasis. A history of pipe smoking and the relatively greater prevalence of nicotine stomatitis gives it a higher rank in the differential diagnosis than atrophic candidiasis barring the presence of decreased immunocompetence.

ERYTHROPLAKIA, CARCINOMA IN SITU, AND RED MACULAR SQUAMOUS CELL CARCINOMA

The term *erythroplakia* (EP) is used in this book as a clinical term for a specific red lesion much as *leukoplakia* is used for white lesions of a specific spectrum. Therefore EP can be defined as a persistent velvety red patch that cannot be identified as any other specific red lesion such as inflammatory erythemas or those produced by blood vessel anomalies or infection. Etiology is that described for oral cancer in Chapter 35. EP is often regarded as the earliest sign of asymptomatic oral cancer. It is reported that invasion may occur in small lesions of less than 1 cm in diameter.[9,10] Indeed, the term erythroplakia carries a more serious implication than its white counterpart because almost all EPs show malignant changes. In a study of 58 cases by Shafer and Waldron, 51% were invasive carcinoma and 41% were carcinoma in situ or severe epithelial dysplasia.[11]

EP's reddish color results from the absence of a surface keratin layer and occurs because the connective tissue papillae, containing enlarged capillaries, project close to the surface.[11] There is a general failure of the epithelial cells to achieve significant maturation (keratinization). Cellular maturation may commence when actual invasion occurs.[11]

Features

EP usually appears as a velvety red or granular red macule (patch) that may be slightly raised (Fig. 5-10 and Plates H, 1 and H, 2). This painless lesion varies greatly in size, and the borders may be well circumscribed or may blend imperceptibly with the surrounding normal mucosa. Small lesions are easily overlooked, but the chances for their detection are greatly enhanced by first drying the mucosa with a gauze, since this intensifies the red color. The use of toluidine blue rinse is discussed in Chapter 2. This method may be helpful in rendering small red lesions or those that have minimal red color more noticeable during the soft tissue examination.

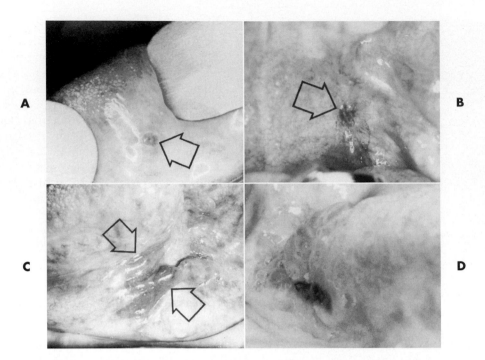

Fig. 5-10. Homogeneous erythroplakia. **A,** Very small red lesion on ventral surface of tongue, which showed invasion microscopically. **B,** Small red lesion on the soft palate at upper extent of pterygomandibular raphe. Lesion was barely discernible until the tissue was dried with a gauze. **C,** Red macule involving the sublingual papilla on the right side. **D,** small red lesion at posterolateral border of tongue. Excisional biopsy revealed early invasion in some sections and carcinoma in situ in others. (**B** courtesy R. Lee, Findlay, Ohio; **D** courtesy P. O'Flaherty, Chicago, Ill.)

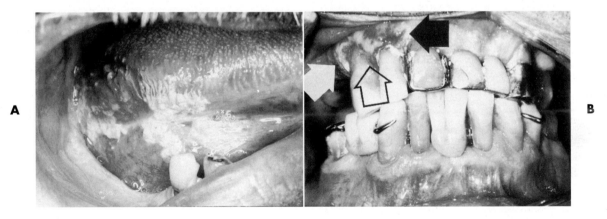

Fig. 5-11. Erythroplakic patches and leukoplakic patches in the same lesion. **A,** Lateral border of the tongue in a 64-year-old man. The red patch showed carcinoma in situ. **B,** Facial gingiva in a 57-year-old man. Some of the red areas showed invasive squamous cell carcinoma. (**A** courtesy R. Crum, Hines, Ill; **B** courtesy E. Seklecki, Tucson, Ariz.)

Three different clinical appearances were described by Shear[12]: (1) the *homogeneous form*, which is completely red in appearance (Fig. 5-10 and Plate G, 1); (2) *patches* of EP and leukoplakia occurring together (Fig. 5-11 and Plate G, 12); and (3) *speckled* EP, in which small leukoplakic specks are scattered over an area of EP (Fig. 5-12 and Plate G, 7 to G, 9). The term *speckled leukoplakia* used in Chapter 8 is synonymous with the term *speckled EP* used here. Homogeneous EP is generally much more aggressive than leukoplakia or speckled EP.[13] There is no gender predilection and the peak age of occurrence falls between 50 and 70 years.[11] The floor of the mouth is the most common site in men, whereas the mandibular gingival–alveolar mucosa–mandibular sulcus is the most common site in women. The retromolar region is the second most common site in both genders.[11]

Differential Diagnosis

The lesions to be considered in the differential diagnosis of erythroplakia are listed in the box on the next page.

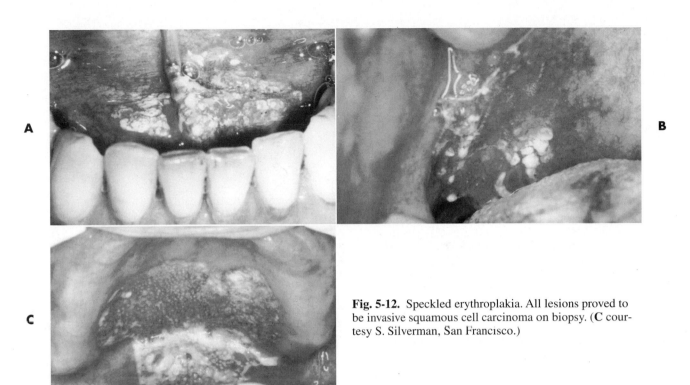

Fig. 5-12. Speckled erythroplakia. All lesions proved to be invasive squamous cell carcinoma on biopsy. (**C** courtesy S. Silverman, San Francisco.)

DIFFERENTIAL DIAGNOSIS OF EP
• Traumatic erythema
• Atrophic candidiasis
• Purpuric macule (early stage)
• Macular hemangioma
• Contact allergy
• Other infection
• Localized gingivitis
• Kaposi's sarcoma (early stage)

Although all the red macular lesions listed in this chapter should be considered in a differential diagnosis of an EP lesion, the lesions that are obviously *macular hemangiomas* and *telangiectasias* can be readily eliminated on the basis of their characteristic features. In a similar way the *traumatic lesions*, *odontogenic infections*, and *allergies* can be given a low ranking on the basis of their transient nature, pain, and often obvious events in the history. The traumatic erythematous macules of the tongue are often more difficult to differentiate because these may persist for weeks after the irritants have been eliminated. Red lesions of *atrophic candidiasis* may also be indistinguishable clinically. In cases of candidiasis, features in the history suggest susceptibility and a smear is diagnostic. *Tuberculosis* and *fungal lesions* such as *histoplasmosis* should be considered,[12] but their probability is low on the basis of incidence alone.

EP areas on the gingiva may be overlooked or misinterpreted as local areas of gingivitis.[13] Cases of EP squamous cell carcinoma of the gingiva have been initially considered as periodontal disease.[14,15] If a red area of the gingiva has no apparent cause or does not respond to the usual periodontal therapeutic measures, it should be considered to be an EP lesion until proved otherwise.

Management

If a red lesion persists for more than 14 days after all local trauma and infectious foci have been eliminated, a biopsy is mandatory.[9] Obviously, if the suspicion index is moderate to high, arrangements should be made for immediate referral to a practioner competent to manage malignant lesions of the oral cavity. Horch et al[16] discussed the use of laser surgery with oral premalignant lesions.

EXOPHYTIC, RED SQUAMOUS CELL CARCINOMA

Exophytic squamous cell carcinoma (ESCC) is discussed in Chapter 10 without emphasis on color. Macular red SCC is discussed under EP earlier in this chapter. To further develop the differential picture, it is necessary to include and describe an additional clinical lesion: the exophytic, red squamous cell carcinoma. Fig. 5-13 illustrates two examples of this entity. Oral cancer is discussed at length in Chapter 35.

Features

The lesions of ESCC illustrate the rule of thumb (Chapter 10) that a mass arising in the covering epithelial surface has a rough contour and surface. These ESCCs usually have a broad base and are irregular in shape. The

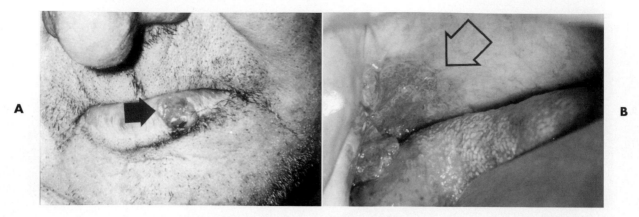

Fig. 5-13. Red exophytic squamous cell carcinoma. **A,** Small lesion on the lower lip. **B,** Large red lesion in the retromolar region. (**A** courtesy James Love, Raleigh, NC.)

DIFFERENTIAL DIAGNOSIS OF ESCC

- Inflammatory hyperplasias
- Papillomas and condylomas (pink to red)
- Hemangiomas (exophytic and reddish)
- Kaposi's sarcoma
- Other malignancies
- Rarities

---

surface may vary considerably in roughness from lesion to lesion and from area to area on the same lesion (Fig. 5-13). The surface may range from granular to pebbly to deeply creviced. The lesion may be completely red, or the red surface may be sprinkled with white necrotic or white keratotic foci. The lesion itself is firm to palpation, and the base usually shows induration and fixation to the deeper structures. Pain is a rare complaint. A major discussion of SCC can be found in Chapter 35.

Differential Diagnosis

The box above lists the lesions to be considered in the differential diagnosis process for ESCC.

Rare infectious proliferating lesions need to be kept in mind: chronic bacterial, such as tuberculosis, gummas, and actinomycosis; and fungal agents, such as histoplasmosis. An *amelanotic melanoma* is also an uncommon possibility.

The chance of the red lesion being either a *metastatic tumor* or a *primary mesenchymal tumor* is unlikely because approximately 90% to 95% of all oral malignancies are primary SCCs, but it must be considered (Plate J, 2). The majority of primary mesenchymal tumors, as well as minor salivary gland tumors, have smooth nonulcerated surfaces, barring injury.

Minor salivary gland tumors are seldom red and have smooth surfaces. Although some examples of exophytic *Kaposi's sarcomas* and other malignancies of blood vessels may be a similar red, their contours are smooth. If

the patient tests positive for the human immunodeficiency virus (HIV), the working diagnosis would likely be Kaposi's sarcoma.

Many of the *hemangiomas* empty or partially empty on digital pressure, which is accompanied by a similar degree of blanching. Consequently these lesions are usually easily identified, and many have a definite bluish tint.

Red IH lesions are more common than exophytic squamous cell carcinoma and are considerably softer to palpation. Pyogenic granuloma with its irregular surface may more closely imitate SCC, especially if enough fibrous content is present to give it some firmness. In most cases of IH the mechanical irritant is evident, and the lesion will shrink after removal of the irritant.

Management

The treatment of oral SCC is discussed in detail in Chapter 35.

CANDIDIASIS
Etiology and Pathogenesis

Candida is a common and harmless dimorphic yeast (Fig. 5-14) that lives without producing disease (commensally) in the oral cavities of up to 68% of normal individuals.[17-19] Although there are several species, *albicans* is the most frequent cause of disease.[20] Within the *albicans* strains, there is a wide variability in characteristics and ability to cause disease.[21] Usually the yeast must change to the pseudohyphal form for a clinical infection to occur, although hyphae can be found on tongue smears in a significant number of normal mouths.[21] Substantial host changes need to occur before *C. albicans* can produce disease.[22] These predisposing factors are presented in various papers[21,23-28] and are listed in the box on the next page.

Recent studies have given more information on pathogenesis. It is possible that a change in phenotype may be required to produce infection.[29] Phenotype switching has been observed during successive episodes of vaginitis.[30]

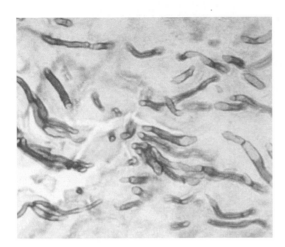

Fig. 5-14. Pseudohyphae of *C. albicans* in tissue. (Courtesy P. Fotos, Iowa City.)

Also, it is interesting that genetically dissimilar commensal strains occur in different anatomic regions of the same healthy women, and it is possible that infection in one region could be caused by the strain from the other region.[31] Another possibility would be that replacement exogenous strains are the causative agent of infection rather than the commensal strain. An exogenous strain would have to be the causative agent when candidal infections occur in noncarriers.[17] These same authors raise the academic possibility that all cases of infection could be caused by exogenous replacement strains. Exogenous replacement strains appear to have been the infectious agent in a cohort of AIDS patients in Leichester, England.[17,32] Another consideration involves the allergenic characteristics of *Candida.* How much of the reaction in clinical infection is the result of allergic response?

Features

The various types of clinical lesions are listed in the box below.

Various sets of circumstances will promote a certain type of clinical lesion. These factors relate to the numbers, virulence, and strains of *C. albicans;* intensity of the tissue reactions; acuteness, chronicity, and duration of the infection; resistance of the patient; presence or absence of treatment; anatomic location; and patient habits.

The pseudomembranous type is the most acute, followed by the erythematous, whereas the atrophic type would be more chronic or else a resolving phase of the first two. The hyperplastic type is chronic also, but the infection may be more deep seated.

At least 50% of patients complain of oral burning and infections. This disease is more common in patients over 40 years of age, and there is a higher incidence in women[33] excluding the younger cohort of AIDS patients. The burning may range in degree from tenderness to pain. The more acute types will more often be painful, whereas the hyperplastic types will be painless.

Diagnostic Procedure

Smears of the pseudomembranous and erythematous types will usually show significant members of pseudohyphae and possibly some yeast forms. Culturing *C. albicans* from

---

PREDISPOSING CONDITIONS TO ORAL CANDIDIASIS

Drugs/Medications

Broad-spectrum antibiotics (e.g., tetracycline)
Multiple antibiotic regimes
Corticosteroids
Cytotoxic agents
Immunosuppressive agents
Anticholinergics (xerostomia-producing)

Endocrinopathies

Diabetes mellitus
Hypoadrenalism
Hypothyroidism
Hypoparathyroidism
Polyendocrinopathy

Hematologic Disorders

Aplastic anemia
Agranulocytosis
Lymphoma
Leukemia

Immunodeficiency

HIV disease
Thymic alymphoplasia (Neselof's syndrome)
Thymic hypoplasia (DiGeorge's syndrome)
Severe combined immunodeficiency syndrome (Swiss type)

Hyperimmunoglobulinemia E syndrome
Chronic mucocutaneous candidiasis

Leukocyte Disorders

Myeloperoxidase deficiency
Agranulocytosis/leukopenia/neutropenia

Malignancy

Leukemia
Lymphoma
Thymoma
Advanced cancer

Nutritional Deficiencies

Iron deficiency
Folic acid deficiency
Biotin deficiency
Vitamin B deficiency
Vitamin C deficiency
Malnutrition
Malabsorbtion

Other

Radiation therapy
Sjögren's syndrome
Pregnancy
Xerostomia
Old age
Infancy
Denture use

From Muzyka BC, Glick M: A review of oral fungal infections and appropriate therapy, *J Am Dent Assoc* 126:63-72, 1995.

CLINICAL LESIONS OF CANDIDIASIS

- Pseudomembranous—white necrotic (Chapter 8)
- Erythematous—red (Chapters 5, 6)
- Atrophic—red (Chapters 5, 7)
- Hyperplastic—white, red raised (Chapter 8)
- Mixed—red/white keratotic/white necrotic
- Mucocutaneous—lip, angle (Chapter 33)
- Esophagitis and other systemic

Modified from Epstein JB: Antifungal therapy in oropharyngeal mycotic infections, *Oral Surg* 69:32-41, 1990.

saliva samples or swabs of lesions does not provide a definitive diagnosis because a large percentage of healthy patients are carriers,[22] although such information may be helpful when integrated with all the other findings.

It is important to consider that any oral lesion with surface debris may harbor candidal organisms to the extent of a secondary candidiasis. Nystatin treatment in such cases would produce some improvement, but full remission must await successful treatment of the primary lesion.

Management

Several appropriate medications are available for the treatment or management of oropharyngeal candidiasis. Both topical and systemic agents are available (Table 5-1), and choices are dictated by specific findings of each case. Drug therapy should be continued at least 1 week after signs and symptoms have disappeared because of the tendency to recur. In one study, 50% of patients that showed initial resolution experienced a recurrence.[34] Postinfection drug therapy should continue for a longer period in patients with serious predisposing conditions.

Topical therapy Generally, topical agents are indicated for milder superficial cases where the patient's resistance is relatively good and there is immunocompetency. Another topical agent can be tried in cases where the disease is refractory to the first topical drug used. Otherwise, therapy can be switched to a systemic agent. Topical and systemic medications can be used jointly.

Topical medications are available in the following forms: capsules, oral troches, pastilles, vaginal tablets, creams, and rinses.[35] To be successful, these agents must remain in contact with the infected mucosal surface for a significant period. Therefore solid agents that must dissolve will have more prolonged contact than rinses. Sufficient saliva must be present to aid the dissolution of the solid types. Sipping water may be used in cases of xerostomia as a salivary substitute, or oral rinses or creams may be used instead of the solid agents. Sucrose is the sweetening agent used in some preparations, and caries-prone individuals should use fluoride gels with prolonged administration of the antifungal. Vaginal troches are unsweetened and so are not cariogenic, but the unpleasant taste may affect patient compliance. Topical agents should be continued for at least 14 days and in some cases 2 to 3 weeks after resolution of symptoms.[36]

Nystatin. Nystatin pastilles are probably the most widely used form. Each pastille carries 200,000 units, and 1 to 2 should be dissolved slowly in the mouth 4 to 5 times per day. Side effects with nystatin products are unusual, and the agent is not absorbed through the gastrointestinal tract. MOTS-Nystatin contains 200,000 units of nystatin in a controlled-release system and is found to be more effective in AIDS patients than regular nystatin.[37] This polyene drug destroys the cell membrane by binding to ergosterol in the cell membrane. It is also available in oral suspension, ointment/creams, vaginal troches, powder, and tablets.

Table 5-1 Drugs used in treatment of fungal disease

Drug	Form	Activity
Amphotericin B	IV	Aspergillosis, cryptococcus, systemic candidiasis
	Topical cream Topical lotion Topical ointment	Cutaneous candidiasis
Nystatin	Oral troche Oral rinse Vaginal tablet	Oral candidiasis
	Topical cream Topical lotion	Cutaneous candidiasis
Clotrimazole	Oral troche Oral suspension	Oral candidiasis
	Topical cream Vaginal cream Vaginal tablet	Cutaneous candidiasis
Miconazole	IV	Histoplasmosis, blastomycosis
	Topical cream	Cutaneous candidiasis
Ketoconazole	Oral tablet	Histoplasmosis Blastomycosis Oropharyngeal candidiasis Chronic mucocutaneous candidiasis
	Topical cream	Cutaneous candidiasis
Fluconazole	Oral tablet IV	Cryptococcus Mucosal candidiasis
Itraconazole	Oral capsule	Blastomycosis Histoplasmosis Aspergillosis* Candidiasis*

*Use is not currently included in the labeling approved by the U.S. Food and Drug Administration.
From Muzyka BC, Glick M: A review of oral fungal infections and appropriate therapy, *J Am Dent Assoc* 126: 63-72, 1995.

Clotrimazole. Clotrimazole is produced in a 10 mg oral troche (Mycelex) that is dissolved slowly in the mouth 5 times a day. Administration should be continued for 2 to 4 weeks and at least 1 week after manifestations have disappeared. This drug is an azole that changes *Candida's* membrane permeability by blocking the production of ergosterol.

Chlorhexidine. Chlorhexidine 0.1%-0.2% mouth rinse has become well established as an agent that reduces the microbial load in the oral cavity. It is active against *Candida* and some bacteria by increasing cell membrane permeability. In addition, chlorhexidine interferes with candidal adhesion to oral mucosal cells.[38] It appears that clotrimazole is of prophylactic use and may also be helpful as an adjunct to other antifungals. Liver profiles must be done in prolonged use.

Gentian violet. This deep-violet alcohol solution is painted directly on the lesions. It has been used with some success over the years. Its main disadvantages are the dehydrating effect of the alcohol and the deep color, which is unsightly and hinders visualization of tissue change.[36] Years ago, it was overutilized for the treatment of white oral lesions of various diagnoses and so fell out of vogue. Perhaps it is now enjoying a resurgence especially in third world countries. In a Zaire AIDS study, it was found to be as effective as ketoconazole and much more effective than nystatin rinse.[39] This agent is economical, can be quickly applied by a clinician, and so does not depend on patient compliance.

Systemic therapy Systemically administered drugs are chosen for chronic deep-seated infections and for superficial cases that are refractory to topical agents. Considerable candidal resistance has developed to individual antifungal agents, and this may occur through phenotype switching, particularly in the azoles.[40] Topical and systemic agents may be used conjointly in difficult cases.

Ketoconazole. Nizoral is available as an orally administered 200 mg systemic tablet and as an intravenous (IV) preparation. One or two tablets are taken daily with food for at least 2 weeks and continued for 1 or 2 weeks after symptoms disappear. This is a very effective drug and is still used. As an azole, it affects the permeability of the fungal cell membrane. Although ketoconazole is not as toxic to the liver as other azoles, liver profile tests should be obtained if chronic administration is considered. During the last few years, usage has shifted from long-term to shorter-term treatment to minimize side effects. IV administration is used with refractory infections in AIDS patients.

Fluconazole. Diflucan is produced as a 50 mg systemically administered tablet. It is an effective triazole antifungal agent with less toxicity than the azoles. Recommended dosage is 50 mg per day as a single dose. This can be raised to 400 mg per day in difficult cases. This is a very useful drug especially in AIDS patients both for prophylaxis and treatment, but significant candidal resistance is occurring.

Amphotericin B. This antifungal agent's major role is as an intravenously administered agent in serious cases of systemic distribution that are resistant to other antifungals. It is significantly toxic to several systems, including the kidney.

Atrophic/Erythematous Candidiasis

This condition is red and may present as a single lesion or else as a generalized mucositis, which is discussed in Chapter 6. This red lesion may be either atrophic (Plate E, 5) or erythematous or a mix. Tenderness, burning, and in some instances significant pain are usual symptoms. Minor bleeding might be observed, and the lesion may blanch somewhat to digital pressure. Some of these cases will represent resolving stages in pseudomembranous infections, whereas others will represent cases that are less acute and did not progress to the more intense necrotic type (Fig. 5-15).

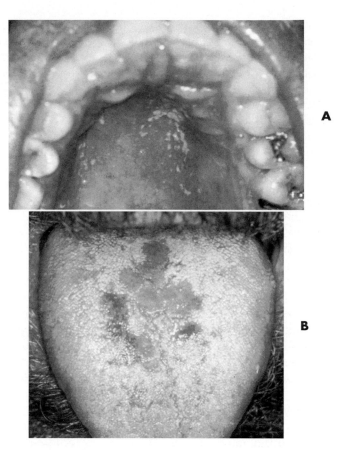

Fig. 5-15. Erythematous candidiasis. **A,** Palatal lesion showing some traces (white) of pseudomembranous type as well. **B,** Lesion on dorsal surface of tongue in HIV positive man. (**A** courtesy S. Fischman, Buffalo, NY; **B** courtesy M. Glick, Philadelphia.)

Although solitary red candidal lesions can occur practically anywhere on the oral mucosa, denture stomatitis and angular cheilitis will be discussed here because they are two of the more common examples.

Denture Stomatitis

The diffuse redness of the palate seen under dentures has posed a diagnostic problem for years. Causes are apparently multifactoral; denture trauma, denture plaque, and candidal infection are the most important.[41] Segal et al demonstrated that various *Candida* species do adhere to denture surfaces.[42] Candidal organisms are almost always found in the smears of the red soft tissue, and even larger quantities are located on the acrylic denture surface,[43] perhaps as residents.

Continual wearing of dentures is thought to be a high risk factor, as is smoking.[44] Ill-fitting dentures may predispose the tissue to infections as well.[44] The inflammatory reaction may be produced by: (1) tissue invasion by organisms,[44] (2) effect of fungal toxins,[44] (3) hypersensitivity to the fungus,[45] (4) bacteria,[46] or (5) carboxylic acids produced by microflora of the denture plaque.[47] In some cases a predisposing systemic condition is present, but diabetes does not seem to be a factor in this regard.[48]

Features Denture stomatitis occurs under either complete or partial dentures and is found more frequently in women. The lesions are usually confined to the palate and seldom if ever involve the mandibular ridge. In approximately 50% of the patients, there is an associated angular cheilitis with or without an inflammatory papillary hyperplasia of the palate. A high correlation has also been established between the occurrence of this condition and wearing dentures at night.

The lesions may be totally asymptomatic, or the patient may complain of a soreness and dryness of the mouth. This soreness may also be described as a burning sensation. The palatal tissue is bright red, somewhat edematous, and granular. Only the tissue covered by the denture is involved. The redness usually involves the entire area covered by the denture but may be focal in its distribution (Fig. 5-16 and Plate A,12).

When seen microscopically, the lesion is rather nonspecific. The epithelium is atrophic and may be ulcerated in areas. An intense chronic inflammatory infiltrate is present in the lamina propria and also involves the epithelium. Usually the *C. albicans* organism is not found in tissue specimens. The most accurate diagnostic test is a smear from the area of the lesion stained with periodic acid—Schiff's reagent. This will show the yeast and hyphal forms of *Candida*.

Differential diagnosis The clinical picture of denture stomatitis is rather specific; few if any other diseases appear the same. Infections by other organisms, however, could be responsible for a similar diffuse redness either alone or in combination with *Candida*. Contact allergy to the denture base acrylic happens occasionally. In such cases, redness will not be restricted to tissue under the denture, but all mucosal surfaces in contact with the acrylic will be red. Epicutaneous tests of the material will usually be diagnostic. From time to time, generalized mucositis conditions will affect the tissue under dentures, but the general distribution of these will differentiate from denture stomatitis. Some of these could be secondarily infected with *Candida*.

Management Treatment of candidiasis is discussed on pp. 62-63. Management of denture stomatitis includes correcting denture faults, improving denture and oral hygiene, and antifungal therapy.[49] Ill-fitting dentures must be adjusted or replaced. The patient must remove the dentures at bedtime and place them in chlorhexidine or nystatin solution at night after proper cleaning, although some clinicians recommend dry storage. One study indicated that a hydrogen peroxide denture cleaner was as effective as using antifungal agents on the denture.[50] (On occasion, fungi will have so thoroughly impregnated the denture that it will have to be discarded and a new denture made.) Antifungal ointments and pastes may be worn with the denture during the day, and oral antifungal rinses or lozenges may be used possibly in combination with a systemic agent. A recent report indicates considerable success utilizing a miconazole lacquer applied to the tissue surface of the denture.[51] Recurrences are common, and it is important to ensure that levels of denture plaque are reduced.[52]

Angular Cheilitis

Angular cheilitis is usually a reddish ulcerative or proliferative condition marked by one or a number of deep fissures spreading from the corners of the mouth. The lesions are most often bilateral, usually do not bleed, and are usually restricted to the vermilion and skin surface

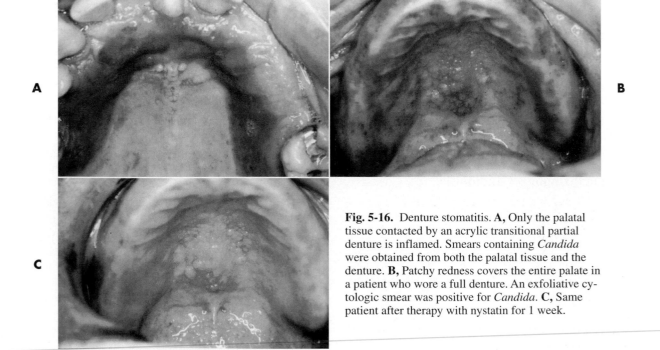

Fig. 5-16. Denture stomatitis. **A,** Only the palatal tissue contacted by an acrylic transitional partial denture is inflamed. Smears containing *Candida* were obtained from both the palatal tissue and the denture. **B,** Patchy redness covers the entire palate in a patient who wore a full denture. An exfoliative cytologic smear was positive for *Candida*. **C,** Same patient after therapy with nystatin for 1 week.

(Fig. 5-17). Although such factors as decreased vertical dimension of dentures, iron deficiency anemia, and vitamin B deficiencies may be predisposing factors or at least associated with the development of this lesion, infection with *C. albicans* and in some cases with a mixture of other microorganisms such as *Staphylococcus aureus* seems to represent a major cause.[53,54] Therefore the lesions usually persist even though the predisposing factors have been eliminated, unless they are treated with an antifungal ointment such as nystatin in conjunction with an *S. aureus* agent or metronidazole.[53,55] Resolution is relatively easily obtained if angular cheilitis is an isolated finding. However, if it is part of a generalized oral/systemic candidal infection, it may be very deep seated and resistant to eradication. That is, major priority of treatment must be directed to the main reservoir of infection in the body.

MACULAR HEMANGIOMAS AND TELANGIECTASIAS

The majority of the oral hemangiomas of soft tissue are exophytic and bluish and are discussed in Chapter 12. However, red macular hemangiomas (Plate A, 3) and exophytic red hemangiomas occur as both nonsyndrome and syndrome manifestations (Figs. 5-18 and 5-19). Red hemangiomas are usually of the capillary rather than the cavernous variety, which are usually more bluish. These reddish macular hemangiomas also occur as port-wine stains or nevus flammeus on the skin. People who have Sturge-Weber syndrome usually have both facial and intraoral macular hemangiomas (Fig. 5-19), although the intraoral hemangiomas may also be of the exophytic variety. An additional characteristic is the "tramline" calcifications seen in lateral skull radiographs.

The macular hemangiomas are readily differentiated from erythemas by the history of long duration, the nontenderness, and the fact that an inflammatory component is not present. They can be differentiated from red purpuric macules by the absence of a recent traumatic episode and the transience of the latter condition.

Telangiectasias represent permanently enlarged end-capillaries that are located superficially just under the skin or mucosa. They are red, seldom over 5 mm in diameter, and blanch readily on digital pressure, which easily differentiates them from red petechiae. They may occur as solitary red macules or multiple lesions. Multiple telangiectasias occur in Rendu-Osler-Weber syndrome, also known as hereditary telangiectasia.

Management

The following methods of treatment have been advocated for the oral hemangioma: conscientious observation, use of radiation, steroids, embolization, sclerosing solutions, antimetabolites, surgical removal, or a combination of sclerosing agents and surgery.[56]

ALLERGIC MACULES

Allergic manifestations in the oral cavity usually occur as a generalized eruption. Occasionally, solitary lesions occur, generally as the result of a contact allergy, and consequently must be differentiated from the other solitary red lesions (Fig. 5-20). When appearing as a red lesion, they may be either an erythema or an erosion. Usually the offending allergen can be identified through history and is quite diagnostic if the lesion disappears after the agent is withdrawn. Lesions have been reported as contact allergies to the following materials: gold alloy,[57] silver amalgam,[58] rubber products,[59] eugenol,[60] orthodontic wire,[61] and cinnamon.[62] A long list of drugs can produce oral lesions, but these allergies would be distributed systemically. Allergic reactions are discussed in greater depth in Chapter 6, p. 86.

Single red lesions caused by contact allergy would need to be differentiated from traumatic erythemas, physical or chemical burns, erythroplakia, macular hemangiomas, ecchymosis, and localized candidiasis.

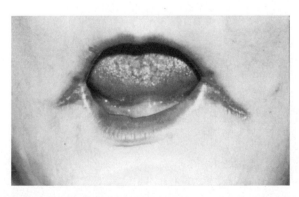

Fig. 5-17. Red lesions of angular cheilitis. *C. albicans* had secondarily infected this condition, which was primarily caused by wearing dentures with decreased vertical dimension.

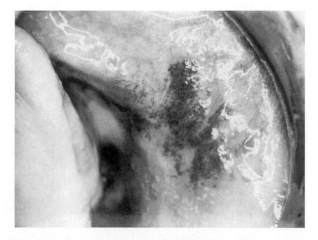

Fig. 5-18. Red macular hemangioma on the buccal mucosa, which had been present since birth. The lesion blanches on digital pressure.

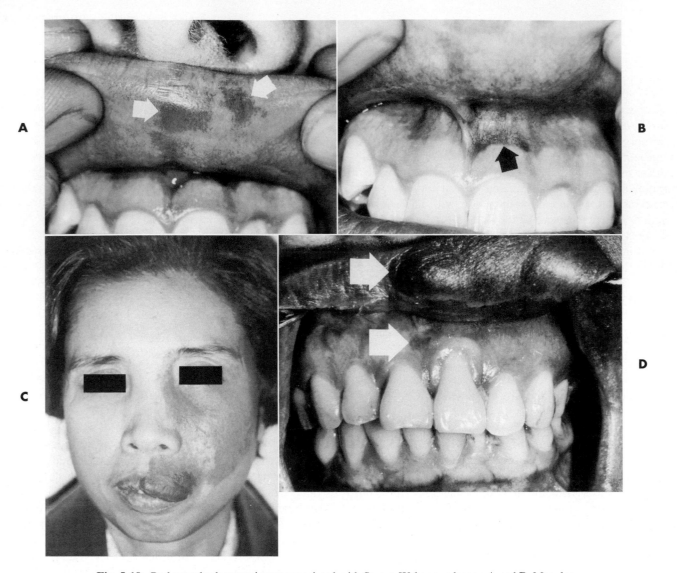

Fig. 5-19. Red macular hemangiomas associated with Sturge-Weber syndrome. **A** and **B,** Macular hemangiomas on the lip and alveolar mucosa in a 17-year-old patient who also had a port-wine stain on the left side of the face. The intraoral lesions blanched readily on digital pressure. **C** and **D,** Another patient with Sturge-Weber syndrome. **C,** Full-face view showing large superficial hemangioma (port-wine stain) on the left side of the face and upper lip terminating at the midline. **D,** Intraoral view of same patient showing the large red macular hemangioma that has involved the maxillary alveolar and gingival mucosa on the left side of the midline. The lip involvement on the left side can also be seen. (Courtesy S. Raibley, River Forest, Ill.)

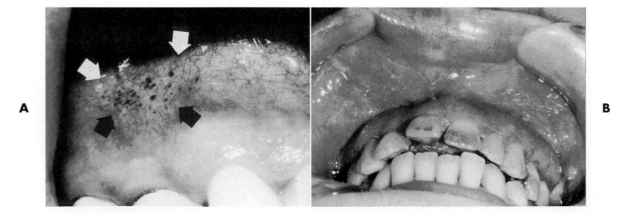

Fig. 5-20. Red allergic manifestations. **A,** Petechiae in red patch *(arrows)*, which was allergic reaction to topical anesthetic (unfortunately, the red patch is not clearly visible in this black-and-white picture). **B,** Allergic reaction to agents in periodontal dressing. Note the deep mostly uniform color of all the mucosa in this picture. (**A** courtesy E. Rainieri, Maywood, Ill.)

HERALD LESION OF GENERALIZED STOMATITIS OR VESICULOBULLOUS DISEASE

Vesiculobullous disease and other conditions that may cause a generalized stomatitis are discussed in Chapter 6. Occasionally, such conditions occur first as a solitary lesion (erythema, bleb, or ulcer) perhaps one or several months before a full-blown attack occurs. Fig. 5-21 illustrates two cases of herald lesions.

METASTATIC TUMORS TO SOFT TISSUE

Metastatic tumors to the oral cavity and jaws are uncommon lesions and represent about 1% of all metastases in humans.[63] These oral metastases represent about 1% of all oral malignancies as well.[64,65] The majority of these are metastatic lesions to bone. Various studies showed soft tissue metastasis in a range of 8% to 16%,[65,66] although one study[63] reported 44% of all metastases to the oral region were to soft tissue. Some metastatic bony lesions involved the oral soft tissues by extension.[67]

Features

Hirshberg et al received 157 cases of soft tissue metastasis to the oral cavity from the English-language literature.[68] These authors reported that 64% occured in the fifth and seventh decade, and that these lesions were more common in men (61.6%) than in women. The primary site differed between genders, but overall the most common primaries in descending order of frequency were from the lung, breast, kidney, genital organs, and skin. The gingiva and alveolar mucosa accounted for 54.8%, followed by the tongue and then much less commonly the tonsil, palate, lip, buccal mucosa, and floor of mouth. The vast majority of these lesions resembled hyperplastic or reactive lesions[68]. This would indicate many of these would be red (NKW).

Exophytic metastatic tumors are usually asymptomatic rapidly growing nodular or polypoid masses. The surfaces may be smooth and covered with intact mucosa, which varies from light pink to normal mucosal pink to red, depending on the integrity of the covering epithelium, the vascularity, the fibrosity, and the amount of inflammation present (Fig. 5-22 and Plates J, 1 to J, 3). Larger tumors frequently develop an ulcerated surface from chronic

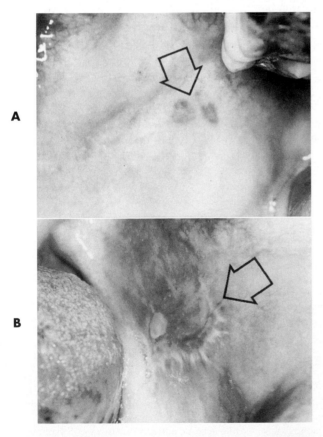

Fig. 5-21. Herald lesion of generalized stomatitis. **A,** Two ruptured vesicles with red rims on the buccal mucosa of a patient. These soon disappeared, but a full-blown case of pemphigus developed in the patient several months later. **B,** Solitary reddish lesion with a keratotic white component that was observed in a 45-year-old woman. Several months later a severe disseminated attack of erosive lichen planus was observed in the patient.

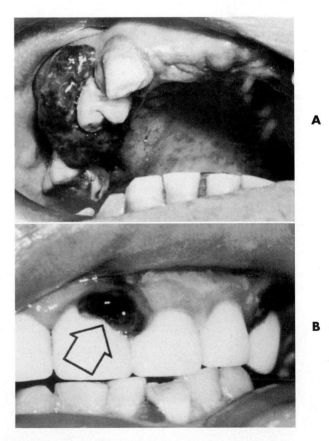

Fig. 5-22. Red metastatic tumors. **A,** Mass of 3 cm on the right maxillary gingiva of a 58-year-old man, which proved to be a metastatic adenocarcinoma from the lung. **B,** Reddish granuloma-like mass on the anterior gingiva of a 27-year-old man, which proved to be metastatic synovial sarcoma. (**A** and **B** from Ellis GL, Jensen J, Reingold IM, et al: Malignant neoplasms metastatic to gingivae, *Oral Surg* 44:238-245, 1977.)

trauma. The resultant appearance will be red or red and white and will ulcerate and bleed easily.

These peripheral lesions may invade adjacent bone and produce a radiographic appearance of a solitary, ragged, poorly marginated radiolucency.

Differential Diagnosis

The most common lesions that have similar clinical appearance to red metastatic tumors are listed in the box below.

Amelanotic melanoma of the oral cavity is a very rare tumor but may occur as a pink or reddish exophytic lesion (see Fig. 10-31, *A*), so it cannot be completely dismissed.

Proliferative chronic infections, for example, hyperplastic/hypertrophic candidiasis and other fungal and chronic bacterial infections, will resemble metastatic tumors and SCC on occasion.

Primary malignant mesenchymal tumors represent less than 1% of all oral malignancies; they are less common than the metastatic variety. Nevertheless, some of these primary tumors are red, especially the vascular variety, and must be considered, although they are assigned a lower ranking in differential diagnosis.

Minor salivary tumors are almost never red, but if the red exophytic tumor in question is located in the posterolateral hard palate, the possibility of a tumor of the minor salivary glands would have to be considered.

Kaposi's sarcoma: This lesion is discussed in detail in Chapter 36.

DIFFERENTIAL DIAGNOSIS OF RED METASTATIC TUMORS

- Inflammatory hyperplasia
- Squamous cell carcinoma
- Kaposi's sarcoma
- Minor salivary tumors
- Primary mesenchymal malignancies
- Proliferative chronic infections
- Amelanotic melanoma

Squamous cell carcinoma: Metastatic tumors and SCC look quite different in the early stages; SCC will have a rough surface, whereas metastatic lesions have smooth surfaces. When the secondary tumor ulcerates, it may be quite similar to SCC.

Inflammatory hyperplastic lesions are the most common by far. They can usually be tentatively identified by finding a chronic irritant associated with the lesion. However, the gingiva is the most common site for soft tissue metastatic lesions and for IH, so the metastatic lesions must always be included in the list. If the underlying bone shows bone resorption, malignancy must be seriously considered.

The suspicion of *metastatic tumor* is enhanced by symptoms of a primary tumor elsewhere or a history of previous treatment of such a tumor. However, the metastatic oral lesion may be the first indication of the presence of a primary tumor in as high as 33% of cases.[69]

Management

Treatment of individual cases of metastatic carcinoma in the oral cavity depends on the general prognosis of the patient. If the patient is terminal as a result of disseminated tumor, observation or palliative measures are the management of choice. On the other hand, if the oral lesion appears to be the only existing metastatic lesion, a serious attempt should be made to eradicate it.

KAPOSI'S SARCOMA (AIDS)

AIDS and associated Kaposi's sarcoma are discussed in Chapter 36. A red color is one of the frequent characteristics of Kaposi's sarcoma. Fig. 5-23 illustrates several nodular red Kaposi's sarcomas on the soft palate of an HIV-positive patient.

RARITIES

The rare oral red lesions are listed on the first page of this chapter.

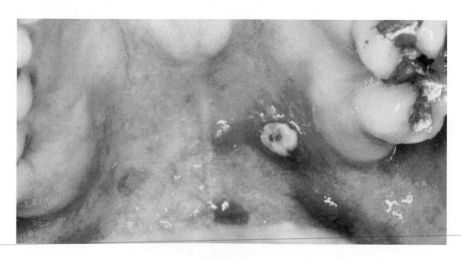

Fig. 5-23. Kaposi's sarcomas. Note the four red nodular lesions on the soft palate of a man with AIDS. One of the more anterior lesions has a white necrotic surface. (Courtesy S. Silverman, San Francisco.)

REFERENCES

1. Damm DD, White DK, Brinker CM: Variations of palatal erythema secondary to fellatio, *Oral Surg* 52:417-421, 1981.
2. Giansanti JS, Craner JR, Weathers DR: Palatal erythema: another etiologic factor, *Oral Surg* 40:379-381, 1975.
3. Lewis MO, MacFarlane TW, McGowan DA: A microbiological and clinical review of the acute dentoalveolar abscess, *Br Dent J* 28:359-366, 1990.
4. Paterson SA, Curzon MEJ: The effect of amoxycillin versus penicillin V in the treatment of acutely abscessed teeth, *Br Dent J* 174:443-448, 1993.
5. Iwu C, MacFarlane TW, MacKenzie D, Stenhouse D: The microbiology of periapical granulomas, *Oral Surg* 69:502-505, 1990.
6. Topazian RG, Peterson LJ: Which antibiotic? letter to the editor, *Oral Surg* 73:621-622, 1992.
7. Gill Y, Scully C: Orofacial odontogenic infections: review of microbiology and current treatment, *Oral Surg* 70:155-158, 1990.
8. Shafer WG, Hine MK, Levy BM: *A textbook of oral pathology,* ed 4, Philadelphia, 1984, WB Saunders.
9. Mashberg A, Morrissey JB: A study of the appearance of early asymptomatic oral squamous cell carcinoma, *Cancer* 32:1436-1445, 1973.
10. Mashberg A: Erythroplakia: the earliest sign of asymptomatic oral cancer, *J Am Dent Assoc* 96:615-620, 1978.
11. Shafer WG, Waldron CA: Erythroplakia of the oral cavity, *Cancer* 36:1021-1028, 1975.
12. Shear M: Erythroplakia of the mouth, *Int Dent J* 22:460-473, 1972.
13. Amagasa T, Yokoo E, Sato K, et al: A study of the clinical characteristics and treatment of oral carcinoma in situ, *Oral Surg* 60:50-55, 1985.
14. Torabinejad M, Rick GM: Squamous cell carcinoma of the gingiva, *J Am Dent Assoc* 100:870-872, 1980.
15. Gallagher CS, Svirsky JV: Misdiagnosis of squamous cell carcinoma as advanced periodontal disease, *J Oral Med* 39:35-38, 1984.
16. Horch HH, Gerlach KL, Schaefer HE: CO_2 laser surgery of oral premalignant lesions, *Int J Oral Maxillofac Surg* 15:19-24, 1986.
17. Soll DR, Morrow B, Srikantha T, et al: Developmental and molecular binding of switching in Candida, *Oral Surg* 78:194-201, 1994.
18. Hauman CHJ, Thompson IOC, Theunissen F, Wolfaardt P: Oral carriage of *Candida* in healthy and HIV-seropositive persons, *Oral Surg* 76:570-572, 1993.
19. Fetter A, Partisani M, Koenig H, et al: Asymptomatic oral candidal albicans carriage in HIV-infection: frequency and predisposing factors, *J Oral Pathol Med* 22:57-59, 1993.
20. Kolnick JR: Oral candidosis: report of a case implicating *Candida paropsilosis* as a pathogen, *Oral Surg* 50:411-415, 1980.
21. Rindum JL, Stenderup A, Holmstrup P: Identification of *Candida albicans* types related to healthy and pathological oral mucosa, *J Oral Pathol Med* 23:406-412, 1994.

22. Cannon RD, Holmes AR, Mason AB, Monk, BC: Oral *Candida:* clearance, colonization, or candidiasis? *J Dent Res* 74:1152-1161, 1995.
23. Al-Tikriti V: Martin MV, Bramley PA: A pilot study on the clinical effects of irradiation on the oral tissues, *Br J Oral Maxillofac Surg* 22:77-86, 1984.
24. Samaranayke LP: Nutritional factors and oral candidosis, *J Oral Pathol* 15:61-65, 1986.
25. Dreizen S, Bodey GP, Valdivieso M: Chemotherapy—associated oral infections in adults with solid tumors, *Oral Surg* 55:113-120, 1983.
26. Muskow BS, Wheaton EA: Severe oral infection associated with prolonged steroid therapy, *Oral Surg* 34:590-602, 1972.
27. Epstein JB, Komiyama K, Duncan D: Oral topical steroids, and secondary oral candidiasis, *J Oral Med* 41:223-227, 1986.
28. Holbrook WP, Rogers GD: Candidal infections: experience in a British dental hospital, *Oral Surg* 49:122-125, 1980.
29. Hellstein JH, Fotos PG, Law SS, et al: Differentation of sugar assimilation characteristics and colony phenotypes in pathogenic and commensal oral candidal isolates, *J Oral Pathol Med* 22:312-319, 1993.
30. Soll DR, Galask R, Isley S, et al: "Switching" of *Candida albicans* during successive episodes of recurrent vaginitis, *J Clin Microbiol* 27:681-690, 1989.
31. Soll Dr, Galask R, Schmid R, et al: Genetic dissimilarity of commensal strains carried in different anatomical locations of the same healthy women, *J Clin Microbiol* 29:1702-1710, 1991.
32. Schmid J, Odds FC, Wiselka MJ, et al: Genetic similarity and maintenance of *Candida albicans* strains in a group of AIDS patients demonstrated by DNA fingerprinting, *J Clin Microbiol* 30:935-941, 1992.
33. Zegarelli DJ, Zegarelli-Schmidt EC: Oral fungal infections, *J Oral Med* 42:76-79, 1987.
34. Fotos, PG, Vincent SD, Hellstein JW: Oral candidosis, clinical, historical and therapeutic features of 100 cases, *Oral Surg* 74:41-49, 1992.
35. Greenspan D: Treatment of oral candidiasis in HIV infection, *Oral Surg* 78:211-215, 1994.
36. Epstein JB: Antifungal therapy in oropharyngeal mycotic infections, *Oral Surg* 69:32-41, 1990.
37. Greenspan D, Dodd CL, MacPhail LA, et al: MOTS-Nystatin for treatment of oral candidiasis in HIV infection, *J Dent Res* 71:172, 1992.
38. Darwazeh AMG, Lamey P-J, Macfarlane TW, McCuish AC: The effect of exposure to chlorhexidine gluconate in invitro and in vivo adhesion of *Candida albicans* to buccal epithelial cells from diabetic and non-diabetic subjects, *J Oral Pathol Med* 23:130-132, 1994.
39. Nyst MJ, Perriens JH, Kimputu L, et al: Gentian violet, ketoconazole and nystatin in oropharyngeal and esophageal candidiasis in Zairian AIDS patients, *Ann Soc Belg Med Trop* 72:45-52, 1992.

40. Gallagher PJ, Bennett DE, Henman MC, et al: Reduced azole susceptibility of oral isolates of *Candida albicans* from HIV-positive patients and a derivative exhibiting colony morphology variation, *J Gen Microbiol* 138:1901-1911, 1992.
41. Arendorf TM, Walker DM: Denture stomatitis: a review, *J Oral Rehabil* 14:217-227, 1987.
42. Segal E, Lehrman O, Dayan D: Adherence in vitro of various *Candida* species to acrylic surfaces, *Oral Surg* 66:670-673, 1988.
43. Davenport JC: The oral distribution of *Candida* in denture stomatitis, *Br Dent J* 129:150-156, 1970.
44. Yulak Y, Arikan A: Aetiology of denture stomatitis, *J Marmara Univ Dent Sch* 1:307-314, 1993.
45. Greenspan JS: Infectious and non-neoplastic diseases of the oral mucosa, *J Oral Pathol* 12:139 166, 1983.
46. Koopmans ASF, Kippow N, de Graaff J: Bacterial involvement in denture-induced stomatitis, *J Dent Res* 67:1246-1250, 1988.
47. Samaranayake LP, Weetman DA, Geddes DAM, et al: Carboxylic acids and pH of dental plaque in patients with denture stomatitis, *J Oral Pathol* 12:84-89, 1983.
48. Phelan JA, Levin SM: A prevalence study of denture stomatitis in subjects with diabetes mellitus or elevated plasma glucose levels, *Oral Surg* 62:302-305, 1986.
49. Bissel V, Felix DH, Wray DW: Comparative trial of fluconazole and amphotericin in the treatment of denture stomatitis, *Oral Surg* 76:35-39, 1993.
50. Walker DM, Stafford GD, Huggett R, et al: The treatment of denture induced stomatitis: evaluation of two agents, *Br Dent J* 151:415-419, 1981.
51. Könsberg R, Axéll T: Treatment of *Candida*-infected denture stomatitis with a miconazole lacquer, *Oral Surg* 78:306-307, 1994.
52. Wilkieson C, Samaranayake LP, MacFarlane TW, et al: Oral candidosis in the elderly in long-term hospital care, *J Oral Pathol Med* 20:13-16, 1991.
53. Ohman SC, Dahlen G, Moller A, Ohman A: Angular cheilitis: a clinical and microbial study, *J Oral Pathol* 15:213-217, 1986.
54. Konstantinidis AB, Hatziotis JH: Angular cheilosis: an analysis of 156 cases, *J Oral Med* 39:199-206, 1984.
55. Lamey P-J, Lewis MAO: Oral medicine in practice: angular cheilitis, *Br Dent J* 167:15-18, 1989.
56. Woods WR, Tulumello TN: Management of oral hemangioma, *Oral Surg* 44:39-44, 1977.
57. Shepherd FE, Moon PC, Grant GC, et al: Allergic contact stomatitis from a gold alloy-fixed partial denture, *J Am Dent Assoc* 106:198-199, 1983.
58. Holmstrup P: Reactions of the oral mucosa related to silver amalgam: a review, *J Oral Pathol Med* 20:1-7, 1991.
59. Cohen DM, Hoffman M: Contact stomatitis to rubber products, *Oral Surg* 52:491-494, 1981.
60. Barkin ME, Boyd JP, Cohen S: Acute allergic reaction to eugenol, *Oral Surg* 57:441-442, 1984.

61. Dunlap CL, Vincent SK, Barker BF: Allergic reaction to orthodontic wire: report of case, *J Am Dent Assoc* 118:449-450, 1989.

62. Miller RL, Gould AR, Bernstein ML: Cinnamon-induced stomatitis venenata, *Oral Surg* 73:708-716, 1992.

63. Cleveland D, Madani F: *Tumors metastatic to the jaws and soft tissue.* Paper presented at annual meeting of the American Academy of Oral Pathology, San Francisco, May 9-13, 1992.

64. Clausen F, Poulsen H: Metastatic carcinoma to the jaws, *Acta Pathol Microbiol Immunol Scand* 57:361-374, 1963.

65. Meyer I, Shklar G: Malignant tumors metastatic to mouth and jaws, *Oral Surg* 20:350-362, 1965.

66. Summerlin D-J, Tomich CE, Abdelsayed R: *Metastatic disease to the jaws.* Paper presented at the annual session of the American Academy of Oral Pathology, Santa Fe, NM, 1994.

67. Hatziotis JC, Constantinido H, Papanayotto PH: Metastatic tumors of the oral soft tissues, *Oral Surg* 36:544-550, 1973.

68. Hirshberg A, Leibovich P, Buchner A: Metastases to the oral mucosa: analysis of 157 cases, *J Oral Pathol Med* 22:385-390, 1993.

69. Bhaskar SN: Oral manifestations of metastatic tumors, *Postgrad Med* 49:155-158, 1971.

CHAPTER 6

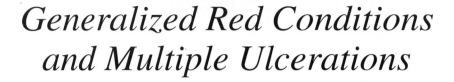

Generalized Red Conditions and Multiple Ulcerations

STUART L. FISCHMAN
RUSSELL J. NISENGARD
GEORGE G. BLOZIS

This chapter deals primarily with the diffuse red conditions, multiple vesicles or blebs, and multiple ulcerations that occur in the oral cavity and affect several oral surfaces simultaneously. The majority of these occur as multiple ulcerations distributed over erythematous mucosal surfaces. They include:

RECURRENT APHTHOUS STOMATITIS
  AND BEHÇET'S SYNDROME
PRIMARY HERPETIC
  GINGIVOSTOMATITIS
EROSIVE LICHEN PLANUS
LICHENOID DRUG REACTION
ERYTHEMA MULTIFORME
ACUTE ATROPHIC CANDIDIASIS
BENIGN MUCOUS MEMBRANE
  PEMPHIGOID
PEMPHIGUS
CHRONIC ULCERATIVE STOMATITIS
DESQUAMATIVE GINGIVITIS
RADIATION AND CHEMOTHERAPY
  MUCOSITIDES
XEROSTOMIA
PLASMA CELL GINGIVITIS
STOMATITIS AREATA MIGRANS
ALLERGIES
POLYCYTHEMIA
LUPUS ERYTHEMATOSUS
RARITIES
  Actinomycosis
  Acute gangrenous stomatitis
  Agranulocytosis

Amyloidosis
Bullous pemphigoid
Cheilitis granulomatosa (Melkersson-
  Rosenthal syndrome)
Crohn's disease
Darier's disease
Diabetic ulcerations
Epidermolysis bullosa
Giardia lamblia infection
Gonococcal stomatitis
Graft-versus-host disease
Granulomatous disease of the newborn
Hand-foot-and-mouth disease
Heavy metal poisoning
Hereditary mucoepithelial dysplasia
Hereditary telangiectasia
Herpangina
Herpes zoster (primary and secondary)
Histoplasmosis
Impetigo
Job's syndrome
Kaposi's sarcoma (multiple)
Leukemia
Major aphthous ulcerations (Sutton's disease)
Maple syrup urine disease

Measles
Metastatic hemangiosarcomas
Monoclonal plasmacytic ulcerative stomatitis
Mycosis fungoides
Paraneoplastic pemphigus
Pernicious anemia
Polyarteritis nodosa
Psoriasis
Psoriasis variants
  Pustular psoriasis
  Acrodermatitis continua
  Impetigo herpetiformis
  Pyostomatitis vegetans
Reiter's syndrome
Scurvy
Streptococcal stomatitis
Thermal and chemical burns (mild, recent)
Ulcerative colitis
Uremic stomatitis
Varicella
Vincent's angina
Vitamin B deficiencies (severe)
Wegener's granulomatosis

Chapter 5 is devoted to solitary red lesions. In contrast, this chapter discusses those diseases that simultaneously produce multiple red lesions and multiple ulcerations on several oral mucous membranes. The lesions may also appear on other mucous membranes and on the skin. Also included are those vesicular lesions that appear red both before the eruption of the vesicles and after their rupture.

For a variety of reasons, these conditions represent the most difficult challenge to clinical diagnosis. There is a wide variation in the degree of severity of individual cases. In many instances the specific cause is unknown, and frequently laboratory and biopsy results are nonspecific. Many of these conditions are relatively uncommon; even the specialist may not have the opportunity to study a sufficient quantity of cases to gain expertise.

Although the initial clinical appearance of the diseases varies, they all appear similar in their later stages. For example, the vesiculobullous group is quite distinctive in the early stages, but after the "blisters" rupture and disappear, the resultant ulcerative stomatitis is quite nonspecific in appearance.

The vesicular diseases are a particular enigma because the "blisters" may form and rupture within 24 hours; consequently the clinician and patient may be unaware that vesicles were even present in a given case. Presentation, remission, and recurrence make up the frequent course of many of these diseases. Treatment is palliative for the vast majority of them.

An overview of the various conditions reveals a considerable divergence; for instance, polycythemia is present as a painless, deep, dusty red color of the mucosa usually without inflammation, blisters, or ulcerations. The stomatitis accompanying xerostomia does not produce bullae and is otherwise nonspecific except for the decrease in salivary pooling. The bullous diseases are similar in that vesicles or blebs are the first lesions to appear. However, these soon rupture to form ulcers on inflamed mucosal surfaces. Diseases such as lichen planus, lichenoid drug reaction, lupus erythematosus, stomatitis areata migrans, and psoriasis form a fifth group frequently demonstrating both white (keratotic) and red lesions.

These conditions have in common the generalized reddened appearance of the oral mucosa. Pain is usually a symptom.

ETIOLOGY

The spectrum of causes of generalized red conditions is especially broad and varied. It includes the following (unfortunately, the specific cause is unknown in many conditions):

Hereditary conditions
Allergic conditions
Autoimmune conditions
Infections (bacterial, fungal, viral)
Altered host state (e.g., diabetes, uremia)
Altered local resistance (e.g., xerostomia)
Trauma
Iatrogenic conditions
Neoplasia
Gastrointestinal conditions
Deficiency states (e.g., vitamin deficiencies)
Idiopathic conditions

RECURRENT APHTHOUS STOMATITIS AND BEHÇET'S SYNDROME

Solitary recurrent aphthous ulcers (RAUs) are discussed in detail in Chapter 11. Their characteristic history and clinical picture permit ready recognition. A patient occasionally is seen with multiple aphthous ulcers distributed over several inflamed mucosal surfaces (Fig. 6-1 and Plate B, 4). The differential diagnosis of this condition, known as recurrent aphthous *stomatitis,* should therefore include those diseases that appear as generalized red ulcers.

Features

The ulcers of recurrent aphthous stomatitis are basically round or ovoid, have yellowish necrotic bases, and are surrounded by a region of inflamed mucosa. When the lesions are less than 1 cm, they are referred to as "minor" ulcers; if larger than 1 cm, they are referred to as "major" ulcers. The lesions are multiple and invariably painful, and they occur most frequently on the labial or buccal mucosa, floor of the mouth, and soft palate (Fig. 6-1). The recurrent attacks each last for about 10 days. If major aphthous ulcers are present, they may persist for months. The patient may then enjoy a disease-free period varying from a few weeks to several months before having a recurrence of aphthous stomatitis. As with all the other stomatitides, a painful lymphadenitis may accompany each ulcerative episode.

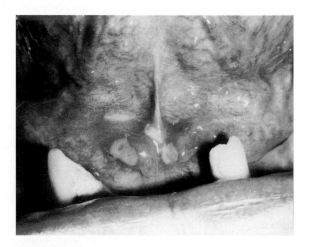

Fig. 6-1. Recurrent aphthous stomatitis. This middle-aged woman had many ulcers scattered throughout the oral mucosa. Note the characteristic reddened (darker) mucosa surrounding these ulcers in the sublingual region.

If extraoral signs and symptoms accompany recurrent aphthous stomatitis, the diagnosis of Behçet's syndrome may be made.[1] Behçet's syndrome is characterized by oral and genital ulcers and ocular inflammation. At least two of these symptoms are required to establish the diagnosis. Behçet's syndrome is further classified as mucocutaneous (oral, genital, or skin lesions, or all three), arthritic (arthritis in addition to mucocutaneous lesions), and neuroocular (neurologic or ocular symptoms or both in addition to the mucocutaneous and arthritic signs).

Differential Diagnosis

All the ulcerative mucosities listed at the beginning of this chapter should be considered. The absence of vesicles and blebs plus the usual healing in 7 to 14 days and well-defined circumscribed appearance of the lesions rules out *benign mucous membrane pemphigoid* and *pemphigus* and partially eliminates *erythema multiforme*. The ulcers in recurrent aphthous stomatitis are quite uniform in appearance and somewhat similar in size. This uniformity differentiates this condition from the lesions of erythema multiforme, which vary greatly from one another in appearance: erythematous macules, blebs, ulcers, and crusted lesions on the lip. The presence of crusted lesions on the vermilion border is not compatible with a diagnosis of recurrent aphthous ulceration. The absence of a white (keratotic) component tends to rule out *lichen planus, lichenoid drug reaction, lupus erythematosus,* and *psoriasis.*

Atrophic candidiasis may also appear red, but predisposing conditions are found in the patient evaluation. Most cases of candidiasis, even the atrophic type, pass through a white necrotic phase or have a minor keratotic component. Negative results on a cytologic test for *Candida albicans* rules out this diagnosis.

Primary herpetic gingivostomatitis must be differentiated from recurrent aphthous stomatitis. Herpetic gingivostomatitis is a systemic herpesvirus infection. The patient usually has a fever and complains of malaise and often nausea. Small vesicles precede herpetic ulceration. The vesicles and subsequent ulcers are pinpoint size, and the attached gingivae are almost invariably involved, whereas in recurrent aphthous stomatitis the gingivae are seldom involved. A history of contact with an active lesion on another person can often be established in primary herpetic infection.

Herpetiform ulcers are characterized by recurrent crops of as many as 100 small (1 to 2 mm) painful ulcers that may involve any part of the oral mucosa. They probably do not represent a herpesvirus infection.

Management

The cause of the aphthous lesion is obscure, and there is no specific treatment. Patients are generally given supportive therapy, including the use of systemic analgesics and topical anesthetic agents. In especially severe cases the use of topical or systemic steroids should be considered. Tetracycline mouth rinse has been reported to be effective in reducing the severity of pain in recurrent aphthous ulcerations.[2]

PRIMARY HERPETIC GINGIVOSTOMATITIS

Primary infections with herpes simplex virus (Herpesvirus hominis) are a relatively common cause of multiple oral ulcerations.

Features

Over 90% of Americans have antibodies to the herpesvirus, presumptive evidence of a prior infection. The initial infection with the herpesvirus may be subclinical or heralded by the appearance of a vesicular lesion on the vermilion border. The primary infection is often characterized by the acute onset of a systemic illness. After an incubation period of 5 to 10 days, the patient complains of malaise, irritability, headache, and fever, and within a few days the mouth becomes very painful. Oral examination reveals widespread inflammation of the marginal and attached gingivae. Numerous small vesicles are seen throughout the oral mucosa and on the lips (Fig. 6-2 and Plate C, 4). These vesicles soon rupture and become pinpoint ulcers, and secondary infection generally occurs. Ulcers on the lips may become bloody and crusted, and saliva may "drool" from the oral cavity. Cervical lymphadenopathy is also a frequent finding. In young children the diagnosis of the infection may be missed because the symptoms may be assumed to result from teething.

Dental personnel should be aware of the possibility of implantation of the virus on the hands. This is one of many reasons to take uniform infection control precautions, including the routine use of gloves. Herpetic whitlow is a primary infection of the finger with this virus. It may be seen in dental personnel who examine mouths of patients with primary herpetic gingivostomatitis or in patients who have a habit of biting the cuticle.

Recurrent herpetic infections develop in about one third of those patients who have had a primary infection. These are discussed in detail in Chapter 11.

Patients with immunodeficiency states such as AIDS or patients undergoing chemotherapy may suffer recurrent herpes attacks as severe as those of primary herpetic stomatitis.

Differential Diagnosis

The aspects of this condition have been reviewed in the Differential Diagnosis section of recurrent aphthous stomatitis. In addition, *hand-foot-and-mouth disease* (Coxsackie A virus etiology) needs to be considered as it presents with multiple pinpoint oral vesicles and ulcers, as well as fever. The absence of lesions on the palms and soles eliminates hand-foot-mouth disease from consideration. *Herpangina* (also Coxsackie A virus) can generally

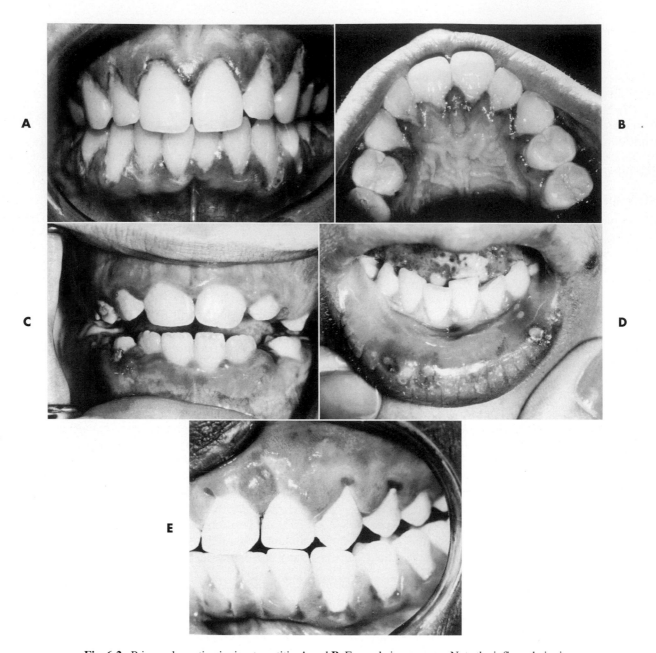

Fig. 6-2. Primary herpetic gingivostomatitis. **A** and **B,** Example in a woman. Note the inflamed gingivae and the ragged appearance with a faint whitish pattern. Close inspection revealed that the ragged white appearance was produced by the rupture and ulceration of the many pinpoint vesicles. **C,** Example in a 9-year-old boy; the primary infection was mostly confined to the gingivae. **D,** Case in which the prominent manifestations involved the mucosa of the lip and the anterior portion of the tongue in a 13-year-old girl. **E,** Gingival inflammation and swelling in leukemia. The ragged appearance with the multiple pinpoint ulcerations is not present in this disease. (**A** and **B** courtesy E. Ranieri, Maywood, Ill; **E** courtesy P. Akers Evanston, Ill.)

be identified by the distribution of the small vesicles and ulcers limited to the soft palate and oropharynx.

Occasionally a very severe intraoral manifestation of *recurrent herpes* occurs (e.g., small pinpoint vesicles and ulcers covering the whole palate). It is important to note that only one surface is involved in the recurrence, whereas multiple surfaces are involved in primary herpetic gingivostomatitis.

Establishment of diagnosis The diagnosis of primary herpetic gingivostomatitis is usually made on a clinical basis. The patient has a number of vesicles or small painful ulcers throughout the oral cavity. A history of systemic signs and symptoms of a viral illness helps to establish the diagnosis.

Confirmation of the viral infection by laboratory methods is available but not routinely used. The virus may be isolated in tissue culture if fluid can be obtained from an intact vesicle. Primary infections are associated with an increase in antibody titer, and paired acute and convalescent sera may be studied. Histologic and cytologic examination of tissue may be done, but identification of the specific virus requires expensive and time-consuming procedures and is generally not indicated.

There are two types of herpes simplex virus that cause disease in humans. The type 1 virus is primarily associated with infections of the skin and oral mucous membrane, and type 2 is associated with infections of the genitalia (although the converse can and does occur).

Management

There is no specific treatment for primary herpetic gingivostomatitis. Acyclovir (Zovirax) is effective in the management of initial herpes genitalis. It is also useful in treating non–life-threatening mucocutaneous herpes simplex virus infections in immunocompromised patients.[3,4] In these patients a decrease in the duration of viral shedding has been reported. There is no reported clinical evidence of benefit in treating herpes labialis in nonimmunocompromised patients.

The usual supportive measures for an acute viral infection should be instituted, including maintenance of proper oral hygiene, adequate fluid intake to prevent dehydration, and the use of systemic analgesics for control of pain. Antipyretic agents are also prescribed when fever is a symptom. In severe cases, it may be necessary to use a topical anesthetic mouth rinse such as viscous lidocaine, dyclonine, or elixir of diphenhydramine. The patient is often able to tolerate cold liquids, which may aid in preventing dehydration. Secondary bacterial infection of the many small punctate ulcers invariably is a major contributor to the pain.

EROSIVE LICHEN PLANUS

The lesions of lichen planus may take several different forms and have been classified into the following types: keratotic, vesiculobullous, atrophic, and erosive. The lesions of the atrophic and erosive forms are somewhat distinct, but they are discussed under the common heading of erosive lichen planus.

Features

The keratotic form of lichen planus is discussed in Chapter 8 along with a review of the epidemiology and etiology. The white lesion of lichen planus has been considered the most common. One report suggests that the erosive form may be seen more often,[5] but this may represent a population skewed towards referral for management of the painful erosive lesions.

Although the keratotic form of lichen planus is usually asymptomatic, the patient with the atrophic or erosive variety usually complains of a burning sensation or pain. The atrophic lesions appear smooth and erythematous and may have a feathery, white, keratotic border. In the erosive form the surface is usually granular and bright red and tends to bleed when traumatized. A pseudomembrane composed of necrotic cells and fibrin covers the more severe areas of erosion. The patterns of involvement change from week to week. However, almost invariably a white keratotic component is clinically apparent in a reticular, feathery, or plaque pattern (Fig. 6-3 and Plate C).

Cases have been reported in which lichen planus was associated with squamous cell carcinoma, and consequently it has been speculated that lichen planus might be a premalignant lesion.[5,6] It is difficult to determine whether there is an increased rate of malignancy in cases of oral lichen planus. The results of most studies are inconclusive, showing a slightly increased risk of malignancy, some of which may be related to tobacco use. In recent follow-up studies the number of patients with lichen planus in whom squamous cell carcinoma developed ranged from less than 1% to 2.5%. These results do not confirm the previous reports and leave the question unresolved.[7] As a matter of precaution, such patients should be observed carefully so that any changes can be detected early and biopsies obtained.

On histopathologic study, the atrophic form of lichen planus shows a thinned epithelium with hydropic degeneration in the basal cell layer. A dense bandlike infiltrate of lymphocytes is confined to the area immediately beneath the epithelium. In the erosive form, either the epithelium is completely missing or only remnants of epithelial tissue are seen. The underlying lymphocytic inflammatory infiltrate becomes mixed with polymorphonuclear leukocytes and loses its distinctive bandlike pattern. The diagnosis of lichen planus can be confirmed only by a biopsy.

The changes are usually characteristic in the atrophic lesions, in which the epithelium is still intact. Unfortunately, an intact epithelium does not exist in erosive lesions and the diagnosis may be difficult if not impossible. A biopsy specimen from the edge of an erosive lesion is usually more helpful than one from the erosive central area in establishing a diagnosis. When more typical lesions are present on other areas of the mucosa or skin, it may be assumed that the red lesions represent lichen planus (Fig. 6-3). However, if the lesions are clinically suggestive of squamous cell carcinoma, biopsy is imperative.

Lichenoid dysplasia Lichenoid dysplasia is the term applied to lichenoid lesions that show dysplastic areas.[8] Specific histologic criteria are used to differentiate epithelial dysplasia, oral lichen planus, and other inflammatory conditions. Lichenoid dysplasia and lichen planus are thought to be biologically distinct lesions. Lovas et al[9] contended that "some, if not most, cases of apparent malignant transformation of lichen planus likely represent red and white lesions that were dysplastic from their inception, but mimic oral lichen planus both clinically and histologically."

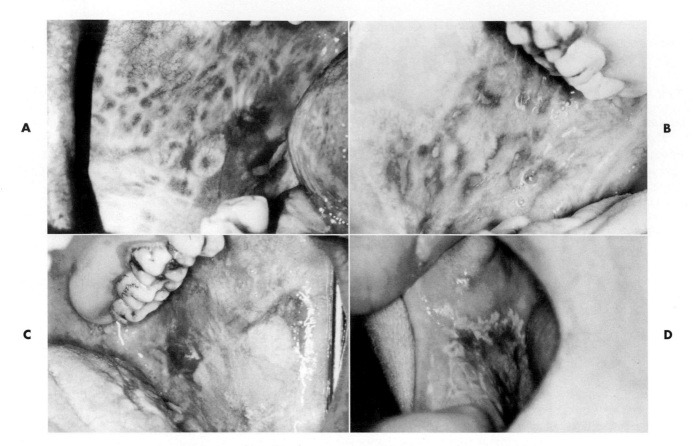

Fig. 6-3. Erosive lichen planus. **A-D,** Four cases of erosive lichen planus. Note the various proportions of keratotic and erythematous involvement in each.

Differential Diagnosis

Other diseases that contain a clinically apparent keratotic component in combination with a mucositis and therefore present lesions similar to those of lichen planus are speckled leukoplakia, squamous cell carcinoma, lichenoid drug reaction, electrogalvanic mucosal lesions, psoriasis, stomatitis areata migrans, atrophic candidiasis with a keratotic border, and discoid lupus erythematosus. Each of these diseases is discussed in detail elsewhere in this chapter.

When red lesions are confined to the gingivae, it is virtually impossible to distinguish atrophic or erosive lichen planus from benign mucous membrane pemphigoid and desquamative gingivitis on the basis of clinical and histologic examination. Immunofluorescence findings in gingival biopsies are diagnostic of benign mucous membrane pemphigoid and some forms of desquamative gingivitis. Kilpi et al[10] summarized the use of this technique.

Special diagnostic procedures In lichen planus, immunofluorescence studies of biopsies reveal characteristic but not diagnostic findings (Table 6-1). Globular deposits, sometimes called cytoid bodies or Civatte's bodies, contain immunoglobulins and fibrin, or they may contain complement and are observed in the papillary dermis along the dermoepidermal junction (Fig. 6-4). Cytoid bodies are more often seen in active stages of the disease and are more common in lesions than in normal tissue. Although cytoid bodies are neither disease specific nor diagnostic, their

identification can be helpful when routine histopathologic studies are inconclusive. Cytoid bodies are seen in biopsy specimens in 97% of lichen planus, 41% of systemic lupus erythematosus, 70% of discoid lupus erythematosus, 75% of dermatomyositis, 50% of erythema multiforme, 50% of pemphigoid, 40% of pemphigus, and 40% of normal specimens. The findings in lichen planus can be partially differentiated from the other diseases and the normal specimens on the basis of size and number of cytoid bodies and other immunologic findings. In addition to revealing cytoid bodies, immunofluorescence studies also reveal fibrin deposits along the basement membrane. These fibrin deposits, found in later stages of lesions, are not disease specific and occur in other diseases, particularly in the healing phase. Diagnostic immunofluorescence findings can also be seen in biopsy specimens of lupus erythematosus, pemphigus, and pemphigoid (Table 6-1). In normal biopsy specimens, smaller and fewer cytoid bodies are observed.

Management

Because of the increased incidence of lichen planus in diabetic patients, it is important to obtain medical consultation for the possibility of this disease. If the patient has diabetes, prompt stabilization of the condition is beneficial to management of the oral condition.

A specific and uniformly successful treatment for erosive lichen planus is not available. Nevertheless, the pa-

Table 6-1   Immunofluorescence findings important in the diagnosis of red conditions

| Disease | Serum | | Tissue | | Significance |
	Types of antibodies	Findings	Pattern of staining	Findings	
Benign mucous membrane pemphigoid or cicatricial pemphigoid	Basement membrane antibodies	− or + (<25%)	Basement membrane	+	Diagnostic
Bullous pemphigoid	Basement membrane antibodies	+(80%)	Basement membrane zone	+(100%)	Diagnostic
Lichen planus	Negative		Globular deposits or cytoid bodies in dermis and epidermis; fibrin deposits along dermoepidermal junctions	+(97%)	Characteristic
Pemphigus, all forms	Intercellular antibodies of epithelium	+(>95%)	Intercellular epithelial deposits	+(100%)	Diagnostic
Discoid lupus erythematosus	Negative or low titer of antinuclear antibodies		Dermoepidermal deposits of immunoglobulins and complement; lesion only	+(80%)	Highly characteristic
Systemic lupus erythematosus	High titer of antinuclear antibodies	+(90%-100%)	Dermoepidermal deposits of immunoglobulins and complement: lesion and normal tissue	+(>95%)	Diagnostic

tient can usually be greatly helped to reduce the degree of pain and produce regression of the lesions with extended drug therapy. A spontaneous remission has been reported in many cases, and the oral lesions are especially prone to recurrence and remission.

Milder cases may be managed successfully with the application of steroid creams such as fluocinonide or Kenalog in Orabase after meals and at bedtime.

For more severe cases the standard treatment has been the oral administration of adequate doses of prednisone for 2 weeks. If the lesions are well into remission by this time, the dosage of systemic corticosteroids may be tapered off and discontinued. If small isolated lesions are still present, these can be managed with the topical application of corticosteroid pastes such as fluocinonide or Kenalog in Orabase. When the systemic administration of corticosteroids must be continued for several weeks, the complications of extended corticosteroid therapy must be considered.

When a remission has been induced and drug therapy discontinued for a variable period of weeks or months, the painful lesions may recur and drug therapy has to be reinstituted.

Lichenoid Drug Reaction

Lichenoid drug reactions resemble lichen planus. Numerous medications have been implicated, and virtually any drug has the potential to provoke this reaction.[11] Various degrees of severity occur, ranging from painless keratotic lesions to painful severely erosive cases. Diagnosis is by clinical appearance and history. Under the physician's supervision, the putative drug is discontin-

ued and alternate therapy prescribed. Healing is usually prompt but may be prolonged in some cases. Severe cases of lichenoid drug reaction may clinically resemble erythema multiforme. The allergic state usually responds to the administration of prednisone or similar steroid agents.

The following are among the drugs that may cause a lichenoid drug reaction:

Bismuth
Captopril
Carbamazepine
Chloroquine
Chlorpropamide
Dapsone
Demeclocycline
Furosemide
Gold
Labetalol
Methyldopa
Nonsteroidal antiinflammatory agents
Para-amino salicylic acid
Penicillamine
Penicillin
Phenothiazines
Propranolol
Quinacrine
Spironolactone
Streptomycin
Tetracycline
Thiazides
Tolbutamide

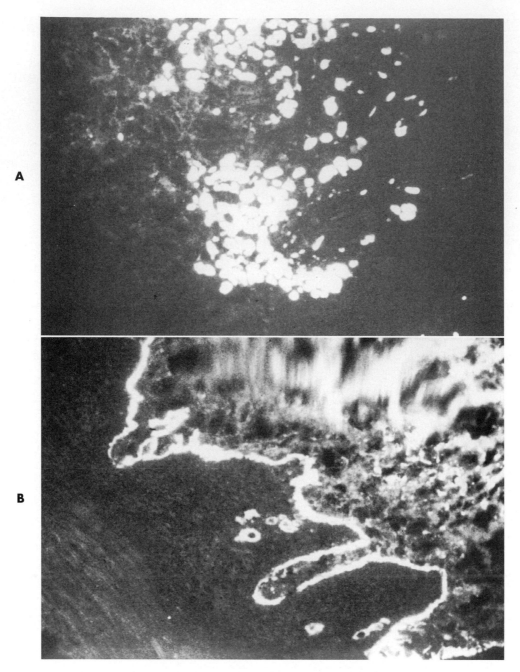

Fig. 6-4. A, Direct immunofluorescence test on oral biopsy specimen from patient with lichen planus demonstrating IgG deposits in cytoid or globular pattern in the dermis. Similar deposits of IgA, IgM, fibrin, and complement can also be seen. Such findings are characteristic. **B,** Direct immunofluorescence test on oral biopsy specimen from patient with lichen planus demonstrating fibrin deposits in a granular pattern along the dermoepidermoid junction.

ERYTHEMA MULTIFORME

Erythema multiforme is a disease of unknown etiology that has many different manifestations. When seen in its classic form, it is easily recognized. Although it is a vesiculobullous disease, vesicles and bullae usually are present for only a limited time.

Although an attack of erythema multiforme usually occurs without apparent reason, certain agents have been identified as precipitating the disease. Among the most common is a herpes simplex infection, but other infections and many drugs have also been implicated.

Features

The disease occurs primarily in young adults, usually men. It has a sudden onset and runs a course of 2 to 6 weeks. Recurrences are common. Lesions may be limited to the oral mucosa and involve, in descending order of frequency, the buccal mucosa, lips, palate, tongue, and

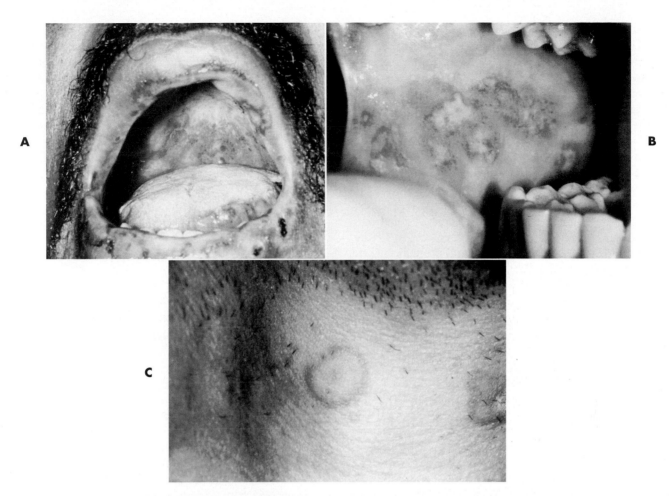

Fig. 6-5. Erythema multiforme. **A,** Extensive lesions of the lips and oral mucous membranes in a 26-year-old man. **B,** A milder case with erythematous patches, blebs, erosions, and ulcers restricted to the mucosa of the cheeks. **C,** Target lesion on the skin of another patient with erythema multiforme. (**A** courtesy W. Heaton, Chicago.)

fauces (Fig. 6-5 and Plates C, 4 and D). The gingivae are rarely involved. In one large study,[12] 70% of cutaneous cases showed oral lesions.

Sloughing of the mucosa and diffuse redness are the most frequent clinical features. The initial lesions are small red macules that may enlarge and show a whitish center. The macules progress to form bullae that soon rupture, leaving a sloughing mucosal surface that appears bright red and raw. In time, the denuded surface becomes covered with a pseudomembrane of fibrin and cells and assumes a grayish appearance. Involvement of the oral tissues may be limited to merely a diffuse redness.

Skin lesions of erythema multiforme are pathognomonic. They may accompany the oral condition, or there may be cutaneous manifestation without oral involvement. Skin lesions have a characteristic "bull's eye" or "target" appearance (Fig. 6-5). Although the palms of the hands are a classic location, these lesions may occur anywhere on the skin. Patients may complain of pruritus.

A microscopic examination of vesicles and bullae reveals a subepithelial cleft. The underlying connective tissue contains a mixed inflammatory infiltrate with numerous eosinophils. The light microscopic changes and immunologic findings seen in immunofluorescence examination of biopsy specimens are not diagnostic but can be used to rule out other diseases. Buchner et al[13] reported on the histologic spectrum of oral erythema multiforme. There are no useful laboratory studies.

The diagnosis is made on the basis of clinical information. Obviously, this can pose a problem if the lesions are limited to the oral cavity. A history of previous attacks that involved other mucous membranes or the skin is most useful in making the diagnosis. *Stevens-Johnson syndrome* is a severe episode of erythema multiforme that involves the mucosa, conjunctiva, and skin.

Differential Diagnosis

Similar oral lesions may be seen in pemphigus vulgaris, benign mucous membrane pemphigoid, allergic reactions, erosive lichen planus, primary herpetic gingivostomatitis, and xerostomia. Oral lesions resulting from drug reactions may appear similar to those of erythema multiforme and may vary from focal or diffuse areas of erythema to areas of erosion and ulceration. At times, it may be difficult to decide whether the drug precipitated an attack of erythema multiforme or the lesions resulted from drug allergy.

Management

Since erythema multiforme is a self-limiting disease, usually only supportive care is necessary. When areas other than the oral cavity are involved, the patient is best managed through a cooperative effort of physician and dentist. If the oral cavity is severely involved, systemic corticosteroids usually bring prompt and dramatic relief. Lozada[14] reported that if 50 to 100 mg of azathioprine were combined with prednisone, a lower dosage of prednisone could be used. A corticosteroid such as dexamethasone elixir used as an oral rinse may provide symptomatic relief in mild cases.

ACUTE ATROPHIC CANDIDIASIS

The lesions of acute atrophic candidiasis (formerly known as acute atrophic candidosis) represent a less common form of *Candida* infection. They may be the sequelae to the typical lesions of acute pseudomembranous candidiasis. When the white plaque of pseudomembranous candidiasis is shed or removed, often a red, atrophic, and painful mucosa remains (Fig. 6-6 and Plate E, 5). At times the lesion may be asymptomatic.

Features

The lesions are seen in the same types of patients as other clinical types of candidiasis (see box on p. 61). Tissue sections show an atrophic epithelium that may contain a few hyphae in the superficial layers. The lamina propria usually has a mild acute inflammatory infiltrate and increased vascularity. An exfoliative cytologic smear of the lesions may be useful in establishing a diagnosis.

Differential Diagnosis

The red lesions of acute atrophic candidiasis are often seen in association with those of the pseudomembranous type and so do not pose a diagnostic problem. When present as multiple red lesions, they are rather nonspecific in appearance. Lesions produced by chemical burns, drug reactions, and other organisms have a similar clinical appearance, as may the predominantly red lesions of erosive lichen planus, mild cases of erythema multiforme, and discoid lupus erythematosus.

Management

This is discussed in Chapter 5, p. 62.

BENIGN MUCOUS MEMBRANE PEMPHIGOID

The specific cause of benign mucous membrane pemphigoid, or cicatricial pemphigoid, is unknown. However, it is known to have an autoimmune component.

Features

Benign mucous membrane pemphigoid is seen twice as frequently in women as in men. The disease affects older individuals, with the highest incidence occurring in those in their late 50s. It is usually reported in the white population. Lesions are found primarily on the mucous membranes, infrequently involving the skin. The mucous membranes of the oral cavity and eyes are most often involved. Lesions occur on the gingiva, buccal mucosa, and palate.

The gingivae, the most common site, become edematous and bright red—a striking feature of the disease. This involvement may be patchy or diffuse. Subsequent to bulla formation or trauma, the surface epithelium may be lost, leaving a raw, red, bleeding surface. The vesiculobullous lesions in other areas of the oral cavity do not appear as red, nor do they bleed as readily. The ulcers that result from the collapse of bullae are surrounded by a zone of erythema (Fig. 6-7 and Plate C, 1) and are relatively asymptomatic. Unless treated, the dis-

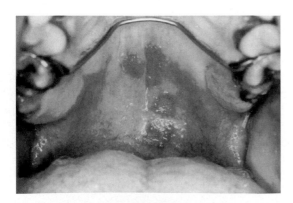

Fig. 6-6. Erythematous papules of candidiasis that were an incidental finding and resolved without treatment. An exfoliative cytologic smear was positive for *Candida.*

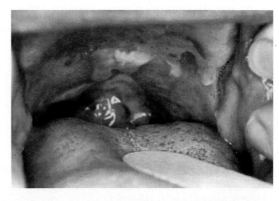

Fig. 6-7. Benign mucous membrane pemphigoid. This illustration shows whitish areas of intact and collapsed bullae and some erythematous and ulcerated areas.

ease follows a chronic course of partial remission and exacerbation.

A clinical feature common to these three diseases is the production of a gingival bleb by a strong jet of air. This occurs because of the defect in the basement membrane region. Manton and Scully[15] emphasized the necessity of using a combination of clinical, histologic, and immunostaining examinations to establish a diagnosis of mucous membrane pemphigoid.

The histologic changes are only characteristic if the epithelium is intact. Frequently the roof of the subepithelial bulla is lost and the histologic changes become nonspecific, characterized by a chronic inflammatory infiltrate of the connective tissue.

Immunofluorescence is an important and useful diagnostic technique because it can help to differentiate the gingival lesions of benign mucous membrane pemphigoid from those of erosive lichen planus and desquamative gingivitis. If the surface is intact, direct immunofluorescence study of the biopsy is particularly important, since the immunofluorescence findings are diagnostic. The basement membrane zone contains a deposition of immunoglobulins and complement (Fig. 6-8). The immunofluorescence

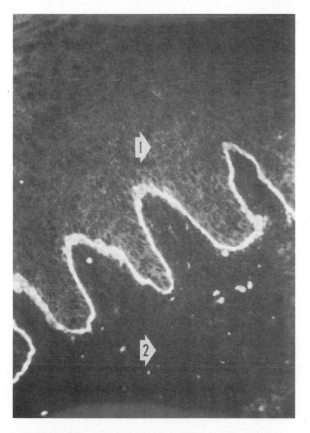

Fig. 6-8. Direct immunofluorescence test on oral biopsy specimen from patient with benign mucous membrane pemphigoid revealing complement deposits along the basement membrane zone in a linear pattern (*1*, epithelium; *2*, lamina propria). Similar deposits of IgG and other immunoglobulins also occur. These findings are diagnostic.

findings can also be observed in the adjacent clinically normal mucosa. The biopsy site of choice for immunofluorescence is the perilesional and the clinically normal mucosa, since these areas have the dermoepidermal relationships necessary for evaluation (see Table 6-1). In approximately 25% of the cases, low titers of serum antibodies to the basement membrane are also observed. When these occur, they are also diagnostic of pemphigoid.

Differential Diagnosis

Other diseases that should be considered in a differential diagnosis of benign mucous membrane pemphigoid are pemphigus vulgaris, bullous pemphigoid, bullous lichen planus, chronic ulcerative stomatitis, and early cases of erythema multiforme.

Benign mucous membrane pemphigoid and *bullous pemphigoid* are clinically, histologically, and immunologically similar but differ in sites of involvement. Benign mucous membrane pemphigoid characteristically involves the mucous membranes, most commonly the oral cavity and next the conjunctiva. Skin lesions are infrequently observed. In bullous pemphigoid, the usual site of involvement is the skin. In approximately 30% of cases the oral mucosa is involved. The immunofluorescence pathologic findings in both diseases are identical, showing immune deposits along the basement membrane. However, the two diseases differ in the incidence and titer of basement membrane zone antibodies in sera. In bullous pemphigoid, basement membrane zone antibodies, generally of high titer (greater than 1:80), occur in approximately 97% of patients. In benign mucous membrane pemphigoid, antibody titers (usually less than 1:40) occur in only approximately 20% to 25% of patients.

Management

The patient with benign mucous membrane pemphigoid may be extremely difficult to treat. Corticosteroids are the only useful form of therapy, but their side effects must be considered. The use of corticosteroids on alternate days has been somewhat successful as a way to prevent these complications. Because the mucous membranes of the eyes are often involved, patients with benign mucous membrane pemphigoid are at risk for blindness and should be referred to an ophthalmologist for examination.

Rogers et al[16] recommended topical corticosteroids for mild cases and dapsone (a bacteriostatic sulfone derivative) for more symptomatic cases. Dapsone therapy must be carefully monitored, since it can cause hemolysis and methemoglobinemia, particularly in patients with glucose-6-phosphate dehydrogenase deficiency.

PEMPHIGUS

Pemphigus is a vesiculobullous disease of unknown cause with an autoimmune etiology that may affect mucous membranes and skin. The four major forms of pemphigus are pemphigus vulgaris, pemphigus vegetans, pemphigus foliaceus, and pemphigus erythematosus. They have similar immunologic findings, which are diagnostic (see Table 6-1).

Features

Pemphigus affects men and women approximately equally, and the vast majority of patients are white. In one report,[17] 74% of the patients with the vulgaris or vegetans type were Jewish, approximately 98% of the patients were over 31 years of age at the time of onset, and 80% of cases of the vulgaris variety (by far the most common type) first occurred intraorally. Laskaris and Stoufi[18] reviewed the rare cases of pemphigus vulgaris in children.

The lesions of pemphigus vulgaris may appear as areas of erosion, but more often they are seen as ulcers, bullae, or areas of sloughing mucosa or skin (Fig. 6-9 and Plate C, 5). Diffuse erythematous involvement of the gingiva has been reported but is not the typical manifestation of the disease. In the typical case, initial lesions occur orally, followed by skin lesions.

The histologic study of intact vesicles or bullae reveals an intraepithelial defect. The individual cells separate from one another, and a pooling of fluid occurs. The basal layer of epithelial cells remains in position on the basement membrane.

Differential Diagnosis

All the vesiculobullous conditions listed at the beginning of this chapter should be considered in the differential diagnosis. As a general rule, the pemphigus bulla is smaller than the bulla in benign mucous membrane pemphigoid and considerably larger than those seen in the viral diseases such as herpes and hand-foot-and-mouth disease.

Special diagnostic procedures Immunofluorescence studies of sera and biopsy specimens reveal antibodies confined to the intercellular substance of epithelium and intercellular deposits of IgG (Fig. 6-9). The sera from more than 95% of pemphigus patients with active disease contain intercellular epithelial antibodies. During early stages of the disease or during remission, the

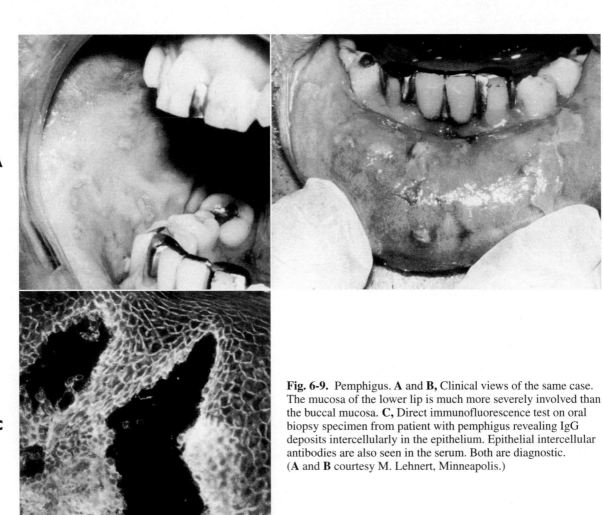

Fig. 6-9. Pemphigus. **A** and **B**, Clinical views of the same case. The mucosa of the lower lip is much more severely involved than the buccal mucosa. **C**, Direct immunofluorescence test on oral biopsy specimen from patient with pemphigus revealing IgG deposits intercellularly in the epithelium. Epithelial intercellular antibodies are also seen in the serum. Both are diagnostic. (**A** and **B** courtesy M. Lehnert, Minneapolis.)

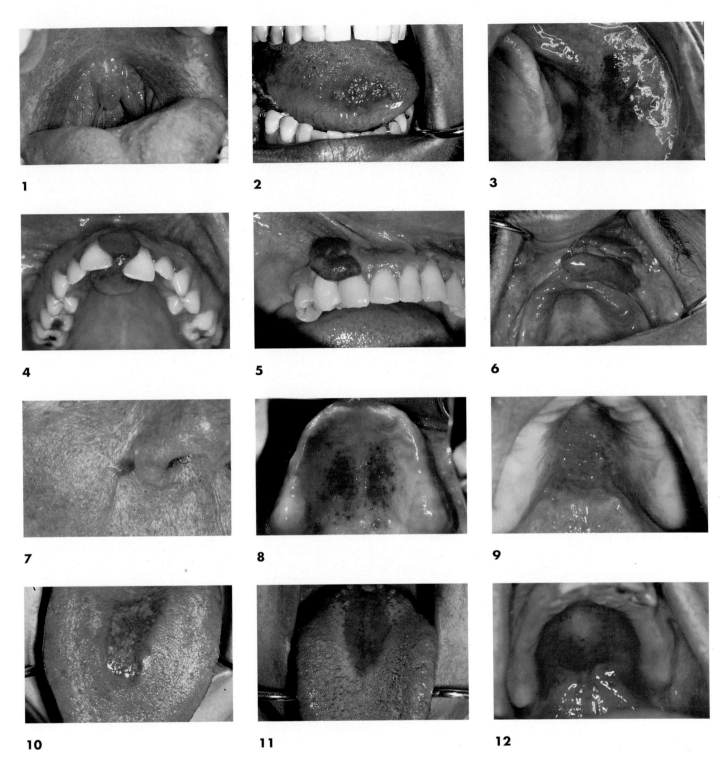

Plate A. **1,** Normal red palatoglossal arch. **2,** Traumatic erythematous macule. **3,** Capillary hemangioma. **4,** Inflammatory hyperplasia. **5,** Inflammatory hyperplasia. **6,** Epulis fissuratum. **7,** Red parulis. **8,** Early papillary hyperplasia. **9,** Papillary hyperplasia. **10,** Pseudomembranous candidiasis. **11,** Healed candidiasis. **12,** Erythematous candidiasis. (**3** courtesy G. Blozis, Columbus, Ohio; **7** courtesy J. Guggenheimer, Pittsburgh.)

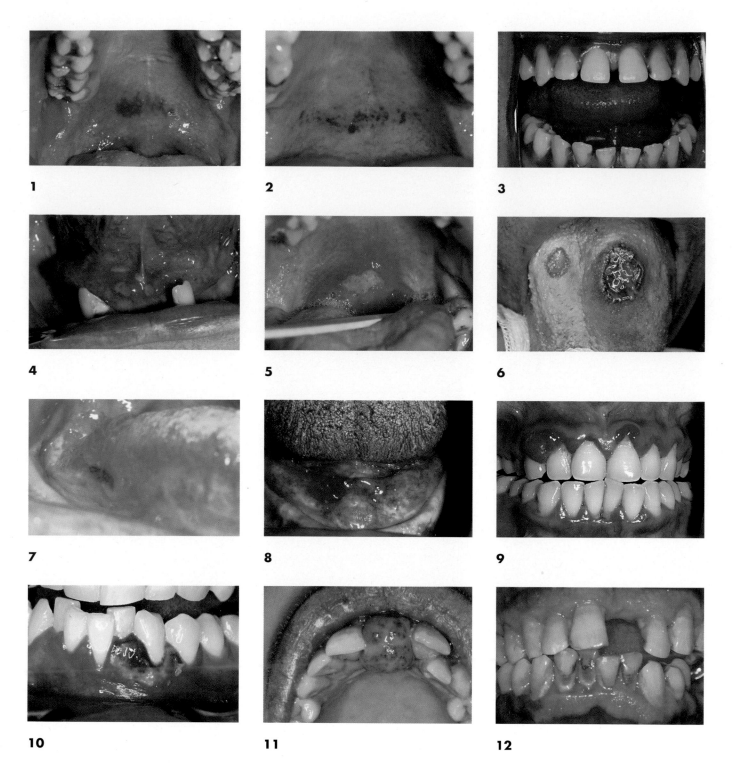

Plate B. 1, Red macule from oral sex. **2,** Red macule from coughing. **3,** Ludwig's angina. **4,** Recurrent aphthous stomatitis. **5,** Major aphthous ulcer. **6,** Two chancres. **7,** Erythroplakia (squamous cell carcinoma). **8,** Erythroplakia (squamous cell carcinoma). **9,** Pregnancy gingivitis. **10,** Cocaine lesion. **11,** Pyogenic granuloma. **12,** Jaundice. (**7** courtesy P. O'Flaherty, Chicago; **10** courtesy A. Gargiolo, Chicago; **11** courtesy G. Mac Donald, San Jose, Calif; **12** courtesy R. Gier, Kansas City, Mo.)

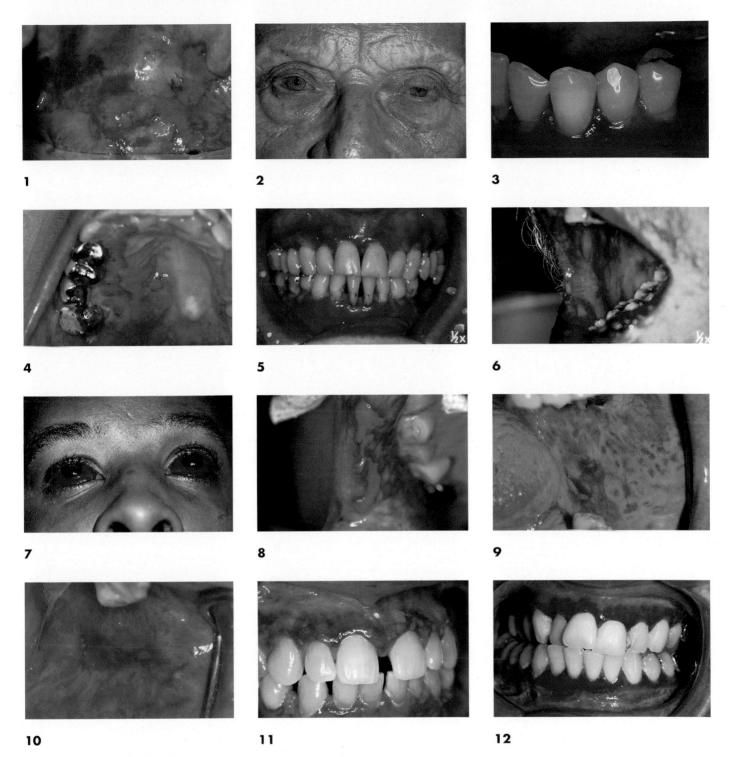

Plate C. **1,** Benign mucous membrane pemphigoid. **2,** Same patient as **1**. **3,** Benign mucous membrane pemphigoid. **4,** Primary herpetic gingivostomatitis. **5,** Pemphigus. **6,** Erythema multiforme. **7,** Stevens-Johnson syndrome. **8,** Bullous lichen planus. **9,** Reticular and erosive lichen planus. **10,** Erosive and reticular lichen planus. **11,** Atrophic lichen planus. **12,** Atrophic and erythematous lichen planus. (**5** and **6** courtesy S. Fischman, Buffalo, NY; **12** courtesy P. Toto, Waukegan, Ill.)

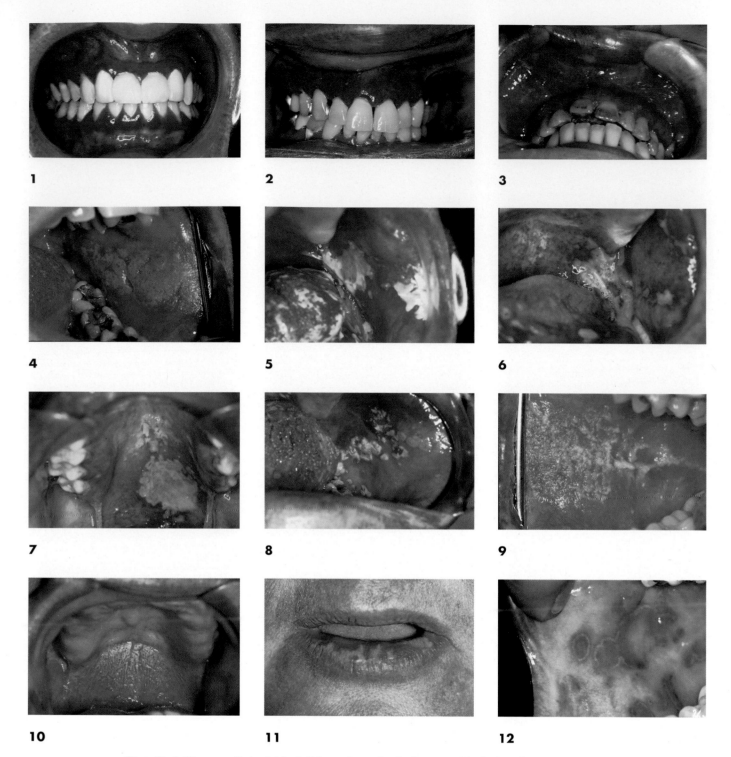

Plate D. **1,** Plasma cell gingivitis. **2,** Primary herpetic gingivostomatitis. **3,** Reaction to periodontal surgical dressing. **4,** Cinnamon reaction. **5,** Drug reaction. **6,** Radiation mucositis. **7,** Candidiasis. **8,** Tylenol burn. **9,** Cheek biting. **10,** Nicotine stomatitis. **11,** Lupus erythematosis. **12,** Ectopic geographic tongue. (**1, 5,** and **6** courtesy G. Blozis, Columbus, Ohio; **4** courtesy M. Bernstein, Louisville, Ky; **12** courtesy S. Fischman, Buffalo, NY.)

antibody titers may be low or negative. The significance of the antibody titer must be considered together with the clinical and histologic findings. Low titers (10 to 20) are significant when there are typical clinical and histologic findings. Low titers of intercellular antibodies with atypical clinical and histologic findings may be termed "pemphigus-like" antibodies rather than true pemphigus antibodies. Pemphigus-like antibodies may occur as a result of extensive burns and after some drug eruptions but do not bind in vivo as do those in true pemphigus.

The intercellular antibody titer frequently relates to disease activity by rising with exacerbations and falling with remissions. In many cases, titer changes of two or more doubling dilutions precede clinical changes and provide a prognostic test for control of drug therapy. Sera should be tested every 2 to 4 weeks until the patient is in remission and then every 1 to 6 months.

Almost all patients with active pemphigus have intercellular deposits of IgG and sometimes IgA, IgM, and complement in biopsy specimens.[19] These findings are diagnostic. Biopsies of oral lesions should be taken from the periphery of the lesion, where the epithelium is still intact. Immunoperoxidase techniques may be an alternative method to immunofluorescence as a diagnostic aid in cases of pemphigus.[20]

Management

Corticosteroid therapy is the preferred treatment for severe pemphigus.[21] Other modes of treatment include alternate-day steroid and gold therapy and immunosuppressive treatment with methotrexate or azathioprine.[17] Favorable results with a combination of levamisole and prednisone, in which lower dosages of prednisone were effectively used, have been reported.[22]

DESQUAMATIVE GINGIVITIS

There is some question whether desquamative gingivitis is a specific disease entity or a clinical manifestation of several different diseases. In a study of 40 patients with clinical desquamative gingivitis, McCarthy and Shklar[23] histologically identified 17 cases of benign mucous membrane pemphigoid, 2 cases of pemphigus, and 4 cases of lichen planus. The remainder were considered hormonal, idiopathic, or abnormal responses to local factors. In an immunofluorescence study of 100 patients with clinical desquamative gingivitis, 35 had benign mucous membrane pemphigoid, 3 had pemphigus, and 1 patient had psoriasis. Of the remaining 61, 28 had findings consistent with lichen planus.[24] Although the cause of desquamative lesions of the gingivae is not always known, it is generally considered to represent a degenerative pathosis of the gingivae. Because it occurs more frequently in postmenopausal women, there may also be an underlying hormonal factor.

Features

Desquamative gingivitis is seen in both genders but is far more prevalent in women. Usually it occurs after the age of 40, but it may occur at any age after puberty. The labial gingivae become bright red and edematous. The palatal and lingual surfaces are not often involved. Changes may be limited to a few small areas (Fig. 6-10), or they may be diffuse and extend throughout the gingivae (Plate C,3). The epithelium is quite friable and can be easily removed from the underlying connective tissue, leaving a red surface that bleeds readily after minimal trauma. Patients may complain of a burning sensation but often are asymptomatic.

On histologic examination, the epithelium is thin and atrophic. The rete ridges are blunted, and there may be clefting below the basement membrane. Edema and a mild chronic inflammatory infiltrate are seen in the underlying connective tissue. The microscopic findings are not diagnostic and serve only to exclude other diseases. Immunofluorescence studies of gingival biopsy specimens are especially valuable in determining if the underlying cause is benign mucous membrane pemphigoid, pemphigus, or lichen planus. The diagnosis is made on the basis of a careful history, physical examination, and laboratory tests.

Differential Diagnosis

Other diseases that produce similar lesions are erosive lichen planus, benign mucous membrane pemphigoid, bullous pemphigoid, chronic ulcerative stomatitis, and, rarely, pemphigus vulgaris.

Management

Treatment of desquamative gingivitis is directed at providing symptomatic relief. It is important that all possible local irritating factors be removed. Different drugs such as estrogens and steroids have been applied topically and do provide variable degrees of improvement. Systemic steroids are also indicated.[25]

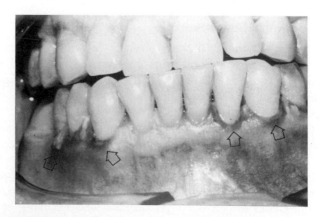

Fig. 6-10. Desquamative gingivitis. Note areas of erosion on the gingiva *(arrows).* (Courtesy E. Ranieri, Maywood, Ill.)

CHRONIC ULCERATIVE STOMATITIS

Chronic ulcerative stomatitis (CUS), a recently identified entity,[26-28] is a subset of desquamative gingivitis. Clinically, it appears similar to lichen planus but with a distinct immunopathology and different response to therapy.

Features

Patients with CUS generally exhibit chronic, painful, burning mouths characterized by erythematous and ulcerative lesions.

Differential Diagnosis

The lesions of CUS most resemble lichen planus, and similar ulcerative and erosive lesions may occur in benign mucous membrane pemphigoid and pemphigus.

Management

On the basis of fewer than 20 patients reported in the literature, it appears that topical and systemic steroid therapy is frequently ineffective. Several patients have reported improvement with the antimalarial hydroxychloroquine (Plaquenil).

Special diagnostic procedures Immunofluorescent findings in perilesional and normal mucosal biopsies reveal a characteristic diagnostic immunopathology of particulate antinuclear antibodies in the basal stratified epithelium. Serum antinuclear antibodies that react primarily on the lower third of stratified epithelial substrates also occur.

RADIATION AND CHEMOTHERAPY MUCOSITIDES

The diagnosis of mucositis occurring as a result of radiation or chemotherapy should be readily established from the patient history. Kolbinson et al[29] discussed the early oral changes after chemotherapy and radiation therapy. The dental management of the patient with cancer has been reviewed by Little and Falace.[30] Since radiation therapy and chemotherapy will adversely affect preexisting periodontal disease, prior periodontal therapy is strongly advised.

Radiation Mucositis

Features Radiation therapy produces characteristic and dramatic changes. During the course of therapy, which may continue for 6 weeks, a diffuse inflammatory change develops in the mucosa. The amount of tissue involved is determined by the portal used for the radiation therapy.

Tissue changes do not become apparent until the last part of the first week or the beginning of the second week of radiation therapy. Distinct blebs may be produced, or a whitish area resulting from decreased cellular division and retention of squamous cells may be seen. In subsequent weeks the surface layers are lost and a thin erythematous mucosa is present. Focal areas may ulcerate and then become covered with a tan-yellow, fibrous exudate (Fig. 6-11 and Plate D, 6). The tissue response varies

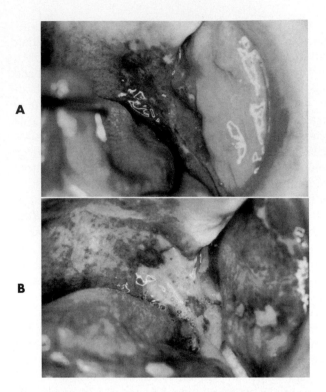

Fig. 6-11. Radiation mucositis. **A,** Squamous cell carcinoma appearing clinically as a large area of erythroplakia in the retromolar and soft palate region. **B,** Same patient approximately midway through radiation therapy. Note the areas of erythema and the fibrinous exudate.

considerably among patients. Profound changes resolve a few weeks after therapy is completed, but there may be some residual redness for variable periods of time.

Management Symptomatic relief is necessary because the pain can be severe, especially when eating. Topical anesthetics such as elixir of diphenhydramine or lidocaine can be combined with milk of magnesia, Maalox, or Kaopectate and used as oral rinse. Analgesics may be necessary.

Chemotherapy Mucositis

Features Oral lesions resulting from chemotherapy may occur during and after the course of therapy. Initially, patients may complain of a burning sensation; lesions may or may not be associated with this sensation. The lesions begin as focal areas of redness that may persist and ultimately ulcerate. Infrequently the ulcerations become numerous and large.

Management Treatment is directed toward providing symptomatic relief. Topical anesthetics such as lidocaine, dyclonine, or diphenhydramine may be prescribed. If the lesions become debilitating, it may be necessary to briefly interrupt chemotherapy. When secondarily infected, the lesions respond well to an oral suspension of tetracycline used as a mouthwash and then swallowed. Chlorhexidine mouth rinses are indicated for prophylaxis and therapy.

XEROSTOMIA

Dryness of the mouth is not a disease but a sign of reversible or irreversible impaired function of the salivary glands. Infectious lesions of the salivary glands such as mumps produce a transient xerostomia. When the primary disease resolves, the flow of saliva returns to normal. Diseases such as Mikulicz's disease or Sjögren's syndrome produce irreversible changes that result in a progressive decrease in the production of saliva. Radiation to the head and neck area causes atrophy of the glands and a decrease in the amount of saliva secreted. Dehydration and senile atrophy of the glands reduce the amount of saliva produced by the glands. Many widely used medications decrease salivary gland activity. Ganglionic blocking agents used to control hypertension, many psychotherapeutic agents (tranquilizers and antidepressants), and antihistamines have this side effect.

Features

In mild short-term cases of xerostomia, the patient may be asymptomatic and the mucosa appears normal. In moderately severe cases the patient may complain of a dry mouth or burning sensation. When these symptoms are intense, patients experience difficulty with speech, mastication, and the retention of artificial appliances. Patches of mucosa appear very atrophic and take on a dark, dusty red appearance. In severe xerostomia, erosion and ulceration of the inflamed mucosa occur.

The combined features of decreased salivary and lacrimal production suggest a diagnosis of Mikulicz's disease. In Sjögren's syndrome, xerostomia, conjunctivitis sicca, rhinitis sicca, and arthritis are seen.

Differential Diagnosis

A lack of saliva is the symptom that enables the clinician to differentiate the mucositis of xerostomia from the other types listed in this chapter.

Historical evidence is useful in establishing the type of xerostomia. A history of radiation treatment, antisialagogue medication, and combinations of features suggesting one of the syndromes associated with xerostomia are clues that direct the clinician to the correct diagnosis.

Management

Artificial saliva preparations may be helpful.[31]

PLASMA CELL GINGIVITIS

Plasma cell gingivitis, also called atypical gingivostomatitis, is a disease that was recognized as a distinct entity in 1968. Studies indicate that the lesions may be caused by some ingredient in chewing gum, and a type of allergic response is the proposed etiology.[32,33] Although this condition was frequently seen in the 1960s and early 1970s, it has been seen much less frequently in recent years.[34]

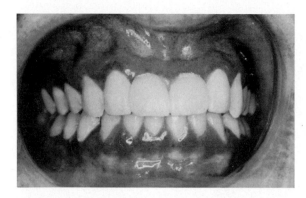

Fig. 6-12. Diffuse and striking erythematous changes of plasma cell gingivitis are confined to the gingiva.

Features

Plasma cell gingivitis occurs much more frequently in women than in men and is seen predominantly in young adults. The patient complains of a sore or burning mouth. The most striking and characteristic feature of the disease is the gingival involvement. The entire free and attached gingivae are edematous and bright red (Fig. 6-12). Frequently, there are associated lesions of the lips, tongue, and buccal mucosa; a scaling of the lips; and an angular cheilitis. The tongue is erythematous and devoid of filiform papillae. The patient may state that the problem has been present for as long as 3 years.

The most spectacular microscopic changes are seen in the lamina propria, which is densely infiltrated by plasma cells. The other changes are nonspecific. A diagnosis is made primarily on the basis of the clinical appearance of the lesions and is supported by a biopsy.

Differential Diagnosis

The clinical features of plasma cell gingivitis are distinctive and are not simulated by other diseases. However, early leukemic infiltrate of the gingiva may appear somewhat similar, as may allergies to toothpaste ingredients.

Management

The patient usually shows a marked improvement shortly after he or she stops chewing gum or changes brands of toothpaste. Complete remission of the disease takes approximately 4 weeks.

STOMATITIS AREATA MIGRANS

Stomatitis areata migrans is also known as migratory mucositis or ectopic geographic tongue.

Features

Most frequently, the lesions of geographic tongue are confined to the dorsal surface and lateral borders of the tongue (see Fig. 7-1, *A*). Occasionally, similar lesions have been reported on other mucosal surfaces of the oral cavity and are considered a more extensive involvement of the same

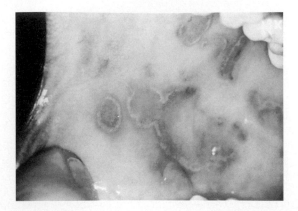

Fig. 6-13. Stomatitis areata migrans on the buccal mucosa.

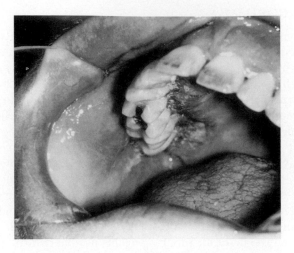

Fig. 6-14. Reaction to periodontal dressing. Note erythematous reaction on superior aspect of buccal mucosa where it was in contact with the dressing. Note severe tissue destruction on lingual gingiva. Plate D shows another view of this case.

process. The basic appearance is that of red patches of various sizes and shapes surrounded by white (keratotic), raised rims (Fig. 6-13 and Plate D, 12). The white rims may show a radiating, feathery appearance as they fade into the surrounding normal mucosa. The patterns change continuously and finally fade completely as the condition enters a remission. Stomatitis areata migrans is usually asymptomatic and found on routine oral examination.

The histopathologic study of stomatitis areata migrans shows a thinning of the surface epithelium in some areas and an epithelial hyperplasia in others. The epithelium may show spongiosis and infiltration by acute and chronic inflammatory cells, often in focal arrangement (Munro's abscesses).

Differential Diagnosis

Lesions that should be differentiated from stomatitis areata migrans are lichen planus, psoriasis, lupus erythematosus, Reiter's syndrome, and electrogalvanically induced lesions.[35]

Management

Most cases of stomatitis areata migrans are asymptomatic. Patients who complain of burning tenderness or pain may be placed on a bland diet and use diphenhydramine mouth rinses until the condition becomes asymptomatic.

ALLERGIES

Diffuse erythematous lesions may be seen on the oral mucosa as a result of allergies or as a toxic effect from drugs. These lesions take a variety of forms and have been classified as "erythema multiforme caused by medication" (stomatitis medicamentosa) or as "lichenoid drug reaction" (lichen planus caused by medication). The clinical presentation is identical to that of erythema multiforme and lichen planus, and the diagnosis is made from a careful history. Cessation of drug therapy with the concurrent administration of antihistaminic agents usually results in prompt resolution.

Reactions to topical agents used in the oral cavity are relatively unusual. Individual idiosyncrasies to agents used in preparations such as surgical dressings, mouth rinses, toothpaste, and chewing gums have been reported[36] (Fig. 6-14 and Plate D). A careful history is usually of assistance in making the diagnosis. The patient frequently reports changing from one brand of oral product to another immediately before development of the symptoms. Prompt withdrawal of the etiologic agent is usually both therapeutic and diagnostic.

Patients and clinicians frequently confuse the irritating effects of poorly fitting prosthetic appliances with allergy to a denture base material. Denture base materials are rarely allergenic, but poorly fitting appliances may produce such pathologic changes as papillary hyperplasia. Appliances that are not kept clean may be associated with an increased incidence of intraoral candidiasis. Improperly cured acrylic materials and improperly used denture relining materials can also cause injury to the oral mucosa, but this injury is a "burn" rather than a true allergy.

POLYCYTHEMIA

Polycythemia, also called *erythremia,* is a chronic and sustained elevation in the number of erythrocytes and level of hemoglobin. One form, primary polycythemia (polycythemia vera), is a neoplastic condition of the erythropoietic system analogous to leukemia. Transition between polycythemia and myelogenous leukemia has been reported.

The other form, secondary polycythemia, is a sustained elevation of erythrocytes and hemoglobin, usually resulting from bone marrow stimulation caused by living at high altitudes or by chronic pulmonary diseases such as emphysema. It is also seen in untreated congenital heart disease.

The entire oral mucosa of patients with polycythemia has a deep red or purple color. This discoloration is particularly noticeable in the gingivae and soft palate. The gingivae usually are prone to easy bleeding, and petechial hemorrhages may be seen on the palate and labial mucosa. These changes are seen much more frequently in polycythemia vera. Infarcts may occur in the smaller vessels because of increased viscosity of the blood and may result in multiple ulcers in the red mucosa. Laboratory tests indicating a marked increase in erythrocytes, hemoglobin concentration, and hematocrit values quickly establish the general diagnosis of polycythemia and thus separate this condition from the other mucosities.

LUPUS ERYTHEMATOSUS

Lupus erythematosus (LE) is a connective tissue disease of unknown cause in which the host produces antibodies to nuclear constituents. Because nearly every organ in the body runs the risk of involvement, the disease produces a vast array of signs and symptoms. Depending on the involvement, two forms of the disease occur—discoid lupus erythematosus (DLE) and systemic lupus erythematosus (SLE). The term *DLE* has been applied to cases in which there is only skin involvement; this is usually a benign disease with a good prognosis. Chances of conversion of DLE to SLE are small.

Features

Lupus erythematosus occurs predominantly in adult women; most are affected before the age of 40. Oral manifestations of DLE occur in about 20% of patients. The oral lesions may occur with or without skin involvement, before skin lesions develop, after skin lesions develop, or simultaneously with the skin lesions. Oral lesions may also be seen in patients with SLE (Plate D, 11).

Schiødt et al[37] studied 32 patients (26 women, 6 men) with LE lesions of the oral mucosa. The age of the patient at onset of the oral lesions ranged from 6 to 75 years with a mean age of 41 years. The mean duration of the oral lesions was 4.2 years. Symptoms such as discomfort, burning, and pain associated with hot spicy food were present in 75% of the patients. The lesions were most often located on the buccal mucosa, gingiva, labial mucosa, and vermilion border. The oral lesions were infected by yeast in more than half the patients.

In Schiødt's study, early lesions were characterized by erythema without striae. The classic well-developed discoid lesions appeared as an area of central erythema with white spots and a 2 to 5 mm border of white striae radiating from the center. Some lesions were white plaques, as in leukoplakia; still others had areas of Wickham's striae, as in lichen planus, usually on a reddish base.

On microscopic examination the epithelium shows hyperorthokeratosis or parakeratosis or both, acanthosis, and pseudoepitheliomatous hyperplasia interspersed with atrophy. The basal layer shows liquefaction degeneration, and keratin plugs can be found. A lymphocytic infiltrate, present beneath the epithelial layer, may concentrate around vessels and extend deeply into the subepithelial tissue. In some cases the microscopic study of lesions may be inconclusive. Schiødt and Pindborg[38] completed a blind study of oral lesions from 21 patients with LE and 21 patients with oral lichen planus and leukoplakia. The correct histologic diagnosis was made in less than half the cases. In one third of the cases, differentiation could not be made between DLE and lichen planus.

Differential Diagnosis

Multiple lesions on several surfaces are the rule in LE. When the lesions are mostly of the red variety, conditions that should be considered are lichen planus, lichenoid drug reaction, ectopic geographic tongue, psoriasis, diffuse leukoplakia with erythroplakic components, and electrogalvanic lesions. Oral lesions of LE may be differentiated from lichen planus on the basis of immunofluorescence studies of sera and biopsy specimens (Table 6-1).

Special Diagnostic Procedures

Serum findings Antinuclear antibodies (ANA) and antibodies to specific nuclear antigens occur in patients with LE, mixed connective tissue disease (MCTD), scleroderma, and other collagen disorders. These antibodies have various specificities for nuclear antigens leading to a variety of nuclear staining patterns in immunofluorescence tests. Antibody tests include ANA, native deoxyribonucleic acid (DNA) antibodies, deoxyribonucleoprotein (DNP) antibodies, antibodies to extractable nuclear antigens (ENAs): Sm, ribonucleoprotein (RNP), SS-A (Ro), SS-B (La), SCL-70, JO-1, PNCA, KU.[39,40]

In suspected SLE, ANA tests are useful as a screen and are usually followed by tests for antibodies to native DNA and Sm, which are specific for SLE. Antibodies to RNP, Sm, SS-A (Ro), SS-B(La), and PCNA are less specific for SLE but are often useful tests because these antibodies occur in a limited number of diseases. Antibodies to SS-A (Ro) also occur in 60% of patients with subacute, cutaneous LE, in almost all patients with neonatal LE, and in two thirds of SLE patients with C_2 deficiency. In addition, a majority (>60%) of SLE patients who are ANA negative are positive for SS-A (Ro) antibodies. The presence of antibodies to native DNA, Sm, and SS-A (Ro) has been associated with an increased incidence of nephritis as compared with patients who have RNP and SS-B (La) antibodies.

Biopsy findings The "lupus" or "IF" band immunofluorescent test is important in the diagnosis of LE. Immunoreactants detected in LE occur at the dermoepidermal junction of the skin. This test also differentiates DLE from SLE in that positive lupus band tests occur only in the lesional but not in the normal skin biopsies of patients with DLE, whereas they appear in both lesional and normal skin biopsies of SLE patients. The incidence of a positive band test is influenced by the site's exposure to sun, its age and location, and treatment.

Management

Treatment of LE consists of the administration of systemic corticosteroids or antimalarials. Topical steroids may be used on symptomatic intraoral lesions.

RARITIES

The rare generalized red conditions are listed at the beginning of the chapter and must be considered in the differential diagnosis. Some rare conditions are illustrated in Figs. 6-15 to 6-17.

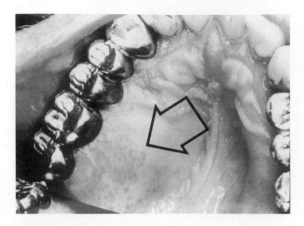

Fig. 6-15. Psoriasis (red macular areas) on palate. (From White DK, Leis HJ, Miller AS: Intraoral psoriasis associated with widespread dermal psoriasis, *Oral Surg* 41(2):174-181, 1976.)

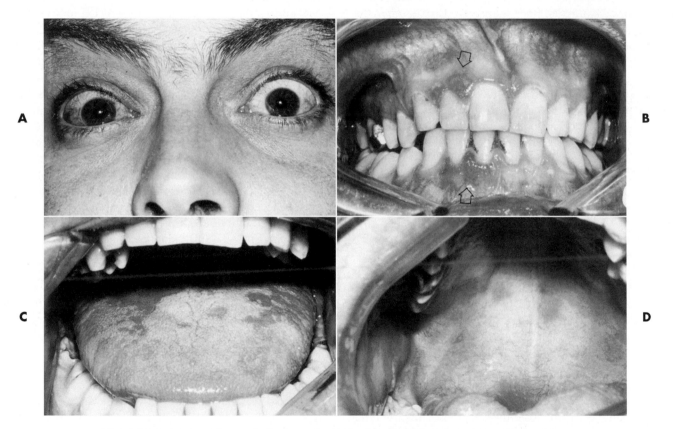

Fig. 6-16. Reiter's syndrome. **A,** Erythema involving the sclera. **B,** Anterior intraoral view. Note small erythematous patches *(arrows).* **C,** View showing reddish macules on tongue. **D,** View of palate showing reddish patches. (Courtesy M. Lehnert, Minneapolis.)

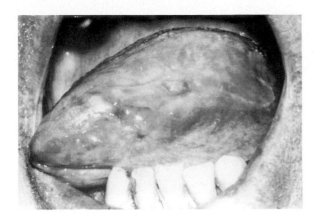

Fig. 6-17. Uremic stomatitis. Note erythematous and eroded areas on the lateral border of the tongue. (Courtesy M. Lehnert, Minneapolis.

REFERENCES

1. Lehner T, Barnes C, editors: Behçet's syndrome, London, 1979, Academic Press.
2. Graykowski E, Hooks J: Summary of workshop on recurrent aphthous stomatitis and Behçet syndrome, *J Am Dent Assoc* 97:599-602, 1978.
3. Myers JD, Wade JC, Mitchell CD, et al: Multicenter collaborative trial of intravenous acyclovir for treatment of mucocutaneous herpes simplex virus infection in the immunocompromised host, *Am J Med* 73(1A):229-235, 1982.
4. Whitley R, Barton N, Collins E, et al: Mucocutaneous herpes simplex virus infections in immunocompromised patients, *Am J Med* 73(1A):236-240, 1982.
5. Silverman S Jr, Griffith M: Studies on oral lichen planus. II. Follow-up on 200 patients, clinical characteristics and associated malignancy, *Oral Surg* 37:705-710, 1974.
6. Fulling HJ: Cancer development in oral lichen planus: a follow-up study of 327 patients, *Arch Dermatol* 108:667-669, 1973.
7. Barnard NA, Scully C, Eveson JW, et al: Oral cancer development in patients with oral lichen planus, *J Oral Pathol Med* 22:421-424, 1993.
8. Krutchkoff DJ, Eisenberg E: Lichenoid dysplasia: distinct histopathologic entity. *Oral Surg Oral Med Oral Pathol* 30:308-315, 1985.
9. Lovas JG, Harsanyi BB, ElGeneidy AK: Oral lichenoid dysplasia: A clinicopathologic analysis, *Oral Surg Oral Med Oral Pathol* 68:57-63, 1989.
10. Kilpi AM, Rich AM, Radden BG, Reade PC: Direct immunofluorescence in the diagnosis of oral mucosal diseases, *Int J Oral Maxillofac Surg* 17:6-10, 1988.
11. Scully C, El-Kom M: Lichen planus: Review and update on pathogenesis, *J Oral Pathol* 14:431-58, 1985.
12. Farthing PM, Margou P, Coates M, et al: Characteristics of the oral lesions in patients with cutaneous recurrent erythema multiforme, *J Oral Pathol Med* 24:9-13, 1995.
13. Buchner A, Lozada F, Silverman S: Histological spectrum of oral erythema multiforme, *Oral Surg* 49:221-228, 1980.

14. Lozada F: Prednisone and azathioprine in the treatment of patients with vesiculoerosive oral diseases, *Oral Surg* 52:257-260, 1981.
15. Manton SL, Scully C: Mucous membrane pemphigoid: an elusive diagnosis? *Oral Surg* 66:37-40, 1988.
16. Rogers RS, Seehafer JR, Perry HO: Treatment of cicatricial (benign mucous membrane) pemphigoid with dapsone, *J Am Acad Dermatol* 6:215-223, 1982.
17. Rosenberg FR, Sanders S, Nelson CT: Pemphigus: a 20-year review of 107 patients treated with corticosteroids, *Arch Dermatol* 112:962-970, 1976.
18. Laskaris G, Stoufi E: Oral pemphigus vulgaris in a 6-year-old girl, *Oral Surg* 69:609-613, 1990.
19. Laskaris G: Oral pemphigus vulgaris: an immunofluorescent study of fifty-eight cases, *Oral Surg* 51:626-631, 1981.
20. Handlers JP, Melrose RJ, Abrams AM, Taylor CR: Immunoperoxidase technique in diagnosis of oral pemphigus vulgaris: an alternative method to immunofluorescence, *Oral Surg* 54:207-212, 1982.
21. Lamey P-J, Rees TD, Binnie WH, et al: Oral presentation of pemphigus vulgaris and its response to systemic steroid therapy, *Oral Surg* 74:54-57, 1992.
22. Lozada F, Silverman S, Cram D: Pemphigus vulgaris: a study of six cases treated with levamisole and prednisone, *Oral Surg* 54:161-165, 1982.
23. McCarthy PL, Shklar G: *Disease of the oral mucosa: diagnosis, management and therapy,* New York, 1964, McGraw-Hill.
24. Nisengard RJ, Neiders M: Desquamative lesions, *J Periodontol* 52:500-510, 1981.
25. Nisengard RJ, Rogers RS: The treatment of desquamative gingival lesions, *J Periodontol* 58:167-172, 1987.
26. Jaremko WM, Beutner EH, Kumar V, et al: Chronic ulcerative stomatitis associated with a specific immunologic marker, *J Am Acad Dermatol* 22:215-220, 1990.
27. Beutner EH, Chorzelski TP, Parodi A, et al: Ten cases of chronic ulcerative stomatitis associated with a specific immunologic marker, *J Am Acad Dermatol* 24:781-782, 1990.

28. Church LF, Schosser RH: Chronic ulcerative stomatitis associated with stratified epithelial specific antinuclear antibodies. A case report of a newly described disease entity, *Oral Surg Oral Med Oral Pathol* 73:579-582, 1992.
29. Kolbinson DA, Schubert MM, Flournoy N, Truelove EL: Early oral changes following bone marrow transplantation, *Oral Surg* 66:130-138, 1988.
30. Little JW, Falace DA: *Dental management of the medically compromised patient,* ed 4, St Louis, 1993, Mosby.
31. Hatton MN, Levine MJ, Margarone JE, Aquirre A: Lubrication and viscosity features of human saliva and commercially available saliva substitutes, *J Oral Maxillofac Surg* 45:496-499, 1987.
32. Kerr BA, McClatchey KD, and Regezi JA: Idiopathic gingivostomatitis, *Oral Surg* 32:402-423, 1971.
33. Perry HO, Deffner NF, Sheridan PJ: Atypical gingivostomatitis, *Arch Dermatol* 107:872-878, 1973.
34. Silverman S, Lozada F: An epilogue to plasma-cell gingivostomatitis (allergic gingivostomatitis), *Oral Surg* 43:211-217, 1977.
35. Bánóczy J, Roed-Petersen B, Pindborg JJ, Inovay J: Clinical and histologic studies on electrogalvanically induced oral white lesions, *Oral Surg* 48:319-323, 1979.
36. Miller RL, Gould AR, Bernstein ML: Cinnamon-induced stomatitis venenata, *Oral Surg Oral Med Oral Pathol* 73:8708-8716, 1992.
37. Schiødt M, Halberg P, Hentzer B: A clinical study of 32 patients with oral discoid lupus erythematosus, *Int J Oral Surg* 7:85-94, 1978.
38. Schiødt M, Pindborg JJ: Histologic differential diagnostic problems for oral discoid lupus erythematosus, *Int J Oral Surg* 5:250-252, 1976.
39. Dahl MV, Gilliam JN: Direct immunofluorescence in lupus erythematosus. In Beutner EH, Chorzelski TP, Kumar V, editors: Immunopathology of the skin, ed 3, New York, John Wiley & Sons. 1987.
40. Halberg P, Ullman, S, Jorgensen F: The lupus band test as a measure of disease of disease activity in systemic lupus erythematosus. *Arch Dermatol* 118:572-576, 1982.

CHAPTER 7

Red Conditions of the Tongue

NORMAN K. WOOD
GEORGE G. BLOZIS

The following red conditions are discussed in this chapter:

MIGRATORY GLOSSITIS	DEFICIENCY STATES	RARITIES
MEDIAN RHOMBOID GLOSSITIS	XEROSTOMIA	

All the single red lesions of the oral mucosa discussed in Chapter 5 occur on the tongue. Likewise, all the generalized reddish conditions of the oral mucosa (see Chapter 6) may involve the tongue. In some cases the tongue is involved first; in others, different mucosal surfaces are initially affected; and in some patients, one or more mucosal surfaces and the tongue are involved simultaneously.

However, this chapter discusses red conditions that occur only on the tongue or that have a predisposition for that structure. Such conditions usually produce one or more bald reddish patches or affect the entire dorsal surface and margins of the tongue.

MIGRATORY GLOSSITIS

A plethora of terms (erythema migrans, glossitis areata migrans, glossitis areata exfoliativa, geographic tongue, wandering rash of the tongue, and annulus migrans) has been used to identify migratory glossitis (MG). Although the cause is unknown, emotional stress may be one of several factors involved in the onset or exacerbation of this lesion.[1,2] Sensitivity to the environment (atopy) has been suggested as another possible cause.[3] Blood antigens HLA-B DR5 and DRw6 are significantly higher in patients with MG whereas the DR2 antigen is lower in patients with MG than it is in normal patients,[4] which suggests that an immunologic factor may be at work. Chronic bacterial or fungal agents have also been suggested as possible causes.

Features

MG is a relatively common condition, occurring in 1% to 2% of the population. The lesions are usually asymptomatic and are discovered as an incidental finding during a routine examination. The patient may complain of a burning sensation made worse by spicy foods or citrus fruits. MG occurs most commonly in young or middle-aged adults but has been seen in patients ranging in age from 5 to 84 years. There is a reported predilection for female patients. The lesions are found more frequently on fissured tongues.[5] An increased incidence of MG has been reported in juvenile diabetes.[6] Another study indicated an increased incidence of MG and ectopic geographic tongue in patients with several regions of cutaneous psoriasis.[7]

Initially, MG appears as irregular, circinate, nonindurated atrophic areas that gradually widen, change shape, and migrate over the tongue (Fig. 7-1). These small red patches are frequently bordered by a slightly elevated, distinct rim that varies from gray to white to light yellow (Fig. 7-1). A more intense redness may be present near the advancing margin of a lesion. Lesions may be single or multiple. Frequently the lesions are confined to the dorsal surface and lateral borders of the tongue, but they may extend to the ventral surface.

The progression of the lesions is usually quite rapid, with the pattern changing in a few days, or the lesions may remain relatively static. The duration of an attack also varies, ranging from a few weeks to months; rarely it may continue for years. However, regression and recurrence is the general pattern.

Lesions similar to those seen on the tongue have been seen occasionally on other mucosal surfaces of the oral cavity.[8] These lesions are considered a more extensive involvement of the same process and have been referred to as *stomatitis areata migrans* or *ectopic geographic tongue.*[9,10] This condition is discussed in Chapter 6 (see Fig. 6-13).

The histopathology of the lesions shows a loss of the filiform papillae and a variable thinning of the mucosa. In some areas, there is an epithelial hyperplasia. The epithelium shows spongiosis and infiltration by acute and chronic inflammatory cells.

Differential Diagnosis

A diagnosis of is made on the basis of the clinical appearance and history of the lesion. Similar-appearing lesions are reported in psoriasis, Reiter's syndrome, ectopic geographic tongue, and occasionally pityriasis rubra pilaris.[8,11,12] These authors report that the clinical and histologic appearances of these conditions are often identical to those of geographic tongue; consequently these conditions may be closely related. If the classic tongue lesions are the only finding, the clinician is correct in establishing a working diagnosis of MG. However, this isolated finding may be the first manifestation of the more generalized diseases included in the second sentence of this paragraph.

In cases of skin, ocular, tongue, and urethral lesions and arthritis, the most likely diagnosis is Reiter's syndrome. If the patient has skin lesions of psoriasis (particularly of the generalized pustular type) or pityriasis rubra pilaris, "geographic tongue" might really be a manifestation of former skin diseases.

Lichen planus may occasionally produce reddish patches on the tongue, which in the healing phase may resemble MG (Fig. 7-2). The absence of raised, whitish-yellow rims in lichen planus helps to differentiate these lesions from those of MG. In addition, it is unusual for lichen planus to affect only the tongue, so at least one white keratotic area can usually be found on one of the oral mucosal surfaces.

The use of strong mouthrinse can produce a variety of clinical lesions, one of which resembles MG.[13] The history of frequent use of mouthrinse followed by the disappearance of the lesions when use is discontinued permits the differentiation of this condition from MG.

Anemic conditions that produce a patchy baldness of the tongue may be confused with MG (see Fig. 7-2). Again the characteristic, raised, yellowish-white borders of MG differentiates this condition from the red patches of anemia. Careful blood studies demonstrate anemia.

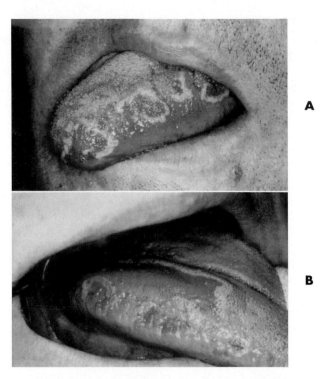

Fig. 7-1. MG. **A,** Multiple lesions with distinct borders and an inflamed atrophic mucosa. **B,** A larger, more diffuse lesion with less inflammatory change and residual fungiform papillae.

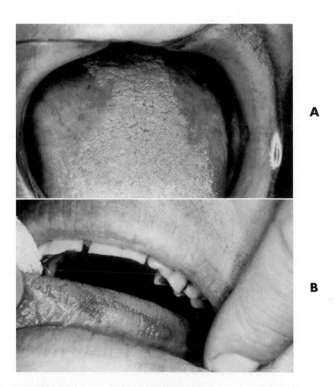

Fig. 7-2. Lesions resembling MG. **A,** Bilateral areas of atrophic lichen planus. **B,** Focal red and white areas on the lateral border of the tongue of an anemic patient.

Management

If there is some discomfort, bland diets and topical corticosteroids provide symptomatic relief while the lesions run the usual course and resolve. The use of topical tretinoin (Retin-A) solution has been advocated for very sensitive cases.[14] Elimination of irritants, mild symptomatic treatment, and psychologic reassurance is advised.[15] Rarely, the clinician encounters painful cases refractory to treatment.

MEDIAN RHOMBOID GLOSSITIS

For years median rhomboid glossitis (MRG) (central papillary atrophy of the tongue) has been considered a developmental and congenital defect causing a segment of the tuberculum impar to persist on the dorsal surface of the tongue, instead of being buried in normal embryonic development. However, the paucity of cases in children[16-19] and some cases of remission has diminished support for this theory. It is thought that a chronic candidal infection plays a leading etiologic role,[18-22,26] and smoking may also act as a promoter.[20,21,23-25] Conflicting reports concern a possible role by diabetes.[22,24,27] A localized defect in immune surveillance may contribute to this persistent fungal infection.[25] Some authorities suggest that the clinical appearance of MRG may be produced by various agents, either singly or in combination, so the etiology may not be the same in all cases.[23,26] Fig. 7-3, A, shows an ulcerative, white necrotic lesion from which smears showed abundant clumps of Candida organisms. The lesion was treated with applications of nystatin ointment. Within a week the lesion became asymptomatic and by 2 weeks was almost completely healed, assuming the reddish macular appearance of MRG (Fig. 7-3, B).

Features

It is unclear whether MRG occurs more frequently in male or female patients.[18,21,25] It has been reported in patients ranging in age from 15 to 84 years. The lesion is located on the dorsal surface of the tongue in the midline and anterior to the circumvallate papillae (Figs. 7-4 and 7-5). The surface is dusky red, completely devoid of filiform papillae, and usually smooth; however, nodular or fissured surfaces have been noted (see Fig. 11-19, E). Rarely, there may be some keratosis. The size and shape of the lesion are somewhat variable, at times causing confusion as to the diagnosis. The lesions are generally asymptomatic, but pain and ulceration have been reported.

An interesting combination or syndrome has been reported by Tuyz and Peters[28]: Frequently, concomitant erythematous areas occur on the palate. These lesions are in contact with the MRG lesion, particularly during swallowing.[28] These authors were unable to find candidal organisms in the palatal lesions and postulated that the lesions resulted from immune or toxic responses to the candidal organisms in the MRG lesions.[28] Presumably in more acute cases the palatal lesions yield candidal organisms as well (NKW). It is interesting that the palate and tongue are the most common sites for candidiasis in HIV patients.[29] The microscopic changes include an epithelium that is devoid of filiform papillae that is slightly thickened and elongation and branching of the rete ridges. The underlying connective tissue shows increased vascularity and a chronic inflammatory infiltrate.

Differential Diagnosis

MRG is easily recognized by its usual asymptomatic nature and its characteristic location. The following lesions need to be included in the differential diagnosis: geographic tongue erythroplakia, carcinoma in situ, squamous cell carcinoma, atypical herpes, another type of fungal infection, lichen planus or lichenoid drug reaction, or deficiency states.

Management

The completely asymptomatic lesion that looks smooth and is not indurated requires no treatment but should be checked periodically in case of change. Burning or painful lesions should be investigated for the presence of candidal organisms; if these are found, the lesion should be treated with topical antifungal agents. The treatment of candidiasis is extensively discussed in Chapter 5.

DEFICIENCY STATES

It has been recognized for years that certain deficiency states can produce a glossitis of a completely bald or a patchy bald type. Diagnosticians of bygone years prided themselves in their ability to diagnose the specific deficiency by recognizing minute differences in appearance. Now it is generally agreed that the glossal changes induced by specific deficiencies are so similar that a definitive diagnosis based on their differentiation is at least unlikely, if not impossible.

Features

Symptoms vary from a tender to burning tongue to extreme glossodynia. In the beginning, the tongue may be intensely red and then becomes smooth as the filiform or both types of papillae atrophy (Fig. 7-6). In some instances, normal papillation returns when the patient's basic problem is successfully treated.[30]

The deficiency states reported to produce the type of glossitides discussed here are iron deficiency anemia; pernicious anemia; Plummer-Vinson syndrome; sprue; and vitamin B–complex deficiencies, especially those of thiamine, riboflavin, nicotinic acid, pyridoxine, pantothenic acid, and vitamin B_{12} (cyanocobalamin).

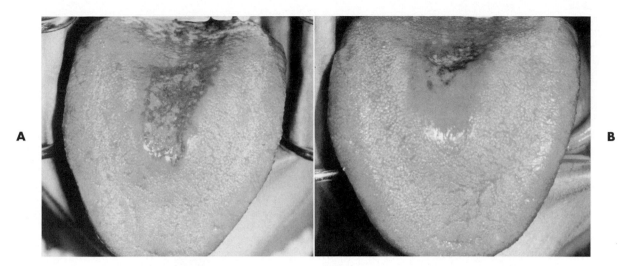

Fig. 7-3. Tongue of a middle-aged woman with pseudomembranous candidiasis of the dorsal surface **(A).** After 2 weeks of nystatin applications, the candidal lesion had almost completely healed **(B).** In 3 weeks the white appearance had completely resolved, and the resultant picture was that of MRG.

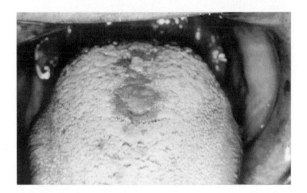

Fig. 7-4. A small but relatively typical lesion of MRG.

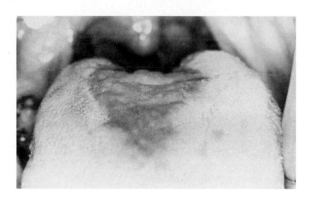

Fig. 7-5. Classic appearance of MRG.

Differential Diagnosis

If the tongue is completely bald, the only other condition that needs to be considered is xerostomia (Fig. 7-7). Xerostomia can usually be recognized by noting the absence of a salivary pool in the floor of the mouth or by sticking a tongue blade to the oral mucosa during the oral examination.

If the tongue shows partial or patchy baldness, all the conditions previously mentioned should be considered; these inlcude MG, psoriasis, Reiter's syndrome, pityriasis rubra pilaris, changes caused by the use of mouthrinse, atrophic lichen planus, and MRG. The differential diagnosis of these entities may be reviewed under the differential diagnosis section of MG. A thorough discussion of the differential aspects of all the deficiency states that may produce a glossitis is well beyond the intended scope of this text.

Management

Once the deficiency state or states have been identified, specific measures may be undertaken for their correction, if such are available.

XEROSTOMIA

The oral changes found in cases of xerostomia are discussed in Chapter 6. The red tongue of xerostomia (see Fig. 7-7) is rather easily differentiated from the other conditions by the absence of a salivary pool in the floor of the mouth.

RARITIES

Many specific infectious diseases can affect superficial red changes in the surface of the tongue, but these are very rare. Fig. 7-8 illustrates a case of syphilitic glossitis.

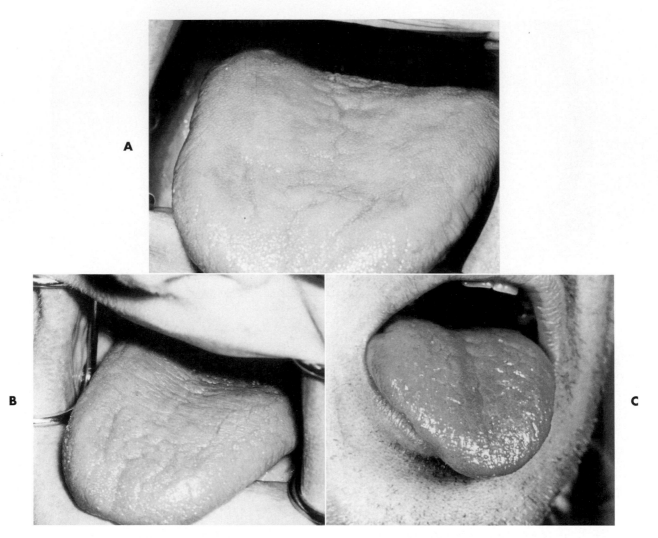

Fig. 7-6. Generalized glossitis. **A,** Patient with iron deficiency anemia. **B,** Patient with an untreated case of pernicious anemia. **C,** Man who was severely malnourished and who had several vitamin deficiencies. (**A** and **B** courtesy M. Lehnert, Minneapolis; **C** courtesy J. Lavieri, Maywood, Ill.)

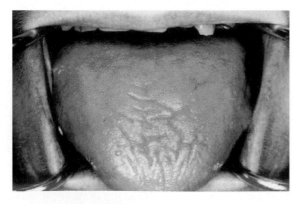

Fig. 7-7. Xerostomia. Tongue changes in a patient with Sjögren's syndrome. The tongue appears dry and is almost completely devoid of papillae.

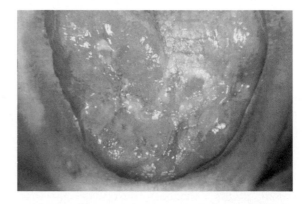

Fig. 7-8. Syphilitic glossitis. (Courtesy R. Gorlin, Minneapolis.)

REFERENCES

1. Redman RS, Vance FL, Gorlin RJ, et al: Psychological component in the etiology of geographic tongue, *J Dent Res* 45:1403-1408, 1966.
2. Sumner MS, Shklar G: Stomatitis areata migrans, *Oral Surg* 36:28-33, 1973.
3. Marks R, Czarny D: Geographic tongue: sensitivity to the environment, *Oral Surg* 58:156-159, 1984.
4. Fenerli A, Papanicolaou M, Laskaris G: Histocompatibility antigens and geographic tongue, *Oral Surg* 76:476-479, 1993.
5. Gorlin RJ, Goldman HM: *Thoma's oral pathology,* ed 6, St Louis, 1970, Mosby.
6. Wysocki GP, Daley TD: Benign migratory glossitis in patients with juvenile diabetes, *Oral Surg* 63:68-70, 1987.
7. Pogrel MA, Cram D: Intraoral findings in patients with psoriasis with a special reference to ectopic geographic tongue (erythema circinata), *Oral Surg* 66:184-189, 1988.
8. Weathers DR, Baker G, Archard HO, Burkes JE: Psoriasiform lesions of the oral mucosa (with emphasis on "ectopic geographic tongue"), *Oral Surg* 37:872-888, 1974.
9. Brooks JK, Balciunas GA: Geographic stomatitis: review of the literature and report of five cases, *J Am Dent Assoc* 115:421-424, 1987.
10. Espelid M, Bang G, Johannessen AC, et al: Geographic stomatitis: report of 6 cases, *J Oral Pathol Med* 20:425-428, 1991.
11. Dawson TAJ: Tongue lesions in generalized pustular psoriasis, *Br J Dermatol* 91:419-424, 1974.

12. O'Keefe E, Braverman IM, Cohen I: Annulus migrans: identical lesions in pustular psoriasis, Reiter's syndrome, and geographic tongue, *Arch Dermatol* 107:240-244, 1973.
13. Kowitz GM, Lucatorto FM, Chernick HM: Effects of mouthwashes on the oral soft tissues, *J Oral Med* 31:47-50, 1976.
14. Helfman RJ: The treatment of geographic tongue with topical Retin-A solution, *Cutis* 24(2):179-180, 1979.
15. Bánóczy J: *Oral leukoplakia,* The Hague, Netherlands, 1982, Martinus Nijhoff.
16. Carter LC: Median rhomboid glossitis: review of a puzzling entity, *Compend Contin Ed J* 11(7):446-451, 1990.
17. Redman R: Prevalence of geographic tongue, median rhomboid glossitis and hairy tongue among 3611 Minnesota school children, *Oral Surg* 31:56-65, 1971.
18. Baughman RA: Median rhomboid glossitis: a developmental anomaly? *Oral Surg* 31:56-65, 1971.
19. Guggenheimer J, Verbin RS: Median rhomboid glossitis in an infant, *J Oral Med* 40:110-111, 1985.
20. Van der Wal N, van der Kwast WAM, van der Waal I: Median rhomboid glossitis: a follow-up study of 16 patients, *J Oral Med* 41:117-120, 1986.
21. Van der Wal N, van der Waal I: *Candida albicans* in median rhomboid glossitis: a postmortem study, *Int J Oral Maxillofac Surg* 15:322-325, 1986.

22. Farman AG: Atrophic lesions of the tongue: a prevalence study among 175 diabetic patients, *J Oral Pathol* 5:255-264, 1976.
23. Farman AG, Van Wyk CW, Staz J, et al: Central papillary atrophy of the tongue, *Oral Surg* 43:48-58, 1977.
24. Mehtafali S, Bhonsle RB, Murti PR: Central papillary atrophy of the tongue among bidi smokers in India: a 10-year study of 182 lesions, *J Oral Pathol Med* 18:475-480, 1989.
25. Walsh LJ, Cleveland DB, Cummings CG: Quantitative evaluation of Langerhans' cells in median rhomboid glossitis, *J Oral Pathol Med* 21:28-32, 1992.
26. Van der Waal I, Bessmster G, van der Kwast WAM: Median rhomboid glossitis caused by *Candida, Oral Surg* 47:31-35, 1979.
27. Farman AG: Atrophic lesions of the tongue among diabetic outpatients: their incidence and regression, *J Oral Pathol* 6:396-400, 1977.
28. Tuyz LZG, Peters, E: Candidal infection of the tongue with non-specific inflammation of the palate: a clinical pathologic entity, *Oral Surg* 63:304-308, 1987.
29. Samaranayake LP, Holmstrup P: Oral candidiasis and human immunodeficiency virus infection, *J Oral Pathol Med* 18:554-564, 1989.
30. Basker RM, Sturdee DW, Davenport JC: Patients with burning mouths: a clinical investigation of causative factors, including the climacteric and diabetes, *Br Dent J* 145:9-16, 1978.

CHAPTER 8

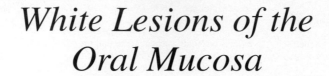

White Lesions of the Oral Mucosa

NORMAN K. WOOD
PAUL W. GOAZ

A list of white lesions of the oral mucosa follows:

KERATOTIC WHITE ENTITIES
LEUKOEDEMA
LINEA ALBA BUCCALIS
LEUKOPLAKIA
NICOTINE STOMATITIS
CIGARETTE SMOKER'S LIP LESION
SMOKELESS TOBACCO LESION
MIGRATORY GLOSSITIS
PERIPHERAL SCAR TISSUE
  (NONKERATOTIC)
LICHEN PLANUS
LICHENOID REACTIONS
ELECTROGALVANIC AND MERCURY
  CONTACT ALLERGY
WHITE HAIRY TONGUE
PAPILLOMA, VERRUCA VULGARIS,
  CONDYLOMA ACUMINATUM
WHITE EXOPHYTIC SQUAMOUS CELL
  CARCINOMA
VERRUCOUS CARCINOMA
  Proliferative verrucous leukoplakia
  Verrucous hyperplasia
HYPERPLASTIC OR HYPERTROPHIC
  CANDIDIASIS
HAIRY LEUKOPLAKIA
WHITE SPONGE NEVUS
SKIN GRAFTS
RARITIES
  Acanthosis nigricans
  Bohn's nodule (Epstein's pearl)
  Candidiasis endocrinopathy syndrome
  Clouston's syndrome
  Condyloma latum
  Cysts—keratin-filled and superficial
    Epidermoid cyst
    Dermoid cyst
    Lymphoepithelial cyst

Darier's disease
Dermatitis herpetiformis
Dyskeratosis congenita
Focal epithelial hyperplasia
Focal palmoplantar and marginal gingival
  hyperkeratosis
Graft-versus-host disease
Granular cell myoblastoma
Grinspan's syndrome
Hereditary benign intraepithelial dyskeratosis
Hyalinosis cutis et mucosae
Hypersplenism and leukoplakia oris
Hypovitaminosis A
Inverted papilloma
Juvenile juxtavermilion candidiasis
Koplik's spots
Larva migrans
Lichen sclerosus and atrophicus
Lupus erythematosus
Molluscum contagiosum
Pachyonychia congenita
Pityriasis rubra pilaris
Porokeratosis
Pseudoepitheliomatous hyperplasia
Pseudoxanthoma elasticum
Psoriasis
Scleroderma (nonkeratotic)
Squamous acanthoma
Submucous fibrosis (nonkeratotic)
Superficial sialolith of minor glands
  (nonkeratotic)
Syndrome of dyskeratosis congenita, dys-
  trophia unguium, and aplastic anemia
Syphilitic interstitial leukoplakial glossitis
Tuberous sclerosis
Verruciform xanthoma
Warty dyskeratoma

**SLOUGHING, PSEUDOMEMBRANOUS,
  NECROTIC WHITE LESIONS**
PLAQUE
TRAUMATIC ULCER
PYOGENIC GRANULOMA
CHEMICAL BURNS
ACUTE NECROTIZING ULCERATIVE
  GINGIVITIS
CANDIDIASIS
NECROTIC ULCERS OF SYSTEMIC
  DISEASE
DIFFUSE GANGRENOUS STOMATITIS
RARITIES
  Allergic reactions
  Candidiasis endocrinopathy syndrome
  Syndrome of familial hypoparathyroidism,
    candidiasis, and retardation
  Syndrome of idiopathic hypoparathyroidism,
    Addison's disease, and candidiasis
  Congenital insensitivity to pain syndrome
  Diphtheria
  Eosinophilic granuloma
  Eosinophilic ulcer
  Graft-versus-host disease
  Heavy metal mucositis
  Henoch-Schönlein purpura
  Mycosis fungoides
  Noma
  Superficial abscess
  Syphilitic chancre and mucous patch
  Tuberculosis
VESICLES AND BULLAE (discussed in
  Chapter 6)

White lesions of the oral mucosa may be conveniently divided into two groups: those that cannot be scraped off with a tongue blade (most are keratotic) and those that can be scraped off with a tongue blade (sloughing, pseudomembranous necrotic types). This chapter is divided into two parts—the first dealing with the keratotic entities, which as a group are the more common, and the second reviewing the sloughing types.

A third type, vesiculobullous lesions, have a white or grayish-white appearance during a stage of their presentation, so they can be considered white lesions, particularly during the examination process (Fig. 8-1). However, for differential diagnosis, it is better to group these lesions by themselves or as generalized reddish conditions (see Chapter 6). This information is introduced at the beginning of this chapter to alert students to the fact that such lesions have a significant white component when the blisters are intact and for a day or two after they rupture. Almost invariably there is an extensive erythematous component.

Another nonkeratotic nonnecrotic lesion is edema of the superficial tissues produced occasionally by chronic mild trauma to the mucosa. Touyz and Hille[1] describe such a case: an extensive white lesion of the gingivae that could not be scraped off. It was caused by excessive use of mouthrinses and acidic fruit juices. Histologically the white appearance was produced by a hyperplasia of the epithelium, marked intracellular edema, and microvesicular formation in the prickle cell layer.

KERATOTIC WHITE ENTITIES

The color of the oral mucosa ranges from a light to a dark pink. This concept is discussed in detail in Chapter 6. Briefly, the masticatory mucosa is light pink because of a thicken epithelial layer of keratin and a more fibrous, less vascular subepithelial layer. On the other hand, the lining mucosa is a reddish-pink because of the absence of a keratin layer and a less fibrous, more vascular subepithelial tissue (Fig. 8-2).

In some regions, normal keratinization, epithelial thickening, or both may be so marked that it appears pathologic. Leukoedema and linea alba are such examples.

The amount of keratin produced by any given stimuli varies from individual to individual. This variation is probably under genetic control and may be influenced by the patient's systemic condition at the time.

LEUKOEDEMA

Leukoedema is a common variation that appears to be related causally to mastication and possibly poor oral hygiene.[2] Although smoking is not believed to be a primary cause, it can intensify the condition.[3] The incidence and intensity increase with age. Some 50% of black teenagers are affected[2] (male incidence is more common[3]), and about 90% of black adults have the condition.[2] Approximately

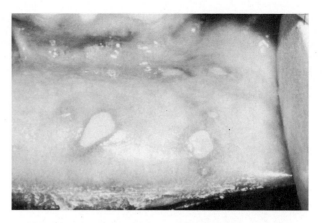

Fig. 8-1. Vesicles of herpes zoster on the mucosa of the lower lip. Note the whiteness of the lesions. They will soon rupture, leaving small ulcers and retaining for a short time whitish remnants of the vesicular covering.

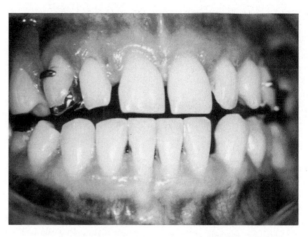

Fig. 8-2. The attached gingiva (masticatory mucosa) is a paler pink than the vestibular (lining) mucosa because of the keratinized surface and less vascularity.

45% of whites were thought to be involved, but with proper lighting, leukoedema could be found in 93% of whites.[4]

Features

Leukoedema is asymptomatic and usually found during routine oral examination. The most frequent site is the buccal mucosa bilaterally, and it also occurs on the labial mucosa and soft palate. The degree of severity varies from a faint, filmy appearance, which requires close inspection for detection, to a much denser opalescence with wrinkling or folding of the surface (Figs. 8-3 and 8-4). Leukoedema cannot be removed with a tongue blade but becomes less prominent or disappears altogether when the tissue is stretched.

Microscopic studies show an increased thickness of the epithelium, usually with marked intracellular edema (ballooning) in the prickle cell layer. A hyperparakeratosis (hyperkeratosis with retention of nuclei) of varying thickness may be present (see Fig. 8-3).

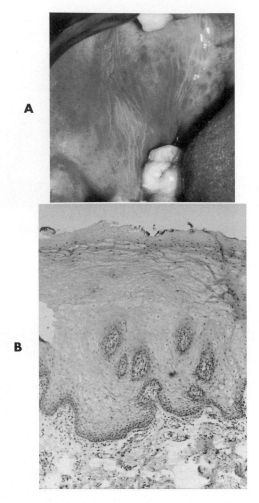

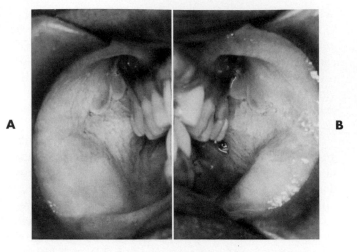

Fig. 8-4. Leukoedema. **A,** The prominent white, wrinkled appearance was present bilaterally in this 52-year-old black woman. Stretching the tissue diminished the white appearance. (Courtesy S. Smith, Chicago.)

Fig. 8-3. Leukoedema. **A,** The white, wrinkled appearance of the buccal mucosa, present bilaterally, occurred in a 45-year-old black man. A faint reticular pattern mimicking lichen planus can be seen. **B,** Photomicrograph showing acanthosis, ballooning in the prickle cells, and parakeratosis.

Differential Diagnosis

The commonly occurring lesions that may be confused with leukoedema are leukoplakia, cheek-biting lesion, lichen planus (LP), and white sponge nevus. A discussion of the differential diagnosis of these lesions is presented under the differential diagnosis of leukoplakia.

Management

Since leukoedema is a normal variant, its recognition is important, and no treatment is required. This condition does not undergo malignant change.

LINEA ALBA BUCCALIS

Linea alba (white line) is a streak on the buccal mucosa at the level of the occlusal plane extending horizontally from the commissure to the most posterior teeth. It is usually seen bilaterally and may be quite prominent in some people (Fig. 8-5). Because it occurs at the occlusal plane and conforms to the space between the teeth, it is

thought to result from slight occlusal trauma to the buccal mucosa.

This impression is strengthened by the observation that linea alba is frequently more prominent in people with little overjet of the molars and premolars. The prominence and pattern of linea alba varies greatly from one individual to another, being especially marked in some people and completely absent in others (see Fig. 8-5).

Histologically an increased thickness or hyperorthokeratosis (hyperkeratosis without retention of nuclei) is seen.

Management requires only the recognition of linea alba as a normal variation.

LEUKOPLAKIA

Leukoplakia is a keratotic plaque occurring on mucous membranes and is considered a premalignant lesion. The World Health Organization defined *leukoplakia* as "a white patch or plaque that cannot be characterized clinically or pathologically as any other disease."[5] As with other keratotic lesions, it cannot be scraped off with a tongue blade.

A variety of local chronic irritations acting alone or in combination produces leukoplakial lesions in certain individuals. Etiologic factors thought to be important in leukoplakia are listed in the box on p. 99.

Leukoplakia and squamous cell carcinoma (SCC) share many of the same etiologic factors. These are discussed in detail in Chapter 35.

The chronic irritation, regardless of type, must be intense enough to induce the surface epithelium to produce and retain keratin but not intense enough to cause a breakdown of the tissue with resulting erosion or ulcer formation. Genetic and systemic factors play a role in preconditioning the mucosa because some people develop a leukoplakic lesion as the result of a relatively minor insult, whereas others show no reaction to the same or more prolonged severe stimulus or suffer tissue destruction and an inflammatory lesion.

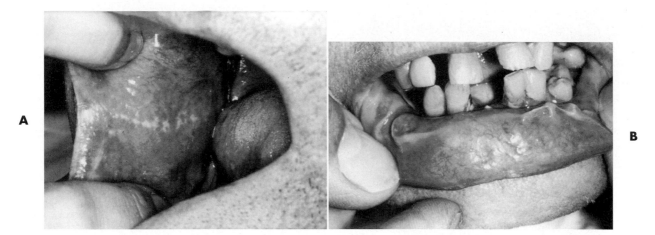

Fig. 8-5. Linea alba. **A,** Prominent example in the classic location. **B,** Unusual location and appearance of linea alba on the mucosal surface of the lower lip. The patient habitually sucked the tissue in against his anterior teeth.

ETIOLOGIC FACTORS OF LEUKOPLAKIA

- Tobacco products
- Ethanol
- Hot, cold, spicy, and acidic foods and beverages
- Alcoholic mouthrinse (Fig. 8-6)
- Occlusal trauma
- Sharp edges of prostheses or teeth
- Actinic radiation
- Syphilis
- Presence of *Candida albicans*
- Presence of viruses

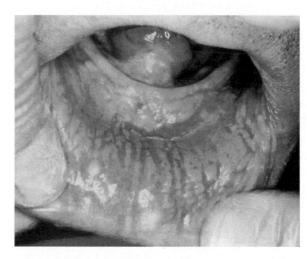

Fig. 8-6. Keratotic condition of the oral mucosa produced by holding Listerine mouthwash in the mouth for 15 minutes once a day. (From Bernstein ML: Oral mucosal white lesions associated with excessive use of Listerine mouthwash: report of two cases, *Oral Surg* 46(6):781-785, 1978.)

Leukoplakia then likely commences as a protective reaction against a chronic irritant. This reaction produces a dense layer of keratin, which is retained to insulate the deeper epithelial components from the deleterious effects of the irritant.

When clinical leukoplakic lesions are studied microscopically, they can be seen to embrace a spectrum of histologic changes that shows only increased keratosis to invasive SCC (Fig. 8-7). These differences cannot be identified clinically, so to establish the specific diagnosis the lesion needs to be examined microscopically.

Features

Leukoplakic lesions are characteristically asymptomatic and are most often discovered during a routine oral examination. Leukoplakia is a common lesion. It represents 6.2% of all oral biopsy specimens[6] and occurs in approximately 3% of white Americans over 35 years of age.[7] Most lesions occur between 40 and 70 years of age and more commonly in men. Frequent sites are the lip vermilion, buccal mucosa, mandibular gingiva, tongue, oral floor, hard palate, maxillary gingiva, lip mucosa, and soft palate. The lesions may vary greatly in size, shape, and distribution. The borders may be distinct or indistinct and smoothly contoured or ragged. The lesions may be solitary, or multiple plaques may be scattered through the mouth.

Classifications

Clinical appearance Lesions may be divided into four basic clinical appearances (see box on p. 100):

1. Homogeneous white plaques have no red component but have a fine, white, grainy texture or a more mottled, rough appearance (Fig. 8-8 and Plate G, 1).
2. Speckled leukoplakias are composed of white and red flecks of fine or coarse variety (see Figs. 8-8, *B*, and 5-12 and Plates G, 7 to G, 9).
3. Combination white and red patches demonstrate segregation of the red and white components and

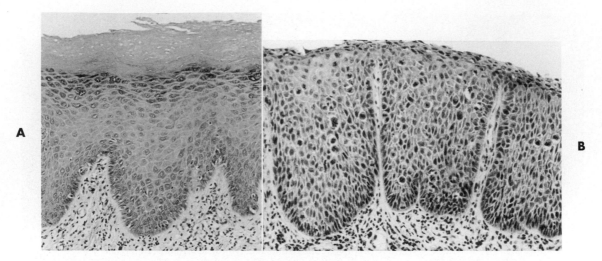

Fig. 8-7. Microscopy of leukoplakia. **A,** Photomicrograph of a completely benign leukoplakic lesion showing acanthosis and hyperkeratosis. **B,** Photomicrograph of a erythoplakic patch showing atypical cells (dysplastic) throughout the epithelial layers. Note the broad rete ridges and the intact basement membrane. The microscopic diagnosis is carcinoma in situ.

are basically erythroleukoplakic lesions (see Fig. 8-8, *C* and Plate G, 12).

4. Verrucous leukoplakias possess red and white components, but the white components are much thicker and protrude above the surface mucosa (see Fig. 8-8).

Red components of leukoplakias represent dysplasias, carcinomas in situs, and invasive carcinomas, providing that the red component is not a traumatic erosion or traumatic ulcer. Bánóczy[8] presented impressive evidence that each of these clinical types has some potential to change from one type to another.

Histologic study Leukoplakias may be histologically divided into two main categories (see Fig. 8-7): those that show no atypia (dysplasia) and those that show different degrees of atypia.[9] From 20% to 25% of leukoplakias show atypia.[6,10] A lesion may show severe atypia with malignant change throughout the depth of the epithelial layer, but its basement membrane may still be intact. Such a lesion is referred to as *carcinoma in situ* or *intraepithelial carcinoma* (see Fig. 8-7).

When an intraepithelial carcinoma breaks through the basement membrane, it becomes an invasive SCC. The investigator must study microscopic sections from various areas of a biopsy of leukoplakia, since the complete spectrum of histopathologic features from increased keratosis to invasive SCC may be found in the surgical specimen from one lesion. Invasive SCC developed in 16% of cases of epithelial dysplasia in a mean of 33.6 months after biopsy.[11]

Reversible or irreversible types Leukoplakia may also be divided into two types according to whether it spontaneously disappears after the chronic irritant has been eliminated. Lesions that disappear are referred to as *reversible leukoplakias,* whereas the persistent lesions are termed *irreversible leukoplakias.* In one large study, 62% of the lesions were completely or partially irreversible.[12]

CLINICAL TYPES OF LEUKOPLAKIA

- Homogeneous type
- Speckled type
- White and red patches
- Verrucous type

Malignant potential It has been reported that the malignant change in leukoplakia ranges between 3% and 7%.[6,7,12] However, it is very difficult to establish a percentage rate for malignant change for leukoplakias in general because so many variables exist. The statistics depend on clinical type, site, etiology, and patient's gender and age.[13] It is helpful to consider just the *homogeneous* type here and assign all lesions with red or verrucous components to a high suspicion index.[13] These latter lesions should be managed with aggressive removal and follow-up. Therefore the *homogeneous* variety, which clearly has a much lower rate of malignant change, is left. Even these vary greatly in the percentage of malignant change. Those situated in the high-risk oval (see Chapter 35), such as the floor of the mouth, ventral surface of the tongue, margins of the tongue, and retromolar region, have a much higher risk[8,14] than those occurring elsewhere, such as the crest of the ridge where the malignant potential may approach zero. The box on p. 101, left, lists the characteristics of high-risk leukoplakias.

Differential Diagnosis

If the homogenously white lesion cannot be scraped off, all the sloughing pseudomembranous types can be eliminated. The keratotic varieties that should especially be considered in the differential diagnosis are listed in the box on p. 101, right.

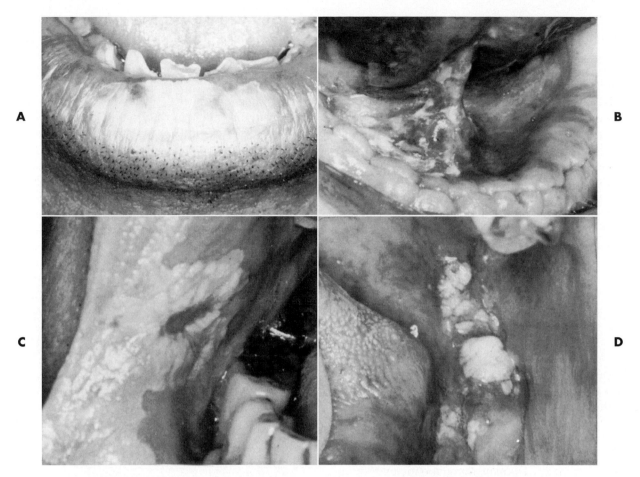

Fig. 8-8. Leukoplakia. **A,** Homogeneous type on the vermilion of the lower lip. The microscopic diagnosis was hyperkeratosis. **B,** Sublingual speckled leukoplakia. The microscopic diagnosis was SCC. **C,** Erythroleukoplakia on the anterior buccal mucosa. The microscopic diagnosis of the erythroplakic patch was carcinoma in situ. **D,** Speckled leukoplakia with a verrucous component in retromolar area. The microscopic diagnosis was SCC. (**B** courtesy M. Lehnert, Minneapolis; **C** courtesy O.H. Stuteville, deceased.)

HIGH-RISK LEUKOPLAKIAS
• Red component • Raised component • Presence in high-risk oval • Tobacco and alcohol use • Nonsmoker and unknown etiology of lesion • Nonreversible type • Microscopic atypia

DIFFERENTIAL DIAGNOSIS OF HOMOGENEOUS LEUKOPLAKIA
• Lichen planus • Leukoedema • Cheek-biting lesion • Smokeless tobacco lesion • Lupus erythematosus • Hyperplastic or hypertrophic candidiasis • Hairy leukoplakia • Electrogalvanic or mercury contact allergy • Verrucous or squamous cell carcinoma • Verruca vulgaris • White sponge nevus

White sponge nevus is the least common of the group. In addition, it occurs soon after birth or at least by puberty and is usually widely distributed over the oral mucous membrane (see Fig. 8-28). In contrast, leukoplakia is seen mostly in patients over 40 years of age and usually is not disseminated throughout the oral cavity. White sponge nevus, furthermore, shows a familial pattern not so characteristic of leukoplakia.

Verruca vulgaris must be differentiated from the verrucous type of leukoplakia. This is usually possible because

verruca vulgaris, uncommon orally, is a small, raised, white lesion seldom more than 0.5 cm in diameter (see Fig. 8-22, *A*). On the other hand, verrucous leukoplakia tends to be much larger and is usually circumscribed by a border of inflamed mucosa, a feature not usually found in verruca vulgaris. In addition, if chronic trauma to the area can be identified, the diagnosis of leukoplakia is further favored.

Since verrucous carcinoma (VC) may develop from a leukoplakic lesion, the clinician must decide whether the lesion's fronds are elevated (exophytic) enough to be suspected as a VC or SCC (see Figs. 8-23 through 8-25).

Electrogalvanic or mercury contact allergy[15-18] perhaps should be considered an entity separate from leukoplakia. The two types of clinical lesions that a microgalvanic current from dissimilar metal restorations can produce on adjacent gingivae, tongue, or buccal mucosa are (1) keratotic plaque lesions like leukoplakia and (2) a variation that mimics LP (see Fig. 8-20). The majority of these lesions disappear when the different metal restorations are replaced with composites or when the teeth are extracted.[15] This is a practical approach to use in differentiating these electrogalvanic white lesions from true leukoplakic lesions, providing that the suspicion index is low (no erythroplakic or verrucous component). Of course, if the suspicion index is high for dysplasia or malignancy, the lesion should be completely excised and studied microscopically; in addition, replacement of the dissimilar metal restorations should occur.

Hairy leukoplakia is usually a corrugated leukoplakic lesion that occurs usually on the lateral or ventral surfaces of the tongue in patients with immunodeficiency (Fig. 8-9). The associated features of this serious disease are usually evident. Human immunodeficiency virus (HIV) tests and biopsy of the lesion in question are helpful in making a definitive diagnosis. This lesion is described in detail in Chapter 36.

Hyperplastic or hypertrophic candidiasis is a somewhat common lesion that occurs as a chronic infection of *C. albicans*. A predisposing factor in the patient history would give this possibility a high ranking. It may be difficult to identify whether the lesion is a primary candidal lesion or a leukoplakia secondarily infected with *Candida* organisms. Multiple lesions favor the diagnosis of candidiasis.

Oral discoid lupus erythematosus lesions are more common than generally thought. They occur frequently in patients who have discoid lupus lesions of the skin and in patients with systemic lupus erythematosus.[19] Oral discoid lesions may initially appear as isolated lesions in a significant number of patients who do not show evidence of discoid lupus or systemic lupus.[20]

The oral discoid lesions share much in common with leukoplakia and LP. The mean patient age at onset is 40 years. Like the lesions of LP, these lesions occur more frequently in women. Buccal mucosa is the most common site of oral discoid lupus lesions, and the gingiva, labial mucosa, and vermilion border are the next most common sites. Also, the lesions are frequently bilateral. In certain cases the clinical appearance of the oral discoid lesions may closely resemble leukoplakia or LP (Fig. 8-10). Discoid lupus erythematosus is discussed in Chapter 32.

It is common for early lesions to be completely red, but after many years, they may slowly change into leukoplakia-like lesions. Oral discoid lesions frequently have a red and white appearance and as such often mimic LP lesions, which have an atrophic, erosive, or ulcerative component

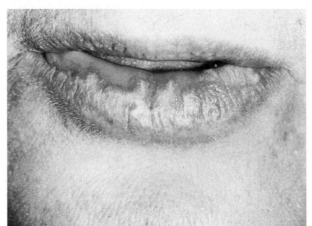

A

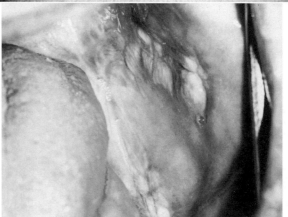

B

Fig. 8-10. Lupus erythematosus. Oral discoid lesions in a woman with systemic lupus. Note characteristic feathery edges of keratotic patches, which have a red component. **A,** Vermilion border. **B,** Buccal mucosa.

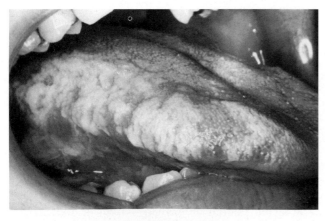

Fig. 8-9. Hairy leukoplakia. (Courtesy S. Silverman, San Francisco.)

(see Fig. 8-10). When an oral discoid lesion has a typical appearance, it is readily identified. Schiødt[19] described the classic oral discoid lesion as "having four outstanding clinical features: (1) a central atrophic area with (2) small white dots and a slightly elevated border zone of (3) irradiating white striae and (4) telangiectasis." However, this researcher explained that considerable variation occurs in about one third of the cases. Some of this latter group mimic leukoplakias, white and red LP lesions, lichenoid drug reactions, and electrogalvanic lesions.

Identifying the cheek-chewing lesion may be a problem for the clinician. In the chronic cheek chewer, the buccal mucosa takes on a roughened, whitish cast because of the increased thickness of the epithelium and keratin (see Fig. 8-30 and Plate D, 9). In periods of heightened stress, the patient may chew away small bits of tissue, producing a plaquelike, whitish lesion with a ragged, eroded surface that may cause the inexperienced clinician to suspect erythroplakic SCC. Paradoxically, true erythroplakic patches characteristically have smoothly contoured borders. Careful questioning of the patient usually elicits the cause and promotes the proper diagnosis. Careful followup reveals regression of the erosions when the habit is modified or eliminated.

Although the smokeless tobacco (ST) lesion resembles regular leukoplakia, it often has a wrinkled pattern and is easily identified by its location in the vestibule and history of ST use (see Fig. 8-12).

Leukoedema is usually easily differentiated from leukoplakia because it classically occurs on the buccal mucosa, frequently covers most of that surface, and extends onto the labial mucosa with a faint milky opalescence (Figs. 8-3 and 8-4). Therefore the definite whiteness that characterizes the leukoplakial lesion is not a feature of the mild case of leukoedema. The characteristic folded and more prominent wrinkled pattern (eliminated by stretching) of the leukoedema, furthermore, distinguishes it from the leukoplakial lesion.

LP is frequently the most difficult lesion to differentiate from leukoplakia. The presence of LP skin lesions tilts the differential diagnosis to oral LP. If the intraoral lesions take the form of Wickham's striae, the diagnosis is also readily discernible. Occasionally, LP is a solitary plaquelike lesion, quite like leukoplakia, but even here borders of the LP plaque are often feathered or perhaps show an annular or a reticular pattern (see Fig. 8-17). Both diseases usually affect patients over 40 years of age; however, leukoplakia more often affects men, whereas LP occurs more frequently in women. Frequently, these plaques have feathering at the margins. If a chronic irritant cannot be identified and an area characteristic of Wickham's striae is discovered, the lesion is probably LP. Definitive diagnosis is made by microscopic study. In addition, cases of disseminated intraoral leukoplakia may be easily mistaken for LP, but again biopsy usually distinguishes between the two. Also, a patient could have two separate diseases at the same time.

Management

Not all leukoplakias are the same. A conservative approach is indicated for those that do not share the characteristics listed in the box on p. 101, left, and thus fall into the low-risk group.

For low-risk lesions, every effort must be made to identify local and chronic causative irritants. The cause may be obvious from the location of the lesion (e.g., a white patch on an edentulous ridge directly beneath an occluding maxillary molar not in direct line with the course of the smoke from a pipe held in the smoker's favorite position or in contact with a fractured crown). These irritants must be eliminated and the patient reexamined biweekly to determine whether the lesion is regressing. If evidence of regression is not detectable within 2 weeks (color photographs are useful as records for comparison), the lesion should be completely excised. A simple procedure for small lesions is, however, a relatively complicated operation if the lesions are large, involve many surfaces, or are in a surgically delicate site. A "ridge callus" is an exception and would not require excision in most cases.

If the lesions are large or widespread, stripping procedures must be used—in stages with free grafts or with allowance for the denuded surface to epithelialize by secondary healing. Approximately 6% of the irreversible leukoplakial lesions undergo malignant transformation to SCC.[21,22] There seems to be little doubt that irreversible leukoplakial lesions should be completely excised with careful postsurgical follow-up. If the microscopic diagnosis is SCC, the patient should be referred to a clinician who is competent in treating oral cancers (see Chapter 35).

High-risk leukoplakias should be referred promptly on detection to a tumor board or clinician who is competent to treat oral cancer (see Chapter 35).

Chemopreventive agents are currently in field trials. Basically researchers are attempting to eliminate leukoplakial lesions with local and systemic agents. This concept is discussed in Chapter 35.

NICOTINE STOMATITIS

Nicotine stomatitis (smoker's palate) is a specific type of leukoplakia seen mostly in men who are pipe smokers. Heat from the pipe smoke may be an important etiologic factor because a case has been recently described in a female patient who did not smoke but admitted to drinking scalding hot beverages.[23] It occurs on the palate, and in most cases the whole mucosal surface of the hard palate is affected. It begins as a reddish stomatitis of the palatal mucosa, and as the irritation is continued, keratotic changes occur and the lesion becomes slightly opalescent and finally white in color. Classically it is described as having a parboiled appearance because of its many transecting fissures, which divide the white mucosal surface into small, flat-topped, nodular areas (Fig. 8-11). A red dot, usually

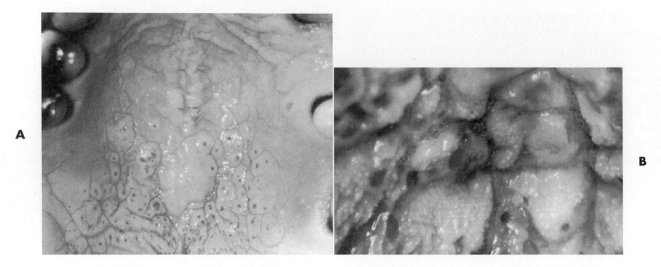

Fig. 8-11. A, Nicotine stomatitis. Both patients were pipe smokers. **B,** Close-up view. (**B** courtesy P.D. Toto, Waukegan, Ill.)

situated in the middle of each nodule, represents the inflamed orifice of a minor salivary gland duct. The lesion usually disappears rapidly after the habit is discontinued. Nicotine stomatitis seldom if ever becomes malignant.

Nicotine stomatitis must be differentiated from all the other conditions of the oral cavity that produce multiple papules: papillary hyperplasia, Darier's disease (see Fig. 10-37), focal epithelial hyperplasia, Goltz' syndrome, Cowden syndrome, acanthosis nigricans, multiple neuroma syndrome, multiple oral fibromas in tuberous sclerosis, multiple papillomas and verrucae (no syndrome), multiple condylomas,[23] and multiple fibroepithelial hyperplasias.[24]

Papillary hyperplasia (see Fig. 10-14) and nicotine stomatitis are the only entities that have a marked predilection for the palate. The small, centrally placed dots and flat nodules of nicotine stomatitis differentiate this condition from papillary hyperplasia, which occurs under an acrylic denture.

CIGARETTE SMOKER'S LIP LESION

This lesion is discussed in Chapter 33.

SMOKELESS TOBACCO LESION

"Oral leukoplakia and smokeless tobacco keratosis are two separate and distinct precancers."[25] They are listed and discussed separately in this textbook.

ST is highly addictive, contains many injurious compounds, and produces similar deleterious systemic effects to smoking.[26] It has enjoyed substantial use in the American South[27] for many years, is used by professional baseball players,[28,29] and more recently has become a widespread fad among young adolescents.[30-34]

ST is available in two basic forms: snuff and chewing tobacco. Snuff is provided as a loose, fine, moist mater-

---

ORAL EFFECTS OF SMOKELESS TOBACCO

- Gingivitis
- Gingival recession
- Periodontitis
- Cervical erosion
- ST mucosal lesion
- Oral cancer*
- Field cancerization*

*Wray A, McGuirt F: Smokeless tobacco usage associated with oral carcinoma: incidence, treatment, outcome, *Arch Otolaryngol Head Neck Surg* 119:929-933, 1993.

---

ial or in a small, portioned bag. Chewing tobacco is manufactured as loose leaf or a plug. A portion of ST is usually placed in the mandibular vestibule in the incisor and canine or molar regions. The patient allows the snuff to dissipate in the saliva, but in the case of chewing tobacco, the patient intermittently removes the quid from its soft tissue location, chews it some, and returns it to its place. Dry snuff was aspirated through the nose by sixteenth-, seventeenth-, and eighteenth century elderly women in England and Europe, but this practice dropped off years ago.

Features

The various oral effects of ST are listed in the box above.

The main oral effects of ST use occur locally where the quid or cud rests, although swallowing ST-inpregnated saliva is reported to induce malignancies of the pharynx and esophagus.[35,36] The asymptomatic mucosal lesion corresponds to the soft tissue area in contact with the quid.

Its earlier stages are white and may range from a mild leukoedema-like opaqueness[37] to a more marked white with a linear, wrinkled (Fig. 8-12), or parboiled appearance.

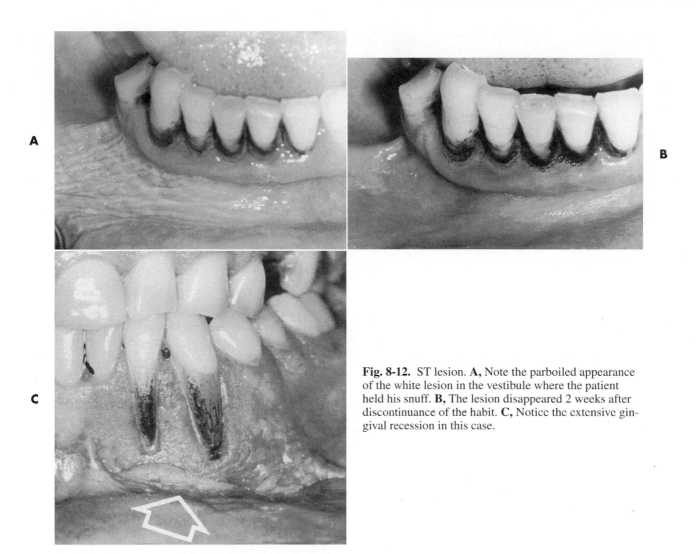

Fig. 8-12. ST lesion. **A,** Note the parboiled appearance of the white lesion in the vestibule where the patient held his snuff. **B,** The lesion disappeared 2 weeks after discontinuance of the habit. **C,** Notice the extensive gingival recession in this case.

The borders are usually vague. These appearances carry a low suspicion index, whereas appearances uncommonly seen show velvet red speckles or patches or elevations on the surface; these should be assigned a high suspicion index. The red patches are erythroplakic, and the elevations would suggest the likelihood of early SCC or VC. The type of ST used as well as the length of exposure per day and duration of the habit all influence the degree of prominence of the changes in each case.[38-40] Snuff users had a higher incidence or more pronounced lesions than those that chewed tobacco.[39,41] Clinical changes in loose snuff users may be more pronounced than those who use portion bag snuff.[39]

Malignant potential The malignancy potential of ST lesions is significantly lower than that for leukoplakial lesions.[24,42] However, both SCC and VC do develop, usually after extensive exposure.[36,43,44] Usually these are lower-grade malignancies but may be rapidly lethal in occasional cases, even with minimal exposure to ST.[45]

Histopathology

The histopathology of snuff lesions is different from that of lesions of chewing tobacco.[37,41] A variety of appear-ances are now recognized,[41,46] but a detailed description is beyond the scope of this text.

Management

The majority of ST lesions may be assigned a low suspicion index on the basis of the clinical appearance. The patient is strongly advised to discontinue the use of all tobacco products and is examined again 2 weeks after discontinuation. If no regression is observed, the lesion should be excised and sent for microscopic study. If the lesion is disappearing (see Fig. 8-12), the patient should be seen periodically to ensure that ST use has not been resumed. Many of these lesions disappear completely after cessation of ST. One study reported that the ST lesions in all patients disappeared after Swedish moist snuff was discontinued.[42] If partial regression is observed at the 2-week visit, the patient should be reexamined after an additional 2 weeks. The persistent lesion should be managed the same as the moderate- to high-risk lesion; the patient should be promptly referred to a professional competent to treat oral cancer.

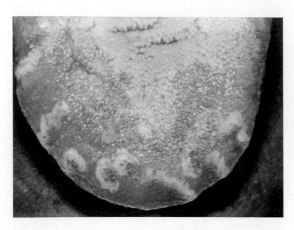

Fig. 8-13. Migratory glossitis. (Courtesy P. Akers, Chicago.)

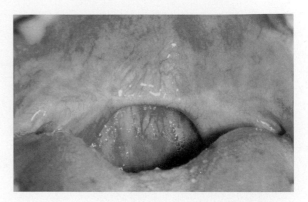

Fig. 8-14. Fibrosed scar appearing as white area across the posterior palate. Notice the pale appearance.

MIGRATORY GLOSSITIS

Migratory glossitis (geographic tongue, ectopic geographic tongue) is discussed in detail in the section on red conditions of the tongue in Chapter 7. Rarely a distinct, white patch of migratory glossitis may look like leukoplakia. The more characteristic red patches with small, raised, white rims identify the condition in such a case (Fig. 8-13).

PERIPHERAL SCAR TISSUE

Peripheral scar tissue (a nonkeratotic lesion) involving the subepithelial layer, the epithelium, or both has been observed in the oral cavity. The condition is uncommon because the rich vascularity of the oral tissue generally ensures good healing after trauma. In some instances, however, the healing of surgical wounds, large traumatic ulcers, and giant aphthae in Sutton's disease produces scarring. Although the scar tissue does not become as light in color as most keratotic lesions, it does appear pale (Fig. 8-14).

The history is important in making the diagnosis. Some patients show a tendency toward keloid formation on the skin, and a few patients are also prone to oral keloid formation, although the oral cases are rare.

Oral scars may be solitary entities but are multiple in cases of Sutton's disease and submucous fibrosis. The area of the scar is firm on palpation, and in some cases the deeper layers are bound to the mucosa.

LICHEN PLANUS

LP is a complex mucocutaneous disease of unknown etiology. It may be an immunologic disturbance, either local or general and perhaps of autoimmune character.[47,48] This area is being very actively researched. Psychologic and emotional stress may play a minor role, but this is unclear.[49-52]

LP patients often have concurrent systemic diseases perhaps related to the older age group affected. Grinspan,

Diaz, Villapol, et al [53] describe a triad of LP, diabetes, and hypertension, but the drugs used to treat the diabetes and hypertension may produce a lichenoid drug reaction instead of LP being present.[54] Reports have indicated an increased incidence of LP in diabetes as well,[55-58] but other authors have not found this association.[59-61] Studies have also reported an increased incidence of liver disease and hepatitis C infection in LP patients.[62,63]

Malignancy Potential

It seems apparent that oral LP carries a slightly increased risk of SCC in 0.5% to 2.5% of cases.[64-68] Not all reports of series of cases indicated examples of malignancy, and this may be related to a short follow-up period or aggressive management.[69] Another school of thought proposes that the examples of malignancy in LP actually represent examples of "lichenoid dysplasia," a separate entity altogether.[70,71] This latter concept is discussed in Chapter 6.

Clinical Features

Approximately 50% of patients with skin lesions (Fig. 8-15) have oral involvement.[72] About 23% of cases only have oral lesions. The prevalence of oral LP is approximately 0.1% to 2.2%.[73] The majority (70% to 80%) occur in female patients, and most patients are over 40 years of age. Lesions are seldom solitary and are frequently bilateral. The buccal mucosa is the most common location (including the vestibules), followed by the tongue and gingivae, although the lesions can occur almost anywhere.

Two basic types of lesions occur: (1) totally white (keratotic), and (2) white (keratotic) and red (atrophic, erosive, bullous) (Fig. 8-16). The second type is discussed in Chapter 6 under generalized red conditions. The keratotic lesions are the most frequent in the general population. However, mixed lesions are the most common in a referral type of practice. The first type is discussed here. The box on p. 107 lists these asymptomatic keratotic patterns.

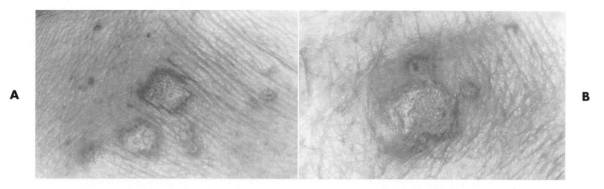

Fig. 8-15. Skin lesions of LP. (Courtesy N. Thompson, Maywood, Ill.)

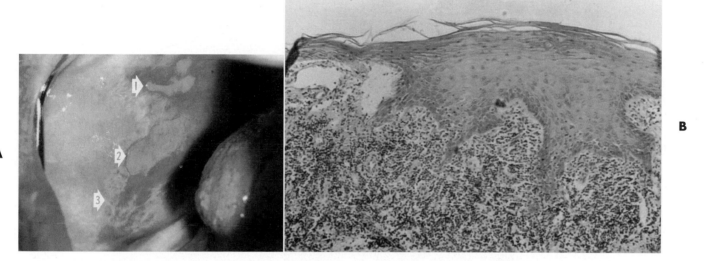

Fig. 8-16. LP. **A,** Three types of lesions on the buccal mucosa: *1,* bullous type; *2,* erosion; *3,* reticular pattern. **B,** Photomicrograph of LP showing the sawtooth rete ridges and chronic inflammation, which is limited to the upper segment of the lamina propria. Note the early formation of microbullae just beneath the epithelium on the left side of the photomicrograph.

CLINICAL PATTERNS OF KERATOTIC LP (FIGS. 8-17 AND 8-18)

- Reticular
- Annular
- Papular
- Linear
- Floral
- Plaquelike

Histopathologic Features

The characteristic microscopic picture reveals a hyperparakeratosis or hyperorthokeratosis with acanthosis. The rete ridges may be saw-toothed in appearance, and there is an eosinophilic amorphous band along the basement membrane.[72] A bandlike distribution of dense infiltrate of lymphocytes lies below the basement membrane, which is usually restricted to the lamina propria in the reticular form.[73] The basal cell layer frequently undergoes hy-

dropic and vacuolar degeneration and may be entirely missing (Fig. 8-16, *B*). If degeneration is severe and restricted to small foci, bullae may form, but if the process is severe and more disseminated, atrophic or erosive lesions develop because of the loss of surface epithelium.

Differential Diagnosis

In addition to the discussion here, see section on differential diagnosis of leukoplakia.

Unusual examples of cheek biting and cheek sucking may mimic LP. Some patients suck their cheeks and tongues into tight contact with their teeth and nibble on the tissue. This may produce patterns that resemble Wickham's striae on the buccal mucosa occlusal (Fig. 8-19). This may be etiologically linked to linea alba.

Electrogalvanic white lesions as well as red and white lesions occur in situations in which similar metals are used and can appear similar to LP (Fig. 8-20).

Lichenoid drug reactions have been reported with increasing frequency, and some are white only, although the majority have a red and white component. In such

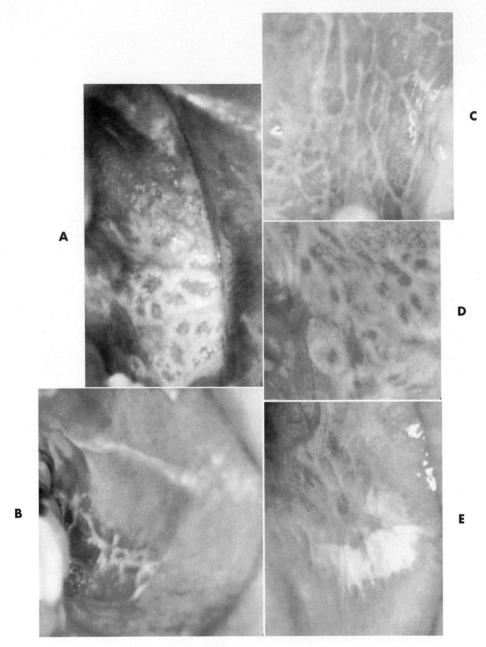

Fig. 8-17. Keratotic types of LP. **A** to **D,** Reticular and oval patterns. **E,** Plaquelike pattern in combination with a reticular flower-petal pattern (**A** courtesy S. Fischman, Buffalo, NY.)

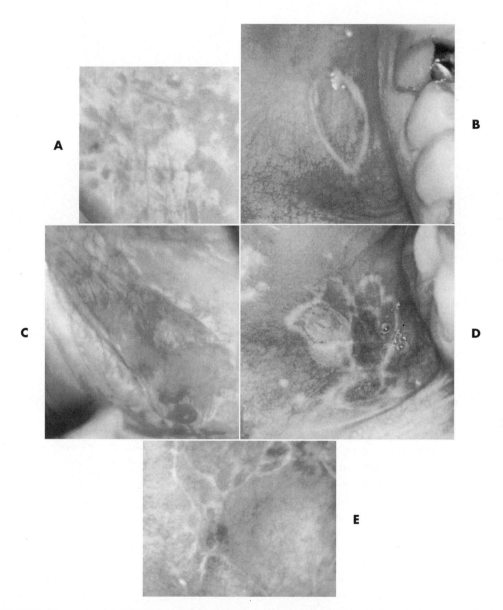

Fig. 8-18. Keratotic types of LP. **A,** Papular. **B,** Annular. **C,** Combination. **D,** Floral. **E,** Reticular and linear.

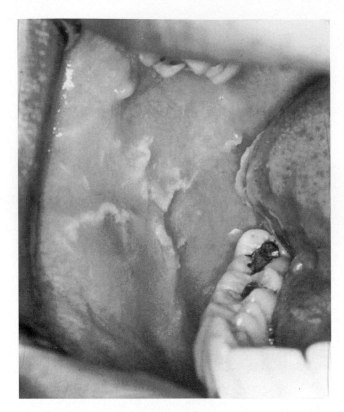

Fig. 8-19. Cheek-biting and cheek-sucking lesion. Note how the white lesions resemble some of the patterns of LP. This was a bilateral finding with the lateral margins of the tongue also involved.

cases, drugs have induced changes that resemble the keratotic clinical variations of LP as well as the mixed red and white types.

Management

The majority (perhaps all) of keratotic LP oral lesions are asymptomatic and do not require active treatment. However, the diagnosis should be established and the patient informed about the nature of the disease. Patients should be reexamined every 6 months to check on the course of the disease so that treatment can be instituted promptly if painful atrophic, erosive, or bullous lesions appear. This also ensures early detection and treatment in the event of malignant change.

If the lesions are present on the gingivae or lateral borders of the tongue or buccal mucosa and seem to be associated with dissimilar metals, consideration should be given to replacement with similar restorative materials. Likewise, if patients are taking medications that can produce lichenoid drug reactions, the diagnosis of the lichenoid drug reaction must be considered. If the physician thinks that it is feasible to change the medication, this should be accomplished, and disappearance of the lesions should be anticipated in a significant number of cases.

LICHENOID DRUG REACTION

This condition is discussed with the generalized red condition in Chapter 6.

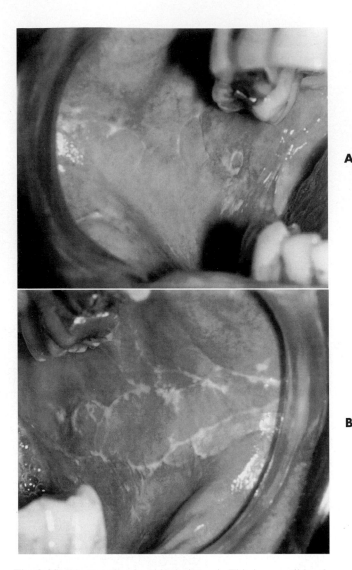

Fig. 8-20. Electrogalvanic white lesions. **A,** This is a possible, although unproven, case. **B,** Notice particularly the patterns that correspond to outlines of marginal gingiva when the molars are in occlusion. Dissimilar metal restorations are present.

ELECTROGALVANIC AND MERCURY CONTACT ALLERGY

Electrogalvanic white and red and white lesions are reported to occur on the attached gingiva by the contact point of the two dissimilar metal restorations and on adjacent mucosa (see Fig. 8-20). A total of 36 patients showed white lesions that could have been attributed to electrogalvanism in a series of 1128 leukoplakic and 326 lichen planus patients.[15] Some 31 of the 36 lesions disappeared completely when the metals were changed or the teeth were extracted.[15] Usually, white lesions caused by electrogalvanism reverse when the dissimilarity of metals is corrected, unless the disparity has been present for over a decade.[15] Clinical corrosion (black, discolored amalgams) in proximity to white lesions suggests electrogalvanic lesions, particularly in the erosive type and less often in the reticular type.[74] The Council on Dental Materials Instruments and Equipment of the American Dental

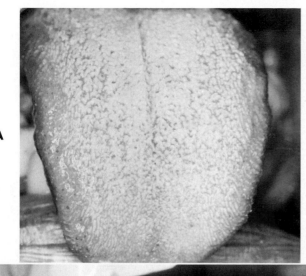

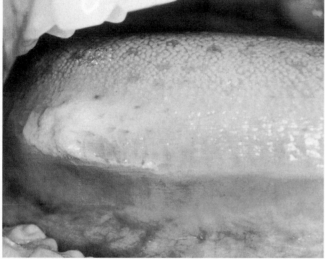

Fig. 8-21. White hairy tongue. **A,** Dorsal surface. **B,** Lateral surface. This white lesion is bilateral and composed of congealed "hairs."

Association[75] reviewed these concerns. Another school of thought suggests that these lesions are mostly the result of a contact allergy or a toxicity to the substances in the restorative material (contact allergy to mercury being the most common[16-18]). Epicutaneous tests for mercury allergy were helpful in making a diagnosis.[17]

WHITE HAIRY TONGUE

White hairy tongue is a condition that occurs on the dorsal surface of the tongue and is of little clinical significance (Fig. 8-21); its cause is unknown. The filiform papillae become elongated because of an increased retention of keratin. It is more common in men and seldom produces symptoms or causes clinical problems. It may cover the whole dorsal surface or just a patch; occasionally the lateral margins may be involved, particularly in the posterior area (see Fig. 8-21). On occasion, patients may become alarmed when they suddenly detect its presence. When the papillae are extremely long, patients may complain of

---

DIFFERENTIAL DIAGNOSIS FOR WHITE EXOPHYTIC SCC
• Large papilloma and condyloma acuminatum • Pyogenic granuloma • VC (nodular) • Other exophytic malignant tumors (necrotic surface) • Hypertrophic or hyperplastic chronic infection

gagging. Under the influences of a varying diet, this lesion may take on different colors. Patients with malignant neoplasia are reported to be more prone to this condition.[76]

White hairy tongue does not present a diagnostic problem, and careful, frequent brushing of the dorsal surface of the tongue is the preferred treatment for milder cases. When the papillae have reached an extreme length, clipping followed by tongue brushing is an effective control measure.

PAPILLOMA, VERRUCA VULGARIS, AND CONDYLOMA ACUMINATUM

Oral papilloma, verruca vulgaris (skin wart), and condyloma acuminatum (veneral wart) are very similar exophytic lesions that appear white if the surface keratin is thick enough (Fig. 8-22). This is usually the case with oral verruca vulgaris, but oral papillomas and veneral warts may have minimal keratin coverings and appear as pink, exophytic masses. These entities are discussed in detail as exophytic lesions in Chapter 10.

WHITE EXOPHYTIC SCC

SCC has been discussed in this chapter as a white plaque or a white and red plaque; in Chapter 5 as a red plaque and as a red exophytic lesion; in Chapter 10 as an exophytic lesion of mucosal coloring; in Chapter 11 as an ulcer; and in Chapter 21 as a radiolucency with ragged, indistinct borders. Pathogenesis and treatment of SCC is discussed in Chapter 35.

Features

The white exophytic SCC is a firm, nodular lesion (Figs. 8-23 and 8-24 and Plate H) but in some cases may be more polypoid. An early lesion shows minor elevation (see Fig. 8-23 and Plate G). The surface is pebbled and in some cases may be multicolored (white, red, and pink) and perhaps partly ulcerated. As with the other clinical varieties of SCC, the lesion usually occurs in the high-risk oval.

Differential Diagnosis

The lesions that should be considered in the differential diagnosis are listed in the box above.

Management

The management of SCC is discussed in Chapter 35.

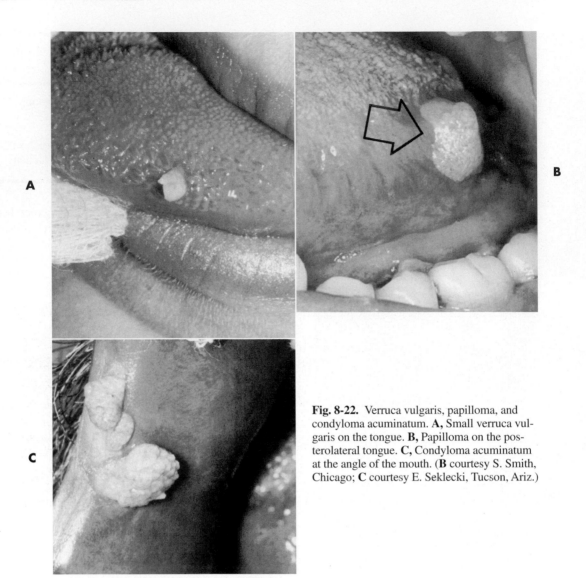

Fig. 8-22. Verruca vulgaris, papilloma, and condyloma acuminatum. **A,** Small verruca vulgaris on the tongue. **B,** Papilloma on the posterolateral tongue. **C,** Condyloma acuminatum at the angle of the mouth. (**B** courtesy S. Smith, Chicago; **C** courtesy E. Seklecki, Tucson, Ariz.)

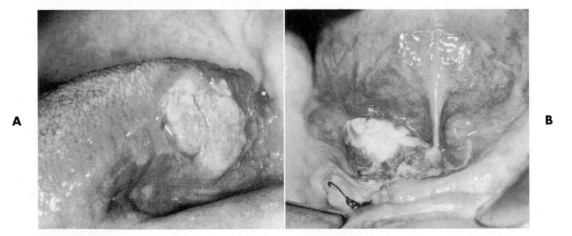

Fig. 8-23. White SCC. **A,** Minimal elevation. **B,** Red and white lesion. (**A** courtesy O.H. Stuteville, deceased; **B** courtesy E. Casper, Maywood, Ill.)

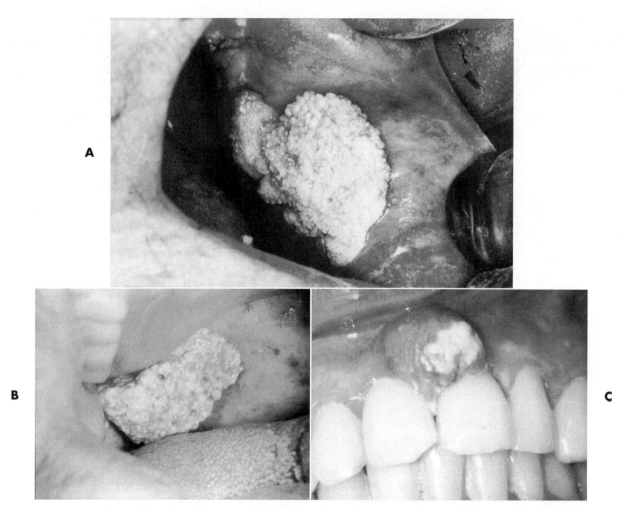

Fig. 8-24. A, White papillary SCC. **B,** VC unusual in somewhat pedunculated base and degree of elevation. **C,** White and pink papillary SCC of gingiva. (**B** from Claydon PJ, Jordan JE: Verrucous carcinoma, *J Oral Surg* 36:564-567, 1978; **C** courtesy S. Silverman, San Francisco.)

VERRUCOUS CARCINOMA

VC is a type of slow-growing, superficial, low-grade carcinoma of the oral cavity and upper aerodigestive tract. The clinical and microscopic appearances are quite characteristic. It is an entity distinct from SCC of the oral cavity because of its unique biologic behavior.[77] VC usually occurs in persons who smoke or use snuff or chewing tobacco. This lesion was first defined as a separate entity by Ackerman[78] in 1948.

Features

VC most often occurs in the buccal mucosa, alveolar ridge and gingivae, tongue, floor of the mouth, and palate of elderly patients (Figs. 8-24 and 8-25). The average age is approximately 65 years for men and 71 years for women.[78] The literature yields conflicting reports on gender preference.[77-82]

Generally the lesion appears initially as a broad leukoplakia, except that the surface is rough, pebbly, and warty with deep crevices that in some instances separate distinct, mamillated folds (see Figs. 8-24 and 8-25 and Plates G, 4 and G, 5). A few lesions are more elevated and even somewhat pedunculated (see Fig. 8-24, *B* and Plate G, 6). The surface is usually white, red, or red and white, depending on the degree of surface keratinization, and ulceration may be present. VC is frequently associated with leukoplakia at its periphery. Clinically the margins are usually well defined and characteristically show a rim of slightly elevated normal mucosa where the tumor has pushed under the edge of the normal tissue and has undermined it slightly.

VC is a slow-growing progressive neoplasm with a clinical phase that lasts several years. Metastasis occurs rarely if ever. However, VC can transform into SCC and adopt a more aggressive behavior.[83] One report indicated that VC coexists or is associated with SCC or epithelial dysplasia in 48% of cases.[81] These other lesions formed part of the VC or occurred separately from the verrucous neoplasm.

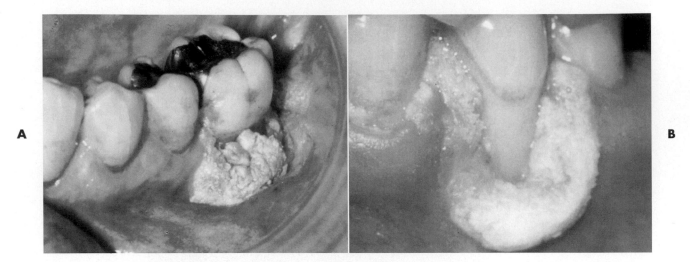

Fig. 8-25. VCs. (**A** courtesy S. Silverman, San Francisco; **B** courtesy R. Priddy, Vancouver, BC, Canada, and Dalhousie University teaching collection.)

Microscopic Features

Microscopically the lesion is deceptively benign. The tumor epithelium is greatly thickened, with outward papillary projections and downward projections of broad, blunt, rete ridges into the connective tissue. The basement membrane is intact. These downgrowths of epithelium into the connective tissue demonstrate a "pushing border" rather than the usual invasive fingers of SCC. Frequently the tumor retracts a margin of normal epithelium down with it into the connective tissue, where a sharp margin exists between the lesion and the normal tissue. An abundance of keratin is generally seen on the surface, and it dips down with the invaginating epithelium and produces keratin plugs. Generally, there is a marked, predominantly lymphocytic infiltrate directly under the invading rete ridges. VC usually lacks the cytologic criteria for malignancy.

Proliferative Verrucous Leukoplakia

Proliferative verrucous leukoplakia is a disease entity first described in 1985.[84] This lesion is uncommon and represents an aggressive form of leukoplakia with a high disposition for malignant change (Fig. 8-26 and Plates G, 2 and G, 9). In the early stage, these lesions clinically are homogeneous leukoplakias that show no worrisome features on biopsy.[85,86] The lesions recur after removal and slowly become more extensive and diffuse and take on rough (warty) projections and at times red components. A later biopsy may show a whole spectrum of changes: hyperkeratosis, dysplasia, carcinoma in situ, VC, and SCC. These lesions were described as slow growing, persistent, progressive, relentless, and irreversible, and they demonstrate regional and distant metastasis at a later stage.[85] Usually the patients are elderly women, a majority of whom had used tobacco. *C. albicans* was often identified in superficial layers of the tissue section. A cytometric analysis may

be able to identify these aggressive lesions during their innocent-looking early stage.[85]

Verrucous Hyperplasia vs. VC

In 1980, Shear and Pindborg[80] introduced the concept of "verrucous hyperplasia," describing how this differed from verrucous carcinoma. They described verrucous hyperplasia as a proliferative epithelial lesion with the epithelial hyperplastic folds extending *above* the margins of the surrounding mucosa, whereas in VC the folds invade down into the connective tissue and *below* the surrounding normal mucosal margins. They believed that verrucous hyperplasia may develop into VC or SCC. Other authorities believe that verrucous hyperplasia and VC are really the same lesion.[81,83] Perhaps the term *proliferative verrucous leukoplakia*[84-86] could be used as an umbrella under which the continuum of lesions, such as verrucous hyperplasia, VC, and SCC that arise from a thickened leukoplakia, could be included.

Differential Diagnosis

Very few lesions could be confused with the broad-based, low-profile variety of VC. Proliferative verrucous leukoplakia, as a concept, seems to cover all of the bases. Multiple biopsies should determine if the lesion in question is a thickened leukoplakia with elevations (verrucous leukoplakia), VC, or SCC. Technically all three could be present in the same lesion.

Smaller, more elevated, and somewhat pedunculated VCs occur on occasion and not associated with thickened leukoplakias with verrucous fronds. These types must be differentiated from large papillomas and veneral warts, large inflammatory hyperplasia lesions, and papillary SCC (see Fig. 8-22 through 8-24). The rough surface contours differentiate it from the smoothly contoured inflammatory hyperplasias. Biopsy is required for definitive diagnosis.

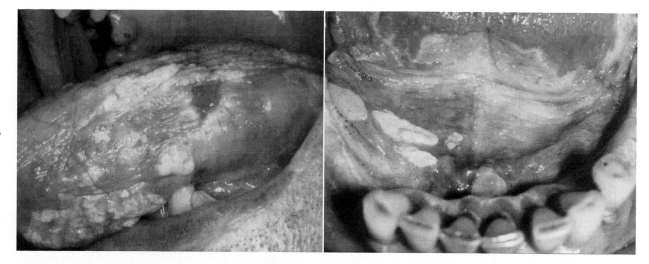

Fig. 8-26. Proliferative verrucous leukoplakia. **A,** Lateral border of tongue. Ulcer represents SCC. **B,** Floor of the mouth. (**A** courtesy S. Silverman, San Francisco.)

Management

It is paramount to establish the correct diagnosis. Toward this end, it helps to have the reporting pathologist examine the lesion clinically. Multiple deep biopsies are recommended to avoid the problem of underdiagnosis.[87] Wide surgical excision has been the recommended treatment for many years. Close and continued postsurgical surveillance is obligatory. It has been suggested that large oral lesions of VC may benefit from a combination of surgery and radiation therapy.[88] Chemotherapy with bleomycin has also been used with some success to shrink the tumor before excision.[89]

HYPERTROPHIC OR HYPERPLASTIC CANDIDIASIS

Candidiasis is discussed in detail in Chapter 5, and the necrotic pseudomembranous type is discussed in this chapter under the section on sloughing white lesions. Hypertrophic or hyperplastic candidiasis is a variety of chronic candidal infection that produces a hyperkeratosis sometimes associated with a hyperplasia of the stratified squamous epithelium. It occurs on the tongue, palate, and other intraoral locations (Fig. 8-27). It can occur as multifocal mucocutaneous lesions at the angles of the mouth and the vermilion[90-92] as well as intraorally.

Microscopically the candidal pseudohyphae can be identified in the hyperkeratin layer. Inasmuch as candidal organisms are found in up to 82% of leukoplakias,[93] the question arises about whether specific cases are primary or secondary candidiasis. The presence of predisposing factors to candidal infection in a case in which multiple lesions are present favors a working diagnosis of candidiasis.

Some lesions may be quite refractory to treatment and require prolonged administration of antifungal drugs.[94] Surgery may be indicated in some cases.[95] Antifungal

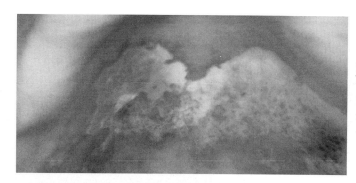

Fig. 8-27. Chronic keratotic (hyperplastic) candidiasis of long standing on the palate. It could not be scraped off.

drugs and the treatment of candidiasis are discussed in Chapter 5.

HAIRY LEUKOPLAKIA

Hairy leukoplakia is a keratotic white lesion that frequently occurs in the mouths of immunodeficient patients. Hairy leukoplakia may resemble "garden variety" leukoplakia clinically because both are keratotic white lesions (see Fig. 8-9 and Plates E, 1 to E, 3). However, hairy leukoplakia predominately occurs on the lateral border of the tongue in immunodeficient individuals and often has a corrugated appearance. Biopsy and microscopic study usually shows keratin hairs and Epstein-Barr virus. This entity is discussed in Chapter 36.

WHITE SPONGE NEVUS

White sponge nevus is a hereditary condition in which white lesions occur on various mucous membranes of the body (e.g., the mucosa of the oral cavity, vagina, and

PLAQUE

Plaque, or materia alba, is included in this group for completeness and because it may be mistaken for a lesion. In some mouths with poor hygiene a mixture of food debris and bacteria may be seen as white plaques on the gingivae, alveolar mucosa, and teeth (Fig. 8-40).

The clinician may notice a slightly inflamed mucosal surface beneath the plaque after the plaque has been removed with gauze.

TRAUMATIC ULCER

On occasion, oral mucosa that has been crushed by mechanical trauma appears as a sloughing white lesion on the gingivae[96] or other oral sites (Fig. 8-41). A history of such a traumatic event is diagnostic. Some of these may be self-inflicted in an effort to secure narcotic drugs or as a result of psychologic problems.[97] Patients with resistance lowered by systemic disease may experience secondary infections or gangrene in these injured areas. Therefore if the severity of a traumatic lesion seems to be out of proportion to the intensity of the precipitating trauma, underlying systemic disease should be suspected.

PYOGENIC GRANULOMA

Pyogenic granuloma is discussed in considerable detail in Chapter 10 with the other exophytic lesions. It is mentioned briefly here because this particular variety of inflammatory hyperplastic lesion almost invariably has a white area of varying size on its surface (Fig. 8-42 and Plate B, 11). This white material is necrotic tissue that can be removed easily with a gauze or a tongue blade. The necrosis is produced by recurrent mechanical trauma and superficial infection of this exophytic lesion.

CHEMICAL BURNS

Chemical burns most often result from the patient applying analgesics, such as aspirin or acetaminophen, to the mucosa adjacent to an aching tooth (Fig. 8-43 and Plate D, 8). Other cases may result from the dentist's applying

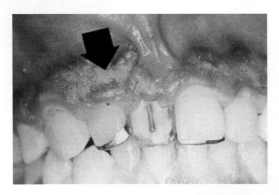

Fig. 8-40. Arrow indicates white plaque (materia alba) that can be easily removed.

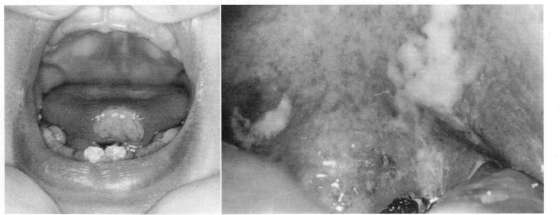

Fig. 8-41. Sloughing traumatic lesions. **A,** Traumatic lesion on the tip of the tongue caused by neonatal incisors. **B,** Sloughing white lesion on the palate produced during a traumatic orotracheal intubation. (Courtesy G. Mac Donald, San Jose, Calif.)

caustic medicaments to a lesion. Addicts who apply drugs, such as cocaine, to a favored location in the oral mucous membrane also have these lesions (Plate B, 10).

A mild, white, filmy desquamation is seen on the oral mucosa of patients who come for dental care after an extended absence. These patients admit to the vigorous use of a strong mouthrinse, dentifrice, and vigorous tooth brushing just before their appointments.[98-100] The strong concentration of various agents has caused a superficial mucosal "burn." The sloughing in such cases would be much milder and more disseminated than the more localized reaction of an analgesic tablet.

The clinical appearance of these burns in most cases depends on the severity of the tissue damage. Chronic mild burns usually produce keratotic white lesions (see Fig. 8-6), whereas intermediate insults cause a localized mucositis. More severe burns coagulate the surface of the tissue and produce a diffuse white lesion. If the coagulation is severe, the tissue can be scraped off, leaving a raw, bleeding, painful surface (see Fig. 8-43). The identi-fication of these lesions is best accomplished by a good history.

The treatment for chemical burns is the application of a protective coating such as oral benzocaine (Orabase) and the initiation of a bland diet. Systemic analgesics may be administered if pain is a problem. The patient should be taught as to the proper use of approved preparations.

ACUTE NECROTIZING ULCERATIVE GINGIVITIS

Acute necrotizing ulcerative gingivitis (ANUG) (Vincent's infection, trench mouth) is a moderately uncommon, infectious, necrotic, and ulcerative disorder of the gingivae. Its etiology is complex, involving genetics, stress, and lowered systemic and local resistance. Pockets often associated with erupting teeth (often third molars) provide a locus for the production of anerobic oral fusiform bacilli and spirochetes. Poor oral hygiene is almost invariably present, and the victim often smokes.

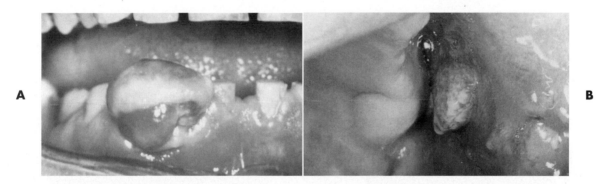

Fig. 8-42. Pyogenic granuloma. Note the white necrotic material on the surfaces of both lesions. **A,** On the labial gingiva. **B,** On the buccal mucosa. (**B** courtesy A.C.W. Hutchinson Collection, Northwestern University Dental School Library, Chicago.)

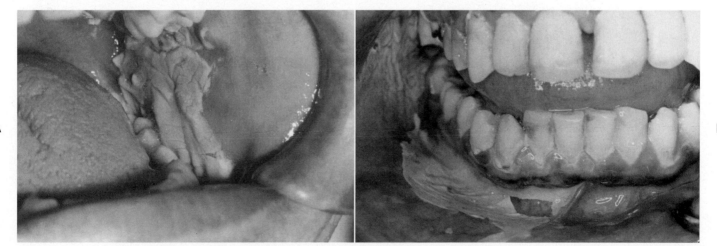

Fig. 8-43. Chemical burns. Both lesions were caused by the topical use of aspirin to relieve toothache. The white material could be removed.

Features

The disease can occur at any age, but the majority of cases affect patients between 17 and 35 years of age, with an average of 23.9 years.[101] ANUG does not show a predilection for either gender and occurs more commonly in whites than blacks.[101] Stress and poor oral hygiene play an etiologic role.[101,102]

The patient frequently complains of tenderness, discomfort, or increasingly intense pain in the gingivae. Lassitude, fever, bad taste, a fetid odor, and an inability to eat properly are also frequent symptoms. The ulcerative and necrotic process commences at the tips of the papillae and expands around the gingival crest. The ulcerative process is covered by a necrotic grayish-white pseudomembrane (Fig. 8-44 and Plates E, 10 and E, 11). ANUG may extend widely, and severe cases have postinfection cratering of the papillae.

Differential Diagnosis

The picture of destructive lesions that have produced punched-out defects of the interdental papillae is practically pathognomonic for ANUG as long as the process has not affected other areas of the mucous membrane.

Somewhat similar lesions may occur in sickle cell anemia (see Fig. 11-14, *B*), but this disease may be readily identified by a special sickle cell blood preparation or by the electrophoretic examination of the hemoglobin. Oral changes in uremia can also be similar to ANUG (see Fig. 11-14, *C-D*). Occasionally, severe contact allergy can mimic ANUG.

If the necrotic gangrenous process expands beyond the gingiva, the diagnosis changes to diffuse gangrenous stomatitis, which is suggestive of serious systemic disease and a weakened defense system.

Management

Severe cases The first phase of treatment calls for the brief use of oxygenating mouthrinses as well as analgesics and amoxicillin or metronidazole. The second phase calls for careful scaling, curetting, and debridement as soon as patient comfort permits. Patient education concerning home care should be given and the patient monitored. Recontouring of the gingiva after regression of the disease may be necessary. *Mild to moderate cases* The first phase of treatment should generally be eliminated, except for the oxygenating mouthrinse, and phase two is implemented immediately.

CANDIDIASIS

Candidiasis is discussed in detail in Chapter 5, but the necrotic, sloughing pseudomembrane type is discussed here. Generally this type is so acute that it destroys the superficial tissue.

Features

The patient with pseudomembranous candidiasis may complain of a burning sensation, tenderness, or sometimes pain in the area of the affected mucosa. Spicy foods cause occasional discomfort because of the increased sensitivity of the affected mucosa. These infections are more common in women and in patients over 40 years of age.[103]

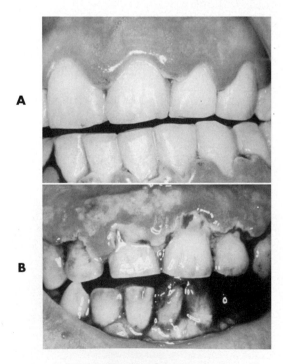

Fig. 8-44. ANUG. **A,** The tips of the interdental papillae are destroyed first. **B,** In this severe case, the necrotizing process has extended to the remaining marginal gingiva and to the alveolar mucosa. (**B** courtesy J. Keene, Omaha.)

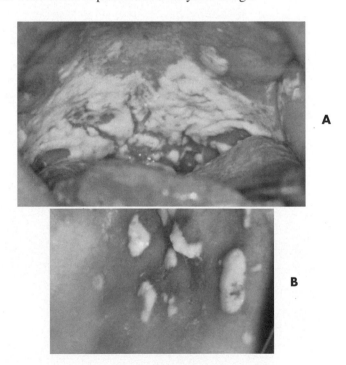

Fig. 8-45. A, Pseudomembranous candidiasis on the soft palate of an HIV-positive patient. **B,** Lesions on the buccal mucosa of a patient who had used tetracycline mouthrinse. (**A** courtesy M. Glick, Philadelphia.)

The pseudomembranous oral infection may present as fine, whitish deposits on an erythematous patch of mucosa or as more highly developed small, soft, white, slightly elevated plaques that closely resemble milk curds (Figs. 8-45 and 8-46 and Plate D, 7). There may be a solitary region or diffuse whitish involvement of several or all the mucosal surfaces. The mucosa adjacent to or between these whitish plaques may appear erythematous. The plaques or pseudomembranes may be stripped off the mucosa, leaving a raw, bleeding surface. The buccal mucosa and vestibule are the most frequent regions affected, followed by the tongue, palate, gingivae, floor of the mouth, and lips.

Microscopically the debrided material is composed of necrotic tissue, pseudohyphae, yeast forms of *Candida* organisms, and bacteria; a smear of these lesions is diagnostic except in cases of secondary candidal infection.

Differential Diagnosis

As a rule, all the keratotic lesions discussed in the first part of this chapter may be readily eliminated from consideration, since they cannot be easily removed by scraping with a tongue blade.

Necrotic white lesions that must be considered in the differential diagnosis are listed in the box at right.

The mucous patch of syphilis is usually a discrete, small, white necrotic lesion on the tongue, palate, or lips (Fig. 8-47), whereas candidiasis is usually more diffuse. The accompanying skin lesions of secondary syphilis and the positive serologic findings readily differentiate the mucous patch from candidiasis.

Necrotic ulcers of debilitating systemic disease may be difficult to differentiate from candidiasis because the latter entity is usually also found in patients with lowered resistance. These lesions are discussed in Chapter 11 (see Fig. 11-14). As a general rule, if the ulcer is deep, candidiasis seldom would be the primary cause, although such an ulcer could indeed be secondarily infected with *C. albicans*.

Traumatic ulcers with necrotic surfaces can in almost all instances be related to a history of specific trauma.

Superficial bacterial infections may occur in patients with debilitating disease and may mimic pseudomembranous candidiasis. Tyldesley, Rotter, Sells, et al[104] described such lesions occurring in renal transplant patients who were receiving combined steroid and immunosuppressive drug therapy. Previously some of these lesions were believed to be caused by antibiotic-resistant *Candida* organisms, but culture yielded abundant bacteria such as staphylococci, *Neisseria,* coliform bacteria, and lactobacilli. On the other

---

DIFFERENTIAL DIAGNOSIS OF PSEUDOMEMBRANOUS CANDIDIASIS

- Chemical burns
- Gangrenous stomatitis
- Superficial bacterial infections
- Traumatic ulcers
- Necrotic ulcers of systemic disease
- Mucous patch

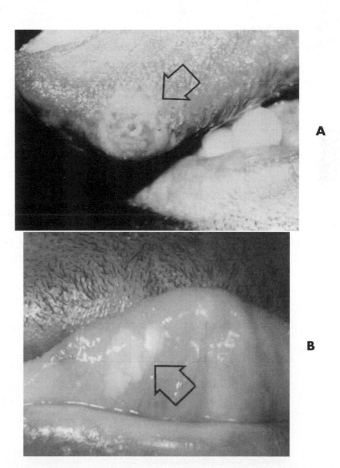

Fig. 8-47. Syphilitic lesions. **A,** Chancre on the anterolateral border of the tongue. It is unusual for a chancre to have a white necrotic surface. **B,** Mucous patch on the tongue of a patient with secondary syphilis. (**A** courtesy T. Wall, Chicago; **B** courtesy R. Gorlin, Minneapolis.)

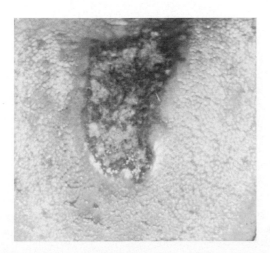

Fig. 8-46. Candidiasis on the dorsal surface of the tongue.

hand, if removable white plaques filled with yeast forms and pseudohyphae are present, the diagnosis is primary or secondary candidiasis.

Because its oral lesions are also covered by pseudomembranes, gangrenous stomatitis may be confused with candidiasis. Its plaques or pseudomembranes are not raised above the mucosa, however, but cover an ulcerating lesion that may extend to bone. Also its pseudomembranes are usually a dirty gray color, in contrast to the whiteness of those that develop in candidiasis. Gangrenous stomatitis may carry a much graver prognosis than candidiasis, since the patient may be seriously ill with an uncontrolled debilitating disease; however, candidiasis also affects terminally ill patients.

Recurrent herpes simplex may resemble pseudomembranous candidiasis. Occasionally candidiasis demonstrates some examples of roundish, white lesions the same size as clusters of recently ruptured herpes simplex vesicles. Herpes lesions are usually more painful. Smears would show candidal organisms.

Chemical burns in some instances closely mimic candidiasis. The distinction is usually made by an accurate history, disclosing that a medicament has been applied to the mucosa.

Management

The management of patients with oral candidiasis is twofold: (1) attempts to identify, correct, or eliminate predisposing or precipitating factors and (2) antifungal therapy. Any oral lesion with surface debris may harbor candidal organisms even to the extent that a secondary candidiasis may become established. Nystatin treatment in such cases produces some improvement, but full remission must await successful treatment for the primary lesion. The treatment of candidiasis is discussed in detail in Chapter 5.

NECROTIC ULCERS OF SYSTEMIC DISEASE

Necrotic ulcers may occur in debilitating systemic diseases such as leukemia, sickle cell anemia, and uremia.

The ulcers are usually deep craters with a white necrotic surface (Fig. 8-48). In most instances they commence as small mucosal injuries that become chronically infected because of the decreased resistance of the patient. These lesions are discussed and illustrated in Chapter 11.

DIFFUSE GANGRENOUS STOMATITIS

Diffuse gangrenous stomatitis is also an oral disease in which a pseudomembrane is formed. Its cause is almost identical to that of ANUG, but it occurs in extremely debilitated patients. It must be differentiated from localized gangrenous stomatitis (cancrum oris or noma), a single localized and very destructive lesion (Fig. 8-49) seldom encountered in the United States. Griffin, Bach, Nespeca, et al[99] described two cases that occurred in young children in the South Pacific.

Features

Diffuse gangrenous stomatitis is usually found in patients with severe debilitating diseases, such as advanced diabetes, uremia, leukemia, blood dyscrasias, malnutritional states, or heavy metal poisoning. The patient complains of sensitive or painful oral lesions and a very unpleasant odor. The lesions are multiple, affecting several mucosal surfaces, and are surrounded by a thin, inflamed margin. The lesions are covered by a dirty gray to yellow pseudomembrane that can be readily removed, leaving a raw, bleeding, painful surface. They may be elliptic, linear, or angular. A tender to painful cervical lymphadenopathy is usually present.

Differential Diagnosis

Differential aspects of diffuse gangrenous stomatitis are discussed in the section on the differential diagnosis of candidiasis.

Management

Local treatment of diffuse gangrenous stomatitis is similar to the regimen described for ANUG: systemic amoxi-

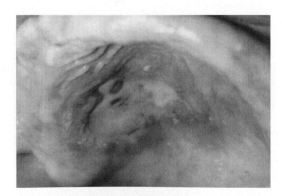

Fig. 8-48. Necrotic ulcer on the palate of a patient with mycosis fungoides. (Courtesy M. Sneed, Los Angeles.)

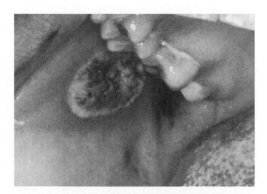

Fig. 8-49. Noma on the buccal mucosa of a patient terminally ill with acute myelogenous leukemia. (From Weinstein RA, et al: *Oral Surg* 38:10-14, 1974.)

cillin and oxygenating mouthrinses 4 times a day. This condition has a graver prognosis than ANUG because of its serious predisposing systemic conditions. Unless the systemic problems can be improved, the oral lesions may be difficult to eliminate completely.

RARITIES

These are listed on the first page of this chapter.

REFERENCES

1. Touyz LZG, Hille JJ: A fruit-mouthwash chemical burn: report of a case, *Oral Surg* 58:290-292, 1984.
2. Martin JL, Crump EP: Leukoedema of the buccal mucosa in Negro children and youth, *Oral Surg* 34:49-58, 1972.
3. Von Wyk CW: An investigation into the association between leukoedema and smoking, *J Oral Pathol* 14:491-499, 1985.
4. Durocher RT, Thalman R, Fiore-Donno G: Leukoedema of the oral mucosa, *J Am Dent Assoc* 85:1105-1109, 1972.
5. Kramer IRH, Lucas RB, Pindborg JJ, Sobin LH: Definition of leukoplakia and related lesions: an aid to studies on oral precancer, WHO Collaborating Centre for Oral Precancerous Lesions, *Oral Surg* 46:518-539, 1978.
6. Waldron CA, Shafer WG: Leukoplakia revisited, *Cancer* 36(4):1386-1392, 1975.
7. Bouquot JE, Gorlin R: Leukoplakia, lichen planus, and other keratoses in 23,616 white Americans over the age of 35 years, *Oral Surg* 61:373-381, 1986.
8. Bánóczy J: *Oral leukoplakia*, The Hague, 1982, Martinus Nijhoff.
9. Waldron CA: Oral epithelial tumors. In Gorlin RJ, Goldman HM, editors: *Thoma's oral pathology*, ed 6, St Louis, 1970, Mosby.
10. Bánóczy J, Csiba A: Occurrence of the epithelial dysplasia in oral leukoplakia, *Oral Surg* 42:766-774, 1976.
11. Lumerman H, Freedman P, Kerpel S: Oral epithelial dysplasia and the development of invasive squamous cell carcinoma, *Oral Surg* 79:321-329, 1995.
12. Pindborg JJ, Jolst O, Renstrup G, Roed-Petersen B: Studies in oral leukoplakia: a preliminary report on the period prevalence of malignant transformation in leukoplakia based on a follow-up study of 248 patients, *J Am Dent Assoc* 78:767-771, 1968.
13. Silverman S, Gorsky M, Lozada F: Oral leukoplakia and malignant transformation: a follow-up study of 257 patients, *Cancer* 53:563-568, 1984.
14. Kramer IRH, El-Labbon N, Lee KW: The clinical features and risk of malignant transformation in sublingual keratosis, *Br Dent J* 144:171-180, 1978.
15. Bánóczy J, Roed-Petersen B, Pindborg JJ, Inovay J: Clinical and histologic studies on electrogalvanically induced oral white lesions, *Oral Surg* 48:319-323, 1979.
16. Holmstrup P: Reactions of the oral mucosa related to silver amalgam: a review, *J Oral Pathol Med* 20:1-7, 1991.
17. Bolewska J, Hansen HJ, Holmstrup P, et al: Oral mucosal lesions related to silver amalgam restorations, *Oral Surg* 70:55-58, 1990.

18. Bolewska J, Holmstrup P, Moller-Madsen B, et al: Amalgam associated mercury accumulations in normal oral mucosa, oral mucosal lesions of lichen planus and contact lesions associated with amalgam, *J Oral Pathol Med* 19:39-42, 1990.
19. Schiødt M: Oral discoid lupus erythematosus. II. Skin lesions and systemic lupus erythematosus in sixty-six patients with 6 year follow up, *Oral Surg* 57:177-180, 1984.
20. Schiødt M: Oral manifestations of lupus erythematosus, *Int J Oral Surg* 13:101-147, 1984.
21. Silverman SJ, Rosen RP: Observations on the clinical characteristics and natural history of oral leukoplakia, *J Am Dent Assoc* 76:772-777, 1968.
22. Bánóczy J, Sugár L: Longitudinal studies in oral leukoplakia, *J Oral Pathol* 1:265-272, 1972.
23. Rossie KM, Guggenheimer J: Thermally induced 'nicotine' stomatitis: a case report, *Oral Surg* 70:597-599, 1990.
24. Buchner A, Sandbank M: Multiple fibroepithelial hyperplasias of the oral mucosa, *Oral Surg* 46:34-39, 1978.
25. Bouquot J, Schroeder K: Oral leukoplakia and smokeless tobacco keratosis are two separate and distinct precancers, Presentation to Annual Meeting of the American Academy of Oral Pathology, Portland, Maine, May 14-19, 1993.
26. Council on Scientific Affairs: Health effects of smokeless tobacco, *J Am Med Assoc* 255:1038-1044, 1986.
27. Christen AG, Swanson BZ, Glover ED, et al: Smokeless tobacco: the folklore and social history of snuffing, sneezing, dipping, and chewing, *J Am Dent Assoc* 105:821-829, 1982.
28. Grady D, Greene J, Daniels TE, et al: Oral mucosal lesions in smokeless tobacco users, *J Am Dent Assoc* 121:117-123, 1990.
29. Wisniewski JF, Bartolucci AA: Comparative patterns of smokeless tobacco use among major league baseball personnel, *J Oral Pathol Med* 18:322-326, 1989.
30. Wood NK: Smokeless tobacco and oral cancer: a summary, *Ill Dent J* 57:334-336, 1988.
31. Greer RO, Poulson TC: Oral tissue alterations associated with the use of smokeless tobacco by teen-agers. I. Clinical findings, *Oral Surg* 56:275-284, 1983.
32. Stewart CM, Baughman RA, Bates RE: Smokeless tobacco use among Florida teenagers: prevalence, attitudes and oral changes, *Fla Dent J* 60:38-42, 1989.
33. Guggenheimer J, Zullot TG, Kruper DC, et al: Changing trends of tobacco use in a teenage population in western Pennsylvania, *Am J Public Health* 76:196-197, 1986.

34. Gottlieb A, Pope SK, Rickert VI, Hardin BH: Patterns of smokeless tobacco use by young adolescents, *Pediatrics* 91:75-78, 1993.
35. Shankaran K, Kandarka SV, Contractor QQ, et al: Ultrastructural changes in esophageal mucosa of chronic tobacco chewers, *Indian J Med Res* 98:15-19, 1993.
36. Winn DM, Blot WJ, Shy C, et al: Snuff dipping and oral cancer among women in the southern United States, *N Engl J Med* 304:745-749, 1981.
37. Axéll T, Andersson G, Larsson Å: Oral mucosal findings associated with chewing tobacco in Sweden: a clinical and histological study, *J Dent Assoc S Afr* 45:194-196, 1992.
38. Creath CJ, Cutter G, Bradley DH, Wright JT: Oral leukoplakia and adolescent smokeless tobacco use, *Oral Surg* 72:35-41, 1991.
39. Andersson G, Axéll T: Clinical appearance of lesions associated with the use of loose and portion-bag packed Swedish moist snuff: a comparative study, *J Oral Pathol Med* 18:2-7, 1989.
40. Sundström B, Mornstad H, Axéll T: Oral carcinomas associated with snuff dipping, *J Oral Pathol* 11:245-251, 1982.
41. Daniels TE, Hansen LS, Greenspan JS, et al: Histopathology of smokeless tobacco lesions in professional baseball players: associations with different types of tobacco, *Oral Surg* 73:720-725, 1992.
42. Larsson Å, Axéll T, Andersson G: Reversibility of snuff dippers' lesion in Swedish moist snuff users: a clinical and histologic follow-up study, *J Oral Pathol Med* 20:258-264, 1991.
43. Wray A, McGuirt WF: Smokeless tobacco usage associated with oral carcinoma: incidence treatment, outcome, *Arch Otolaryngol Head Neck Surg* 119:929-933, 1993.
44. Link JO, Kaugers GE, Burns JC: Comparison of oral carcinomas in smokeless tobacco users and nonusers, *J Oral Maxillofac Surg* 50:452-455, 1992.
45. Fincher J: Sean Marssc's smokeless death, *Reader's Digest*, Oct 1985, pp. 107-112.
46. Andersson G, Axéll T, Larsson Å: Histologic changes associated with the use of loose and portion-bag snuff: a comparative study, *J Oral Pathol Med* 18:491-497, 1989.
47. Lacy MF, Reade PC, Hay KD: Lichen planus: a theory of pathogenesis, *Oral Surg* 56:521-526, 1983.
48. Watanabe T, Ohishi M, Tanaka K, Sato H: Analysis of HLA antigens in Japanese with oral lichen planus, *J Oral Pathol* 15:529-533, 1986.

49. Hampf BGC, Malmstrom MJ, Aalberg VA, et al: Psychiatric disturbance in patients with oral lichen planus, *Oral Surg* 63:429-432, 1987.

50. Lowenthal U, Pisanti S: Oral lichen planus according to the modern medical model, *J Oral Med* 39:224-226, 1984.

51. Allen CM, Beck FM, Rossie KM, Kaul TJ: Relation of stress and anxiety to oral lichen planus, *Oral Surg* 61:44-46, 1986.

52. McCartan BE: Psychological factors associated with oral lichen planus, *J Oral Pathol Med* 24:273-275, 1995.

53. Grinspan D, Diaz J, Villapol LO, et al: Lichen ruber planes de la muquese buccale son association a un diabete, *Bull Soc Fr Dermatol Syphiligr* 72:721, 1966.

54. Lamey P-J, Gibson J, Barkley SC, Miller S: Grispan's syndrome: a drug induced phenomenon? *Oral Surg* 70:184-185, 1990.

55. Lundström IMC: Incidence of diabetes mellitus in patients with oral lichen planus, *Int J Oral Surg* 12:147-152, 1983.

56. Albrecht M, Bánóczy J, Dinya E, Tamás G Jr: Occurrence of oral leukoplakia and lichen planus in diabetes mellitus, *J Oral Pathol Med* 21:364-366, 1992.

57. Christensen E, Holmstrup P, Wiberg-Jørgesen F, et al: Glucose tolerance in patients with oral lichen planus, *J Oral Pathol* 6:143-151, 1977.

58. Bagán-Sebastián JV, Milián-Masanet MA, Peñarraha-Diago M, Jimenez AY: A clinical study of 205 patients with oral lichen planus, *J Oral Maxillofac Surg* 50:116-118, 1992.

59. Lozada-Nur F, Luangjarmekorn L, Silverman S Jr, Karam J: Assessment of plasma glucose in 99 patients with oral lichen planus, *J Oral Med* 40:60-61, 1985.

60. Borghelli RF, Pettinari IL, Chuchurro JA, Stirparo MA: Oral lichen planus in patients with diabetes: an epidemiologic study, *Oral Surg* 75:498-500, 1993.

61. Van Dis ML, Parks ET: Prevalence of oral lichen planus in patients with diabetes mellitus, *Oral Surg* 79:696-700, 1995.

62. del Olmo JA, Bagan JV, Rodrigo JM, et al: Oral lichen planus and hepatic cirrhosis: letter to the editor, *Ann Intern Med* 110:666, 1989.

63. Gandolfo S, Carbone M, Carrozzo M, and Gallo V: Oral lichen planus and hepatitis C virus (HCV) infection: is there a relationship? A report of 10 cases, *J Oral Pathol Med* 23:119-122, 1994.

64. Holmstrup P, Thorn JJ, Rindum J, Pindborg JJ: Malignant development of lichen planus–affected mucosa, *J Oral Pathol* 17:219-225, 1988.

65. Silverman S, Gorsky M, Lozada-Nur F, Giannotti K: A prospective study of findings and management in 214 patients with oral lichen planus, *Oral Surg* 72:665-670, 1991.

66. Voute ABE, deJong WFB, Schulten EAJM, et al: Possible premalignant character of oral lichen planus: the Amsterdam experience, *J Oral Pathol Med* 21:326-329, 1992.

67. Holmstrup P: The controversy of a premalignant potential of oral lichen planus is over, *Oral Surg* 73:704-706, 1992.

68. Barnard NA, Scully C, Evenson JW, et al: Oral cancer development in patients with oral lichen planus, *J Oral Pathol Med* 22:421-424, 1993.

69. Brown RS, Bottomley WK, Puente E, Lavigne GL: A retrospective evaluation of 193 patients with oral lichen planus, *J Oral Pathol Med* 22:69-72, 1993.

70. Eisenberg E, Krutchkoff DJ: Lichenoid lesions of oral mucosa: diagnostic criteria and their importance in the alleged relationship to oral cancer, *Oral Surg* 73:699-704, 1992.

71. Lovas JGL, Harsanyi BB, Elbeneidy AK: Oral lichenoid dysplasia: a clinicopathologic analysis, *Oral Surg* 68:57-63, 1989.

72. Vincent SD, Fotos PG, Baker KA, Williams TP: oral lichen planus: the clinical, historical, and therapeutic features of 100 cases, *Oral Surg* 70:165-171, 1990.

73. Jungell P: Oral lichen planus: a review, *Int J Oral Maxillo fac Surg* 20:129-135, 1991.

74. Lundström IMC: Allergy and corrosion of dental materials in patients with oral lichen planus, *Int J Oral Surg* 13:16-24, 1984.

75. Council on Dental Materials, Instruments, and Equipment: American Dental Association status report on the occurrence of galvanic corrosion in the mouth and its potential effects, *J Am Dent Assoc* 115:783-787, 1987.

76. Farman AG: Hairy tongue (lingua villosa), *J Oral Med* 32:85-91, 1977.

77. McCoy JM, Waldron CA: Verrucous carcinoma of the oral cavity: a review of 49 cases, *Oral Surg* 52:623-629, 1981.

78. Ackerman LV: Verrucous carcinoma of the oral cavity, *Surgery* 23:670-678, 1948.

79. Shafer WG: Verrucous carcinoma, *Int Dent J* 22:451-459, 1972.

80. Shear M, Pindborg JJ: Verrucous hyperplasia of the oral mucosa, *Cancer* 46:1855-1862, 1980.

81. Slootweg PJ, Müller H: Verrucous hyperplasia or verrucous carcinoma: an analysis of 27 patients, *J Oral Maxillofac Surg* 11:13-19, 1983.

82. Tornes K, Bang G, Koppang HS, Pedersen KN: Oral verrucous carcinoma, *Int J Oral Surg* 14:485-492, 1985.

83. Batsakis JG, Hybels R, Crissman JO, et al: The pathology of head and neck tumors: verrucous carcinoma. XV. *Head Neck Surg* 5:29-35, 1982.

84. Hansen LS, Olson JA, Silverman S Jr: Proliferative verrucous leukoplakia, *Oral Surg* 60:285-298, 1985.

85. Kahn MA, Dockter ME, Hermann-Petrin JM: Proliferative verrucous leukoplakia: four cases with flow cytometric analysis, *Oral Surg* 78:469-475, 1994.

86. Murrah VA, Batsakis JG: Pathology consultation: proliferative verrucous leukoplakia and verrucous hyperplasia, *Ann Oto Rhinol Laryngol* 103:660-663, 1994.

87. Bohmfalk C, Zallen RD: Verrucous carcinoma of the oral cavity, *Oral Surg* 54:15-20, 1982.

88. McClure DL, Gullane PJ, Slinger RP, et al: Verrucous carcinoma: changing concepts in management, *J Otolaryngol* 13:7-12, 1984.

89. Kapstad B, Bang G: Verrucous carcinoma of the oral cavity treated with bleomycin, *Oral Surg* 42:588-590, 1976.

90. Collins JR, Van Sickles JE: Chronic mucocutaneous candidiasis, *J Oral Maxillofac Surg* 41:814-818, 1983.

91. Holmstrup P, Bessermann M: Clinical, therapeutic, and pathogenic aspects of chronic oral focal candidiasis, *Oral Surg* 56:388-395, 1983.

92. Bouquot JE, Fenton SJ: Juvenile juxtavermilion candidiasis: yet another form of an old disease? *J Am Dent Assoc* 116:187-192, 1988.

93. Krogh P, Holmstrup P, Thorn JJ, et al: Yeast species and biotypes associated with oral leukoplakia and lichen planus, *Oral Surg* 63:48-54, 1987.

94. Lamey PJ, Lewis MAO, MacDonald DG: Treatment of candidal leukoplakia with fluconazole, *Br Dent J* 166:296-298, 1989.

95. Bjorlin G, Palmer B: Surgical treatment of angular cheilosis, *Int J Oral Surg* 12:137-140, 1983.

96. Pattison GL: Self-inflicted gingival injuries: literature review and case report, *J Periodontol* 54:299, 1983.

97. Shiloah J, Lee WB, Binkley LH: Self-inflicted oral injury to secure narcotic drugs, *J Am Dent Assoc* 108:977-978, 1984.

98. Gagari G, Kabani S: Adverse effects of mouthwash use: a review, *Oral Surg* 80:432-439, 1995.

99. Kowitz GM, Lucatorto FM, Cherrick HM: Effects of mouthwashes on the oral soft tissues, *J Oral Med* 31:47-50, 1976.

100. Rubright WC, Walker JA, Karlsson UL, Diehl DL: Oral slough caused by dentifrice detergents and aggravated by drugs with antisialic activity, *J Am Dent Assoc* 97:215-220, 1978.

101. Cogen RB, Stevens AW, Cohen-Cole SA: Stressed whites especially prone to "trench mouth": medical news, *JAMA* 249:157-158, 1983.

102. Taiwo J: Oral hygiene status and necrotizing ulcerative gingivitis in Nigerian children, *J Periodontol* 63:1071-1074, 1993.

103. Zegarelli DJ, Zegarelli-Schmidt EC: Oral fungal infections, *J Oral Med* 42:76-79, 1987.

104. Tyldesley WR, Rotter E, Sells RA: Oral lesions in renal transplant patients, *J Oral Pathol* 8:5359, 1979.

105. Griffin JM, Bach DE, Nespeca JA, et al: Noma: report of two cases, *Oral Surg* 56:605-607, 1983.

CHAPTER 9

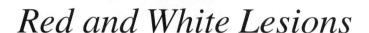

Red and White Lesions

NORMAN K. WOOD

HENRY M. DICK

Solitary red lesions, generalized red conditions, and white lesions compose the spectrum of conditions discussed in Chapters 5 through 8. These chapters group and discuss red lesions and white lesions in the pure sense. In the clinical situation, however, many of these may have both red and white components, and some may be considered mixed types.

Mixed red and white lesions can be separated into three distinct clinical groups, depending on whether their white components are keratotic, necrotic, or vesiculobullous. The red component is produced by thinning or loss of the surface epithelium (atrophy, erosion, or ulceration), by increased capillary blood supply just beneath the epithelium, or by combinations of these (inflammation, congenital hyperplasia, hypertrophy, and hemangioma).

RED WITH KERATOTIC COMPONENT
MIGRATORY GLOSSITIS
CHRONIC MECHANICAL TRAUMA
NICOTINE STOMATITIS
EROSIVE LICHEN PLANUS AND
   LICHENOID REACTION
SPECKLED LEUKOPLAKIA AND
   ERYTHROLEUKOPLAKIA
SQUAMOUS CELL CARCINOMA
HYPERTROPHIC AND HYPERPLASTIC
   CANDIDIASIS
LUPUS ERYTHEMATOSUS
RARITIES
   Contact allergy
   Darier's disease
   Lichen sclerosus and lichen planus atrophicus
   Migratory stomatitis
   Oral psoriasis
   Papilloma
   Proliferative verrucous leukoplakia
   Smokeless tobacco lesions
   Verrucous carcinoma

RED WITH NECROTIC COMPONENT
CHEMICAL AND DRUG BURNS
THERMAL BURNS
APHTHOUS ULCERS AND STOMATITIS
CRUSHING TYPES OF TRAUMA
PSEUDOMEMBRANOUS CANDIDIASIS
ACUTE NECROTIC ULCERATIVE
   GINGIVITIS
PYOGENIC GRANULOMA
ALLERGIC MUCOSITIS
XEROSTOMIA
RADIATION MUCOSITIS
CHEMOTHERAPY MUCOSITIS
RARITIES
ACTINOMYCOSIS
AGRANULOCYTOSIS
ANEMIA (SEVERE)
GANGRENOUS STOMATITIS
INFLAMED SOFT TISSUE AROUND
   DENUDED BONE
LEUKEMIA
MIDLINE GRANULOMA

MUCOUS PATCH
MYCOSIS FUNGOIDES
MYCOTIC LESIONS
CYCLICAL NEUTROPENIA
NONSPECIFIC ULCERS
VESICULOBULLOUS LESIONS
PRIMARY AND SECONDARY HERPES
   SIMPLEX
BENIGN MUCOUS MEMBRANE
   PEMPHIGOID
ERYTHEMA MULTIFORME
LICHEN PLANUS
PEMPHIGUS
RADIATION MUCOSITIS
RARITIES
   Childhood viral diseases
   Drug allergies
   Hand-foot-and-mouth disease
   Herpangina
   Herpes zoster
   Stevens-Johnson syndrome

RED AND WHITE LESIONS WITH KERATOTIC COMPONENTS

Lesions in this group have a white component that cannot be removed with a tongue blade.

Migratory glossitis is usually identified by its classic features: location on the tongue, red patches with raised whitish rims, the changing patterns, and its usual asymptomatic course (see Figs. 7-1 and 8-13). On rare occasions, migratory stomatitis accompanies this condition, with lesions involving various mucosal surfaces and the tongue (Plate D).

Mechanical trauma of a chronic and mild nature produces whitish leukoplakial patches. Chronic cheek or lip chewing is a good example. Periodically the chewing habit may become more severe, perhaps as a result of increased stress. Thus small bites may be taken out of the white patch, producing a red and white lesion (see Fig. 8-30). The condition may look worrisome and reminiscent of speckled leukoplakia. However, close inspection reveals rough tissue tags that surround red areas. These tissue tags are not characteristic of speckled leukoplakia.

Nicotine stomatitis characteristically occurs on the hard palate of smokers, usually pipe smokers. This condition is painless. The white keratotic component may have a cobblestone appearance speckled with red dots that may be the size of pinpoints in some cases and much larger in others (see Fig. 8-11). These red dots are inflamed ducts of minor salivary glands. This appearance is pathognomonic for the condition. Occasionally the soft palate also has an appearance similar to the reticular pattern of lichen planus with reddened mucosa between the striae. This appearance may be difficult to differentiate from speckled leukoplakia and atrophic or erosive lichen planus. A cobblestone appearance with dots in any area of the lesion, most commonly near the junction of the hard palate, permits the diagnosis. A definitive diagnosis can be made if the lesion disappears on discontinuation of smoking.

Erosive lichen planus and lichenoid reaction in the classic presentation and in a bilateral or generalized distribution in the mouth are usually readily identifiable (Plate C), although lupus erythematosus can mimic it (Plate D). When this condition occurs as a single lesion, it can easily be confused with speckled leukoplakia and hyperplastic, hypertrophic, erythematous, or atrophic candidiasis. Biopsy usually is necessary to distinguish among them.

Speckled leukoplakia and erythroleukoplakia are, as the names imply, lesions with a mix of erythroplakia and leukoplakia (Plate G). Considering that almost all erythroplakial lesions histologically demonstrate extensive dysplasia, carcinoma in situ, or early invasive carcinoma, diagnosis and treatment must be established quickly. In the authors' experience the red components are usually smoothly marginated, which distinguishes them from leukoplakias, which have roughly marginated red areas

resulting from episodes of chronic trauma. The characteristic white feathering at the borders of lichen planus lesions is usually not seen in these lesions; they also do not exhibit the reticular pattern of lichen planus.

Frank squamous cell carcinoma may have red and white components in a plaque lesion. The lesion usually soon shows raised components as shown in Plates G, H, and I.

Hypertrophic and hyperplastic candidiasis are conditions in which leukoplakial lesions are associated with or caused by low-grade candidiasis. A red component is frequently part of the clinical picture. Hyperplastic candidiasis is most commonly seen at the oral commissures as angular cheilosis or mucocutaneous candidiasis.

Lupus erythematosus produces variable red and white lesions, which may be similar to those of lichen planus but usually adopt a broader, less linear pattern with feathered borders (Plate D). Like the lesions in lichen planus, these lesions have a wide distribution in the oral cavity and lips and may involve the skin. Systemic workup and biopsy are usually necessary to establish the diagnosis.

RED LESIONS WITH NECROTIC COMPONENT

Chemical or drug burns may produce red and necrotic white areas on an erythematous background, depending on the severity of injury. Aspirin and acetaminophen burns, for example, are produced when patients hold these analgesics in their mouths to relieve toothache (Plate D, 8). Occasionally a clinician accidentally spills chemicals in a patient's mouth, and the chemicals produce burns. Some patients apply addictive drugs to the oral mucosa, and these drugs may produce red and white necrotic lesions (Plate B, 10). Facts from the patient's history help establish the diagnosis.

Thermal burns may result when patients ingest food or beverages that are very hot. Depending on the severity of the burn, the lesion may be red (erythematous) and white (deeply necrotic) or white (mildly necrotic).

Aphthous ulcers and stomatitis characteristically show ulcers with serofibrinous yellow or white necrotic centers with well-defined red borders. (Plate B, 4).

Crushing types of trauma produce various clinical appearances, one of which is a combined necrotic and erythematous reaction (see Fig. 8-41). Red patches or rims may be apparent when inflammation or gross loss of surface tissue occurs. Exophytic lesions are subject to trauma and may demonstrate surface necrosis.

Pseudomembranous candidiasis characteristically shows a necrotic surface with red inflammatory components surrounding the necrotic pseudomembrane. Bleeding areas occur when the necrotic curds are stripped away (Plate D, 7).

Acute necrotic ulcerative gingivitis involves principally the interdental papillae and the marginal gingiva. Although necrosis is the most prominent aspect of the condition, varying degrees of erythema (redness) are seen around the necrotic margins (see Fig. 8-44 and Plates E, 10 and E, 11).

The pyogenic granuloma is frequently reddish with a necrotic white patch of variable size on the surface. Identifying a chronic irritant usually helps to establish the working diagnosis.

In mild to moderate cases, allergic mucositis, shows as an inflammatory red plaque. In severe cases, it also has a necrotic white component (Plates C and D).

Xerostomia varies in severity and may lead to a generalized erythematous mucositis. In severe cases, necrosis may occur and give a disseminated red and white appearance.

Radiation mucositis, also depending on stage and severity, may show erythematous and necrotic components disseminated as patches throughout the oral mucosa (Plate D, 6). Frank blebs that appear white before and after rupture may also be present. The history is usually diagnostic.

Chemotherapy mucositis usually shows patches of red scattered throughout the mouth. Although necrosis may also be present, it is not usually as prominent in chemotherapy mucositis as in radiation mucositis.

VESICULOBULLOUS LESIONS

These lesions are discussed in detail in Chapter 6. Originally surrounded by red rims, these lesions appear white, and the vesicles, or blebs, are intact. When coalesced vesicles rupture, they may retain a white appearance for a while. When the blebs fully rupture and become emptied, their white appearance usually disappears, although the torn fragments of their roof tissue may persist as whitish flaps for a time. Some vesiculobullous conditions that the clinician might expect to see are herpes simplex, both primary and secondary; benign mucous membrane pemphigoid; erythema multiforme; pemphigus and its variants; and occasionally radiation mucositis (see Figs. 6-1, 6-2, 6-5, 6-7, 6-9, and 6-11 and Plates C and D).

CHAPTER 10

Peripheral Oral Exophytic Lesions

NORMAN K. WOOD

PAUL W. GOAZ

Peripheral exophytic structures and lesions of the oral cavity include the following:

EXOPHYTIC ANATOMIC STRUCTURES
ACCESSORY TONSILLAR TISSUE
BUCCAL FAT PADS
CIRCUMVALLATE PAPILLAE
FOLIATE PAPILLAE
GENIAL TUBERCLES
LINGUAL TONSILLAR TISSUE
PALATINE RUGAE
PALATINE TONSILS
PAPILLA PALATINA
RETROCUSPID PAPILLA
RETROMOLAR PAPILLA
STENSEN'S PAPILLAE
SUBLINGUAL CARUNCLES
TONGUE
UVULA
EXOPHYTIC LESIONS
TORI AND EXOSTOSES
INFLAMMATORY HYPERPLASIAS
  Fibrous hyperplasias
  Pyogenic granuloma
  Hormonal tumor
  Epulis fissuratum
  Parulis
  Papillary hyperplasia of palate
  Peripheral giant cell granuloma
  Pulp polyp
  Epulis granulomatosum
  Acquired hemangioma
  Peripheral fibroma with calcification
MUCOCELE AND RANULA
HEMANGIOMA, LYMPHANGIOMA, AND
  VARICOSITY
CENTRAL EXOPHYTIC LESIONS
ORAL PAPILLOMA, VERRUCA VULGARIS,
  AND CONDYLOMA ACUMINATUM
EXOPHYTIC SQUAMOUS CELL
  CARCINOMA
VERRUCOUS CARCINOMA

MINOR SALIVARY GLAND TUMORS
PERIPHERAL BENIGN MESENCHYMAL
  TUMORS
NEVUS AND MELANOMA
PERIPHERAL METASTATIC TUMORS
PERIPHERAL MALIGNANT
  MESENCHYMAL TUMORS
RARITIES
SOLITARY LESIONS
  Actinomycosis
  Adenomatoid hyperplasia of the minor sali-
    vary glands
  Adenomatoid squamous cell carcinoma
  Alveolar soft part sarcoma
  Ameloblastoma (peripheral)
  Angiolymphoid hyperplasia
  Antral neoplasms
  Basaloid squamous cell carcinoma
  Benign lymphoid hyperplasia
  Blastomycosis
  Blue nevus (Jadassohn-Tièche)
  Bohn's nodule (Epstein's pearl)
  Calcifying odontogenic cyst, peripheral
  Calcinosis
  Chondroma of soft tissue
  Chordoma
  Choristoma
  Condyloma acuminatum
  Condyloma latum
  Congenital epulis of the newborn
  Early chancre
  Early gumma
  Eruption cyst
  Extraosseous odontogenic tumor
  Focal mucinosis
  Follicular lymphoid hyperplasia
  Foreign body granuloma
  Gastrointestinal cyst (heterotopic)
  Giant cell fibroma

Gingival cyst
Glomus tumor
Granular cell lesion
Granulomatous fungal disease
Hamartoma
Herpes proliferative lesion
Histiocytosis X
Inflammatory pseudotumor, intraoral
Intravascular papillary endothelial hyperplasia
Inverted ductal papilloma
Juvenile nasopharyngeal angiofibroma
Juvenile xanthogranuloma
Kaposi's sarcoma
Kaposi's sarcoma (AIDS)
Keratoacanthoma
Labial artery—caliber persistent
Lead poisoning
Leukemic enlargement
Lichen sclerosus and lichen planus atrophicus
Lingual thyroid gland
Lymphoma
Median nodule of the upper lip
Median rhomboid glossitis (nodular variety)
Midline nonhealing granuloma
Molluscum contagiosum
Myofibroma
Myxoma of soft tissue
Necrotizing sialometaplasia (nodular)
Neuroectodermal tumor of infancy
Neuroendocrine carcinoma
Nodular fasciitis
Nodular leukoplakia
Odontogenic fibroma, peripheral
Odontogenic keratocyst, peripheral
Oral focal mucinosis
Plasmacytoma of soft tissue
Pseudosarcomatous fasciitis
Pulse granuloma
Rhabdomyoma

Rhabdomyosarcoma
Rheumatoid nodule
Rhinoscleroma
Sarcoidosis
Sebaceous adenoma
Sebaceous cyst
Sebaceous hyperplasia
Sialolith
Skin cysts and tumors
Spindle cell carcinoma
Squamous acanthoma
Sturge-Weber syndrome
Teratoma
Traumatic granuloma
Tuberculosis
Tuberculum impar, persistent
Verruciform xanthoma
MULTIPLE LESIONS
Acanthosis nigricans
Acrokeratosis verruciformis of Hope
Amyloidosis
Bohn's nodules
Calcinosis
Chronic granulomatous disease
Condyloma acuminatum
Condyloma latum
Cowden disease
Crohn's disease
Cysticercosis
Darier's disease
Eruption cysts

Focal dermal hypoplasia (Goltz' syndrome)
Focal epithelial hyperplasia
Gardner's syndrome
Giant cell fibromas
Graft-versus-host disease
Gummata
Hereditary telangiectasia
Histiocytosis X
Idiopathic gingival fibromatosis
Kaposi's sarcoma
Kaposi's sarcoma (AIDS)
Leishmaniasis
Leprosy
Leukemic enlargements
Lichenoides chronica
Lymphangiomas of neonates
Lymphomas (extranodal)
Lymphomatoid papulosis
Lymphoproliferating disease of the palate
Maffucci's syndrome
Melkersson-Rosenthal syndrome
Molluscum contagiosum
Multinucleate cell angiohistiocytoma
Multiple endocrine neoplasias type IIb
Multiple exophytic metastatic carcinomas
Multiple exostoses
Multiple fibroepithelial hyperplasias
Multiple gingival cysts
Multiple granular cell tumors
Multiple hamartoma neoplasia syndrome
Multiple lipomas

Multiple melanomas
Multiple mucoceles
Multiple myeloma
Multiple papillomas
Multiple peripheral brown giant cell lesions (hyperparathyroidism)
Multiple peripheral metastatic carcinomas
Multiple superficial mucoceles
Multiple teratomas
Multiple verrucae
Murray-Puretic-Drescher syndrome
Noonan's syndrome
Oral florid papillomatosis
Orofaciodigital syndrome (multiple hamartomas of the tongue)
Palisaded encapsulated neuroma
Phenytoin hyperplasia
Pyostomatitis vegetans
Sarcoidosis
Subacute necrotizing sialadenitis
Syphilitic papules
Thrombocytopenic purpura
Tuberous sclerosis
Tumoral calcinosis
Urticaria pigmentosa
von Recklinghausen's disease, types I and II
Xanthoma disseminatum

The term *exophytic lesion* in the context of the following discussion means "any pathologic growth that projects above the normal contours of the oral surface."

Hypertrophy, hyperplasia, neoplasia, and the pooling of fluid are four mechanisms by which exophytic lesions may be produced. *Hypertrophy* refers to an enlargement caused by an increase in the size but not in the number of cells. *Hyperplasia* is generally defined as an enlargement caused by an increase in the number of normal cells. Combinations of these two processes occur with some frequency. *Neoplasia* is defined as the formation of a neoplasm, which is identical to a tumor and may be benign or malignant.

The terms used to describe the shapes of exophytic lesions are often confusing. The descriptive terms used in this discussion to identify the specific shapes are as follows: *papillomatous, verrucous, papular, nodular* (a papule more than 0.5 cm in diameter), *dome shaped, polypoid,* and *bosselated* (Fig. 10-1). As a general rule, exophytic lesions with a papillomatous or verrucous shape originate in the surface epithelium (e.g., verrucae vulgaris, papillomas, squamous cell and verrucous carcinomas, and keratoacanthomas), whereas those with a smoothly contoured shape originate in the deeper tissues and are beneath and separate from the stratified squamous epithe-lium (e.g., tori, fibromas, lipomas, and early malignant mesenchymal tumors.)*

The surfaces of the lesions may become eroded (red), keratinized (white), necrotic (white), or ulcerated, depending on the reaction of the epithelial surface to varying degrees of trauma. Mild trauma may cause the epithelial surface to become eroded or keratinized, whereas severe trauma may cause the surface to become ulcerated.

When an exophytic lesion is found on an area of oral mucosa that is overlying bone, it must be identified as originating in the soft tissues or the bone. Such a distinction helps in developing the differential diagnosis. Careful visual, digital, and radiographic examinations usually indicate whether the origin is in soft tissue or bone.

If the lesion and accompanying soft tissues can be moved over the underlying bone and a radiograph fails to show bony changes, the lesion probably originated in the soft tissue. However, the mucosa over the anterior hard palate and alveolar gingivae is normally fixed to bone. As a result, this test is not helpful in determining whether the lesion originated in soft tissue or bone in these locations. Difficulty in identifying the tissue of origin may be experienced

---

*This concept is discussed in detail in Chapter 3.

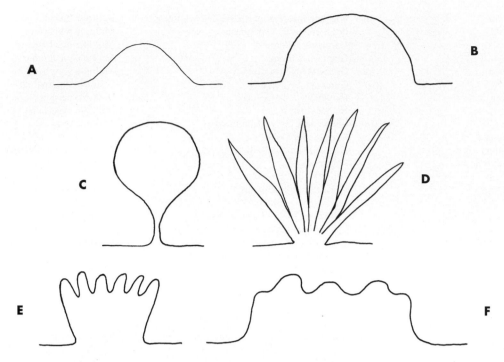

Fig. 10-1. Various shapes of exophytic lesions. **A,** Nodular. (A papular mass is a nodule measuring less than 0.5 cm.) **B,** Dome shaped. **C,** Polypoid. **D,** Papillomatous. **E,** Verrucous. **F,** Bosselated.

EXOPHYTIC ANATOMIC STRUCTURES

- Accessory tonsillar tissue
- Buccal fat pads (Fig. 10-2)
- Circumvallate papillae
- Foliate papillae
- Genial tubercles
- Lingual tonsillar tissue
- Palatine rugae
- Palatine tonsils
- Palatine papillae
- Retrocuspid papillae
- Retromolar papillae
- Stensen's papillae
- Sublingual caruncles
- Tongue
- Uvula

when changes occur in both tissues. This circumstance prompts the inclusion of a large number of possibilities in the differential diagnosis and multiple entities in the working diagnosis.

Lesions originating within bone may become exophytic lesions and are discussed in Part III. The reported incidence of exophytic lesions in people over 35 years of age was found to be 6.1%.[1]

EXOPHYTIC ANATOMIC STRUCTURES

Although exophytic anatomic oral structures are not likely to be confused with pathologic lesions, the former are listed in the box at left for completion. Occasionally some of these structures attain such a size that they are mistaken for pathoses. The anatomic location of the structures, however, usually enables immediate recognition.

The foliate papillae are located on the posterolateral borders of the tongue. They vary greatly in size, being absent in some patients and prominent in others. Frequently they are nodular, with deep vertical fissures appearing to divide them into several closely associated exophytic projections (Fig. 10-3). They are normally pink unless traumatized and have approximately the same consistency as the rest of the tongue. The great variation in size and occasionally appearance is frequently troublesome for the inexperienced clinician. Furthermore, lingual tonsillar tissue is also frequently seen in the area of the foliate papillae and may be confused with the foliate papillae or similar-appearing pathoses.

The genial tubercles may become exophytic in patients who have experienced extreme resorption of their edentulous mandibular ridges. In some cases the genial tubercles project into the anterior floor of the mouth under the mucosa just posterior to the lingual surface of the mandible; in others, they project superiorly above the level of the anterior portion of the ridge. If an exophytic mass is bony hard

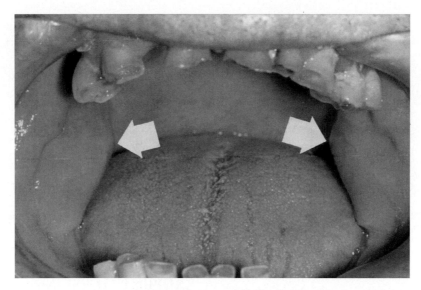

Fig. 10-2. Buccal fat pads.

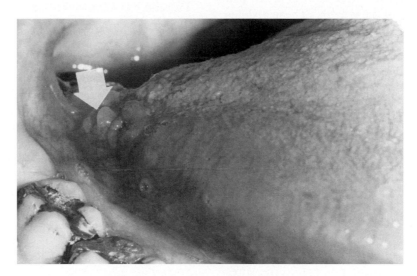

Fig. 10-3. Foliate papillae.

on palpation and is attached to the lingual surface of the mandible in the midline, it should be recognized as a genial tubercle; if the genial tubercles interfere with the construction of dentures, they should be surgically reduced.

Lingual tonsillar tissue forms part of Waldeyer's ring, which is composed of the pharyngeal tonsil (adenoids), palatine tonsil, and lingual tonsil. These large aggregates of lymphatic tissue are linked by isolated tonsillar nodules; consequently, they encircle the entrance to the oropharynx. The lingual tonsillar tissue is on the pharyngeal surface of the tongue and frequently extends over the posterolateral borders into, or just posterior to, the location of the foliate papillae (Fig. 10-4, *A*).

The portion of the lingual tonsil in the area of the foliate papillae may vary greatly in size. It may be just a small deposit of tonsillar tissue appearing as a single, discrete pink papule or nodule with a smooth, yellowish-pink, glossy surface, or it may be larger accumulations of tonsillar tissue giving the appearance of an aggregation of papules and consequently recognizable as a nodular or dome-shaped mass with a coarse, pebbly (papular) surface (see Fig. 10-4). In some cases the grooves between the individual papules are deep and impart a papillomatous appearance to the structure (see Fig. 10-4). Lingual tonsillar tissue is usually moderately firm on palpation.

Accessory tonsillar tissue may occur in various locations in the oral cavity (floor of the mouth, ventral surface of the tongue, soft palate, and most often, posterior pharyngeal wall) (Fig. 10-5). Some patients seem to have a relative abundance of lymphoid tissue; in these people, the small, usually smooth-surfaced papules and nodules are most commonly found in various sites throughout the oral cavity. The glossy, yellowish-pink sheen often permits the ready identification of small deposits of tonsillar tissue.

Studies indicate a higher prevalence of accessory oral tonsillar tissue than was previously believed.[2,3] One

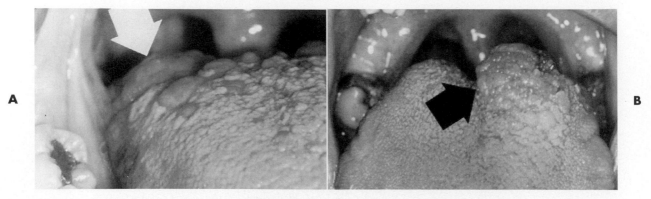

Fig. 10-4. Lingual tonsillar tissue. **A,** Classic position for the tonsil *(arrow)*. **B,** Unusually large tonsil located more anteriorly than usual.

report on male patients indicated that 21% of the patients had tonsillar aggregates on the soft palate, 12% had tonsillar aggregates on the floor of the mouth, and 5% had them on the ventral surface of the tongue.[3] These nodules varied from 1 to 3 mm in size, and their number in individuals ranged from 1 to 25.[3]

Concerning pathosis of oral tonsillar tissue, Adkins[2] described in some detail the changes observed in lymphoid hyperplasia. In a more comprehensive study,[4] three types of pathoses most commonly found in these aggregates were described: hyperplasia—pink, pseudocyst—yellow (lymphoepithelial cyst), and hyperemia—red. These entities should be included in the differential diagnosis of exophytic, yellow, and red lesions.[4]

• • •

The retrocuspid papilla is a pink papule or nodule that may be present on the alveolo lingual gingivae by the mandibular canine teeth (Fig. 10-5, *C*).[5] This normal anatomic variation usually occurs bilaterally, measures approximately 0.4 cm in width, and occurs more frequently in children and adolescents.[5] It seems to disappear with age: almost 40% occur in children and adolescents compared with just over 11% in patients ranging in age from 18 to 60 years.[6]

The histopathology in 80% of cases shows loosely arranged, delicate connective tissue fibers with stellate and multinucleated fibroblasts. Increased vascularity and/or elongated rete ridges are also seen in a considerable number of cases.[5]

The retromolar papillae are normal structures located just behind the most posterior molar teeth on the crest of the ridge of both arches. In the maxilla, these structures correspond to the crestal mucosa covering the tuberosities. The retromolar papillae in the mandibular arch extend posteriorly from the free gingival margins of the most posterior molars to blend into the retromolar pads bilaterally.

Although each of the exophytic anatomic structures can undergo pathologic change, this rarely occurs.

EXOPHYTIC LESIONS

TORI AND EXOSTOSES

Tori and exostoses are the most common oral exophytic lesions and are discussed in Chapters 27 to 29 as radiopacities of the jaws. They are peripheral, benign, slow-growing bony protuberances of the jaws. These readily recognizable lesions usually appear symmetrically as nodular or bosselated lesions that have smooth contours and are covered with normal mucosa. They are hard on palpation and are attached by a broad, bony base to the underlying jaw. Growth occurs mainly during the first 30 years of life.

Palatine tori are located on the hard palate, usually in the midline (Fig. 10-6), and are almost twice as common (42%) in female as in male patients.[7,8] Mandibular tori are found in about 12% of adults and are located on the lingual aspect of the mandible above the mylohyoid ridge, most often bilaterally in the premolar region (see Fig. 10-6). No differences in occurrence between genders have been noted. Patients from the United Kingdom have a markedly lower incidence and smaller tori than patients from the United States.[7]

Another study investigated Florida whites, Florida blacks, and Kentucky whites.[8] No significant difference was found in the incidence of maxillary tori (twice as common in female patients) among the three groups. Concerning mandibular tori, no gender preponderance was found, but Florida blacks had a lower incidence than Florida and Kentucky whites.[8]

Similar bony protuberances that occur in other locations around the jawbones are simply termed *exostoses* (see Fig. 10-6). The radiographic images of tori and exostes are discussed in Chapter 27.

Differential Diagnosis

Tori and exostoses are usually readily identifiable by their distinguishing features. Ulcerated mucosa over these bony protuberances may pose a diagnostic problem. In most

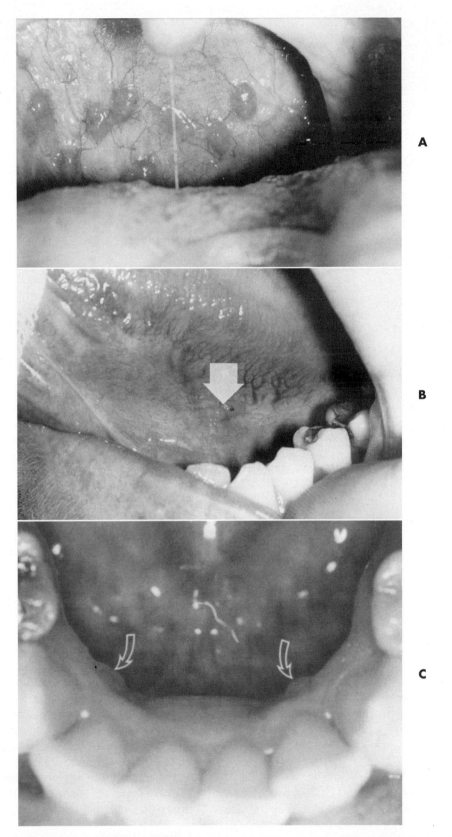

Fig. 10-5. Accessory tonsillar tissue. **A,** Several nodules on the posterior pharyngeal wall. **B,** Small deposit of tonsillar tissue on the ventral surface of the tongue *(arrow).* **C,** Retrocuspid papillae situated bilaterally *(arrows)* on the lingual gingivae. (**C** courtesy D. Weathers, Atlanta, Ga.)

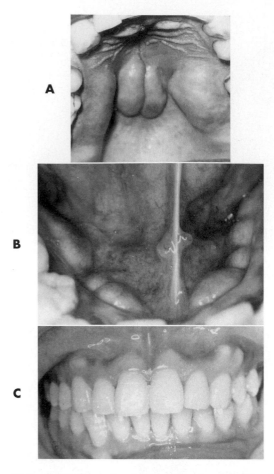

Fig. 10-6. A, Palatine tori and lingual exostoses. **B,** Mandibular tori. **C,** Buccal exostoses.

cases, however, the ulcers are traumatic in origin, and the history and clinical examination disclose the cause.

Occasionally the following lesions may closely resemble a torus or exostosis on clinical and radiologic examinations: a mature cementifying or ossifying fibroma that has caused a bulge on the cortical palate (Fig. 28-2), an ossified subperiosteal hematoma, a nonresolved bony callus, an osteoma, an early osteosarcoma, and an early chondrosarcoma.

Management

Removal is usually considered unnecessary unless prompted by psychologic, prosthetic, phonetic, or traumatic considerations.

INFLAMMATORY HYPERPLASIAS

An oral inflammatory hyperplastic (IH) lesion is a common entity and may be defined as "an increase in the size of an organ or tissue due to an increase in the number of its constituent cells, as a local response of tissue to injury."[9] It can be considered as an overexuberant reparative response.

Traumatic irritants include calculi, overhanging margins of restorations, foreign bodies, chronic biting, mar-

gins of caries, sharp spicules of bones, and overextended borders of appliances. The initiating chronic injury, regardless of type, produces an inflammation, which in turn stimulates the formation of granulation tissue that consists of proliferating endothelial cells; a very rich, patent capillary bed; chronic inflammatory cells; and a few fibroblasts (Fig. 10-7, *B*). The granulation tissue (granuloma) soon becomes covered with stratified squamous epithelium.

Clinically at this stage the lesion is asymptomatic and smoothly contoured or lobulated with a very red appearance because of the rich vascularity and transparency of the nonkeratinized epithelial covering (see Fig. 10-7, *A*). It is moderately soft and spongy and blanches on careful digital pressure. Most lesions are sessile (broad based), although some may be polypoid.

If the recurring insult is eliminated at this stage, the lesion shrinks markedly as the inflammation subsides, and the vascularity is reduced. If the insult is permitted to continue, however, the granulomatous lesion continues to increase in size, although some fibrosis may occur in the regions farthest from the areas being irritated. These fibrotic areas appear as pale pink patches on the reddish surface of the lesion (see Fig. 10-7, *C*). In time, the complete lesion may fibrose, resulting in a pale pinkish, smooth or lobulated, firm lesion: fibrous hyperplasia (FH) (traumatic or irritating fibroma).

If the instigating factor is eliminated at the mixed stage, the decrease in the size of the lesion is directly proportional to the amount of inflammation present; in other words, if the lesion is composed mostly of fibrous tissue, there is little shrinkage, but if considerable granulation tissue and inflammation exist, there is marked shrinkage. Usually these lesions show a fairly consistent pattern of injury, healing, and reinjury.

Clinical Terms

Various clinical terms have been used on the basis of the anatomic site and traumatic agent involved or on the basis of an ulcerated or necrotic surface (see box above). Some of these terms are fading from use.

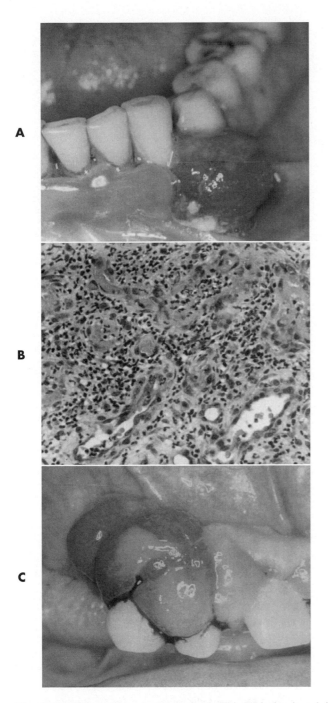

Fig. 10-7. IH and fibrous hyperplasia. **A,** This IH lesion is red; it is composed mostly of granulation tissue and inflammatory components. **B,** Photomicrograph of IH lesion in **A. C,** This lesion is a combination of IH and fibrous hyperplasia. Note the fibrosed regions (pale patches) in the red IH lesion. (**A** courtesy P.D. Toto, Waukegan, Ill.)

Differential Diagnosis

The IH lesions are common and generally distinctive. Their locations suggest the cause, and the causative traumatic factors are easily identified. However, the lesions listed in the box above must be considered in the differential diagnosis.

DIFFERENTIAL DIAGNOSIS OF IH

- Acquired hemangioma
- Kaposi's sarcoma
- Metastatic tumors
- Benign mesenchymal tumors
- Malignant mesenchymal tumors
- Squamous cell carcinoma (unusual)

On occasion, squamous cell carcinoma (SCC) may commence at a small location on the surface, burrow, and undermine the subepithelial tissue in such a manner that the lesion appears mostly as a smooth-surfaced exophytic lesion. This is a very unusual presentation. The mass would be firm, painless, and nonhemorrhagic with perhaps a small, rough patch on its top.

Benign and malignant mesenchymal tumors are rare but can mimic the IH lesions, especially if there is a generous vascular component. This possibility should be considered if an irritant cannot be identified.

Metastatic tumors also can mimic IH lesions, especially in the early stages (see Fig. 10-31, *A*). Again, these are uncommon and receive a low ranking unless there are symptoms or a history of a primary lesion.

Kaposi's sarcoma is common in AIDS and sometimes in other immunodeficient conditions and may look very similar to IH (see Fig. 10-10, *A*). Positive AIDS tests and indicative signs and symptoms indicate a high ranking for Kaposi's sarcoma.

Acquired hemangioma is really a converted type of IH and is discussed on p. 143.

Management

The management of IH lesions is determined by the clinical appearance of the lesion, which in turn is governed by the microstructure. Basically, if the lesion is red and soft and the irritating cause can be eliminated, a significant reduction in size may be observed, perhaps even to the point of eliminating the need for excision. If excision is required, the procedure is easier and less blood is lost if the lesion is permitted to regress (sclerose) before it is removed.

When the lesion is pale pink and quite firm, almost no reduction can be expected because its bulk is predominantly fibrous tissue (FH). Excision followed by microscopic examination of the specimen is the procedure indicated.

FIBROUS HYPERPLASIA

Again FH (traumatic or irritation fibroma) is the healed end product of an IH lesion and is not a true neoplasm. Consequently it is really an aggregate of scar tissue covered with a smooth layer of stratified squamous epithelium (Fig. 10-8). FH is the second most common oral exophytic lesion found in a large study.[1]

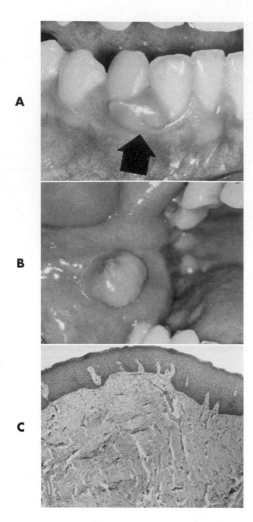

Fig. 10-8. FH (traumatic fibroma). **A,** This lesion represents a fibrosed IH lesion. **B,** FH on the buccal mucosa. **C,** Photomicrograph of FH. Note the dense avascular collagen.

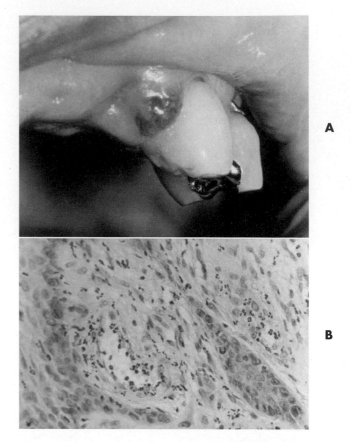

Fig. 10-9. Pyogenic granuloma. **A,** Clinical view. Note small ulcer on lesion. **B,** Photomicrograph. Polymorphonuclear leukocytes are distributed throughout the granulation tissue.

The lesions are most often sessile or slightly pedunculated with a smooth contour, pale pink, and firm to palpation; they occur on the gingiva, tongue, buccal mucosa, and palate. An excisional biopsy is the indicated treatment. Clearly an intermediate-type or mixed lesion occurs[10] and is composed of cellular or granulation elements and collagen.

Differential diagnosis The fibroma may be confused with benign tumors such as minor salivary gland neoplasms, neurofibroma, neurilemoma, rhabdomyoma, leiomyoma, and giant cell fibroma.

The giant cell fibroma is reported to be a small, firm, papular or polypoid lesion that occurs on the gingiva, tongue, buccal mucosa, and palate and is not more than 1 cm in diameter. These lesions are said to be characterized histologically by large, multinucleated, active fibroblasts.[9] Some clinicians prefer not to classify it as separate from IH or FH lesions.[9] These should be included in the differential diagnosis of fibroma.[11]

The fibroma is ranked above any of these lesions, however, because of its relatively high incidence in the oral cavity.

Pyogenic Granuloma

Pyogenic granuloma is an IH lesion that becomes ulcerated. The ulceration occurs usually because of trauma during mastication, and this IH lesion then becomes contaminated by the oral flora and liquids. As a result, an acute inflammatory response occurs.

Clinically the asymptomatic reddish papule, nodule, or polyp usually shows at least part of its surface to be rough, ulcerated, and necrotic (Figs. 8-42 and 10-9 and Plate B). The fact that this necrotic white material clinically resembles pus prompted early clinicians to refer to the lesion as a *pyogenic granuloma;* however, there is no pus in the lesion.

The most common location by far is the gingiva,[12-16] particularly the anterior segment. Other locations are the lips, tongue, buccal mucosa, palate, vestibule, and alveolar mucosa in edentulous regions. Female patients are affected more than male patients.[12,13] This lesion has been reported after allogenic bone marrow transplants.[16]

On microscopic examination, clusters of polymorphonuclear leukocytes are present in some areas of the granulation tissue, especially areas adjacent to the necrotic or ulcerated surface (see Fig. 10-9).

Differential diagnosis The only additional considerations to the differential diagnosis entities listed in the box on p. 136 is that ulcerated exophytic lesions are stressed.

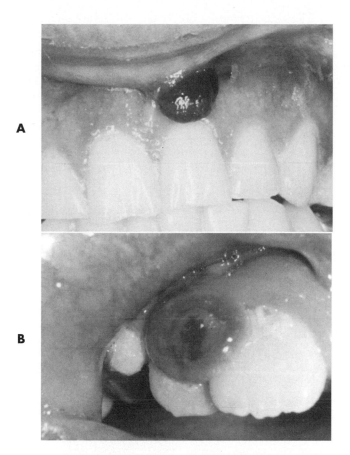

Fig. 10-10. **A,** Hormonal tumor. This IH lesion was present in a girl at puberty. Poor hygiene was evident, and a distal caries was present on right central incisor. **B,** Kaposi's sarcoma in the labial gingiva of a patient with AIDS. This reddish polypoid to nodular lesion may mimic the clinical appearance of IH lesions. (**B** courtesy S. Silverman, San Francisco.)

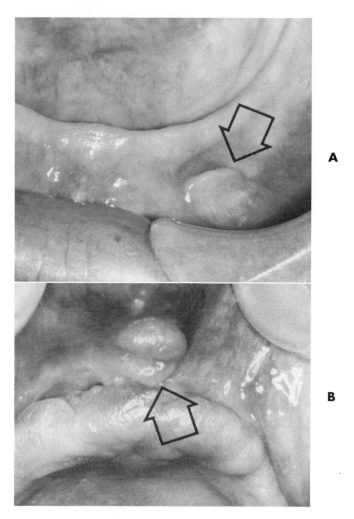

Fig. 10-11. Epulis fissuratum.

Management See the section on the management of IH lesions.

Hormonal Tumor

Some clinicians believe that IH lesions occurring during puberty and pregnancy are a special group. It is thought that the increased incidence during these periods may be related to the higher levels of sex hormones. Other researchers lump the tumors with all the IH lesions or with pyogenic granuloma.

These IH lesions of the gingivae characteristically involve the interdental papillae and are usually deep red (Fig. 10-10, *A* and Plate B). One study involving gingival lesions during puberty concluded that oral hygiene is probably a more important causative factor than steroid hormone levels.[17]

There is a significant increase of these lesions during pregnancy, particularly during the first and second trimester.[18] The physiologic changes induced by increased levels of estrogen and the markedly increased levels of progesterone may be responsible.[18-20] These hormones may exert their greatest effect on the en-

dothelium and not on special receptors, which are quite sparse.[18]

Proper management dictates professional cleaning and scaling and supervised home care. This effects a marked shrinkage in the lesion. The resultant FH lesion can be excised after parturition.

Epulis Fissuratum

Epulis fissuratum is an IH lesion observed at the borders of ill-fitting dentures. In most instances the dental flanges overextend secondary to alveolar bone resorption and settling of the denture.

Features The exophytic, often elongated lesion usually has at least one cleft into which the denture flange fits, with a proliferation of tissue on each side (Figs. 10-11 and 10-12, *A* and Plate A).

Most of these lesions are asymptomatic; there is a greater incidence in the maxilla than in the mandible, and the anterior regions of both jaws are more often affected than the posterior regions.[21] The lesions occur most often under the buccal and labial flanges and are seen predominantly in female patients.[21] Epulides fissurata are found

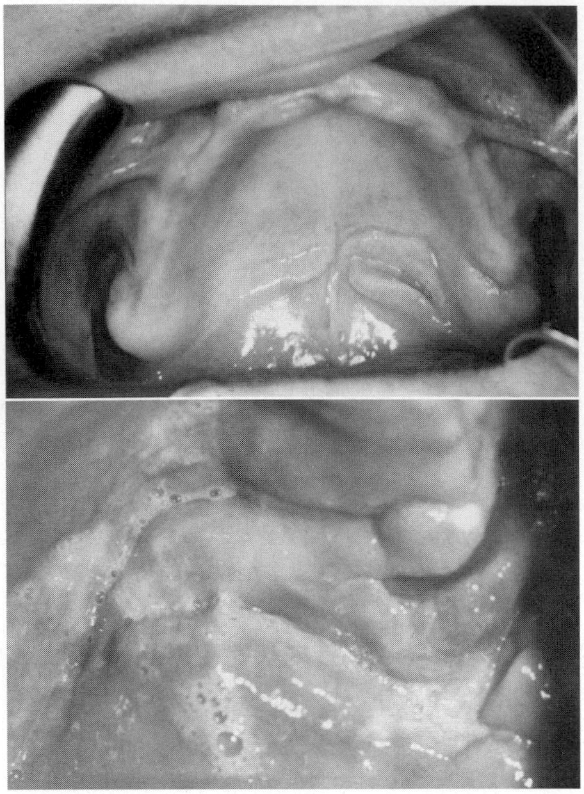

Fig. 10-12. Palatal growths posterior to denture flanges. **A,** Epulis fissuratum. **B,** Malignant SGT. Note the progressive fissuring.

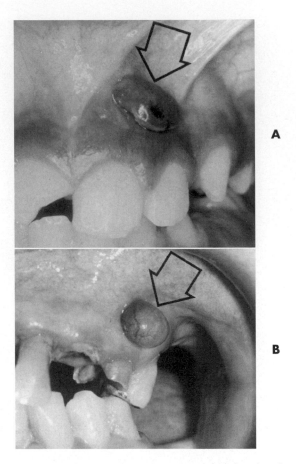

Fig. 10-13. **A,** Parulis. IH lesion at the mucosal draining site of a chronic alveolar abscess. **B,** The lesion contains pus and is really a soft tissue abscess.

in patients from childhood to old age but are seen more often in patients over 40 years of age.

Differential diagnosis The frequency of occurrence of the epulis fissuratum far exceeds that of any other exophytic lesion at the periphery of dentures. However the possibility of malignancy must be considered in each case: squamous and verrucous carcinomas, minor salivary gland tumors (SGTs), metastatic tumors, osteosarcoma, and down-reaching maxillary sinus malignancies (Figs. 10-12 and 10-25).

Management Small, red lesions composed mostly of inflamed tissue and some hyperplasia may subside in 2 or 3 weeks if the denture flange is reduced without further treatment. Larger, more fibrosed lesions will require excision, perhaps combined with a sulcus-deepening procedure. In either case a new, well-adapted denture should be fabricated, or at least the current appliance should be adjusted and rebased. Microscopic examination of excised tissue is always mandatory.

Parulis

A parulis is a small, IH type of lesion that develops on the alveolar mucosa at the oral terminus of a draining sinus (Fig. 10-13 and Plate A). This lesion usually accompanies a draining chronic alveolar abscess in children. The maxillolabial and buccoalveolar mucosae are the most frequent sites (see Fig. 10-13), but the mandibuloalveolar mucosa and palate may also be involved (see Fig. 13-6).

Slight digital pressure on the periphery of a parulis may force a drop of pus from the sinus opening, and this is almost pathognomonic.

The lesion usually regresses spontaneously after the chronic odontogenic infection has been eliminated. If size is considerable and there is a substantial amount of fibrosis, however, the lesion regresses somewhat and then persists as FH.

Rarely, a draining osteomyelitis or infected malignant tumor may produce a similar appearance.

Papillary Hyperplasia of the Palate

The IH lesion known as *papillary hyperplasia of the palate (PHP)* (palatine papillomatosis) occurs almost exclusively on the palate beneath a complete or partial removable denture. It is more commonly associated with a flipper-type partial denture or a full denture. Approximately 10% of the people who wear maxillary dentures have this condition,[9] and most wear their dentures continuously. Although its cause is not well understood, PHP appears to be related to the frictional irritation produced

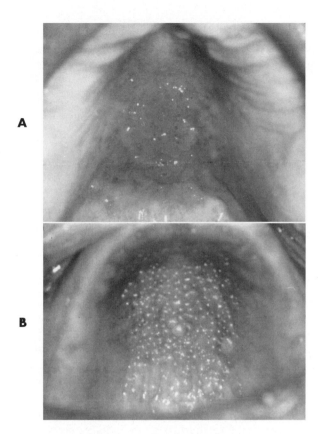

Fig. 10-14. PHP. **A,** Early inflammatory stage. **B,** Later, fibrosed stage. (**B** courtesy S. Fischman, Buffalo, NY.)

by loose-fitting dentures on the palatine tissue. *Candida albicans* may play an etiologic role. Cases of dentate PHP have been reported in homosexual AIDS patients; these were associated with candidal infection.[22]

Features A small region in the vault or perhaps the whole palatine mucosa under the denture may be covered with numerous small, painless papular or polypoid masses that are seldom over 0.3 cm in diameter (Fig. 10-14 and Plate A). As with all the other IH lesions, these masses are red and soft and bleed easily in the inflammatory stage, when they become fibrosed; however, they are firm and pale pink.

Differential diagnosis Since PHP occurs almost exclusively on the palate under a full or partial removable denture, it can seldom be confused with other lesions.

Nicotine stomatitis may also feature multiple small nodules on the palate, which are reddish before hyperkeratosis develops. The following observations aid in the differentiation of this condition from inflammatory papillary hyperplasia:

1. Nicotine stomatitis on the hard palate occurs almost exclusively in pipe smokers who do *not* wear full maxillary dentures.
2. The pattern in nicotine stomatitis is linear and angular, and the segments are flatter and broader but less elevated.

3. The segments in nicotine stomatitis have a characteristic red dot in their approximate center, which is not seen in PHP (see Fig. 8-11).

In unusual cases the clinician may consult the list of rare entities catalogued at the beginning of this chapter, in the column of rare multiple lesions. Darier's disease, multiple fibroepithelial hyperplasia, focal epithelial hyperplasia, and candidal proliferation[22] especially need to be considered (see Figs. 10-37 and 10-39).

Management The patient must be persuaded to remove the denture at night to rest the tissues. If the condition is in the IH stage, the placement of a soft tissue–conditioning liner in the denture may curb the inflammatory response and reduce the size and extent of the polypoid masses, possibly to such a degree that surgery is not necessary.

In fibrosed (FH) cases, surgical removal is usually required, and the denture containing a surgical dressing may be used as a stent. Methods of removal include surgical curettage, electrosurgery, cryosurgery, and mucobrasion.[23]

The following procedure has been recommended: loop-knife surgery, that requires a modified razor blade attached in a bow shape to a holder. The cutting edge is drawn from the back to the front of the site in continuous strokes, removing strips of hyperplastic tissue with clean incisions.[24-26] Although inflammatory papillary hyperplasia does not show malignant tendencies, any excised tissue should be examined microscopically. A new denture that is well adapted to the oral tissues should then be fabricated.

Peripheral Giant Cell Lesion

The peripheral giant cell lesion (granuloma) is an IH type of lesion that probably involves a reactive response in the periosteum, periodontal ligament, and gingiva. It is set apart from other IH lesions by the presence of multinucleated giant cells whose origin is yet undetermined.[9]

Features Microscopic examination shows varying degrees of inflammation and vascularity with a scattering of the aforementioned giant cells. Extravasated erythrocytes and varying amounts of hemosiderin exist. The lesion may be bluish because of this pigment or unoxygenated erythrocytes near the periphery (Fig. 10-15), or the lesion may be red to pale pink, depending on the proportions of collagen and vascular components present. Red is the predominant color.[27]

The lesions are polypoid or nodular;[13,27] located on the gingiva or edentulous alveolar ridge; rubbery to soft on palpation;[27] found predominantly in whites;[28] and more common in the mandible,[27-29] where the premolar or molar region predominates.[27] Although all ages may be affected, there is a relative predilection for the 30 to 70 age-group,[27] and a greater number of women are affected.[29] There may be a cupping type of resorption in the underlying bone.

Differential diagnosis The differential diagnosis of pink or red lesions is identical to that of IH lesions (see p. 196). The differential diagnosis for the bluish variety is discussed in Chapter 12.

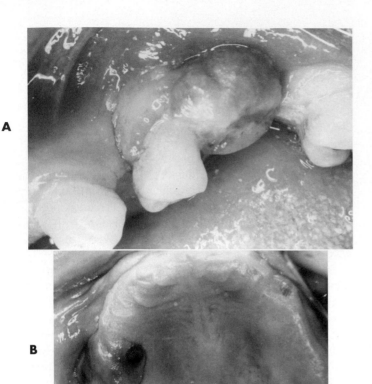

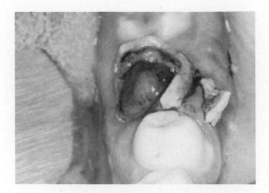

Fig. 10-16. Pulp polyp.

Fig. 10-15. Bluish IH and peripheral giant cell lesions (granulomas). **A,** Lesions on the gingiva distal to the second premolar. **B,** The pressure of the maxillary denture caused the lesion to be flatter than usual. (Courtesy S. Svalina, Maywood, Ill.)

Management All lesions clinically identified as peripheral giant cell lesion should be excised with a border of normal tissue, and the specimen should be examined microscopically. Since there is some inclination to suspect the role played by chronic trauma in the formation of this lesion, all chronic irritants should be eliminated. Because of the recurrence rate of approximately 10%,[27] close follow-up is indicated. Also, peripheral giant cell lesions of hyperparathyroidism may manifest as exophytic giant cell granulomas.[30,31] As a result, hyperparathyroidism and central giant cell granuloma should be considered in the workup (see Chapter 23).

Pulp Polyp

An IH lesion of the pulp tissue occurs when caries have destroyed part or all the tooth crown covering the pulp chamber (Fig. 10-16). The pulp polyp (chronic hyperplastic pulpitis, pulpitis aperta) is an uncommon lesion observed mostly in the deciduous and permanent first molars of children and young adults. The lesion acquires a stratified squamous covering, apparently as the result of a fortuitous grafting of vital exfoliated epithelial cells from the adjacent oral mucosa. Its histologic

characteristics are identical to those of the other types of IH lesions.

Differential diagnosis Occasionally a flap of adjacent gingiva extends into a large proximal carious lesion and appears to be a chronic hyperplastic pulpitis. Careful examination, however, discloses that the exophytic growth is continuous with the gingiva rather than the pulp. The occurrence of any other type of lesion growing from the pulp is too rare to be considered in this text.

Management The two ways of treating a pulp polyp are conservation of the tooth (through endodontic procedures followed by a full coverage) and extraction of the tooth.

Epulis Granulomatosum

Epulis granulomatosum is the specific IH type of lesion that grows from a tooth socket after the tooth has been extracted or otherwise lost (Fig. 10-17). The precipitating cause in most cases is a sharp spicule of bone left in the walls of the socket. The growth may become apparent in a week or two after the loss of the tooth, and the clinical characteristics are similar to those of other IH lesions.

Differential diagnosis The two other lesions that might be confused with an epulis granulomatosum are an antral polyp protruding into the oral cavity through a maxillary molar or premolar socket and a malignant tumor growing from a recent extraction (see Fig. 10-17). In addition, herniation of the antral membrane through an extraction site has been reported.[32] In most cases a radiograph helps the clinician identify either entity.

In the case of a malignant mesenchymal lesion growing out of a recent extraction wound, a radiograph usually shows bony destruction or a combined radiolucent-radiopaque lesion.

The oroantral fistula that permits the extrusion of an antral polyp often is evident as a well-defined loss of bone from the antral floor. If antral polyps are present, the patient should be referred to a surgical specialist for management and for confirmation that the "polyp" is not an antral malignancy.

Management Careful inspection of the socket and removal of any bony spicules at the time the tooth is ex-

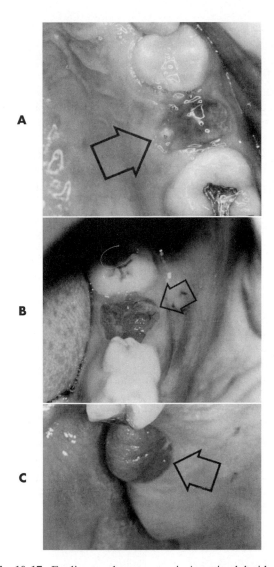

Fig. 10-17. Epulis granulomatosum. **A,** A retained deciduous root was the irritating factor in this case. **B,** Sharp, bony spicules remaining in an extraction socket caused this lesion. **C,** This lesion proved to be an antral polyp that had extruded through a socket with an oroantral fistula. (**B** courtesy P. Akers, Chicago; **C** courtesy P.D. Toto, Waukegan, Ill.)

tracted prevent the formation of an epulis granulomatosum. Treatment requires the excision of the lesion and a careful curettage of the alveolus to ensure the elimination of irritating bony spicules. Because the growth might be malignant, the excised tissue should be examined microscopically.

Acquired Hemangioma

A majority of hemangiomas are congenital, but some are acquired later in life. Some of the acquired capillary hemangiomas of the oral cavity may develop from IH lesions mostly on the gingivae. The conditions may be right for certain IH lesions with many patent capillaries to develop significant blood flow during the IH stage. Such capillary systems remain after the irritant has been

eliminated and the inflammation subsides. The resultant lesion is usually nodular and bluish-red, usually bleeds easily, and may blanch on pressure.

Indicated treatment is sclerosis, excision, or perhaps a combination of these modalities after determination of the blood supply to the lesion.

Peripheral Fibroma with Calcification

The peripheral fibroma with calcification (PFC) (peripheral ossifying fibroma) is a benign overgrowth of gingival tissue that most oral pathologists consider to be a type of IH lesion. It is thought to involve the periodontal ligament superficially, and it often contains calcified deposits resembling cementum, or osteocementum,[9] scattered throughout a background of fibrous tissue. If the calcified element is significant, radiopaque foci within the soft tissue tumor mass are observed on radiographs (Fig. 10-18). Papers have clearly differentiated its characteristic features from those of the central odontogenic fibroma, which on rare occasions may occur peripherally and is referred to as the *peripheral odontogenic fibroma, WHO-type.*[33,34] The latter lesion contains odontogenic epithelium.[35,36] One study indicates that PFC is more common than previously realized: 46.5% of fibrous epulides contained calcifications.[37]

This lesion is also included with the mixed radiolucent-radiopaque lesions in Chapter 25, in the section on the differential diagnosis of osteosarcoma.

Features PFC occurs on the gingiva and usually involves the interdental papillae (see Fig. 10-18). The lesion may cause a separation of the adjacent teeth, and occasionally minimal bone resorption can be seen beneath the lesion. Some 50% occur in patients between the ages of 5 and 25 years, predomintly female patients. A total of 80% of the lesions occur anteriorly to the molar areas,[38] over 50% occur in the incisor and canine region,[9] and 60% occur in the maxilla.[34]

As with other IH lesions, causative irritants can usually be identified, and early inflammatory and late fibrotic stages are typical. The fibrotic PFC may be more common.

Differential diagnosis The lesions that need to be considered in the differential diagnosis of PFC are listed in the box above.

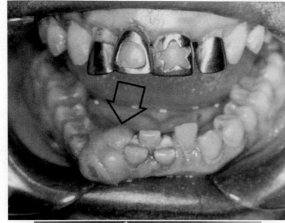

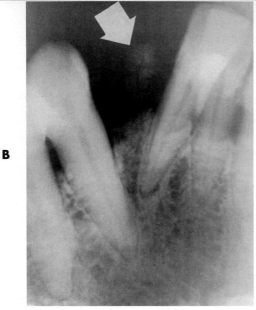

Fig. 10-18. Peripheral fibroma with calcification. **A,** The lesion *(arrow)* has caused a separation of the lateral incisor and canine. **B,** Radiograph. The arrow indicates calcification within the mass.

Chondrosarcoma and osteogenic sarcoma, considered together, are less frequent gingival lesions than PFC. Although a slight bony resorption may occur beneath the PFC, more worrisome bony changes typically are seen with malignant lesions. A bandlike asymmetric widening of the periodontal ligaments of involved teeth is another finding suggestive of chondrosarcoma and osteogenic sarcoma but is not a feature of PFC (see Fig. 21-12).
Management PFC should be excised and special care taken to remove the lesion's attachment in the periodontal ligament and alveolar bone. As a rule, the adjacent teeth do not have to be extracted. Although the recurrence rate is 13% to 16%,[33,34,39] management is not a problem. All excised tissue should be examined microscopically.

MUCOCELE AND RANULA

The mucocele and ranula are retention phenomena of the minor salivary glands and the sublingual (major) salivary glands, respectively. They are discussed in detail in Chapter 12 as bluish lesions.

Differential Diagnosis

When the mucosal covering is thicker than usual or the lesion is not superficial, the appearance is pink, not bluish. It is soft to rubbery in consistency and is fluctuant but not emptiable.

In such instances it must be differentiated from a superficial cyst, lipoma, plexiform neurofibroma, relatively deep cavernous hemangioma, lymphangioma, and mucus-producing salivary gland tumor.

If aspiration of the lesion produces a sticky, viscous, clear, mucuslike fluid, all the preceding lesions can be eliminated except the mucus-producing salivary gland tumors (SGTs). These lesions are uncommon.

Mucoceles occur almost 80% of the time on the lower lip[40] and rarely on the palate. Mucus-producing malignant SGTs (e.g., mucoepidermoid tumor, mucous adenocarcinoma) occur most often on the posterior hard palate, retromolar area, and posterolateral aspect of the floor of the mouth. An induration at the base of a retention phenomenon may be just fibrous tissue, but it should alert the clinician to the possibility of a malignant tumor.

Management

If the conservative approach of marsupialization is followed, the base of the lesion must be examined carefully for pathosis, and cautious periodic follow-up must be maintained. Clinicians may choose complete excision. Specimens must be examined microscopically.

HEMANGIOMA, LYMPHANGIOMA, AND VARICOSITY

Hemangiomas, lymphangiomas, and varicosities are discussed as bluish lesions in Chapter 12.

If a hemangioma, lymphangioma, or varicosity is deep in the tissue, its bluish color is masked, and it is seen as a pink, smooth, nodular or dome-shaped lesion.

The differential diagnosis of such lesions is similar to that of the mucocele and ranula in that significant information can be obtained by sampling the material within the lesion by aspiration, whether the aspirate be mucus; pus; red blood; blue blood; or foamy, colorless lymph fluid.

CENTRAL EXOPHYTIC LESIONS

Central lesions of the jawbones frequently produce exophytic masses as the result of expansion, erosion, or invasion. Consequently, for the differential diagnosis of oral lesions, the possibility that an exophytic mass could be central in origin must always be considered. Usually a complete examination, including a history and clinical and radiographic surveys, indicates whether the lesion is central in origin. Since lesions of bone are discussed in

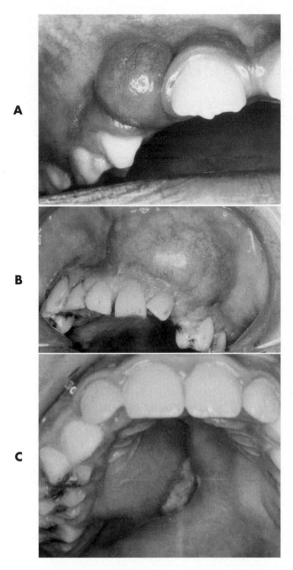

Fig. 10-19. Exophytic lesions that are central in origin. **A,** Eruption cyst. **B,** Dentigerous cyst. **C,** Palatine space abscess from a maxillary molar. (**A** courtesy D. Bonomo, Flossmoor, Ill; **B** courtesy R. Nolan, Williston, ND.)

detail in Part III, only the more common pathoses that may produce these exophytic growths are listed here (Fig. 10-19):

- Benign tumors
- Cysts
- Infections
- Malignant tumors
- Odontogenic tumors

Soft tissue abscesses, resulting from odontogenic infection, are central in origin, but because their peripheral manifestations are usually exophytic dome-shaped masses (see Fig. 10-19), they must often be considered in the differential diagnosis of peripheral lesions. Such abscesses are readily recognized by their location; by the fact that they are rubbery, fluctuant, painful, and hot; and by the fact that they yield pus on aspiration. Their odontogenic origins can usually be

---

HPV STRAINS ASSOCIATED WITH CLINICAL LESIONS

- Verruca vulgaris—types 2 and 57[42,43]
- Oral papilloma—types 6 and 11[44]
- CA—types 6 and 11[45]

---

traced by careful examination. Gingival abscesses are included here.

Oral Papilloma, Verruca Vulgaris, and Condyloma Acuminatum

Oral papilloma, verruca vulgaris and condyloma acuminatum (CA) are benign, rough-surfaced exophytic hyperplasias of epithelial tissue (see Fig. 10-1) purportedly caused by human papillomavirus (HPV): These belong to the papovavirus group.[41-44] Verruca vulgaris, the common wart of the skin, is not a common oral lesion when it is invariably white. Fig. 10-1, *E* shows its characteristic verrucous shape with a base almost as wide as its greatest diameter. The superior surface is a firm, horny, rough plateau. The oral papilloma has long been recognized as a relatively common oral lesion (Fig. 10-20). CA is known as the *common venereal wart* that now is frequently seen in the oral cavity. Oral CAs are particularly common in HIV-positive individuals.[41] Although skin warts, papillomas, and CAs can be solitary lesions, multiple lesions often develop as a result of autoinnoculation (Fig. 10-21). Clinically and microscopically, oral papillomas and oral CAs cannot always be differentiated, although if genital warts are present this would suggest that the oral lesion is probably a CA. The box above indicates the different strains of HPV associated with the three lesions using in situ hybridization and polymerase chain reaction techniques.

Features

Oral papillomas and CAs are papillomatous in shape, although multiple CAs may clump and share a sessile base (see Figs. 8-22, *C* and 10-1, *D* and Plate F). They show slender fronds or arms of surface epithelium that have undergone hyperplasia often in a clumplike manner; secondary branching occurs as well. These rough-surfaced lesions have a pebbled surface, often with prominent clefting (see Figs. 10-20 and 33-3). A thin core of mesenchymal tissue supports the epithelial fronds (see Fig. 10-20). CAs may have extensive acanthosis.[45] Usually surface keratinization is mild, so the lesions are pink. Lesions that retain a significant thickness of keratin are white (see Fig. 8-22). Oral verrucae vulgarus occur on the palate 50% of the time, and the next most common site is the commissures.[43] Mean age is approximately 15 years.[43]

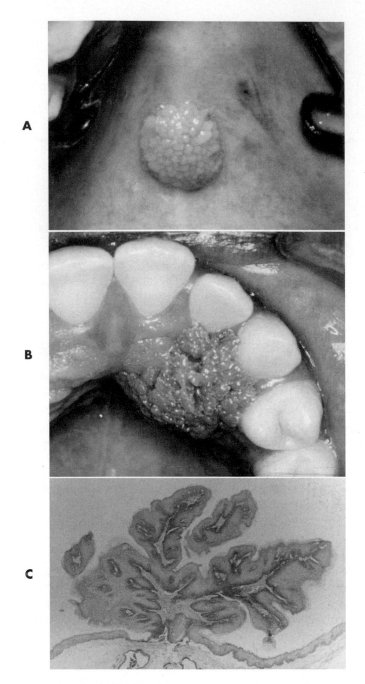

Fig. 10-20. Pink papillomas and CAs. Both lesions were pedunculated. Also note the overall symmetry and homogeneous surface pattern. **A,** Midline of the palate. **B,** Maxillo lingual alveolus (pedunculated). **C,** Low-power microscopy of papilloma.

The oral papilloma is seldom larger than 1 cm in diameter. Approximately a third of these lesions occur on the tongue; the remaining sites, in order of descending frequency, are the palate, buccal mucosa, gingivae, lips, mandibular ridge, and floor of the mouth.[46] Most cases occur in patients ages 21 through 50 years with an average age of 38 years.[46] Oral papillomas do not show a tendency for malignant change.

Papillomas, verrucae vulgaris, and CAs are symmetric lesions that have a uniform pattern, whether the surface is

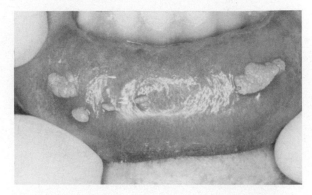

Fig. 10-21. Multiple CAs on the mucosa of the lower lip. (Courtesy S. Smith, Chicago.)

hornified, is tight pebbly (see Fig. 10-20, *A*), or has longer fronds with deeper recesses (see Fig. 10-20, *B*).

Differential Diagnosis

See the section on differential diagnosis of SCC.

Management

Single lesions are best removed by surgery, including blade excision, laser, heat cautery, or cryosurgery. Any excised tissue *must* be submitted for microscopic study. Fig. 10-22 shows a miniature lesion that was assigned a working diagnosis of papilloma and CA but proved to have carcinoma in situ. Podophyllin resin can be used to manage multiple lesions. One or two topical applications may be given per week over 4 to 8 weeks.[47] Although interferon-α is very effective against HPV with intralesional injection, this costly and painful procedure should be used only as a last resort.

EXOPHYTIC SQUAMOUS CELL CARCINOMA

SCC is discussed in Chapter 5 as a red lesion, in Chapter 8 as a white lesion, in Chapter 9 as a red and white lesion, in Chapter 11 as an ulcerative lesion, and in Chapter 21 as a radiolucent lesion. Chapter 33 gives an extensive discussion of SCC. In this chapter the exophytic variety of SCC is described.

Features

Approximately 55% of all the SCCs of the tongue are exophytic-type lesions.[48] Exophytic carcinoma occurs most often on the lateral borders of the tongue, the floor of the mouth, and the soft palate.

All exophytic SCCs have a rough surface. They are usually irregular in shape and, if not totally white, are usually pink to red with possibly some white. Low-grade lesions, especially early ones, may have a pebbly surface not unlike a papilloma. However, SCC is *not* symmetric, and the surface pattern is not uniform but rather varies considerably (Figs. 10-22 and 10-23 and Plates H and I). Ulceration may be present (Fig. 10-24), especially in larger fungating lesions in which the sur-

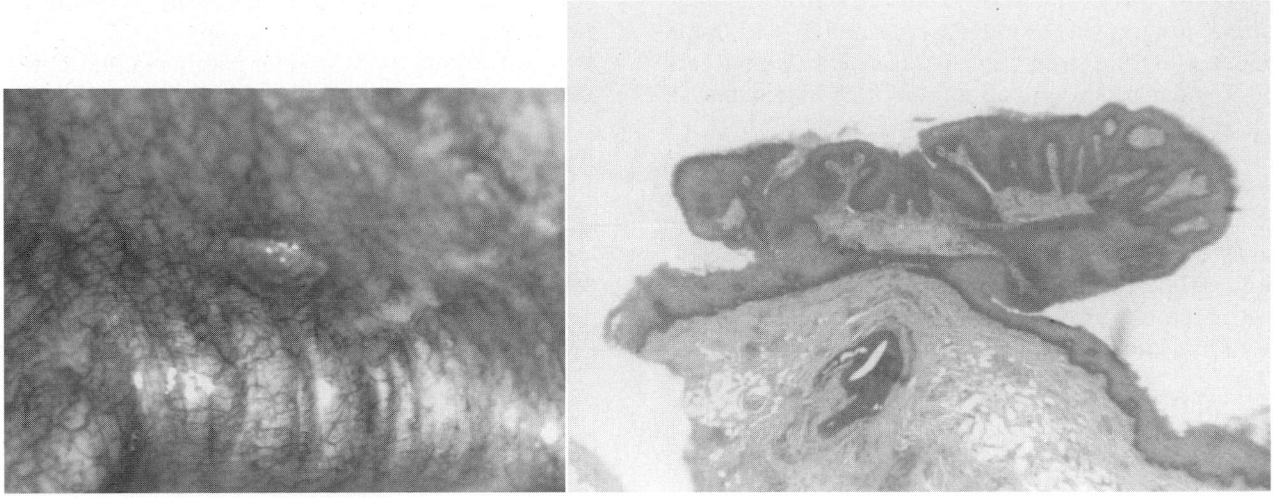

Fig. 10-22. Miniature exophytic lesion not more than 0.4 cm across, showing carcinoma in situ. **A,** Clinical photograph of lesion on mucosa of upper lip. **B,** Low-power microscopy of excisional biopsy. Note the definite asymmetry, which suggests that the lesion may not be benign.

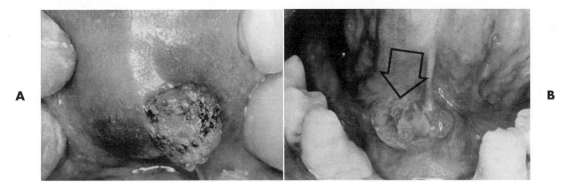

Fig. 10-23. "Papillary" SCC. **A,** SCC on the maxillary lip mucosa. Notice the asymmetry and uneven pebbly pattern. Early invasion was observed microscopically. The smooth swelling under the lesion represents a pool of local anesthetic solution. **B,** Small lesion in floor of the mouth. Note the asymmetry and the lack of uniformity in the surface pattern.

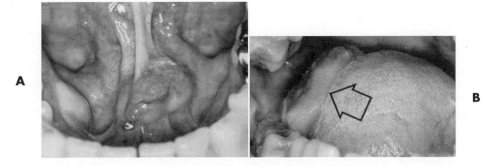

Fig. 10-24. Unusual exophytic SCC with partially *smooth* surfaces. Near the bases the peripheries are smooth, whereas the "crown" surfaces are rough and ulcerated. The smooth contours near the bases represent a shell of noncancerous surface epithelium. **A,** Floor of the mouth. **B,** Lateral margin of the tongue.

face may be necrotic and multicolored. Occasionally, exophytic SCC has a smooth collar at the base, where peripheral margins of the mass are formed by nontumor, surface epithelium (see Fig. 10-24). The lesions are painless and firm on palpation, and bleeding is not an early characteristic.

It is generally believed that the majority of exophytic carcinomas are less aggressive than the purely ulcerative varieties, but all lesions must be evaluated on an individual basis. (Prognosis is affected mostly by the histodifferentiation at the invading margin of the neoplasm, rather than at its crown.) Cervical lymph node involvement is the usual route of metastasis.

Differential Diagnosis

The lesions that need to be considered in the differential list of exophytic SCC are found in the boxes. The box below, left, lists lesions that resemble small (early) exophytic SCC, whereas the box below, right, lists large fulminating lesions that may resemble large, ulcerated, necrotic exophytic SCC.

The list in the box below, left, is not surprising, considering the rule that rough-surfaced exophytic lesions have their origins on or in the surface epithelium and those that originate deep to the surface have smooth profiles until they are large enough to be traumatized.

Verrucous carcinoma, although well illustrated as exophytic in Fig. 10-25, is predominantly a flat, wide-based lesion. It has a somewhat uniform surface pebbling. Verrucous carcinoma is less common and slower growing than SCC.

Keratoacanthoma, although common on the skin and even the vermilion border, is a rare oral lesion. It may present as a rough symmetric exophytic lesion with horny keratin occupying a cupped depression on the top of the lesion. When occurring on the lips, it may look clinically identical to well-differentiated exophytic SCC (see Fig. 32-4). Its period of rapid growth followed by stagnation is a helpful differentiating feature.

Pyogenic granuloma may resemble an SCC because it usually has an ulcerated patch on its surface (see Fig. 8-42).

It is softer on palpation and bleeds readily, and usually its instigating irritant can be found. Usually its overall contour is smooth.

Small exophytic SCC, like papilloma and CA, has a rough, often pebbly surface, but unlike papilloma and CA, the surface pattern is *not* uniform, and the shape is asymmetric (see Figs. 10-22 and 23). Consequently an elongated dimension or other irregularities rather than a circular or ovoid one should initiate suspicion. Multiple lesions suggest papilloma and CA; also, these latter entities are softer on palpation than SCC.

Oral verruca vulgaris is an uncommon oral lesion, and its small size and characteristic verrucous appearance with a horny "crown" distinguishes it from SCC.

At the early stage, all of the tumors in the box below, right, (except SCC) are smoothly contoured, nodular or dome-shaped masses covered with normal-appearing mucosa. When these cancers are permitted to grow large and are biopsied or become ulcerated by oral trauma, they can become fulminating and resemble large exophytic SCCs.

Amelanotic melanoma is a rare oral tumor that, when ulcerated, is clinically indistinguishable from an exophytic carcinoma. Because of its low frequency of occurrence, however, it has a low rank in the differential diagnosis.

Peripheral malignant mesenchymal tumors (e.g., fibrosarcoma, myosarcoma, neurosarcoma, liposarcoma) are also rare oral lesions. These malignant mesenchymal tumors become ulcerated in more advanced stages and mimic large exophytic SCCs. Evidence of metastatic involvement of the cervical lymph nodes is unusual in most mesenchymal tumors and strongly supports a diagnosis of SCC. A clinician must conclude, on the basis of the lesion's low incidence, that an ulcerated exophytic lesion is more likely a SCC than a peripheral malignant mesenchymal tumor.

Peripheral metastatic tumors have a relatively low incidence, so they are assigned a low rank in the list of possible entities, unless evidence from the history or examination suggests the presence of a parent tumor elsewhere.

DIFFERENTIAL LIST OF SMALL, ROUGH-SURFACED EXOPHYTIC LESIONS

- Papilloma, verruca vulgaris, and CA
- Pyogenic granuloma
- Exophytic SCC
- Keratoacanthoma
- Exophytic verrucous carcinoma
- Rarities
  - Condyloma latum
  - Raised pseudoepitheliomatous hyperplasia
  - Sialadenoma papilliferum

DIFFERENTIAL LIST OF LARGE, FULMINATING MASSES

- Exophytic SCC
- Minor SGTs
- Soft tissue metastatic tumors
- Peripheral malignant mesenchymal tumors
- Amelanotic melanoma
- Rarities

Malignant SGTs are second to SCCs as the most common oral malignancy. The firm types are considered here. The fluctuant, mucus-producing varieties have necessarily been grouped in the differential diagnosis with retention phenomena. Like the early secondary tumors and early peripheral malignant mesenchymal tumors, the malignant SGTs originate in tissue situated deep to and separate from the surface epithelium. Consequently, in their early stages, they are nodular or dome shaped, have a smooth contour, and are covered with normal-appearing epithelium. Later, when their surfaces become ulcerated because of the trauma of mastication or biopsy or perhaps because of the rupture of retained fluid, they may appear to be malignant (i.e., have ulcerated, necrotic, friable surfaces). At this stage the malignant SGTs may not be readily differentiated from exophytic SCCs. The following clues, however, are helpful:

1. SCC is not as common on the posterior hard palate as malignant SGTs.
2. SGTs occur more frequently in women, whereas SCC occurs 2 to 4 times as frequently in men. The significance of this difference must be modified, however, because approximately 95% of the oral malignancies are SCCs, whereas only about 4% are malignant minor SGTs.
3. Malignant minor SGTs frequently maintain their overall nodular or dome shape even after their surfaces become ulcerated (see Fig. 10-26, *C*).

Many rare oral exophytic lesions, including syphilis, fungal diseases, sarcoidosis, and tuberculosis, may be confused with exophytic SCC, but discussion of these possibilities is beyond the scope of this text.

Management

The management of intraoral SCC is discussed in detail in Chapter 35.

VERRUCOUS CARCINOMA

Verrucous carcinoma frequently has a white keratotic surface (see Fig. 8-25) and is discussed in detail with the white lesions in Chapter 8.

On occasion, verrucous carcinoma develops as a nodular lesion or may present with a reddish, pinkish, and whitish surface (Fig 10-25 and Plate G). Its differential diagnosis in this context is discussed in the differential diagnosis section of exophytic SCC.

MINOR SALIVARY GLAND TUMORS

Most of the minor SGTs are exophytic lesions. The intraoral minor salivary glands are predominantly of the mucous type and are normally distributed throughout the oral mucosa except for the anterior hard palate, attached gingivae, and anterior two thirds of the dorsal surface of the tongue. Unusual cases of SGTs occurring in the latter locations have been reported and are considered to have arisen in ectopic minor salivary glands.

The mucous glands are not attached to the surface mucosa except by the common ducts that drain a cluster of glands. These clusters of mucous glands are situated deep to the surface and usually lie just superficially to the loose connective tissue layer. Consequently, as a tumor originates in these glands and enlarges, it becomes a nodular or dome-shaped exophytic mass with a smooth surface (see Chapter 3).

Because of the great variety of neoplasms that occur in the salivary glands, the establishment and adoption of a uniform classification and nomenclature have been difficult. The boxes on p. 150 give a current classification for benign and malignant SGTs. (With only one or two exceptions, all the tumors occurring in the major salivary glands are also found in the minor salivary glands.)

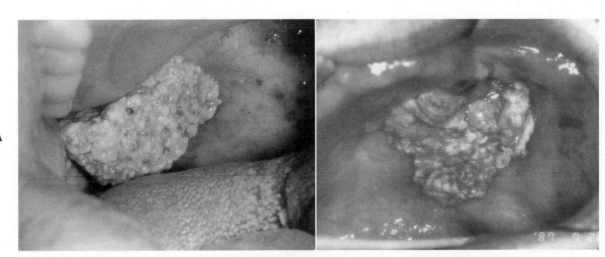

Fig. 10-25. Exophytic verrucous carcinoma. **A,** Note the somewhat uniform, *pebbly,* whitish-pink surface of this slow-growing lesion, which has a relatively pedunculated base. **B,** Broader-based lesion on the palate of an elderly patient. (**A** from Claydon RJ, Jordan JE: Verrucous carcinoma of Ackerman, a distinctive clinicopathologic entity: report of two cases, *J Oral Surg* 36:564-567, 1978; **B** courtesy B. Barker, Kansas City, Mo.)

CLASSIFICATION OF BENIGN SGTS AND ADENOMAS

- Benign mixed tumor (pleomorphic adenoma)
- Monomorphic adenoma
  - Basal cell adenoma
  - Canalicular adenoma
  - Myoepithelioma
  - Sebaceous adenoma
  - Oncocytoma
  - Papillary cystadenoma lymphomatosum
- Ductal papilloma
  - Sialadenoma papilliferum
  - Inverted ductal papilloma
  - Intraductal papilloma

Modified from Seifert G, Brocheriou C, Cardesa A, Eveson JW: WHO international classification of tumors. Tentative histological classification of salivary gland tumors, *Pathol Res Pract* 186:555-581, 1990; as adapted from Regezi J, Sciubba J: *Oral pathology: clinical-pathologic correlations,* ed 2, Philadelphia, 1993, Saunders.

CLASSIFICATION OF SALIVARY GLAND ADENOCARCINOMAS

- Mucoepidermoid carcinoma
- Adenoid cystic carcinoma
- Acinic cell carcinoma
- Carcinoma ex mixed tumor and malignant mixed tumor
- Epimyoepithelial carcinoma
- Polymorphous low-grade adenocarcinoma
- Salivary duct carcinoma
- Basal cell adenocarcinoma
- Sebaceous adenocarcinoma
- Oncocytic adenocarcinoma
- Adenocarcinoma (not otherwise specified)

Classification According to Biologic Behavior

- Low grade
  - Mucoepidermoid carcinoma (low grade)
  - Acinic cell carcinoma
  - Polymorphous low-grade adenocarcinoma
  - Basal cell adenocarcinoma
- Intermediate grade
  - Mucoepidermoid carcinoma (intermediate grade)
  - Epimyoepithelial carcinoma
  - Sebaceous adenocarcinoma
- High grade
  - Mucoepidermoid carcinoma (high grade)
  - Adenoid cystic carcinoma
  - Carcinoma ex mixed tumor and malignant mixed tumor
  - Salivary duct carcinoma
  - SCC
  - Oncocytic adenocarcinoma

Modified from Seifert G, Brocheriou C, Cardesa A, Eveson JW: WHO international classification of tumors. Tentative histological classification of salivary gland tumors, *Pathol Res Pract* 186:555-581, 1990; as adapted from Regezi J, Sciubba J, *Oral pathology: clinical-pathologic correlations,* ed 2, Philadelphia, 1993, Saunders.

Benign vs. Malignant

There are no clinical features of SGTs that helps the diagnostician determine whether the masses are malignant or benign, although the box on p. 151, top, lists features that are nevertheless helpful. The clinical appearances of both lesions are so similar that in most cases they cannot be ranked in the working diagnosis according to its malignancy or lack of malignancy.

Early benign and malignant minor SGTs are usually nodular or dome-shaped elevations with smooth contours, and the overlying mucosa is normal or appears smoother and glossier because of the tension created by the underlying expanding tumor (Figs. 10-26 and 10-27, *E* and *G* and Plate I, 11). As the overlying mucosa becomes thinned by the expanding tumor and traumatized during mastication, the pooled mucus ruptures, or a biopsy of the growth is made, an ulcer appears that is persistent and usually becomes necrotic, so ulceration is not a criterion for malignancy of minor SGT.

Likewise, the firmness (induration) of a lesion is no more help than ulceration in the differential diagnosis because the majority of malignant and benign tumors are firm. The fact that some malignant and benign SGTs are moderately soft and fluctuant or have soft and firm areas further emphasizes this point.

The minor SGTs that are almost categorically firm to palpation are listed in the box on p. 151, middle. They are ranked, as much as possible, in order of frequency of occurrence.

The firmness in these tumors results from the presence of dense aggregates, nests, and cords of closely packed tumor cells, fibrous tissue, and hyaline areas, as well as cartilage-like and bonelike tissue (mixed tumor).

The moderately soft and frequently fluctuant minor SGTs are listed in the box on p. 151, bottom. Again, an attempt has been made to arrange them in descending order of incidence.

The softness of these tumors results from the lack of dense cell aggregates, the fluid produced, and the consequent retention phenomena. Mucus is produced in well-differentiated mucoepidermoid tumors and in mucous adenocarcinomas, whereas other fluid is produced in Warthin's tumor. The tumors in this group may be fluctuant because of the enclosed fluid in a superficial location.

Features

Minor SGTs are often fully movable, spherical or ovoid masses when they occur in the lining mucosa. Irregular, fixed masses in these locations suggest fibrosis or malignancy. Minor SGTs situated in masticatory mucosa are usually nodular or dome shaped and usually immobile. The posterior palate is the most common site of minor SGTs by far. From 47% to 83% of all neoplasms reported

BENIGN VS. MALIGNANT FEATURES

- Malignant SGT occurs in older patients: 49.8 years vs. 36.5 years.[49]
- Margins as described by magnetic resonance imaging are poorly defined (malignant) vs. well defined (benign).[50]
- Erosion of bone is ragged and vague vs. well defined and smooth.
- Highly malignant types have a faster growth or a sudden spurt.

FIRM MINOR SGTS

- Benign mixed tumor
- Adenoid cystic carcinoma
- Mucoepidermoid carcinoma of high-grade malignancy
- Acinic cell carcinoma
- Carcinoma ex mixed tumor and malignant mixed tumor
- Oncocytoma
- Oncocytic adenocarcinoma

MODERATELY SOFT MINOR SGTS

- Well-differentiated mucoepidermoid carcinoma
- Mucus-producing adenocarcinoma
- Papillary cystadenoma lymphomatosum (Warthin's tumor)

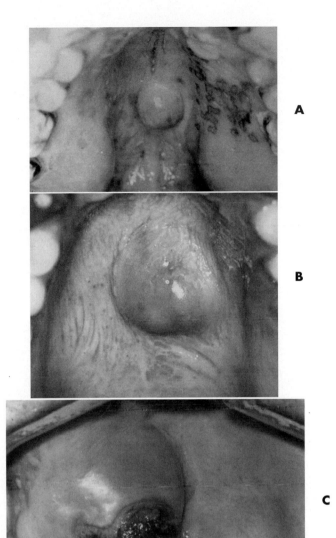

Fig. 10-26. Minor SGTs. **A** and **B**, Benign mixed tumors. **C**, Adenoid cystic carcinoma that became ulcerated after an incisional biopsy. (**B** and **C** courtesy E. Kasper, Maywood, Ill.)

in large studies were found in this location.[49,51-59] Most of the remainder occurred in the buccal mucosa or retromolar region and the upper lip, whereas a few were located on the tongue, gingivae, bone, lower lip, and floor of the mouth.[49,52-54] The upper lip is 10 times more likely to be involved than the lower lip.[60]

Most studies indicate that female patients are affected more frequently than male patients, a ratio of 1.6 or 1.2 to 1.[49-52] One study showed male and female patients equally affected.[57] Patients with benign minor SGTs are younger than those with the malignant variety: 36.5 vs. 49.8.[49]

Benign tumors are more common: The study results range from 54% to 72%.[53,54,56-59] Two studies reported that malignancy was more common: 52% and 66.3%.[49,53]

The mixed tumor is the most common benign type by far. The majority of malignant tumors are of these types: mucoepidermoid carcinoma, adenoid cystic carcinoma, and adenocarcinoma. Ranking according to frequency varies from study to study.[49,51-59]

These tumors may be present and tolerated for several months or even years because they are characteristically asymptomatic. A sudden growth spurt suggests malignant change. The adenoid cystic carcinoma may be painful, especially if it has extended into a perineural space.

Benign minor SGTs may produce a well-defined saucerlike depression in the underlying bone. In contrast, malignant tumors may invade the bone and produce a ragged radiolucent defect with poorly defined borders (see Fig. 21-9). Such tumors positioned on the lateral aspect of the posterior hard palate may destroy the alveolar or palatine bone and invade the maxillary sinus.

The malignant types may spread by hematogenous routes to distant organs and perhaps less often through lymphatic vessels to the cervical lymph nodes. The lungs are the most common site of distant metastasis. In addition

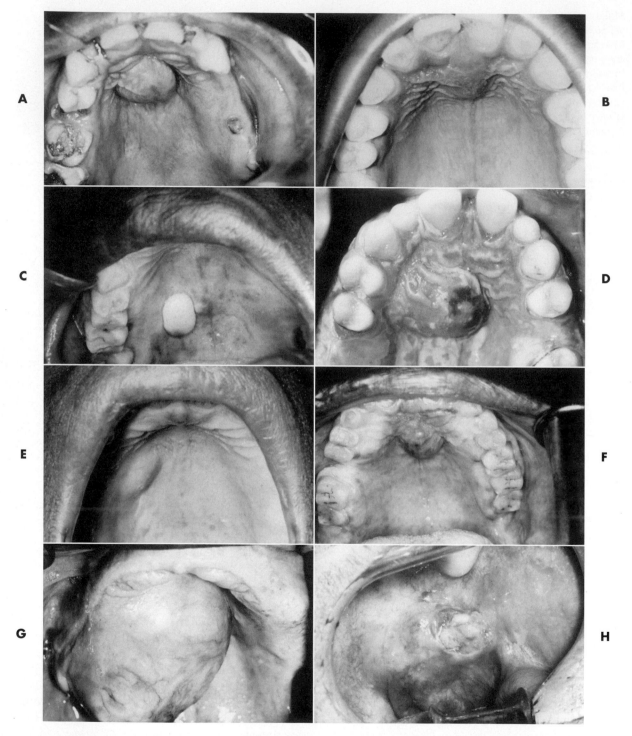

Fig. 10-27. Palatine masses. **A,** Palatine space abscess from an infected lateral incisor tooth. **B,** Nasopalatine cyst. **C,** Fibrous hyperplasia. **D,** Palatine space abscess from the periapical abscess of the first premolar tooth. **E,** Benign mixed tumor. **F,** Small midline fissural cyst of the palate. **G,** Large benign SGT. **H,** Large SCC of the soft palate. Most of the lesion surface is smooth, a very unusual feature. (**B** courtesy W. Heaton, Chicago; **E** courtesy W. Heaton, Chicago; **H** courtesy M. Lehnert, Minneapolis.)

DIFFERENTIAL LIST FOR FIRM MINOR SGT

- Fibrous hyperplasia (see Fig. 10-27, *C*)
- Lingual torus or exostosis (see Fig. 10-6, *A*)
- Benign lymphoid proliferative disease[61,62]
- Lymphoma[63,64]
- Firm mesenchymal tumors
- Necrotizing sialometaplasia
- Metastatic tumor
- Malignancy of maxillary sinus
- Tuberculosis
- Syphilitic gumma
- Rare fungal infections

DIFFERENTIAL LIST FOR SOFT MINOR SGT

- Space abscess (see Fig. 10-27, *D*)
- Inflammatory hyperplasia
- Buccal fat pads
- Retention phenomenon
- Cavernous hemangioma
- Plexiform neurofibroma (see Fig. 10-29, *B* and *C*)
- Amputation neuroma (see Fig. 10-28, *B*)
- Lipoma
- Adenomatoid hyperplasia of minor salivary glands (see Fig. 10-35, *B*)[65-67]

to hematogenous and lymphatic spread, the adenoid cystic carcinoma frequently extends locally along the perineural spaces, and other types also occasionally do this.

Differential Diagnosis

See the section on differential diagnosis of exophytic SCC and the boxes on p. 151.

Firm minor SGTs The lesions that should be considered in the differential diagnosis of firm minor salivary gland tumors are listed in the box above, left.

Soft minor SGTs Several lesions must be considered in the differential diagnosis for a soft fluctuant minor SGT. These are listed in the box above, right.

Adenoid hyperplasia of the minor salivary glands is a rare lesion but mimics soft minor SGTs quite closely (see Fig. 10-35, *B*); over 80% occur on the palate, the predominant age ranges from 26 to 67, and the majority are soft or firm sessile masses covered with normal epithelium.[65,66] Chronic local trauma may play an etiologic role.[66] Although there is a slight male predominance, the other features correspond so closely to minor SGT that they should be included in all differential lists that include minor SGT.

With lipoma, superficial varieties are easily recognized by their softness and yellow color, which is usually overlaid with a clear pattern of minuscule arterial blood vessels. Lipomas are rare in the oral cavity.

Amputation neuromas are soft, smooth lesions that rise from surgery in the area. They may be quite painful.

The plexiform neurofibroma (Fig. 10-29, *C*) is uncommon except in patients with von Recklinghausen's disease. It and the submerged lipoma cannot be differentiated from minor SGT through palpation or visual examination. Aspiration, however, may be productive in the case of soft and fluctuant minor SGT, although not with plexiform neurofibromas or lipomas. A yellow color suggests superficial lipoma.

Cavernous hemangiomas are bluish, whereas deeper ones appear pink. These usually can be emptied by carefully applied digital pressure, and this fact differentiates hemangiomas from mucoceles and soft SGTs.

Retention phenomenona mucoceles) are encountered more often than minor SGTs, but approximately 82% of the former occur on the lower lip, which is not a common site for a minor SGT.[40] Mucoceles are uncommon on the palate, the most common site for minor SGT. In practical terms, mucoceles cannot be clinically differentiated from some malignant tumors containing a superficial pool of mucus, which may show as mucocele-like masses (e.g., mucoepidermoid tumor, mucus-producing adenocarcinoma). Consequently, it is important to remove the base of mucoceles and submit all the tissue for microscopic study. Very close surveillance is necessary if the mucocele is marsupialized.

Ulcerated minor SGTs Ulceration can occur on the usual smooth contours of minor SGT masses resulting from trauma (see Fig. 10-26, *C*). All the masses listed in the boxes can become ulcerated and should be considered in the differential diagnosis of ulcerated minor SGT. In addition, the following should be added: SCC, midline granuloma, and Wegener's granulomatosis.

Management

The recurrence rates for minor SGTs vary greatly from series to series but are relatively high even in the case of benign tumors. This is probably because the original tumor was incompletely excised and residual tumor cells left. Consequently, it is expedient to include a wide margin of normal tissue in the removal of benign or malignant lesions. Frozen sections completed at surgery indicate whether the margins are free of tumor and whether a wider excision should be undertaken. One study reported that 67% of adenoid cystic carcinomas and 18% of benign mixed tumors recurred.[51]

Magnetic resonance imaging yields a better picture of the margins of the adenoid cystic carcinomas and their characteristics than computed tomography.[50] Benign tumors invariably have well-defined margins, whereas malignant neoplasms (minor SGT) usually have irregular ones.[50]

Glandular tumors have a better prognosis than solid ones. A tumor size larger than 4 cm is correlated with a poor prognosis, and an atypical histogram also indicates a shorter survival time.[68] The long-term prognosis for this tumor is generally very poor.[68] Malignant tumors are treated by surgery or a combination of surgery and radiation.

Close posttreatment surveillance should be maintained to detect early recurrences. In malignant cases, chest radiographs every 6 months are imperative to detect the earliest pulmonary metastasis.

PERIPHERAL BENIGN MESENCHYMAL TUMORS

Individual types of oral peripheral mesenchymal tumors are uncommon lesions, but when considered as a group, they demonstrate a more impressive incidence. Such a group would include the following:

- Lipomas
- Myomas (rhabdomyoma and leiomyoma)

- Peripheral nerve tumors (neurofibroma, plexiform type of neurofibroma, schwannoma, traumatic neuroma)

Features

All the peripheral benign mesenchymal tumors are oval, nodular, polypoid, or dome shaped with smooth contours and are characteristically covered with normal mucosa unless chronically traumatized. They may be located on the tongue, buccal mucosa, lips, hard and soft palates, floor of the mouth, and vestibule. They usually are asymptomatic, grow slowly, and can be moved over the deeper tissue. When situated within loose connective tissue, they are often exceptionally movable.

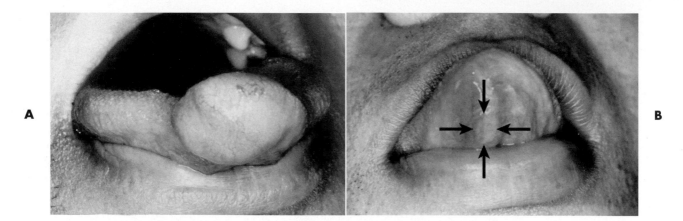

Fig. 10-28. Mesenchymal tumors. **A,** Leiomyoma of the tip of the tongue. **B,** Amputation neuroma on the ventral surface of the tongue *(arrows)*. (From Kelly DE, Harrigan WF: Leiomyoma of the tongue: report of case, *J Oral Surg* 35:316-318, 1977.)

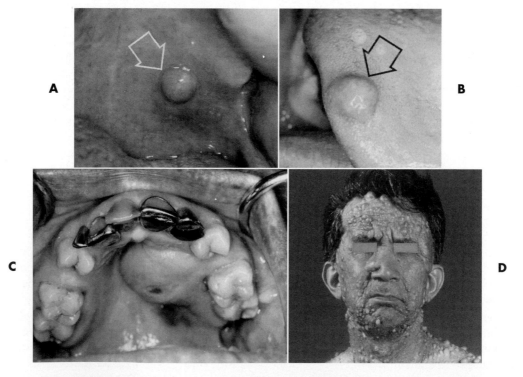

Fig. 10-29. Benign mesenchymal tumors. **A** and **B,** Lipomas. **C,** Neurofibroma on the palate. **D,** Multiple neurofibromatosis. (**C** courtesy R. Nolan, Williston, ND; **D** courtesy P.D. Toto, Waukegan, Ill.)

Although the most frequently occurring true peripheral mesenchymal tumor, the lipoma is an uncommon oral lesion (Fig. 10-29). The lipoma is discussed in detail in Chapter 14.

The remainder of the benign mesenchymal tumors (such as myomas, schwannomas, firm neurofibromas, traumatic neuromas) seldom occur in the oral cavity, although some have been reported on the tongue, lip, buccal mucosa, floor of the mouth, and posterior palate (Figs. 10-28 and 10-29). They are usually firm with discrete borders and, if situated in the loose connective tissue layer, are freely movable.[69,70] Amputation neuromas and plexiform neurofibromas may be soft and fluctuant.

Differential Diagnosis

See the section on differential diagnosis of minor SGTs.

Management

The recommended treatment for peripheral benign mesenchymal tumors is excision, microscopic examination of the tumor tissue, and postoperative surveillance.

NEVUS AND MELANOMA

Nevus and melanoma are uncommon intraoral tumors discussed in detail in Chapter 12 as macular and exophytic brownish, bluish, or black lesions (Fig. 10-30 and Plate J).

An amelanotic melanoma appears as a firm, smoothly contoured, nodular or somewhat polypoid mass covered with normal-appearing mucosa (Fig. 10-31, *A*). The list of possible lesions then must include fibrous hyperplasia and benign mesenchymal tumors. If its surface is ulcerated as the result of trauma, it may mimic a pyogenic granuloma.

As the intraoral amelanotic melanoma grows and is traumatized, its surface ulcerates and becomes necrotic. At this stage, it has the clinical appearance of a malignant tumor. Then based on the incidence of similar-appearing lesions, the possible diagnoses would be ranked as follows: SCC, malignant SGT, peripheral metastatic tumor, malignant primary mesenchymal tumor, and amelanotic melanoma.

PERIPHERAL METASTATIC TUMORS

Peripheral metastatic tumors have been discussed in detail in Chapter 5 as red and exophytic tumors (Plate J). Those with a normal pink surface (see Fig. 10-31 and Plate J) would be included in the differential diagnosis of many of the lesions discussed in this chapter.

Differential Diagnosis

See the section on the differential diagnosis of minor SGTs.

A patient with a history of a tumor elsewhere should prompt the clinician to consider the possibility that the oral lesion is a metastatic tumor. If there is no history of a primary tumor or suggestive symptoms, however, the

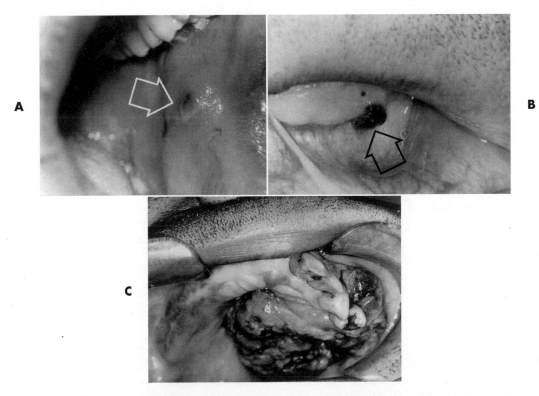

Fig. 10-30. Nevus and melanoma. **A,** Intramucosal nevus. **B,** Melanoma. **C,** Large melanoma. (**A** courtesy E. Kasper, Maywood, Ill; **B** courtesy D. Skuble, Hinsdale, Ill; **C** courtesy R. Oglesby, Stroudsburg, Pa.)

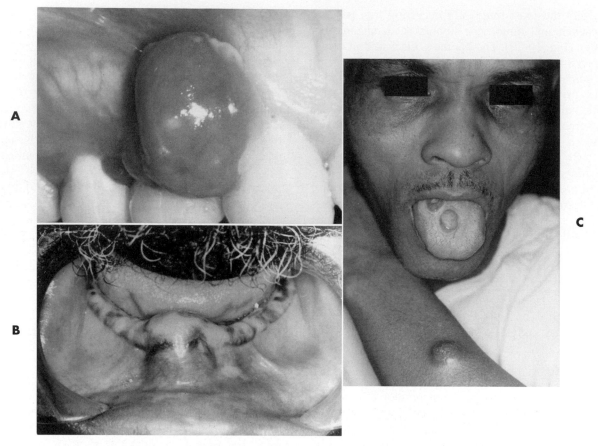

Fig. 10-31. Exophytic metastatic tumors. **A,** Metastatic melanoma. **B,** Metastatic adenocarcinoma from the lung. **C,** Three metastatic lesions from a carcinoma of the esophagus in a 46-year-old man. (**A** from Mosby EL, Sugg WE Jr, Hiatt WR: Gingival and pharyngeal metastastis from a malignant melanoma: report of a case, *Oral Surg* 36:6-10, 1973; **B** courtesy R. Kallal, Chicago; **C** courtesy E. Robinson, Toledo, Ohio.)

incidence of these tumors would prompt the clinician to pursue the possibility of more common entities. If the patient is younger than 20 years old, the probability that the lesion is an SCC, a malignant SGT, or a metastatic tumor is considerably lessened.

Management

The rationale of the management of metastatic tumors is considered in Chapter 20.

PERIPHERAL MALIGNANT MESENCHYMAL TUMORS

Since reports of intraoral peripheral malignant mesenchymal tumors (e.g., neurosarcomas, malignant schwannomas, fibrosarcomas, rhabdomyosarcomas, hemangiosarcomas, liposarcomas) are found only occasionally in the literature, it must be concluded that this group of lesions is uncommon. The intraoral osteogenic sarcoma and chondrosarcoma occur relatively more frequently (Plate J), but these usually are central in origin and consequently are discussed in Part III.

Very little differentiates mesenchymal tumors from any of the clinically benign or malignant-appearing lesions (Fig. 10-32), except possibly the age factor. These tumors usually affect a considerably younger age-group than SCC.

RARITIES
Solitary Lesions

The rare solitary exophytic lesions are listed at the beginning of this chapter and represent a formidable number of entities. Several are illustrated in Figs. 10-33 to 10-35. In spite of the rarity of these lesions, the clinician must at least be aware, when examining a specific lesion, of the possibilities that they represent. Circumstances and special characteristics may prompt the clinician to include one or more of these lesions in the differential list.

Multiple Lesions

The many rare exophytic pathoses that occur as multiple lesions are impossible to rank according to frequency and are listed in alphabetical order at the beginning of this chapter. Figs. 10-36 to 10-39 illustrate some of these.

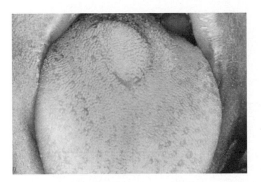

Fig. 10-32. Rhabdomyosarcoma of the dorsal surface of the tongue. (Courtesy N. Choukas, Barrington, Ill.)

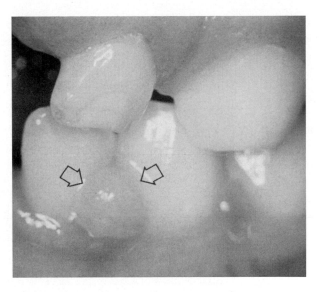

Fig. 10-33. Giant cell fibroma *(arrows)* situated on the interdental papilla area. (Courtesy D. Weathers, Atlanta.)

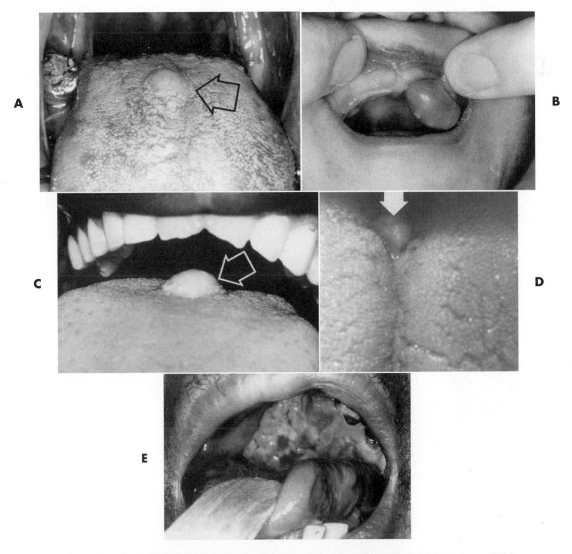

Fig. 10-34. Rare exophytic lesions. **A,** Granular cell myoblastoma. **B,** Epulis of the newborn. **C,** Lingual thyroid gland. **D,** Persistent tuberculum impar. **E,** Lymphosarcoma in the pharynx. (**A** courtesy R. Kallal, Chicago; **C** and **D** courtesy E. Kaspar, Maywood, Ill; **E** courtesy E. Evans, St Cloud, Minn.)

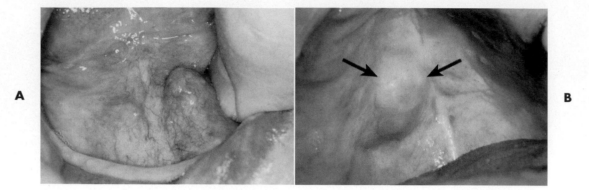

Fig. 10-35. Rare exophytic lesions. **A,** Sialolith in Wharton's duct. **B,** Adenomatoid hyperplasia of the minor salivary glands of the posterolateral palate. (**B** from Buchner A, Merrell PW, Carpenter WM, Leider AS: Adenomatoid hyperplasia of minor salivary glands, *Oral Surg* 71:583-587, 1991.)

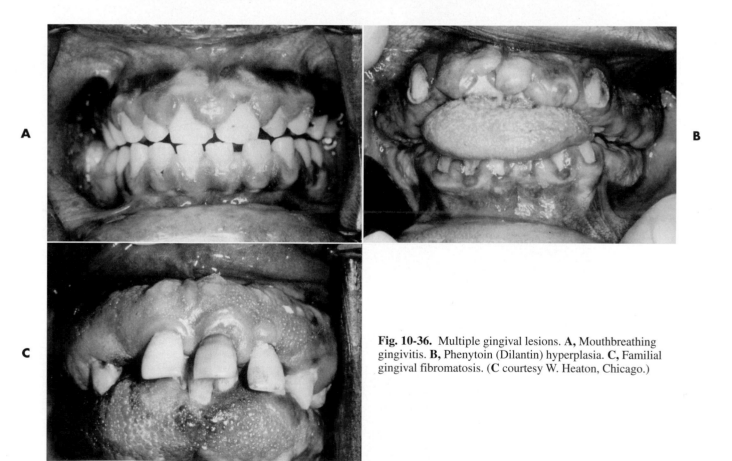

Fig. 10-36. Multiple gingival lesions. **A,** Mouthbreathing gingivitis. **B,** Phenytoin (Dilantin) hyperplasia. **C,** Familial gingival fibromatosis. (**C** courtesy W. Heaton, Chicago.)

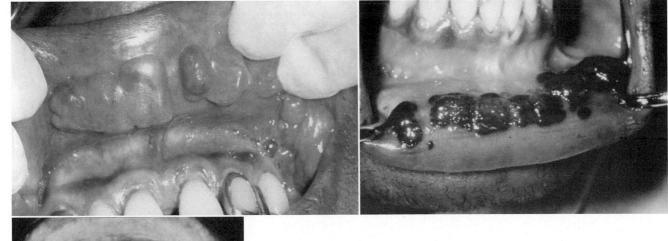

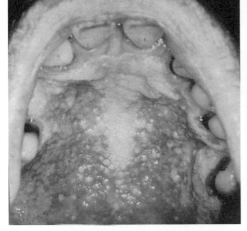

Fig. 10-37. Multiple exophytic lesions. **A,** Amyloidosis in multiple myeloma. **B,** Multiple blood clots in heroin-induced thrombocytopenic purpura. **C,** Multiple papules of palate in a patient with Darier's disease. (**A** from Kraut RA, Buhler JE, LaRue JR, Acevedo A: Amyloidosis associated with multiple myeloma, *Oral Surg* 43:63-68, 1977; **B** from Kraut RA, Buhler JE: Heroin-induced thrombocytopenic purpura, *Oral Surg* 46:637-640, 1978; **C** courtesy M. Bernstein, Louisville.)

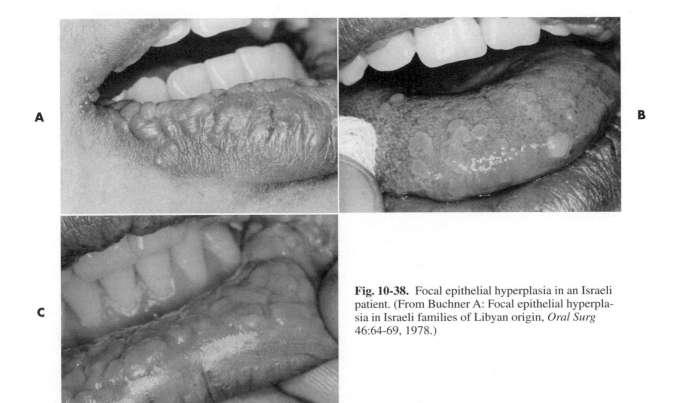

Fig. 10-38. Focal epithelial hyperplasia in an Israeli patient. (From Buchner A: Focal epithelial hyperplasia in Israeli families of Libyan origin, *Oral Surg* 46:64-69, 1978.)

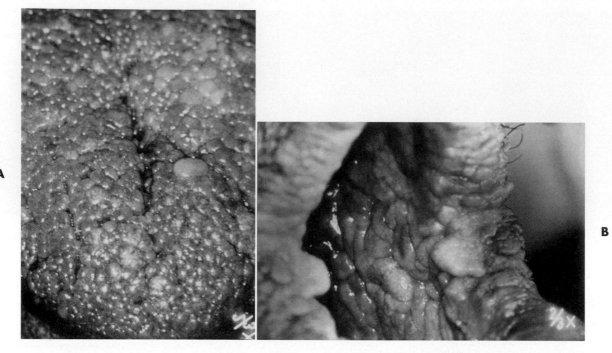

Fig. 10-39. Multiple fibroepithelial hyperplasia seen on the tongue, buccal mucosa, and lips of a patient. (From Buchner A, Sandbank M: Multiple fibroepithelial hyperplasias of the oral mucosa, *Oral Surg* 46:34-39, 1978.)

REFERENCES

1. Bouquot JE, Gundlach KKH: Oral exophytic lesions in 23,616 white Americans over 35 years of age, *Oral Surg* 62:284-291, 1986.
2. Adkins KF: Lymphoid hyperplasia in the oral mucosa, *Aust Dent J* 18:38-40, 1973.
3. Knapp MJ: Oral tonsils: location, distribution, and histology, *Oral Surg* 29:155-161, 1970.
4. Knapp MJ: Pathology of oral tonsils, *Oral Surg* 29:295-304, 1970.
5. Buchner A, Merrell PW, Hansen LS, Leider AS: The retrocuspid papilla of the mandibular lingual gingiva, *J Periodontal* 61:586-590, 1990.
6. Gorsky M, Begleiter A, Buchner A, Harel-Raviv M: The retrocuspid papilla in Israeli Jews, *Oral Surg* 62:240-243, 1986.
7. King DR, Moore GE: An analysis of torus palatinus in a transatlantic study, *J Oral Med* 31:44-46, 1976.
8. King DR, King AC: Incidence of tori in three population groups, *J Oral Med* 36:21-23, 1981.
9. Priddy RW: Inflammatory hyperplasias of the oral mucosa, *J Can Dent Assoc* 58:311-321, 1992.
10. Zain RB, Fei YJ: Fibrous lesions of the gingiva: a histopathologic analysis of 204 cases, *Oral Surg* 70:466-470, 1990.
11. Weathers DR, Callihan MD: Giant-cell fibroma, *Oral Surg* 37:374-384, 1974.
12. Angelopoulos AP: Pyogenic granuloma of the oral cavity: statistical analysis of its clinical features, *J Oral Surg* 29:840-847, 1971.
13. Eversole LR, Rovin S: Reactive lesions of the gingiva, *J Oral Pathol* 1:30-38, 1972.
14. Vilmann A, Vilmann P, Vilmann H: Pyogenic granuloma: evaluation of oral conditions, *Br J Oral Maxillofac Surg* 24:376-382, 1986.
15. Macleod RI, Soames JV: Epulides: a clinicopathological study of a series of 200 consecutive lesions, *Br Dent J* 163:51-53, 1987.
16. Lee L, Miller PA, Maxymin WG, et al: Intraoral pyogenic granuloma after allogenic bone marrow transplant: report of three cases, *Oral Surg* 78:607-610, 1994.
17. Tiainen L, Asikainen S, Saxen L: Puberty-associated gingivitis, *Comm Dent Oral Epidemiol* 20:87-89, 1992.
18. Daley TD, Nartey NO, Wysocki GP: Pregnancy tumor: an analysis, *Oral Surg* 72:196-199, 1991.
19. Whitaker SB, Bouquot JE, Alimario AE, Whitaker TJ: Identification and semiquantification of estrogen and progesterone receptors in pyogenic granulomas of pregnancy, *Oral Surg* 78:755-760, 1994.
20. Raber-Durlacher JE, van Steenbergen TJM, van der Velden V, et al: Experimental gingivitis during pregnancy and post-partum: clinical, endocrinological, and microbiological aspects, *J Clin Periodont* 21:549-558, 1994.
21. Cutright DE: The histopathologic findings in 583 cases of epulis fissuratum, *Oral Surg* 37:401-411, 1974.
22. Reichart PA, Schmidt-Westhausen A, Samaranayake LP, Philipsen HP: *Candida*-associated palatal papillary hyperplasia in HIV infection, *J Oral Pathol Med* 23:403-405, 1994.
23. Miller EL: Clinical management of denture-induced inflammations, *J Prosthet Dent* 38:362-365, 1977.
24. Uohara GI, Federbusch MD: Removal of papillary hyperplasia, *J Oral Surg* 26:463-466, 1968.
25. Bergendal T, Heindahl A, Isacsson G: Surgery in the treatment of denture related inflammatory hyperplasia of the palate, *Int J Oral Surg* 9:312-319, 1980.
26. Rathofer SA, Gardner FM, Vermilyea SG: A comparison of healing and pain following excision of inflammatory papillary hyperplasia with electrosurgery and blade-loop knives in human patients, *Oral Surg* 59:130-135, 1985.
27. Katsikeris N, Kakarantza-Angelopoulou E, Angelopoulos AP: Peripheral giant cell granuloma: clinicopathologic study of 224 new cases and review of 956 reported cases, *Int J Oral Maxillofac Surg* 17:94-99, 1988.
28. Bhaskar SN, Cutright DE: Giant cell reparative granuloma (peripheral): report of 50 cases, *J Oral Surg* 29:110-115, 1971.
29. Giansanti JS, Waldron CA: Peripheral giant cell granuloma: review of 720 cases, *J Oral Surg* 27:787-791, 1969.
30. Burkes EJ, White RP: A peripheral giant cell granuloma manifestation of primary hyperparathyroidism: report of case, *J Am Dent Assoc* 118:62-63, 1989.

31. Smith BR, Fowler CB, Svane TJ: Primary hyperparathyroidism presenting as a "peripheral" giant cell granuloma, *J Oral Maxillofac Surg* 46:65-69, 1988.

32. Shultz RE, Theisen FC, Dunlap CL: Herniation of the antral membrane through an extraction site, *Oral Surg* 71:280-282, 1991.

33. Gardner DG: The peripheral odontogenic fibroma: an attempt at clarification, *Oral Surg* 54:40-48, 1982.

34. Buchner A, Ficcarra G, Hansen LS: Peripheral odontogenic fibroma, *Oral Surg* 64:432-438, 1987.

35. Slabbert HD, Altini M: Peripheral odontogenic fibroma: a clinicopathologic study, *Oral Surg* 72:86-90, 1991.

36. Daley TD, Wysocki, GP: Peripheral odontogenic fibroma, *Oral Surg* 78:329-336, 1994.

37. Zain RB, Fei YJ: Fibrous lesions of the gingiva: a histopathologic analysis of 204 cases, *Oral Surg* 70:466-470, 1990.

38. Cundiff EJ: Peripheral ossifying fibroma: a review of 365 cases, MSD thesis, Indiana University, 1972. Cited in Shafer WG, Hine MK, Levy BM: *A textbook of oral pathology,* ed 3, Philadelphia, 1974, WB Saunders.

39. Mulcahy JV, Dahl EC: The peripheral odontogenic fibroma: a retrospective study, *J Oral Med* 40:46-48, 1985.

40. Cohen L: Mucoceles of the oral cavity, *Oral Surg* 19:365-372, 1965.

41. Scully C, Epstein J, Porter S, Cox M: Viruses and chronic disorders involving the human mucosa, *Oral Surg* 72:537-544, 1991.

42. Padayachee A: Human papilloma virus (HPV) types 2 and 57 in oral verrucae demonstrated by *in situ* hybridization, *J Oral Pathol Med* 23:413-417, 1994.

43. Premoli-de-Percoco G, Galindo I, Ramirez JL, et al: Detection of human papillomavirus–related oral verruca vulgaris among Venezuelans, *J Oral Pathol Med* 22:113-116, 1993.

44. Ward KA, Napier SS, Winter PC, et al: Detection of human papilloma virus DNA sequences in oral squamous cell papillomas by the polymerase chain reaction, *Oral Surg* 80:63-66, 1995.

45. Eversole LR, Laipis PJ, Merrell P, Choi E: Demonstration of human papillomavirus DNA in oral condyloma acuminatum, *J Oral Pathol Med* 16:266-272, 1987.

46. Greer RO, Goldman HM: Oral papillomas, *Oral Surg* 38:435-440, 1974.

47. Flaitz CM, Nichols CM, Hicks MJ, Adler-Storthz K: Oral human papilloma virus infection in HIV seropositive males: diagnosis and therapeutic management, paper presented to the annual meeting of the American Academy of Oral Pathology, Portland, Maine, May 14-19, 1993.

48. Whitaker LA, Lehr HB, Askovitz SI: Cancer of the tongue, *Plast Reconstr Surg* 30:363-370, 1972.

49. van Heerden WFP, Raubenheimer EJ: Intraoral salivary gland neoplasms: a retrospective study of seventy cases in an African population, *Oral Surg* 71:579-582, 1991.

50. Kaneda T, Minami M, Ozawa K, et al: Imaging tumors of the minor salivary glands, *Oral Surg* 77:385-390, 1994.

51. Pogrel MA: Tumors of the salivary glands: a histological and clinical review, *Br J Oral Surg* 17:47-56, 1979.

52. Waldron CA, El-Mofty S, Gnepp DR: Tumors of the intraoral salivary glands: a demographic and histologic study of 426 cases, *Oral Surg* 66:323-333, 1988.

53. Main JHP, McGurk FM, McComb RJ, Mock D: Salivary gland tumors: review of 643 cases, *J Oral Pathol* 5:88-102, 1976.

54. Eveson JW, Cawson RA: Tumors of the minor (oropharyngeal) salivary glands: a demographic study of 336 cases, *J Oral Pathol* 14:500-509, 1985.

55. Chaudhry AP, Labay GR, Yamane GM, et al: Clinicopathologic and histogenetic study of 189 intraoral minor salivary gland tumors, *J Oral Med* 39:58-78, 1984.

56. Chaudhry AP, Vickers RA, Gorlin RJ: Intraoral minor salivary gland tumors, *Oral Surg* 14:1194-1226, 1961.

57. Chau MNY, Radden BG: Intraoral salivary gland neoplasms: a retrospective study of 98 cases, *J Oral Pathol* 15:339-342, 1986.

58. Soskolne A, Ben-Amar A, Ulmansky M: Minor salivary gland tumors: a survey of 64 cases, *J Oral Surg* 31:528-531, 1973.

59. Isacsson G, Shear M: Intraoral salivary gland tumors: a retrospective study of 201 cases, *J Oral Pathol* 12:57-62, 1983.

60. Krolls SO, Hicks JL: Mixed tumors of the lower lip, *Oral Surg* 35:212-217, 1973.

61. Bradley G, Main JHP, Birt BD, From L: Benign lymphoid hyperplasia of the palate, *J Oral Pathol* 16:18-26, 1987.

62. Wright JM, Dunsworth AR: Follicular lymphoid hyperplasia of the hard palate: a benign lymphoproliferative process, *Oral Surg* 55:162-168, 1983.

63. Eisenbud L, Sciubba J, Mir R, et al: Oral presentations in thirty-one cases of non-Hodgkin's lymphoma. I. Data analysis, *Oral Surg* 56:151-156, 1983.

64. Blok P, van Delden L, van der Waal I: Non-Hodgkin's lymphoma of the hard palate, *Oral Surg* 47:445-452, 1979.

65. Buchner A, Merrell PW, Carpenter WM, Leider AS: Adenomatoid hyperplasia of minor salivary glands, *Oral Surg* 71:583-587, 1991.

66. Barrett AW, Speight PM: Adenomatoid hyperplasia of oral minor salivary galnds, *Oral Surg* 79:482-487, 1995.

67. Arafat A, Brannon RB, Ellis GL: Adenomatoid hyperplasia of mucous salivary glands, *Oral Surg* 52:51-55, 1981.

68. Hamper K, Lazar F, Dietel M, et al: Prognostic factors for adenoid cystic carcinoma of the head and neck: a retrospective evaluation of 96 cases, *J Oral Pathol Med* 19:101-107, 1990.

69. Sist TC, Greene GW: Traumatic neuroma of the oral cavity: report of thirty-one new cases and review of the literature, *Oral Surg* 51:394-402, 1981.

70. Wright BA, Jackson D: Neural tumors of the oral cavity: a review of the spectrum of benign and malignant oral tumors of the oral cavity and jaws, *Oral Surg* 49:509-522, 1980.

CHAPTER 11

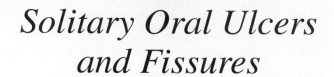

Solitary Oral Ulcers and Fissures

NORMAN K. WOOD
PAUL W. GOAZ

Ulcers and fissures of the oral cavity include the following:

ULCERS
TRAUMATIC ULCER
RECURRENT ORAL ULCERS
  Recurrent aphthous ulcer
  Recurrent intraoral herpes simplex
  Herpetiform oral ulcers
  Major aphthous ulcer
ULCERS FROM ODONTOGENIC
  INFECTIONS
SLOUGHING, PSEUDOMEMBRANOUS
  ULCERS
GENERALIZED MUCOSITIDES AND
  VESICULOBULLOUS DISEASES
SQUAMOUS CELL CARCINOMA
SYPHILIS
  Chancre
  Gumma
ULCERS SECONDARY TO SYSTEMIC
  DISEASE
TRAUMATIZED TUMORS (TYPES
  USUALLY NOT ULCERATED)
MINOR SALIVARY GLAND TUMORS
RARITIES
  Actinomycosis
  Adenoid squamous cell carcinoma
  Animal diseases
  Basal cell carcinoma

Basidiobolus haptosporus infection
Botryomycosis hominis
Cancrum oris
Child abuse
Contact allergy
Crohn's disease
Eosinophilic ulcer
Foot-and-mouth disease
Fungal infections
  Aspergillosis, blastomycosis, coccidioido-
    mycosis, cryptococcosis, histoplasmosis,
    paracoccidioidomycosis sporotrichosis
Gastrointestinal disease
Glycogen storage disease
Gonococcal stomatitis
Graft-versus-host disease
Granuloma inguinale
Granulomatous disease of the newborn
Hand-foot-and-mouth disease
Helminthic infection
Herpangina
Herpes zoster infection
Keratoacanthoma
Leishmaniasis
Leukemia
Lymphoma
Median rhomboid glossitis—ulcerative variety

Metastatic tumor
Midline nonhealing granuloma (midline
  malignant reticulosis)
Mucormycosis
Mycosis fungoides
Necrotizing sialometaplasia
Neurotrophic ulcer
Phycomycosis
Sarcoidosis
Self-mutilation wounds
Sutton's disease
Syringomyelia
Tuberculosis
Waldenström's macroglobulinemia
Warty dyskeratoma
FISSURES
ANGULAR CHEILOSIS
CONGENITAL CLEFT
EPULIS FISSURATUM
FISSURED TONGUE
MEDIAN RHOMBOID GLOSSITIS—
  FISSURED VARIETY
MELKERSSON-ROSENTHAL SYNDROME
SQUAMOUS CELL CARCINOMA—
  FISSURED VARIETY
SYPHILITIC RHAGADES

ULCERS

Oral ulcers represent a variable and impressive group of lesions. A cursory examination of the previous list reveals that some of these lesions are caused by local influences (e.g., traumatic ulcers), whereas others are manifestations of systemic problems (e.g., oral ulcers).

Also, some oral ulcers are primary, with early manifestations such as erosions or ulcers (e.g., traumatic ulcers); others are secondary[1] because they are subsequent to other clinical forms, which become ulcerated (e.g., vesicles and blebs). Exophytic lesions frequently illustrate this secondary change when they become ulcerated from chronic mechanical injury or as the result of an incisional biopsy.

The terms *erosion* and *ulcer* are often confused and mistakenly used interchangeably. An *erosion* has been defined as a shallow crater in the epithelial surface that appears on clinical examination as a very shallow erythematous area and implies only superficial damage.[1] *Ulcer* has been defined as a deeper crater that extends through the entire thickness of surface epithelium and involves the underlying connective tissue.[1] These terms have become somewhat interchangeable today (e.g., lichen planus).

Oral ulcers are unique: They have diverse causes but frequently show similar histologic changes; therefore they cannot be differentiated by routine microscopy. This uniformity derives from the irritating effect of oral liquids and flora as soon as an ulcer is formed; consequently, an acute or chronic inflammation is immediately initiated. The resultant inflammatory changes may mask the more subtle and diagnostic histologic changes that are a feature of the basic pathosis.

The intraoral herpes simplex lesion is a good example of an oral ulcer that loses its microscopic identity because of secondary contamination. In the early vesicular stage, pathognomonic features include the ballooning of the epithelial cells and the presence of giant cells in the vesicular fluid. After the vesicle ulcerates, these definitive features are soon lost, and all that remains is the histologic picture of a nonspecific ulcer.

The following changes are inferred when the clinician encounters a microscopic diagnosis of "nonspecific" ulcer:

1. The complete thickness of the surface epithelium is missing, and the exposed connective tissue often is necrotic on the surface and covered by a fibrinous exudate (Fig. 11-1).
2. Depending on its age and the circumstances relating to its development, the ulcer has acute inflammation with polymorphonuclear leukocytes in the connective tissue at its borders.
3. A less acute phase of the ulcer shows a greater concentration of chronic inflammatory cells, such as lymphocytes, plasma cells, and possibly macrophages with some fibroblastic proliferation.

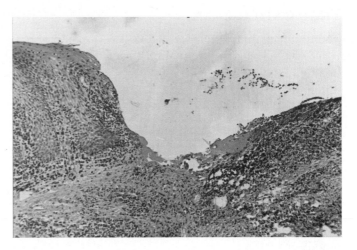

Fig. 11-1. Nonspecific ulcer. Photomicrograph reveals loss of the surface epithelium and the upper portion of the lamina propria. Inflammatory cells are abundant.

4. In the healing phase of the ulcer, granulation tissue with fibroblastic proliferation predominates, and a few macrophages, plasma cells, and lymphocytes may also be present.

In spite of the foregoing list, some of the ulcers discussed in this chapter can be diagnosed by routine light microscopy when they are stained with hematoxylin and eosin or special stains.

For example, histologic changes in squamous cell carcinoma and ulcerative mesenchymal minor salivary gland tumors are diagnostic as long as the biopsy includes a section of tumor underlying the ulcer. Lesions such as chancres, herpetic ulcers, and tuberculous, sarcoid, and fungal lesions may produce tissue changes that indicate a definitive diagnosis, but usually, special staining procedures must be used to assist in making a definitive microscopic identification.

When a clinician is attempting to complete a differential diagnosis of a clinical ulcer, it helps to separate oral ulcers into two groups: short-term ulcers (those that persist no longer than 3 weeks and regress spontaneously or as a result of nonsurgical treatment) and persistent ulcers (those that last for weeks and months). The majority of traumatic ulcers, recurrent aphthous ulcers (RAUs) (except major aphthae), recurrent intraoral herpetic ulcers, and chancres fall into the category of short-term ulcers.

Occasionally, traumatic ulcers, major aphthae, ulcers from odontogenic infection, malignant ulcers, gummas, and ulcers secondary to debilitating systemic disease are classified as persistent ulcers and may remain for months and even years. Persistent ulcers should be considered malignant until proved otherwise.

This chapter is devoted to conditions that have single ulcers or a localized cluster of ulcers. The generalized ulcerative conditions are dealt with in Chapter 6.

TRAUMATIC ULCER

The traumatic ulcer is by far the most common oral mucosal ulcer. The cause may be mechanical, chemical, or thermal; the traumatic incident may be accidentally self-inflicted or iatrogenic.

Features

The patient with a traumatic ulcer complains of tenderness or pain in the area of the lesion, and usually the traumatic agent can be readily identified. A variety of causes need to be considered: lip, tongue, and cheek biting (sometimes after the administration of a local anesthetic); a toothbrush that slipped; a child who fell with an object in the mouth while running; and a mouth burned by hot liquids or toothache drops.

Some long-standing ulcerations of the attached gingivae are caused by repeated trauma from toothbrushing.[2] Cases of self-inflicted oral ulcerative lesions have been reported in patients who were seeking prescriptions for narcotic drugs.[3] Denture-induced traumatic ulcers are observed in 5.5% of people aged 65 to 74 years.[4] Self-inflicted trauma of the tongue is a problem in decerebrate and comatose patients.[5] The placement of a fixed acrylic tongue stent is recommended in some of these cases.[5] Lingual frenum ulcers may be related to orogenital sex.[6]

Traumatic ulcers are most common on the tongue, lips, mucobuccal fold, gingivae, and palate. They may persist for just a few days or may last for weeks (especially ulcers of the tongue). They vary greatly in size and shape but seldom are multiple or recurrent, unless they result from ill-fitting dentures. Their borders are somewhat raised and reddish, and their bases may have a yellowish-white necrotic surface that can be readily removed (Figs. 11-2 and 11-3). Ulcers on the vermilion border, unlike those on the oral mucosa, usually have a crusted surface because of the absence of saliva. In some instances the ulcers conform nicely to the shape of a tooth cusp or a denture flange, or they may be positioned against a sharp edge of a tooth.

A cause-and-effect relationship must be established not only to make a definitive diagnosis of traumatic ulcer, but also to identify and eliminate the traumatizing agent. Frequently a tender or painful regional lymphadenitis occurs as a result of contamination of the ulcer by the oral flora.

Differential Diagnosis

The history of the traumatic injury in most cases enables the clinician to identify the traumatic ulcer and establish a working diagnosis. The history of a traumatic incident may be misleading, however, and cause the true identity of a more serious lesion to be overlooked. Since traumatic ulcers may be short-term or persistent, both varieties must be considered in the differential diagnosis. For a more thorough discussion,

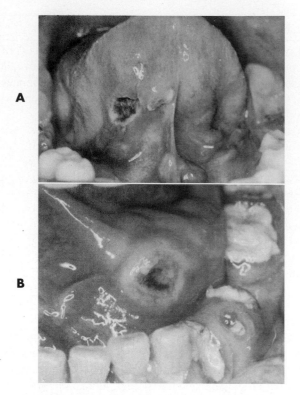

Fig. 11-2. Traumatic ulcers. **A,** Traumatic ulcer on the ventral surface of the tongue resulting from a self-inflicted bite. **B,** Ulcer caused by a sharp premolar root.

see the differential diagnosis section at the end of this chapter.

Management

Most traumatic ulcers become painless within 3 or 4 days after the injury-producing agent has been eliminated, and most heal within 10 days. Occasionally, a lesion persists for some weeks because of continued traumatic insults, continued irritation by the oral liquids, or development of a secondary infection. The last occasion may indicate the presence of lowered resistance from an underlying systemic disease.

Coating the ulcerated surface of the persistent traumatic ulcers and the less serious varieties with fluocinonide or triamcinolone acetonide in an emollient base before bedtime and after meals usually relieves the pain and hastens healing. The base protects the denuded connective tissue from continued contamination by oral liquids, and the corticosteroid component tends to arrest the inflammatory cycle (which may become self-perpetuating). Oral bandage materials such as hydroxypropyl methylcellulose also help promote healing.[7,8] Chlorhexidine mouthrinses are also helpful if occluding bandages are not used.[9]

Persistent ulcers not responding to this regimen should be surgically excised and closed primarily; the excised tissue must always be microscopically examined, since a persistent ulcer could be a malignant lesion.

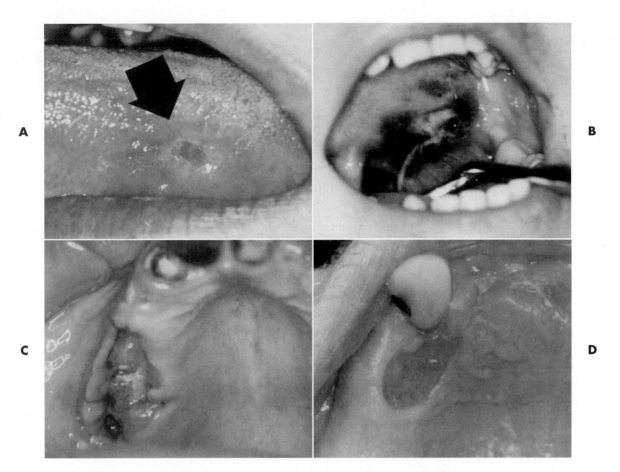

Fig. 11-3. Traumatic ulcers. **A,** Ulcer on the lateral margin of the tongue. **B,** Ulcerated and ecchymotic lesion on the posterior palate of a boy who was holding a Popsicle stick in his mouth when he fell. **C,** Ulcer on the maxillary ridge caused by a traumatic extraction. **D,** Ulcer on the maxilloalveolar crest caused by trauma from the lower canine. (**C** courtesy D. Bonomo, Flossmoor, Ill; **D** courtesy of P.D. Toto, Waukegan, Ill.)

RECURRENT ORAL ULCERS

Four conditions present as recurrent oral ulcers: RAU, recurrent intraoral herpes simplex (RIHS), major aphthous ulcer (major AU), and herpetiform aphtha (HA). RAU is also one of the features of Behçet's syndrome. Approximately 10% of the adult population suffer from these recurrent ulcerations, not counting RIHS. Each of these conditions are discussed, but RAU and RIHS are stressed because of their frequency of occurrence and also because it may be difficult to distinguish these two lesions at times.

Recurrent Aphthous Ulcer

Pathogenesis Three subgroups may be included under RAU: (1) minor RAU, (2) major RAU, and (3) herpetiform ulcers. The minor RAU are the most common by far.

Current concepts of RAU and recurrent aphthous stomatitis (see Chapter 6) indicate a multifactoral etiology, but the overall disorder is immunologic. The etiology may be stated as follows: Certain mononuclear peripheral blood cells target and destroy oral epithelial cells that possess class I and II major histocompatibility complex antigens.[10]

Once this process occurs, ulceration of the oral mucosa may permit additional local factors to come into play.[11] Conceptually the problematic antigens in or on the target epithelial cells could result from (1) autoalteration or (2) foreign antigens from ingested materials or viruses.[10] Certain food and flavoring agents have been suspected for some time as promoting factors.[12,13] Incidentally, gluten withdrawal is ineffective in the treatment of patients with RAU.[14]

A number of studies have validated systemic T-cell imbalances in RAU patients.[10,15-17] The possible roles of $CD4^+$ and $CD8^+$ in the process are being investigated.[10,15-17] In addition, the production of leukocyte tumor necrosis factor is increased in RAU, so this cytokine could be associated with destruction of epithelial cells.[18] Apparently immunoglobulin G subclass levels are not a feature in minor RAU, and this would shift suspicion from bacterial promoters.[19]

It is possible that the epithelial antigen change has been produced by viruses such as herpes simplex virus (HSV),[20] varicella-zoster,[20,21] cytomegalovirus,[21] and human herpesvirus type 6.[22,23]

Table 11-1 RAU and RIHS: dissimilar features

RAU	RIHS
Preferred location*	
Lesion occurs on movable mucosa (nonkeratinized), lips, buccal mucosa, tongue, mucobuccal fold, floor of mouth, and soft palate (see Fig. 11-4).	Lesion occurs on fixed mucosa; it is tightly bound to periosteum (keratinized), hard palate, gingivae, and alveolar ridge (see Fig. 11-5).
Initial lesion	
Erythematous macule or papule presents; lesion undergoes central blanching followed by necrosis and ulceration.	Cluster of small, discrete, gray or white vesicles without red erythematous halo present; vesicles quickly rupture, forming small, punctate ulcers 1 mm or less in diameter.
Mature lesion	
Shallow ulcer is 0.5 to 2 cm in diameter; has yellow necrotic center; has smooth, contoured border; and has constant red halo; lesion is usually more symmetric and circular.	Shallow ulcer is no larger than 0.5 cm in diameter with red halos. A number of vesicles may occur in tight cluster. When these rupture, a much larger ulcer, up to 1.5 cm in diameter, is formed. Border is scalloped, and red halo is present.
Number of lesions	
Lesions usually occur singly; occasionally, two or three are widely distributed (see Fig. 11-4).	Usually, several small, punctate ulcers occur in cluster in small, localized area (see Fig. 11-5); they have regular border and are usually round; there is variable erythematous halo.
Site of recurrence	
There is no preference.	Lesion often returns to same location.
Histopathology	
Mature lesion is nonspecific ulcer.	With *early lesion,* vesicular fluid contains epithelial cells with ballooning degeneration, multinucleated giant cells, and viral particles. With *mature lesion,* after vesicle ruptures, ulcer is nonspecific.

Modified from Weathers DR, Griffin JW: Intraoral ulcerations of recurrent herpes simplex and recurrent aphthae: two distinct clinical entities, *J Am Dent Assoc* 81:81-87, 1970.
*Under certain conditions, both lesions can occur anywhere on the mucosa.

RAU AND RIHS: COMMON FEATURES

- Frequent occurrence
- Fact that any age can be affected
- Proneness to recur
- Lack of seasonal pattern
- Lesion that can occur on most mucosal surfaces, especially in certain conditions
- Duration of 7 to 10 days
- Prodromal tenderness
- Pain (RIHS more of a "smarting" pain)
- Red-rimmed ulcer borders and lack of induration
- Ulcers that are contaminated by oral flora
- Ulcers that may be the same size
- Spontaneous healing without sequelae
- Painful cervical lymphadenopathy

Studies on folate levels are equivocal,[24,25] and psychologic stress has been deemphasized.[26] RAU may be an inherited disorder,[27] and the condition has been reported to be more common in menstruating female patients,[28] which would suggest a role played by female sex hormones. RAU is more common in celiac disease.[14] Mucosal injury may play a role in initiating RAU in some cases.[11,29] It is interesting that smoking and smokeless tobacco use have an inhibiting effect on RAU, possibly through increased keratinization or through the systemic effects of nicotine.[30] Recurrent aphthous stomatitis is discussed in detail in Chapter 6.

Features Clinical characteristics of RAU are listed in the box above and Table 11-1 and are illustrated in Fig. 11-4. The mean age is approximately 36 years. A slight female preponderance is possible and frequent sites are the buccal mucosa and vestibule, lateroventral area of the tongue, floor of the mouth, soft palate, and oropharynx.[31] The box lists the similarities that RAU and RIHS share, whereas Table 11-1 lists their differences.

Differential diagnosis The information in the box and Table 11-1 usually enables differentiation between RAU and RIHS ulcers.[32] For more complete differential diagnosis, see the section on p. 178.

Management Whereas aphthous stomatitis with its many ulcers is often managed by general applications of agents to the whole oral mucosa in the form of rinses, one or two RAUs are usually treated by direct local application to the ulcer. RAU generally heals in 7 to 10 days, and much of the pain after initiation seems to be related to secondary contamination by oral flora. Placement of a tetracycline solution or a 0.12% chlorhexidine solution by cotton applicator to the dried lesion, which is then covered by an oral bandage material, gives quick pain relief and prevents further contamination for a period. Bandage or barrier material includes cyanoacrylate, Orabase, or hydroxypropyl cellulose (Zilactin).[7,8] These materials

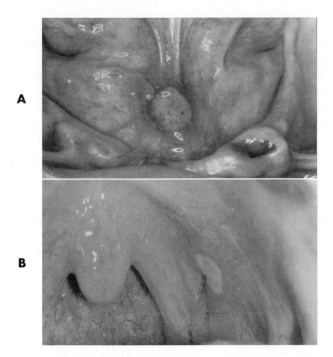

Fig. 11-4. RAUs. **A,** Floor of the mouth. **B,** Palatoglossal arch.

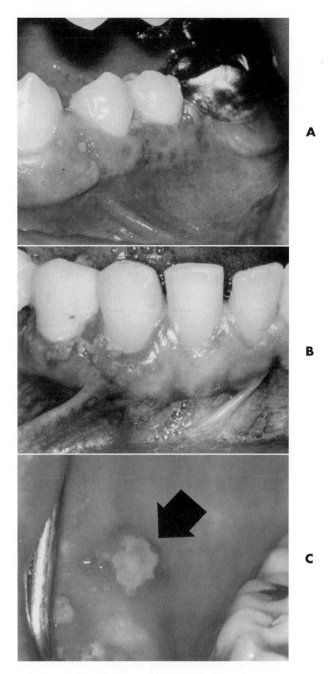

Fig.11-5. **A** and **B** RIHS lesions on attached gingivae. Both occurred after dental treatment. In **A,** note three intact vesicles in the anterior area and a cluster of small punctate ulcers distally. In **B,** note the white rims of pinpoint ulcers and the tracklike white pattern. The white areas are the remnants of the vesicle roofs. Considerable erythematous reaction can be seen also in association with the lesions. **C,** RIHS lesion of the buccal mucosa. Note the large lesion *(arrow)* formed by a close cluster of small vesicles, which are rupturing to form a large ulcer with scalloped borders.

may be used by themselves or as vehicles for topical corticosteroids such as triamcinolone or fluocinolone. Triamcinolone and chlorhexidine applications before bandaging with cyanoacrylate are equally effective in relieving pain.[33] Regarding prevention, rinsing with Listerine or a 5% hydroalcoholic solution twice daily reduces the occurrence of RAU in susceptible patients.[34]

Recurrent Intraoral Herpes Simplex

Pathogenesis RIHS vesicles and ulcers are secondary lesions, as are those that occur on the vermilion border and skin. These patients have been primarily infected with this deoxyribonucleic acid virus previously, the majority of manifestations being subclinical or minor vesiculoulcerative lesions. Approximately 10% of patients experience major manifestations of infection, a severe primary herpetic gingivostomatitis. This condition is described in Chapter 6. More detail on HSV is given in Chapter 36.

After primary infection, the HSV enters a latent state and later becomes reactivated by various stimulae (e.g., sunburn on the lips, trauma to the soft tissue during dental work, influenza attack, menstruation) and recurs[35] as a vesiculoulcerative lesion on the skin, perioral tissue, and oral mucosa, usually the fixed mucosa. Although it has been known for years that the virus resides in latency in the sensory ganglia, it is now thought to reside also in the gingivae and other extraneural tissues.[35]

HSV type 1 has been associated with oral and perioral lesions and HSV type 2 with genital lesions. Both types produce lesions indistinguishable at both sites.

Features The box on p. 166 and Table 11-1 detail the clinical features of RIHS lesions, and examples are illustrated in Fig. 11-5. Usually, small vesicles occur in a cluster on the gingiva or hard palate and soon rupture, producing punctate ulcers with erythematous rims (see Fig. 11-5). If the vesicles are close when they rupture, a solitary ulcer with scalloped borders and an erythematous rim results (see Fig. 11-5, *C*). In such cases the resultant ulcer can easily measure 1 cm or more. Cervical lymph nodes may be swollen and painful. Unlike RAU, RIHS lesions often recur in the same location, particularly in cases that have only occasional occurrences.[36]

The herpetic whitlow is an occupational disease of practicing dentists and dental workers.[37,38] This HSV infection of the fingers may be contracted by working on a patient who has a herpetic lesion of the lips or oral cavity. Lesions of the fingers may be recurrent and may also spread to the rest of the hand.[37] As a preventive measure, it is recommended that dental treatment be delayed until the patient's active herpetic lesion is healed;[38] if this is not possible, the use of a rubber dam and disposable rubber gloves and autoclaving of both these items before discarding is advised.[38] Safety glasses are strongly recommended to guard against herpetic infections of the eye and other contaminants as well.

The difficulty with all diagnostic techniques is that the viruses are shed quickly after vesicles rupture. HSV can be cultured from intact vesicles, and cytologic smears from freshly ruptured vesicles show typical multinucleated giant cells. Serum antibody titers are positive in a large percentage of adults.

Differential diagnosis Application of the criteria in the box on p. 166 enables the clinician to differentiate between RAU and RIHS in most cases. Of course, if other body surfaces are involved, the various syndromes mentioned previously must be considered.

Herpangina and hand-foot-and-mouth disease are two other conditions that must be differentiated from RIHS lesions. Herpangina is caused by coxsackie A virus (ribonucleic acid virus) that usually affects children in the late summer and early fall. Patients experience fever, general malaise, and multiple vesicles distributed over a reddened soft palate and fauces. Like the vesicles of herpes simplex, they rupture quickly. Localization to the soft palate usually distinguishes them from herpes, which seldom involves the soft palate except in patients who are experiencing immunosuppression.

Hand-foot-and-mouth disease is also caused by a coxsackie A virus (various strains). Children under 10 years of age are usually affected. Characteristic symptoms of a systemic viral disease, such as fever, malaise, nausea, and diarrhea, occur. The feature that distinguishes hand-foot-and-mouth disease from intraoral herpes simplex is that the vesiculoulcerative lesions occur simultaneously in the oral cavity (hard palate, gingiva, and tongue) and on the hands and feet.

A further discussion of the distinguishing features of similar-appearing intraoral ulcers is presented in the differential diagnosis section at the end of this chapter. For a discussion of generalized oral ulcerations and mucositides, see Chapter 6.

Atypical RIHS Lesions

Several atypical clinical appearances and behaviors can be observed with RIHS (see box below).

RIHS of the gingival papillae frequently shows one or two very red, swollen papillae that are very painful (Fig. 11-6). Often the patient first notices the lesion when floss is drawn through the indicated contact point and an intense "smarting" type of pain ensues. Close examination may yield a mild, ragged appearance of the contours of the engorged papilla (see Fig. 11-6). A magnifying lens shows minute vesicles and ulcers throughout the surface of the

---

ATYPICAL RIHS

- RIHS of gingival papilla
- Persistent infection of gingivae
- Persistent enlarged ulcers
- RIHS in immunoincompetence

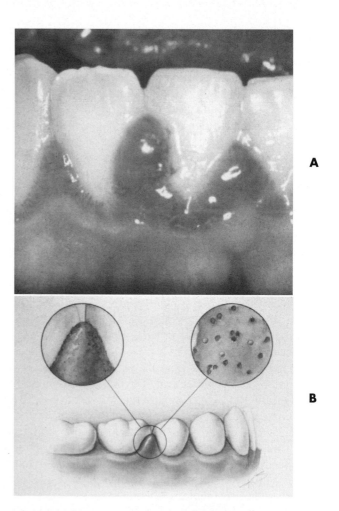

Fig. 11-6. A, Swollen, red interdental papilla is a clinical manifestation of RIHS. **B,** Diagram showing miniature punctate ulcers under magnification.

enlarged gingiva, which prompts the working diagnosis of RIHS. If the patient continues to floss as usual, adjacent gingiva papillae become infected in turn. RIHS lesions of gingival papillae usually heal within 7 to 10 days.

Persistent RIHS infection of the gingiva may persist for months if the patient with RIHS lesions of the interdental papilla brushes and uses floss in a regular manner. These patients may move the infection around the entire arch with a contaminated brush and floss. A protracted course of continued development and healing of lesions occurs in these patients. Careful examination with a magnifying lens again shows the true identity of the disease. The long-term course of the disease in otherwise healthy patients often obscures the diagnosis. Flossing should be

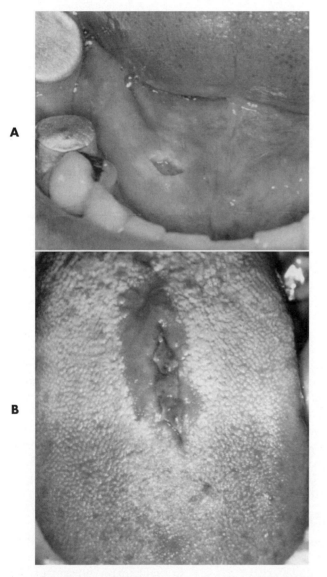

Fig. 11-7. Atypical RIHS lesions that have become large, persistent ulcers. **A,** Four-week ulcer on the oral floor that was originally diagnosed as a traumatic ulcer secondary to the second premolar temporary crown. **B,** Three-week elongated ulcer on the dorsal surface of the tongue.

discontinued and a new brush used in such a fashion that it does not contact the gingiva until complete regression has occurred. A tetracycline mouthrinse used and expectorated 3 times a day may help resolution.

Persistent single ulcers of RIHS occur in some situations in which the patient is otherwise healthy (Fig. 11-7). These ulcers may measure more than 1 cm across, continue indefinitely, and require excision and closure for secondary healing to occur. Such lesions have a tendency to recur at the same site. Diagnosis is difficult because the classic vesiculoulcerative phase has usually disappeared before examination.

RIHS is frequent and persistent in the *immunocompromised* individual[39-41] and may take two forms: (1) disseminated erythrematous involvement of the oral mucosa with scattered small vesiculoulcerative lesions or (2) one, two, or three larger, destructive ulcers sometimes marginated with small vesicles.[39] Herpes and acquired immunodeficiency syndrome are discussed in Chapter 36.

Management Usually, RIHS lesions do not require treatment. The troublesome lesion may be dried and swabbed with a tetracycline solution or 0.12% solution of chlorhexidine and covered with an oral bandage material. This can be used with triamcinolone or fluocinolone in the otherwise healthy patient. Continuing persistent active lesions benefit from systemic administration of acyclovir.[42] Care should be taken to avoid contacting these lesions during brushing and flossing. Large doses of lysine may be helpful in shortening the duration of lesions and suppressing recurrences.[43]

Major Recurrent Aphthous Ulcer

Major RAU has also been called *Sutton's disease* or *periadenitis mucosa necrotica recurrens.* Approximately 80% of RAUs are minor RAUs, and 10% are major RAUs.[9] Major RAUs are considered a more severe form of minor RAU. Usually major RAU lesions are single, or at the most there are three. They become much larger than the minor type, sometimes up to 2 cm across; they are quite deep, are very painful, and persist for months. They often occur in the posterior of the mouth (Fig. 11-8 and Plate B). They frequently heal with scar formation because of their depth.

Major RAUs are difficult to treat. Patients often suffer from these painful nonhealing ulcers for months. The following modalities have been used with some success: excision with primary closure, cryosurgery, topical application of tetracycline followed by cortisone ointment, and injection of corticosteroids directly into the lesion alone or in combination with systemic administration of prednisone. Other immunosuppressive drugs have been used with corticosteroids with good results.[44]

The antiinflammatory actions of corticosteroids include: (1) a reduction in the exudation of the leukocytes and plasma

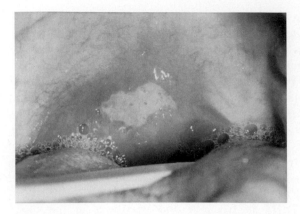

Fig. 11-8. Major RAU of the soft palate. This painful lesion had been present for 3 months.

constituents; (2) maintenance of cellular membrane integrity with prevention of cellular swelling; (3) inhibition of lysozyme release from granulocytes and inhibition of phago-cytosis; (4) stabilization of the membranes of the intracellular lysozomes containing hydrolytic enzymes; (5) decreased scar formation by inhibiting proliferation of fibroblasts; and (6) possible effect on antibody formation when administered in large doses. Corticosteroids have also been shown to suppress T-cell formation.[31]

Herpetiform Aphtha

HA account for approximately 10% of all cases of aph-thous ulceration.[31] This condition is more common in fe-male patients, and the cause is unknown. Many small, painful punctate ulcers occur over the mucosal surfaces, sometimes in clusters (Fig. 11-9). The duration is similar to minor RAU.

The widespread distribution calls for management by mouthrinse instead of treatment of individual ulcers.

Behçet's Syndrome

Behçet's syndrome involves the following types of ul-cers: (1) oral ulcers (aphthouslike); (2) recurrent ulcers of the genital region; and (3) ocular lesions, including con-junctivitis, retinitis, and uveitis.[31]

ULCERS FROM ODONTOGENIC INFECTIONS

Ulcers resulting from the drainage of pus from odonto-genic infections are easily recognized. Two similar clini-cal situations can cause them: The ulcer may serve as the cloacal opening of a sinus draining a chronic alveolar ab-scess, or the ulcer may be the site of a superficial space abscess that has spontaneously ruptured.

Features

In most cases of chronic alveolar abscess, the ulcer is on the alveolar ridge on the buccal or the lingual surface, usually near the mucobuccal fold but occasionally on the palate (Figs. 11-10 and 13-6). The majority of chronic

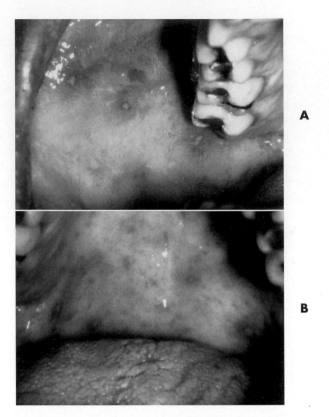

Fig. 11-9. Herpetiform aphthous ulceration. Small vesiculoulcera-tive lesions of the buccal mucosa (**A**) and posterior palate (**B**). (Courtesy J. Guggenheimer, Pittsburgh.)

alveolar abscesses are seen in children younger than 14 years of age. Such draining sinuses and similar pathoses are discussed in detail in Chapter 13.

Other ulcers may represent the ruptured surface of an odontogenic space abscess situated on the palate or in the sublingual or vestibular areas (see Fig. 11-10). Pres-sure on the adjacent soft tissue, which causes pus to exude from the ulcer, identifies the condition. If odonto-genic infection is suspected, a thorough clinicoradio-logic examination of the teeth and supporting structures is indicated.

A gutta-percha point may be placed in the ulcer and passed into the tract as far as it will go without undue force. A radiograph is taken, and if the point is seen to reach the apex of an infected tooth, the diagnosis is ensured.

Differential Diagnosis

The odontogenic ulcer can be misdiagnosed only as the result of a cursory or careless examination. When a small ulcer (0.2 to 1 cm in diameter) is present on the mucosa of the palate, alveolus, or vestibule, an odonto-genic ulcer must always be considered. Other, less likely conditions are sinus openings from osteomyelitis and in-fected malignant tumors. A thorough discussion may be

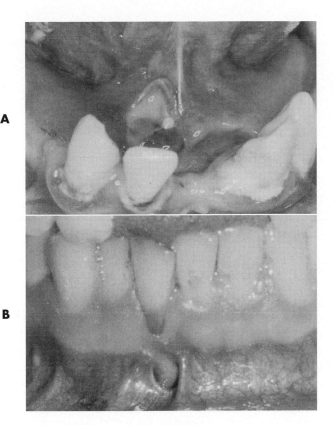

Fig. 11-10. Odontogenic ulcers. **A,** Sublingual abscess from the infected lateral incisor ruptured to produce this ulcer. **B,** Ulcer represents the oral opening of a draining chronic alveolar abscess from the pulpless lower incisor.

found in the differential diagnosis section at the end of this chapter.

Management

Endodontic therapy or extraction, which on occasion may have to be accompanied by the administration of antibiotics, usually results in the healing of the ulcer.

SLOUGHING, PSEUDOMEMBRANOUS ULCERS

Sloughing, pseudomembranous ulcers, described in detail in Chapter 8, are mentioned here because they have an ulcerated surface easily seen when the membrane is removed. Such lesions include crushing types of traumatic ulcers, acute necrotic ulcerative gingivitis, candidiasis, and gangrenous stomatitis.

Acute necrotic ulcerative gingivitis is the most common example of such lesions, and the fact that the necrotic and ulcerative process involves one or more of the tips of the interdental papillae is practically pathognomonic for the disease. However, similar lesions may be seen on the gingivae accompanying other oral lesions such as diffuse gangrenous stomatitis (see Chapter 8).

GENERALIZED MUCOSITIDES AND VESICULOBULLOUS DISEASES

Generalized mucositides and vesiculobullous diseases have been included here for completion. Although these diseases produce oral ulcerations, the ulcerations may be secondary to vesicular and bullous lesions. In most cases the whole mucosal surface of the oral cavity is a mass of ulcers, blebs, and erosive erythematous areas. A list of such diseases follows:

1. Behçet's syndrome
2. Erosive lichen planus
3. Erythema multiforme
4. Gangrenous stomatitis
5. Stevens-Johnson syndrome
6. Vesiculobullous lesions (benign mucous membrane pemphigoid, bullous lichen planus, cat-scratch disease, epidermolysis bullosa, herpangina, primary herpetic gingivostomatitis, herpes zoster, pemphigus and its variants, foot-and-mouth disease, hand-foot-and-mouth disease)

Some of these more common diseases are discussed in detail in Chapter 6. Their usually wide dissemination in the oral cavity precludes their being taken for one of the discrete, frequently solitary ulcers discussed in this chapter. However, a solitary lesion may precede the disseminated manifestations and may therefore be confused with the solitary ulcers that are the subject of this chapter.

SQUAMOUS CELL CARCINOMA

Squamous cell carcinoma is the most common oral malignancy and represents approximately 90% to 95% of all malignant tumors that occur in the mouth and jaws. It is discussed as a red lesion in Chapter 5, a white lesion in Chapter 8, a red and white lesion in Chapter 9, and an exophytic lesion in Chapter 10. In this chapter the ulcerative variety is stressed. Etiology, epidemiology, and management are discussed in detail in Chapter 35.

Features

Squamous cell carcinoma is the most common persistent ulcer in the oral cavity or on the lips. The patient usually is not aware of its presence until it has become relatively advanced because it is usually painless. Consequently the smaller ulcerative tumors are found during routine oral examinations.

The classic ulcerative squamous cell carcinoma is described as a craterlike lesion having a velvety red base and a rolled, indurated border (Fig. 11-11 and Plates H and I). If situated on the vermilion border, it may be covered with a crust because of the absence of saliva (see Fig. 11-11, *A*). The intraoral ulcer is usually devoid of necrotic material and is situated in the high-risk oval (see Fig. 35-1 and Plates H and I). This region includes the lower lip, floor of the mouth, ventral and lateral borders

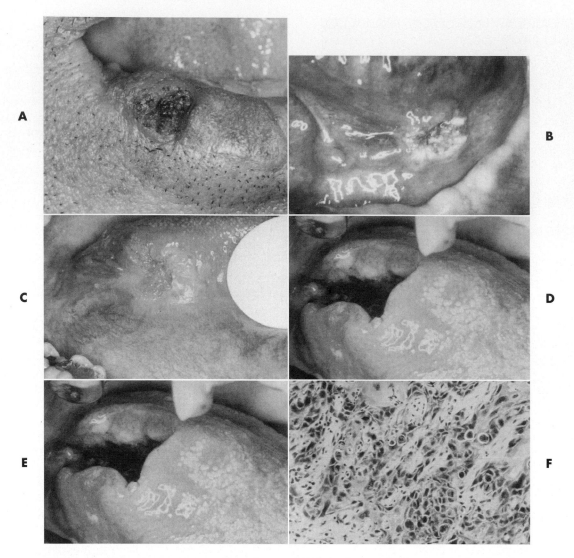

Fig. 11-11. Ulcerative squamous cell carcinomas. **F,** Photomicrograph of an invasive border of squamous cell carcinoma. (**A** courtesy R. Oglesby, East Stroudsburg, Pa; **B** courtesy S. Silverman, San Francisco.)

of the tongue, retromolar areas, tonsillar pillars, and lateral soft palate. Lesions are usually solitary but in some cases have been multifocal.

When the tumor has infiltrated the surrounding connective tissue, the base and borders of the lesion are firm on palpation. When deep infiltration occurs and the tumor is on "movable" mucosa, the mucosa becomes fixed to the deeper structures. When this occurs in specific locations, such as the undersurface of the tongue, the function of the organ may be impaired, with an alteration in speech and food management.

Differential Diagnosis

Ulcerative squamous cell carcinoma is classified as a persistent ulcer; a discussion of its distinguishing features may be found in the section on differential diagnosis of persistent ulcers at the end of this chapter.

Management

See Chapter 35.

SYPHILIS (CHANCRE AND GUMMA)

Syphilis is a venereal disease caused by the motile spirochete *Treponema pallidum;* it may be congenital or acquired. The untreated acquired form has the following easily recognizable stages:

1. The primary lesion is the chancre, which is usually solitary.
2. The secondary lesions are numerous macules, papules, mucous patches, condylomas, or combinations of these.
3. The tertiary (oral) lesions are gummas and interstitial glossitis.

The mucous patch is a grayish-white, sloughing lesion and has been included in the list of rarities in the section on sloughing, pseudomembranous, nonkeratotic white lesions in Chapter 8. Both the chancre and the gumma are ulcerated lesions, so they are included here.

Congenital syphilis may include findings of Hutchinson's incisors, mulberry molars, saddle nose, interstitial keratitis, and deafness. Hutchinson's incisors are bell- or screwdriver-shaped central incisors with notches in the middle of their incisal edges. Mulberry molars are first permanent molars that are a little smaller than normal with hypoplasia so severe on the occlusal one third of the teeth that the cusps are dwarfed and the resultant biting surface has a mulberry appearance. Interstitial keratitis is a diffuse chronic inflammation of the cornea involving the whole thickness of the cornea and is associated with superficial and deep vascularization.

Chancre

Chancres are found on the genitalia in 90% of syphilis patients but may occur on the oral mucous membrane. They develop at the site of inoculation, usually where a defect in the surface continuity of the skin or mucosa exists. The *T. pallidum* organisms are transferred by direct contact with primary or secondary lesions of an infected individual. The chancres develop approximately 3 weeks after inoculation and persist for 3 weeks to 2 months.

Features Chancres on the genitalia are characteristically painless. Oral lesions, on the other hand, almost invariably become painful soon after they ulcerate because of contamination by the oral fluids and flora. A tender and painful cervical lymphadenitis is almost always present.

The primary oral lesions occur most often on the lips, on the tip of the tongue, in the tonsillar region, or on the gingivae, commencing as small erythematous macules that become papules or small nodules and then ulcerate. Mature chancres measure from 0.5 to 2 cm in diameter and have narrow, copper-colored, slightly raised borders with a reddish-brown base or center (Figs. 11-12 and 11-13 and Plate B). The lesions are ulcerated over nearly their entire surface and have bases that are shiny and usually clear of necrotic material and debris. Occasionally chancres retain white, sloughy material (see Fig. 8-47, *A*) and have to be differentiated from the other white pseudomembranous ulcers. Chancres occurring on the vermilion border may be crusted.

The chancres are extremely contagious. They are teeming with spirochetes, which may be detected by dark-field microscopy or phase microscopy, the usual methods for examining material from the lesions. These methods are not diagnostic for oral lesions, however, because of the probable contamination of the ulcers by nonpathogenic oral spirochetes; *T. pallidum* can be positively identified if immobilized by syphilis antiserum.

Screening tests (Kahn, Wassermann, reactive plasma reagin) are used routinely, and although not specific, they

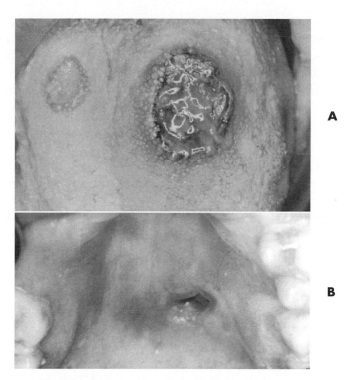

Fig. 11-12. Chancre. **A,** Two lesions on the dorsal surface of the tongue. **B,** Lesion at the junction of the hard and soft palates.

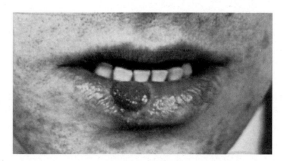

Fig. 11-13. Chancre of the lower lip. (Courtesy R. Gorlin, Minneapolis.)

are quite sensitive. Consequently, when a screening test gives a positive result, a specific test for the diagnosis of syphilis (e.g., the fluorescent treponemal antibody test or the microhemagglutinin antibody test, both of which are usually available from the state department of health) should be performed. Results of serologic tests are usually negative until the chancre has been present for 2 or 3 weeks. If the disease is not treated, the antibody levels rise slowly and remain elevated for the life of the patient. If the patient receives successful treatment in an early stage, antibody levels soon return to normal.

Since the lesions are contaminated by the oral flora, the microscopic examination of a mature oral chancre seldom yields information specific enough to identify the chancre. Consequently the microscopic diagnosis is usually "nonspecific" ulcer. Sometimes, however, the characteristic obliterative endarteritis and perivascular cuffing by lymphocytes are apparent deep in the tissue. Silver stain also reveals the presence of retained spirochetes in the inflamed areas of the biopsy specimen.

Differential diagnosis Because chancres may be present for 3 weeks to 2 months, they must be classified as both short-term and persistent ulcers. The distinguishing features are discussed in the differential diagnosis section at the end of this chapter.

Management Systemic penicillin initiated during the primary stage of the disease successfully eliminates syphilis in several days in most cases.

The multiple secondary lesions of syphilis appear 5 to 6 weeks after the disappearance of the chancres in untreated cases and undergo spontaneous remission within a few weeks, but recurrences may be manifested periodically for months or several years.

Gumma

Although a variety of lesions may occur in different locations during the tertiary stage of untreated syphilis, gummas develop in 33% to 66% of such cases. They are the most common syphilitic lesion seen in the oral cavity and appear to be the result of a type of sensitivity, since the severity of the lesion is vastly out of proportion to the few *Treponema* organisms present.[45]

Features Intraoral gummas occur most often in the midline of the palate or tongue, starting as small, firm, nodular masses and often growing to become several centimeters in diameter. Necrosis commences within the nodules and produces an ulceration of the surface epithelium. The painless lesions are sharply demarcated, and the necrotic tissue at the base of the ulcers may slough away, leaving a punched-out defect. The semifirm type of necrosis imparts a rubberlike consistency to the nodular, ulcerative masses. On occasion the necrosis is destructive, causing perforation of the palate and formation of a persistent oronasal fistula. The nodular ulcers heal after several months.

On microscopic examination a nonspecific ulcer with an extraordinary amount of necrosis is seen, and occasionally a few giant cells are present. The result of serologic examination at this stage is usually positive and often at a high titer.

Differential diagnosis Gummas may be confused easily with tubercular lesions, sarcoidosis, granulomatous fungal (mycotic) infections, oral malignancies, necrotizing sialometaplasia, and midline granuloma. The differential features are discussed in the differential diagnosis section at the end of this chapter.

Management Patients with gummas should be managed by clinicians who have been trained in all aspects of syphilitic disease because intraoral gummas imply the presence of additional gummas in other locations, which may cause more serious complications, and treatment must be tailored to minimize the possibility and intensity of the Jarisch-Herxheimer reaction.

ULCERS SECONDARY TO SYSTEMIC DISEASE

The incidence of ulcers that occur secondary to a particular noninfectious systemic disease is not high enough to warrant the assignment of separate categories to the individual ulcers. However, when all the ulcers that result from such systemic diseases are considered as a group, their combined incidence is high enough to preclude listing them among the rarities.

Such ulcers most often occur in patients with uncontrolled diabetes, uremia, blood dyscrasias (i.e., pancytopenia, leukemia, neutropenia,[46] and sickle cell anemia), and gastrointestinal disease. Ulcers occurring in immunocompromised individuals are discussed in Chapter 36.

Except in the cases of sickle cell anemia and uremia, the pathogenesis of ulcer formation is similar. The resistance of the host tissue and the leukocytic defense is so diminished that a small break in the integrity of the mucosa becomes superficially infected by the oral flora and an ulcer results. Although a diffuse gangrenous stomatitis may also occur in these diseases (see Chapter 8), the discrete ulcers are emphasized in this chapter.

Features

The ulcers are tender or painful, usually well demarcated, and shallow with a narrow erythematous halo; they may contain some yellowish or gray necrotic material (Fig. 11-14). They may vary in size from 0.5 to 2 or 3 cm in diameter. A painful regional cervical lymphadenitis is almost invariably present.

In sickle cell anemia the ulcers form in regions of ischemic infarcts caused by the plugging of small blood vessels by sickle cell thrombi; this plugging occurs during sickle cell crisis. Such ulcers are usually painless and frequently involve the marginal gingivae and interdental papillae (see Fig. 11-14, *A*).

Ulcers that occur in patients with uremia may also involve the marginal gingivae (see Fig. 11-14, *C* and *D*) or other regions of the oral mucosa. These ulcers are related to the bacterial breakdown of urea (present in high concentrations in the saliva) to ammonia, mouth-breathing acidosis, dehydration, and bacterial or fungal infection.

Differential Diagnosis

The distinguishing features of these ulcers secondary to systemic disease are discussed in the section on differential diagnosis at the end of this chapter.

Management

In the management of oral ulcers secondary to a systemic disease, it is important that the dental clinician recognize the predisposing condition that is basic to the oral problem. It is especially important that the dentist seek medical consultation. The dentist and physician can manage the problem as a team, whereas the oral condition is un-

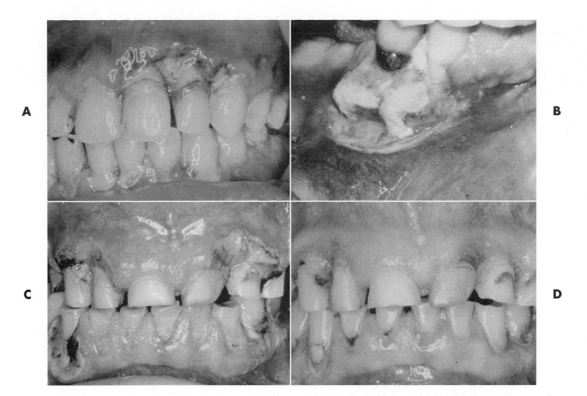

Fig. 11-14. Ulcers in systemic disease. **A,** Gingival ulcer in a patient with sickle cell anemia. **B,** Gingival ulcer in a patient with acute leukemia. **C** and **D,** Ragged, sloughing gingival ulcers in a uremic patient. (**D** was taken 2 weeks after **C.** The uremia had been corrected, and a brief regimen of hydrogen peroxide mouthwashes was instituted.) (**A** courtesy R. Dixon, Chicago; **B** courtesy G. MacDonald, San Jose, Calif.)

likely to respond satisfactorily to local treatment alone. While the physician treats the systemic disease, the dental clinician initiates procedures to ensure the establishment of the best possible oral hygiene. Toward this end, a brief regimen of hydrogen peroxide mouthrinses several times a day is recommended (see Fig. 11-14). The hydrogen peroxide debrides the necrotic tissues. In addition, the systemic administration of antibiotics (amoxicillin) compensates for the patient's diminished defenses and helps sterilize the oral ulcers. If resolution does not occur within a few days, culture and sensitivity tests should be attempted.

TRAUMATIZED TUMORS (TYPES USUALLY NOT ULCERATED)

As described in Chapter 3, exophytic growths originating in tissues beneath the surface epithelium characteristically have smoothly contoured, nonulcerated surfaces. Such lesions include benign and malignant mesenchymal tumors, inflammatory hyperplasias, metastatic tumors (not superficial), most types of minor salivary gland tumors, and odontogenic tumors. Most of these entities are discussed in detail in Chapter 10 as exophytic lesions. Some of these exophytic lesions become ulcerated, so they are included as a group in this chapter. The cause of the ulceration is usually obvious but should always be identified so that the lesion is not confused with a primarily ulcerative lesion. Fortunately, most of these lesions retain part of their smooth surface contour (Fig. 11-15).

The ulceration is often the result of mechanical trauma from mastication. Fig. 11-15, *C,* illustrates a case in which a central ameloblastoma became ulcerated when an extruded upper third molar repeatedly traumatized the posterior mandibular swelling that was produced by the ameloblastoma. Even malignant mesenchymal tumors usually have a smooth surface until some traumatic episode causes a surface erosion or ulceration. Such a surface ulceration is frequently the result of an incisional biopsy. Fig. 11-15, *A* and *B,* show a smooth-surfaced chondrosarcoma of the maxilla that became necrotic and ulcerated after an incisional biopsy.

In other instances, masses of tumor cells interfere with the blood supply of the surface epithelium to such an extent that the epithelium becomes necrotic and ulcerative. Occasionally a tumor mass extrudes from a recent extraction wound, and since the growth does not have an epithelial covering, it soon becomes necrotic and ulcerated because of the oral environment.

It is helpful to recognize that these ulcerated lesions are primarily exophytic; their classification as such facilitates their identification.

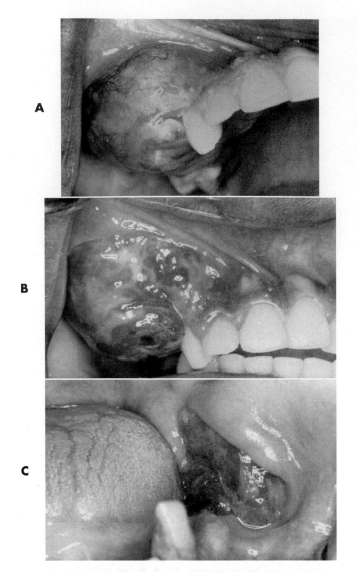

Fig. 11-15. Ulcerated tumors. **A** and **B,** Chondrosarcoma. (**B** was taken 2 weeks after an incisional biopsy of the lesion in **A.**) **C,** Ameloblastoma with an unusual surface ulceration inflicted by an upper molar. (**A** and **B** courtesy R. Nolan, Willison, ND.)

MINOR SALIVARY GLAND TUMORS

Most salivary gland tumors are firm exophytic lesions (see Chapter 10) that seldom ulcerate except as a result of the trauma described in the preceding section (Fig. 11-16, *B*). Some types of salivary gland tumors, however, contain quantities of pooled liquid and are relatively soft and fluctuant. Such lesions include low-grade mucoepidermoid carcinoma, mucous adenocarcinoma, and papillary cystadenoma lymphomatosum (Warthin's tumor). If the collection of fluid is near the surface, the pool may rupture with ensuing ulceration. These tumors may ulcerate at a relatively early stage, even before they have attained sufficient mass to produce much of an exophytic lesion. They therefore appear as shallow persistent ulcers that can easily be mistaken for a squamous cell carcinoma (Fig. 11-16, *A*).

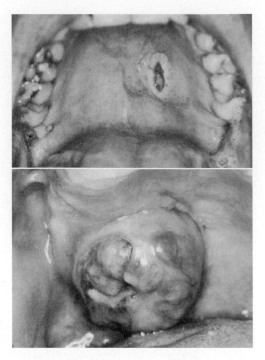

Fig. 11-16. Ulcerated minor salivary gland tumors. **A,** Low-grade mucoepidermoid tumor. **B,** Benign mixed tumor 1 week after incisional biopsy. Before the biopsy, the surface was smooth and nonulcerated. (**A** courtesy D. Bonomo, Flossmoor, Ill.)

A further discussion is included in the section on differential diagnosis at the end of this chapter.

Differential Diagnosis

Lesions that should be considered in the differential diagnosis with ulcerated minor salivary gland tumors of the posterior hard palate are squamous cell carcinoma, necrotizing sialometaplasia (Fig. 11-17), midline nonhealing granuloma (see Fig. 11-17), chancre, gumma, leukemic ulcer, malignancy of the maxillary sinus, neurotrophic ulcer, traumatic ulcer, and major aphthous ulcer (see Fig. 11-8).

RARITIES

A multitude of rare lesions may occur as oral ulcers. A suggested list is located at the beginning of this chapter. Some rare oral ulcers are shown in Figs. 11-17 and 11-18.

DIFFERENTIAL DIAGNOSIS OF ORAL ULCERS

Since oral ulcers may be conveniently divided into two groups, short term (those that usually disappear within 3 weeks) and persistent (those that usually last longer than 3 weeks), it is convenient to discuss the differential diagnosis of these two groups separately. Nonetheless, both groups have the following in common:

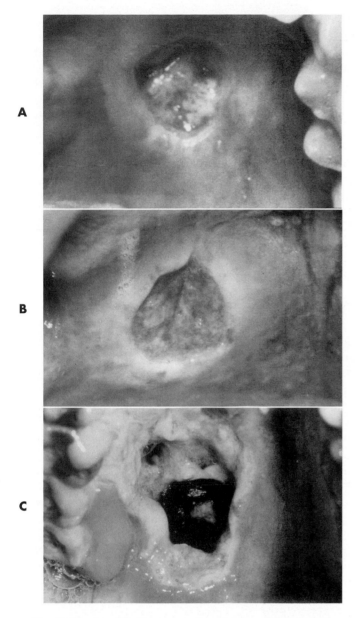

Fig. 11-17. **A** and **B,** Two cases of necrotizing sialometaplasia on the palate. **C,** Midline nonhealing granuloma. (**A** courtesy A. Abrams, Los Angeles; **B** courtesy C. Dunlap, and B. Barker, Kansas City, Mo; **C** courtesy S. Goldman, Hinsdale, Ill.)

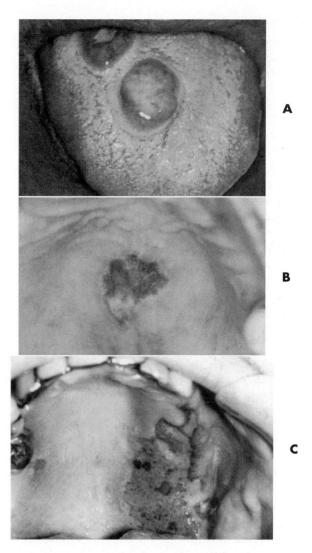

Fig. 11-18. Rare oral ulcers. **A,** Metastatic carcinoma from squamous cell carcinoma of the esophagus in a 46-year-old man. **B,** Palatine lesion of psoriasis. **C,** Benign mucous membrane pemphigoid. (**A** courtesy E. Robinson, Toledo, Ohio; **B,** courtesy P.D. Toto, Waukegan, Ill; **C** courtesy D. Bonomo, Flossmoor, Ill.)

1. The complaint of pain in an oral ulcer does not permit a definite identification of the ulcer, since the majority of oral ulcers, regardless of their cause, may soon become painful from contamination by the oral liquids and flora.
2. Because of contamination by oral fluids, a painful regional lymphadenitis almost always accompanies oral ulcers.

Consequently the presence or absence of pain in the ulcer or the associated enlarged nodes is not a conclusive diagnostic feature. Exceptions to this rule are squamous cell carcinoma and other peripheral malignancies, which are characteristically painless early in their course because most of the peripheral sensory nerve endings are destroyed or their surfaces are covered by tumor epithelium. These malignant lesions often do not become painful until they have attained a large size. When metastatic spread to regional lymph nodes has occurred, the enlarged nodes are likewise characteristically painless, as well as quite firm.

Again, it should be emphasized that these characteristics are not diagnostic because entities such as benign lymph node hyperplasias and enlarged fibrosed nodes are usually firm and painless.

Short-term ulcers are shallow lesions; they are not raised above the mucosal surface. In contrast, persistent ulcers frequently are associated with extensive borders and bases (see Fig. 11-11, *B*).

Short-Term Ulcers

The more common short-term ulcers, ranked according to their approximate frequency of occurrence in the general population, are listed in the box below, left.

Ulcers secondary to systemic disease may be short or long term. Helpful leads are often obtained from the patient's history, if the disease has been previously detected. If the patient is not aware of the predisposing disease, however, a careful history should reveal information that suggests the possibility of a specific disease or group of diseases. For instance, the patient may complain of fatigue, dizziness, and nausea with some of the anemias or of the polydipsia and polyuria with diabetes. The patient may have a fever, a paleness of the mucosa, or both, which should alert the clinician to the possibility of one of the anemias, leukemias, or pancytopenias. Appropriate laboratory procedures are invaluable in helping identify the specific disease. Since there is nothing specific about the appearance of these oral ulcers, the clinician must obtain a complete history and rely on it in every case.

The single ulcer that heralds the arrival of any of the generalized mucositides or vesiculobullous diseases appears perhaps a few days or weeks before the diffuse nature of the disease manifests itself. A discussion of the differential diagnosis of the oral mucositides is included in Chapter 6.

Ulcers resulting from odontogenic infection are easily diagnosed if the clinician remembers to include them in the differential diagnosis. Although there is no fluctuant, painful swelling at this stage, a careful systematic approach identifies the involved tooth from which the infection is draining. The clinician should suspect any small ulcer on the alveolus or palate of being associated with an odontogenic infection. He or she should then attempt to demonstrate the presence of a sinus with a gutta-percha cone, and, if successful, should take a radiograph of the area with the cone in place to determine whether the tract leads to the apex of a tooth. Sometimes, digital pressure on the involved tooth or the alveolus causes a drop of pus to exude from the opening in the ulcer, which helps the clinician determine the correct diagnosis.

The RAU and RIHS lesions can be differentiated, in most cases, by the criteria listed in the box on p. 166 and Table 11-1. As a general rule, RIHS lesions involve a cluster of small, punctate ulcers, none of which is more than

0.5 cm in diameter, and occurs on mucosa that is fixed to periosteum. (Hand-foot-and-mouth disease shows these small ulcers in the three locations.) On the other hand, RAU involves a yellowish ulcer with smoothly contoured borders measuring between 0.5 and 2 cm in diameter with a narrow erythematous halo and occurring on a loose mucosal surface. This conclusion is drawn if trauma cannot be implicated and the patient does not have an underlying systemic disease associated with stomatitis or if an odontogenic infection cannot be identified.

Traumatic ulcers are easily recognized if the clinician can establish the cause of the physical injury. In some cases the origin or nature of the trauma is obscure; consequently the diagnosis is difficult to establish. Occasionally, traumatic lesions, especially those occurring on the tongue, may persist for weeks; these lesions are discussed in the section on the differential diagnosis of persistent ulcers.

Persistent Ulcers

The most common persistent ulcers, ranked according to their approximate incidence in the general population, are listed in the box below, right.

Systemic mycosis with oral lesions is very uncommon in most of the United States and Canada. Nevertheless, when considered as a group, the general practitioner could be faced with one of these. Oral lesions in systemic mycoses have been recently reviewed for the practitioner.[47] Metastatic tumors of the oral soft tissues are quite uncommon and occur usually in the lower half of the oral cavity. In the absence of a primary tumor elsewhere or symptoms of such, secondary tumors are assigned a low rank on the differential list.

If a cystic area in a low-grade mucoepidermoid tumor ruptures, the resemblance to a squamous cell carcinoma may be striking, since both tumors may appear as deep ulcers with firm, raised, rolled borders (see Fig. 11-16, *A*). Al-

---

DIFFERENTIAL LIST OF SHORT-TERM ULCERS

- Traumatic ulcer
- RAU, RIHS, and herpetiform ulcers
- Ulcer occurring as a result of odontogenic infection
- Ulcer occurring as a herald lesion of generalized mucositis or vesiculobullous disease
- Ulcer secondary to noninfectious systemic disease

DIFFERENTIAL LIST OF PERSISTENT ULCERS

- Traumatic ulcer
- Ulcer from odontogenic infection
- Major aphthous ulcer
- Squamous cell carcinoma
- Ulcer secondary to systemic disease
- Ulcer in human immunodeficiency virus disease
- Traumatized tumor that does not usually ulcerate
- Low-grade mucoepidermoid tumor
- Metastatic tumor
- Keratoacanthoma
- Necrotizing sialometaplasia
- Systemic mycosis
- Chancre
- Gumma
- Other rarities

though the squamous cell carcinoma is a more common oral malignancy, if the questionable lesion is situated in the posterolateral region of the hard palate, it is most likely to be a minor salivary gland tumor, since the hard palate is an unlikely site for a squamous cell carcinoma. If a mucocele-like lesion was reported to be in the same location a few days earlier, mucoepidermoid tumor must be given a high priority in the differential diagnosis. If the lesion in question is painless, the possibility that it is a traumatic ulcer, a chancre, an ulcer secondary to systemic disease, or major aphthae is eliminated. If an odontogenic infection cannot be found, the probability that it is an odontogenic ulcer is lessened. Intraoral gummas occur most often in the midline of the palate or tongue and are rare in industrialized countries.

Tumors and growths originating in tissues separate from and beneath the stratified squamous epithelial surface do not characteristically ulcerate, but they may do so because of a mechanical injury or as the result of an incisional biopsy. If such ulcers are the result of an incisional biopsy, they should be easily identified in the history; on the other hand, if they have resulted from mechanical trauma, a careful intraoral examination discloses the cause. The differential diagnosis of exophytic lesions is discussed in detail in Chapter 10.

Ulcers secondary to systemic disease are usually short term, but they may persist if the predisposing systemic disease is not corrected. They may be confused with any of the shallow persistent ulcers—traumatic ulcer, early squamous cell carcinoma, chancre, and early mucoepidermoid tumor. Usually the systemic problem becomes apparent through the history or clinical examination and prompts the proper diagnosis. These ulcers secondary to systemic disease are usually painful and have minimal bases in contrast to early squamous cell carcinoma or early mucoepidermoid tumors. A traumatic ulcer can generally be ruled out by establishing the absence of physical injury. Although serologic tests of a patient who appears to have an ulcer secondary to a systemic disease may have positive findings, a chancre can usually be ruled out if a smear of the lesion does not provide spirochetes that are immobilized by syphilitic antiserum.

Ulcers in human immunodeficiency virus disease are discussed in Chapter 36. A positive human immunodeficiency virus test would prompt inclusion of these ulcerations in the diagnostic list.

Gummata are uncommon oral lesions that occur mostly in the midline of the palate or the midline of the dorsum of the tongue. Similar-appearing pathoses rarely develop at these sites. A traumatic ulcer on a palatine torus or a midline nonhealing granuloma might be considered, but the ulcerated torus should be recognized, and the latter entity is so rare as to be an unlikely diagnosis. Also, the rubbery consistency of the gumma eliminates the torus and the midline nonhealing granuloma from consideration. The serologic findings are usually strongly positive in the case of gummata.

Tests for chancres usually result in positive serologic findings, especially after the lesion has been present for 2 or more weeks. If the patient states that he or she was recently in contact with a person who may have had syphilis, this establishes a high priority for chancre in the differential diagnosis. If the ulcer is reddish brown, has a copper-colored halo, and is shallow and if there is no history of mechanical trauma, the diagnosis is strengthened; this is especially true if the patient is under 40 years of age because the lesion is less likely to be an early squamous cell carcinoma or mucoepidermoid tumor. If spirochetes immobilized by syphilitic antiserum are found in the ulcer, the diagnosis of chancre is firmly established.

Necrotizing sialometaplasia is a benign, inflammatory process of the minor salivary glands, which is primarily found in the posterior hard palate[48-53] (see Fig. 11-17, *A* and *B*). The cause is unknown. Infarction has been suggested, although the underlying predisposing factors are not clear. The lesion is usually a nodule of slight elevation, and the surface may be ulcerated. Average age of patients is 46 years, and it is more common in men. These lesions, although uncommon, mimic minor salivary gland tumors in appearance and location and must thus always be considered as a possible diagnosis when a soft tissue mass is observed in the posterior hard palate. Necrotizing sialometaplasia is basically a self-limiting disease that usually heals in 6 to 12 weeks. During its ulcerated stage (see Fig. 11-17), it very much resembles a squamous cell carcinoma and an ulcerated mucoepidermoid carcinoma. Biopsy is indicated to establish the diagnosis and to differentiate between necrotizing sialometaplasia and other, similar lesions.

Keratoacanthoma is similar to ulcerative types of squamous cell carcinoma (see Figs. 32-3 and 33-19). It rarely occurs in the oral mucosa but often is seen on the lower lip, where it may look identical to a squamous cell carcinoma.[54-55] Its rapid growth may help differentiate it from carcinoma, but excision is necessary. Although there are some histopathologic (histochemical) differences between keratoacanthomas and squamous cell carcinomas, the differences are not significant and are not reliable for differentiation.[55]

Major RAU is a persistent ulcer that may closely resemble a squamous cell carcinoma on clinical examination (see Fig. 11-8). However, two striking features help the clinician rule out the malignancy and make the identification of major RAU: the severe pain and the broad inflammatory (nonvelvety red) border.

Squamous cell carcinoma is the most common malignant ulcer of the oral mucosa. The early lesion may be a painless, shallow ulcer with a velvety red base and a firm, raised border. The healing traumatic ulcer, because its base may be filled with reddish-pink granulation tissue, may resemble this early lesion. A lesion is most likely a squamous cell carcinoma, however, if (1) the patient is over 40 years of age, is male, and smokes or drinks heavily; (2) there is no evidence that the lesion is related to trauma or systemic disease; (3) the serologic findings are negative, and the presence of spirochetes cannot be demonstrated; and (4) the lesion is not located on the posterolateral region of the hard palate.

Ulcers from odontogenic infection are discussed in the section on the differential diagnosis of short-term ulcers.

Traumatic ulcers, especially on the tongue, may persist for several weeks after the traumatic factor has been eliminated. Such ulcers cannot be differentiated from malignancies on a clinical basis alone and often require complete excision and primary wound closure before they resolve. This procedure is indicated because it permits the microscopic examination of the ulcerated tissue, as well as healing and resolution of the lesion.

FISSURES

Fissures represent a distinct clinical entity and should be grouped separately. The more common fissures that occur in the oral region, ranked according to approximate frequency, include the following (Fig. 11-19):

1. Angular cheilosis
2. Congenital cleft
3. Epulis fissuratum
4. Fissured tongue
5. Median rhomboid glossitis—fissured variety
6. Melkersson-Rosenthal syndrome
7. Squamous cell carcinoma—fissured variety
8. Syphilitic rhagades

The differential diagnosis for these entities is not included in this text.

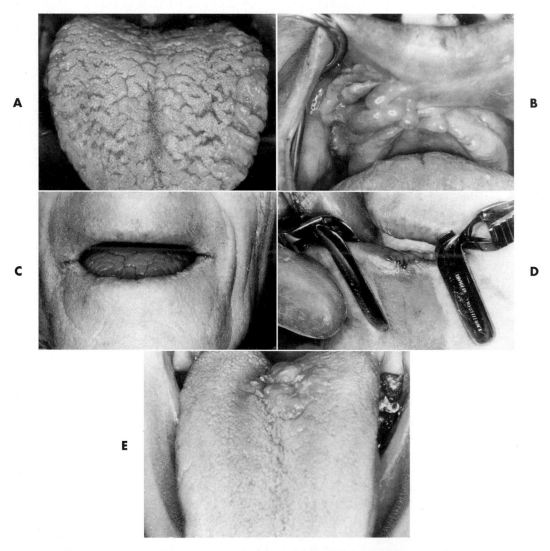

Fig. 11-19. Oral fissures. **A,** Fissured tongue. **B,** Large inflammatory hyperplasia (epulis fissuratum). **C,** Angular cheilosis. **D,** Squamous cell carcinoma. **E,** Fissured type of median rhomboid glossitis.

REFERENCES

1. Spouge JD: *Oral pathology,* St Louis, 1973, Mosby.
2. Schiødt M: Traumatic lesions of the gingiva provoked by tooth brushing, *Oral Surg* 52:261, 1981 (letter to the editor).
3. Pattison GL: Self-inflicted gingival injuries: literature review and case report, *J Periodontol* 54:299, 1983.
4. Budtz-Jorgensen E: Oral mucosal lesions associated with the wearing of removable dentures, *J Oral Pathol* 10:65-80, 1981.
5. Peters TED, Blair AE, Freeman RG: Prevention of self-inflicted trauma in comatose patients, *Oral Surg* 57:367-370, 1984.
6. Mader CL: Lingual frenum ulcer resulting from orogenital sex, *J Am Dent Assoc* 103:888-890, 1981.
7. Rodu B, Russell CM: Performance of a hydroxypropyl cellulose film former in normal and ulcerated mucosa, *Oral Pathol* 65:699-703, 1988.
8. Rodu B, Russell CM, Desmarais AJ: Clinical and chemical properties of a novel mucosal bioadhesive agent, *J Oral Pathol* 17:564-567, 1988.
9. Lamey P-J, Lewis MAO: Oral medicine in practice: oral ulceration, *Br Dent J* 167:127-131, 1989.
10. Savage NW, Seymour GJ: Specific lymphocytotoxic destruction of autogenous epithelial cell targets in recurrent aphthous stomatitis, *Aust Dent J* 39:98-104, 1994.
11. Damm D: A theory unifying the pathogenesis of recurrent aphthous ulcerations, *Oral Surg* 76:588, 1993.
12. Nolan A, Lamey P-J, Milligan KA, Forsyth A: Recurrent aphthous ulceration and food sensitivity, *J Oral Pathol Med* 20:473-475, 1991.
13. Hay KD, Reade PC: The use of an elimination diet in the treatment of recurrent aphthous ulceration of the oral cavity, *Oral Surg* 57:504-507, 1984.
14. Hunter IP, Ferguson MM, Scully C, et al: Effects of dietary gluten elimination in patients with recurrent aphthous stomatitis and no detectable enteropathy, *Oral Surg* 75:595-598, 1993.
15. Pedersen A, Pedersen BK: Natural killer cell function and number of peripheral blood are not altered in recurrent aphthous ulceration, *Oral Surg* 76:616-619, 1993.
16. Pedersen A, Hougen HP, Kenrad B: T-lymphocyte subsets in oral mucosa of patients with recurrent aphthous ulceration, *J Oral Pathol Med* 21:176-180, 1992.
17. Landesberg R, Fallon M, Insel R: Alterations of T helper/inducer and T suppressor/inducer cells in patients with recurrent aphthous ulcers, *Oral Surg* 69:205-208, 1990.
18. Taylor LJ, Bagg J, Walker DM, Peters TJ: Increased production of tumor necrosis factor by peripheral blood leukocytes in patients with recurrent oral aphthous ulceration, *J Oral Pathol Med* 21:21-25, 1992.
19. Porter SR, Scully C, Bowder J: Immunoglobulin G subclasses in recurrent aphthous stomatitis, *J Oral Pathol Med* 21:26-27, 1992.
20. Scully, C: Are viruses associated with aphthae or oral vesiculoerosive disorders? *Br J Oral Maxillofac Surg* 31:173-177, 1993.
21. Pedersen A, Hornsleth A: Recurrent aphthous ulceration: a possible clinical manifestation of reactivation of varicella zoster or cytomegalovirus infection, *Oral Pathol Med* 22:64-68, 1993.
22. Siegel RD, Granich, R: Letter to the editor, *Oral Surg* 76:406, 1993.
23. MacPhail L, Greenspan D, Greenspan JS: Letter to the editor, *Oral Surg* 76:406-407, 1993.
24. Tyldesley WR: Stomatitis and recurrent oral ulceration: is a full blood screen necessary? *Br J Oral Surg* 21:27-30, 1983.
25. Olson J, Feinberg I, Silverman S, et al: Serum vitamin B_{12}, folate, and iron levels in recurrent aphthous ulceration, *Oral Surg* 54:517-520, 1982.
26. Pedersen A: Psychological stress and recurrent aphthous ulceration, *J Oral Pathol Med* 18:19-22, 1989.
27. Miller MF, Garfunkel AA, Ram CA, et al: The inheritance of recurrent aphthous stomatitis: observations on susceptibility, *Oral Surg* 49:409-412, 1980.
28. Ferguson MM, Carter J, Boyle P: An epidemiological study of factors associated with recurrent aphthae in women, *J Oral Med* 39:212-217, 1984.
29. Wray D, Graykowski EA, Notkins AL: Role of mucosal injury in initiating recurrent aphthous stomatitis, *Br Med J* 283:1569-1570, 1981.
30. Grady D, Ernster VL, Stillman L, Greenspan J: Smoking tobacco use prevents aphthous stomatitis, *Oral Surg* 74:463-465, 1992.
31. Vincent SD, Lilly GE: Clinical, historic, and therapeutic features of aphthous stomatitis: literature review and open clinical trial employing steroids, *Oral Surg* 74:79-86, 1992.
32. Weathers DR, Griffin JW: Intraoral ulcerations of recurrent herpes simplex and recurrent aphthae: two distinct clinical entities, *J Am Dent Assoc* 81:81-87, 1970.
33. Miles DA, Bricker SL, Rasmus TF, Potter RH: Triamcinolone acetonide versus chlorhexidine for treatment of recurrent stomatitis, *Oral Surg* 75:397-402, 1993.
34. Meiller TF, Kutcher MJ, Overholser CD, et al: Effect of an antimicrobial mouthrinse on recurrent aphthous ulcerations, *Oral Surg* 72:425-429, 1991.
35. Amit R, Morag A, Ravid Z, et al: Detection of herpes simplex virus in gingival tissue, *J Periodontol* 63:502-506, 1992.
36. Davis LE, Redman JC, Skipper BJ, McLaren LC: Natural history of frequent recurrences of herpes simplex labialis, *Oral Surg* 66:558-561, 1988.
37. Merchant VA, Molinari JA, Sabes WR: Herpetic whitlow: report of a case with multiple recurrences, *Oral Surg* 55:568-571, 1983.
38. Rowe NH, Hëine CS, Kowalski CJ: Herpetic whitlow: an occupational disease of practicing dentists, *J Am Dent Assoc* 105:471-473, 1982.
39. Cohen SG, Greenberg MS: Chronic oral herpes simplex virus infection in immunocompromised patients, *Oral Surg* 59:465-471, 1985.
40. Flaitz CM, Hammond HL: The immunoperoxidase method for the rapid diagnosis of intraoral herpes simplex virus infection in patients receiving bone marrow transplants, *Spec Care Dent* 8:82-85, 1988.
41. Barrett AP, Buckley DJ, Greenberg ML, Earl MJ: The value of exfoliative cytology in the diagnosis of oral herpes simplex infection in immunosuppressed patients, *Oral Surg* 62:175-178, 1986.
42. Peterson DE, Greenspan D, Squier CA: Oral infections in the immunocompromised host, *J Oral Pathol Med* 21:193-198, 1992.
43. Thein DJ, Hurt WC: Lysine as a prophylactic agent in the treatment of recurrent herpes simplex labialis, *Oral Surg* 58:659-666, 1984.
44. Braun RS, Bottomley WK: Combination immunosupressant and topical steroid therapy for treatment of recurrent major aphthae: a case report, *Oral Surg* 69:42-44, 1990.
45. Meyer I, Shklar G: The oral manifestations of acquired syphilis: a study of eighty-one cases, *Oral Surg* 23:45-57, 1967.
46. Porter SR, Scully C, Standen GR: Autoimmune neutropenia manifesting as recurrent oral ulceration, *Oral Surg* 78:178-180, 1994.
47. de Almeida OP, Scully C: Oral lesions in systemic mycoses, *Curr Opin Dent* 1:423-428, 1991.
48. Abrams AM, Melrose RJ, Howell FV: Necrotizing sialometaplasia: a disease simulating malignancy, *Cancer* 32:130-135, 1973.
49. Grillon GL, Lally E: Necrotizing sialometaplasia: literature review and presentation of five cases, *J Oral Surg* 39:747-753, 1981.
50. Samit AM, Mashberg A, Greene GW: Necrotizing sialometaplasia, *J Oral Surg* 37:353-356, 1979.
51. Brannon RB, Fowler CB, Hartman KS: Necrotizing sialometaplasia: a clinicopathologic study of sixty-nine cases and review of the literature, *J Oral Surg* 72:317-325, 1991.
52. Russel JD, Glover GW, Friedmann: View from beneath: pathology in focus-necrotizing sialometaplasia, *J Laryngol Otol* 106:569-571, 1992.
53. Anneroth G, Hanson LS: Necrotizing sialometaplasia, *Int J Oral Surg* 11:283-291, 1982.
54. Bass KD: Solitary keratoacanthoma of the lip, *J Oral Surg* 38:53-55, 1980.
55. Ellis GL: Differentiating keratoacanthoma from squamous cell carcinoma of the lower lip: an analysis of intraepithelial elastic fibers and intracytoplasmic glycogen, *Oral Surg* 56:527-531, 1983.

CHAPTER 12

Intraoral Brownish, Bluish, or Black Conditions

NORMAN K. WOOD

PAUL W. GOAZ

DANNY R. SAWYER

The intraoral conditions classified as brownish, bluish, or black may be categorized according to whether they produce distinct and discretely circumscribed lesions or a generalized and diffuse discoloration of the patient.

DISTINCT CIRCUMSCRIBED TYPES
MELANOPLAKIA
SMOKER'S MUCOSAL MELANOSIS
VARICOSITY
AMALGAM TATTOO
PETECHIA AND ECCHYMOSIS
EARLY HEMATOMA
LATE HEMATOMA
HEMANGIOMA
ORAL MELANOTIC MACULE
MUCOCELE
RANULA
SUPERFICIAL CYST
GIANT CELL GRANULOMA
BLACK HAIRY TONGUE
LYMPHANGIOMA
"PIGMENTED" FIBROUS HYPERPLASIA
MELANOMA
ORAL NEVUS
MUCUS-PRODUCING SALIVARY GLAND
  TUMORS
VON RECKLINGHAUSEN'S DISEASE
ALBRIGHT'S SYNDROME
HEAVY METAL LINES
KAPOSI'S SARCOMA
RARITIES
  Acanthosis nigricans
  Acromegaly
  Addison's disease (distinct circumscribed
    lesions)
  Acquired immunodeficiency syndrome–
    related pigmentation
  Ameloblastoma, peripheral
  Amyloidosis
  Angioma bullosa haemorrhagica
  Angiosarcoma

Blue nevus
Blue rubber bleb nevus syndrome
Chewing of *Catha edulis* leaves[1]
Child abuse
Chronic obstructive pulmonary disease
Cushing's syndrome
Drug administration
  Chlorpromazine
  Minocycline
  Oral contraceptives (high estrogen)
  Quinidine
Fabry's disease
Gaucher's disease
Giant cell lesion of hyperparathyroidism
Hemangioendothelioma
Hemangiopericytoma
Henoch-Schönlein purpura
Hereditary hemorrhagic telangiectasia
Incontinentia pigmenti
Kaposi's sarcoma (not related to acquired
  immunodeficiency syndrome)
Lentigo
Lichen planus
Lupus erythematosus
Lymphangiomas of neonates
Lymphoma
Maffucci's syndrome
Melanocytic hyperplasia[2]
  Lentigo simplex
  Junctional lentigo
  Malignant melanoma in situ
  Intraoral melanoacanthoma
McCune-Albright Syndrome[3]
Melanotic neuroectodermal tumor of infancy
Multinucleate cell angiohistiocytoma[4]
Necrotizing fasciitis

Nelson's syndrome
Oral focal mucinosis[5]
Oral intravascular papillary endothelial
  hyperplasia[6]
Oral psoriasis
Pernicious anemia
Peutz-Jeghers syndrome
Pheochromocytoma
Quinidine pigmentation
Radiotherapy, external beam
Rheumatic fever
Scleroderma
Squamous cell carcinoma, pigmented[7]
Submucous fibrosis
Superficial cartilaginous tumor in patient
  with ochronosis or alkaptonuria
Superficial *Pseudomonas aeruginosa* infec-
  tion
Tattoo (other than amalgam)
Thyrotoxicosis
Tooth cleaning with *Juglans regia* bark[1]
Uremia (petechiae)
Wegener's granulomatosis
Xeroderma pigmentosa
**GENERALIZED BROWNISH, BLUISH,
  OR BLACK CONDITIONS**
CYANOSIS
CHLOASMA GRAVIDARUM
ADDISON'S DISEASE
HEMOCHROMATOSIS
ARGYRIA
RARITIES
  Aniline intoxication
  Arsenic poisoning
  Carotenemia
  Chloroquine therapy

Dermatomyositis
Idiopathic familial juvenile hypoparathyroidism, Addison's disease, superficial
   candidiasis

Minocycline therapy
Pellagra
Porphyria
Sprue

Wilson's disease

The brownish, bluish, or black color that serves as the basis for this category of disorders originates from one of two sources: the accumulation of colored material in abnormal amounts or locations in the superficial tissues or a pooled, clear fluid just beneath the epithelium. The amassed material that effects these color changes may be exogenous or endogenous.

The exogenous substances that produce the brownish, bluish, or black conditions usually include heavy metals not normally found in the body, commercial dyes, vegetable pigments, and various other stains that have been ingested or introduced directly into the tissues. The point of introduction may be at the site of or remote from the lesion in question.

The endogenous chromatic materials that produce the brownish, bluish, or black conditions usually result from increased melanin states or are derived from blood pigments or abnormal aggregations of metals normally found in the body. The color imparted by such exogenous or endogenous materials is a function of not only the amount of pigment, but also the depths at which the pigments have been deposited in the tissues. For example, superficial melanin deposits appear browner, whereas deeper melanin deposits seem bluish.

Refraction phenomena cause abnormal coloration in superficial cavities filled with clear fluid, such as some cysts. They also cause retention phenomena of the intraoral salivary glands. Although in these pathoses the distinctive bluish color might appear to be caused by pigment in the area, it is actually the result of altered reflection and absorption of light in the area.

DISTINCT CIRCUMSCRIBED TYPES

MELANOPLAKIA

All people except those with albinism* have a discernible degree of melanin pigmentation distributed throughout the epidermis of the skin; this distribution is under genetic control. Produced by the dendritic melanocytes in the basal layer of the epidermis (Fig. 12-1), melanin is formed by the oxidation of tyrosine, a reaction that is catalyzed by the copper-containing enzyme tyrosinase and mediated by melanocyte-stimulating hormone (MSH) from the anterior pituitary. The melanin is secreted by melanocytes and picked up by the adjacent basal cells of the epithelium.

---

*Melanin formation is impaired by a congenital decrease in tyrosinase in albinism.

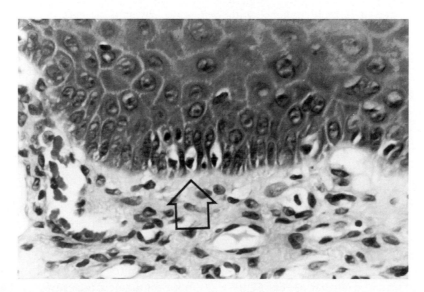

Fig. 12-1. The clear cells in the basal cell layer of the epithelium are melanocytes. The arrow indicates three melanocytes.

Melanocytes originate from neural crest cells. Barrett and Scully[8] discuss the physiology and pathology of oral mucosal melanocytes.

Features

The clinical appearance of melanin varies from light brown through blue to black, depending on the amount present and its depth in the tissues. The deeper (within certain limits) and heavier the deposit of melanin in the skin or mucosa, the darker it appears. There is great variation in the degree of pigmentation of the skin among the races and individuals of the same race. Although much of this variation is genetically controlled, the remainder is caused by various degrees of tanning from exposure to sunlight.

Most light-skinned individuals have a relatively even coloration throughout the oral cavity; however, dark-complexioned people, especially blacks, frequently have macules of pigmentation (melanoplakia) of various configurations and sizes on their oral mucosae, particularly on the gingivae (Fig. 12-2). Variations in gingival pigmentation have been reported in various ethnic groups.[9] In Israel, oral physiologic pigmentation was reported to be more common in adults than in children (35.6% vs. 13.5%) and varied significantly among ethnic groups.[9,10] Almost all Malay and Indian populations of Thailand and Malaysia had genetically acquired oral pigmentation.[11]

Such areas of melanoplakia on the oral mucous membranes in blacks are not usually a cause for concern, but if they are known to be of recent origin, they may complicate the formulation of a differential diagnosis and prompt a biopsy.

Differential Diagnosis

The differential list for melanoplakia is highlighted in the box at right. A condition similar to melanoplakia (melanosis) has been reported in female patients with light complexions.[12] All these patients were taking the combination (high-estrogen) type of oral contraceptives. In addition, chlorpromazine, minocycline, and quinidine can cause melanosis.

On microscopic examination the increased pigmentation in the basal layer is the only significant observation in melanoplakia. The number of melanocytes is not increased.

Management

The diagnosis of melanoplakial patches in blacks is seldom a problem, and after correct identification, this entity requires no further attention. However, it is not always possible to differentiate between a patch of melanoplakia and a superficial spreading melanoma on a clinical basis. Therefore the pigmented patch should be excised with an adequate border of normal-appearing tissue and submitted for microscopic study if the pigmented

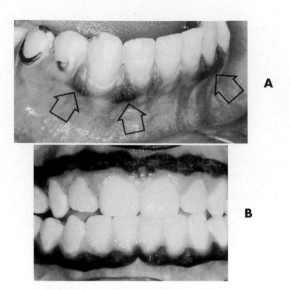

Fig. 12-2. Melanoplakia. **A,** Arrows indicate areas of involvement. **B,** Unusual, ribbonlike appearance of melanoplakia is shown.

DIFFERENTIAL LIST FOR MELANOPLAKIA

- Smoker's melanosis
- Oral melanotic macule
- Resolving ecchymosis
- Amalgam tattoo
- Addison's disease
- Peutz-Jegher's syndrome
- Drug administration (see under list of rarities)
- Superficial spreading melanoma

---

patch has (1) appeared recently rather than at birth or during childhood, (2) decreased or increased in size, (3) become elevated in part or whole, (4) undergone color changes of any type, or (5) undergone surface ulceration or fissuring.

The clinician and patient may decide to remove melanoplakic patches in the anterior gingiva for aesthetic reasons. This may be readily accomplished by deepithelialization (gingiabrasion).[13,14]

SMOKER'S MUCOSAL MELANOSIS

Tobacco smoking is another major cause of oral melanin pigmentation in both white[11,15] and Asian patients.[11,16] Agents in tobacco smoke apparently stimulate the melanocytes to produce more melanin.[11]

Features

Tobacco smokers, at least in some populations, have more pigmented oral surfaces than nontobacco users.[11] The percentage of pigmented individuals is significantly

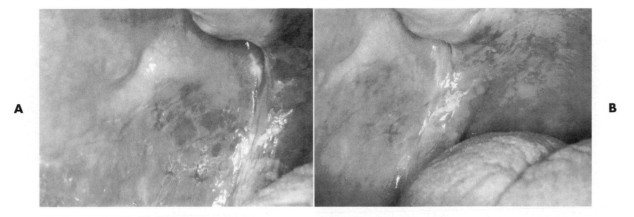

Fig. 12-3. Smoker's melanosis on the buccal mucosa. **A,** Note the pigmentation and other changes related to smoking. **B,** Some 6 months after cessation of smoking. Note decreased pigmentation.

higher (11.4% vs. 3%) among tobacco smokers as well.[11] These brown, gray, or black areas are located on the gingiva or other oral mucosa and are indistinguishable from areas of melanoplakia (Fig. 12-3). The anterior labial gingiva is a frequent location.

Differential Diagnosis

See the section on melanoplakia. Reduction or complete disappearance of smoker's melanosis is observed when the patient reduces or discontinues smoking.[11]

Treatment

This pigmentation is harmless and may even be protective.[11] Unfortunately, it may mask the presence of a more serious pigmented pathologic condition.

VARICOSITY

A varicosity, a distended vein, is a common occurrence in the oral cavity, especially in older individuals. It may also result from partial blockage of the vein proximal to the distension, either by a structure causing external pressure or from a plaque that has formed on the luminal side of the vessel wall because of an injury.

Features

The varicosities most frequently observed by the clinician are superficial, painless, and bluish; they appear somewhat congested and accentuate the shape and distribution of the vessel. The most frequent site is the ventral surface of the tongue (Fig. 12-4).

When many of the sublingual veins are involved, this condition is called *caviar tongue* (phlebectasia linguae) (see Fig. 12-4). The clinician should know that varicosities in the oral cavity, although occurring normally for the most part, may on rare occasions be caused by a tumor pressing on the superior vena cava at a proximal site, such as in the mediastinum. Congested veins in the head and neck region are also seen in apprehensive individu-

---

DIFFERENTIAL LIST FOR BULBOUS VARICOSITY
• Hemangioma
• Aneurysm
• Mucocele
• Ranula
• Superficial nonkeratotic cyst

als, in children who are holding their breath, and sometimes in patients with congestive heart failure.

Differential Diagnosis

The clinical identification of a lesion as a varicosity usually does not present a problem, but occasionally one is found with a bulbous shape (see Fig. 12-4, *C*). This lesion must be differentiated from all other fluid-filled, bluish lesions of the oral cavity, such as those listed in the box above.

In contrast to the superficial nonkeratotic cyst, ranula, and mucocele, which are fluctuant and cannot be emptied by digital pressure because they contain fluid in a closed chamber, the varicosity, the hemangioma (especially the cavernous variety), and the aneurysm generally do not demonstrate fluctuation and usually can be emptied by digital pressure.

An aneurysm is exceedingly rare in the oral cavity and demonstrates a pulse, as does an arteriovenous shunt. An angiogram may help in the identification of an arteriovenous lesion.

Although the cavernous hemangioma can be readily emptied into the afferent and efferent vessels by digital pressure, the capillary hemangioma cannot be as readily emptied because the vascular spaces and the afferent and efferent vessels are so small that they may be immediately sealed when pressure is applied to the lesion. Also, the capillary hemangioma, like its cavernous counterpart, is seldom a bluish-domed mass but may be more reddish.

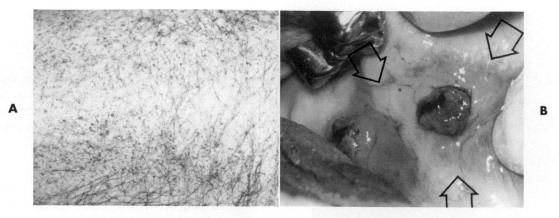

Fig. 12-6. A, Petechiae on the arm of a patient with thrombocytopenic purpura. **B,** Ecchymosis *(arrows)* surrounding an exophytic blood clot in the same patient. (Courtesy S. Svalina, Maywood, Ill.)

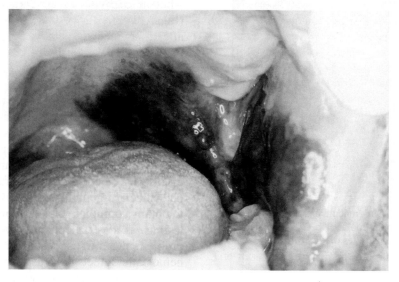

Fig. 12-7. Large purpuric lesion in the buccal and palatine mucosae after a mandibular fracture. (Courtesy D. Bonomo, Flossmoor, Ill.)

Early petechial lesions must be differentiated from telangiectasis in patients with Rendu-Osler-Weber syndrome (hereditary hemorrhagic telangiectasia). This syndrome manifests as small, reddish, macular-papular lesions that are dilated capillaries situated just under the epithelium; the lesions blanch on pressure. They can therefore be differentiated from petechiae.

Palatine petechiae and ecchymotic patches require further differentiation when they occur as a solitary lesion at or near the junction of the hard and soft palates. The possibilities for the differential diagnosis are listed in the box at right.

When a reddish or bluish macule is detected on the posterior palate and has been produced by extravasated blood, the dentist must first consider the possibility of trauma from oral sexual practices (see Fig. 5-4). If the lesion is indeed caused by fellatio, the bruise disappears in a few days after passing through changes from blue to

---

DIAGNOSTIC LIST FOR PALATINE PETECHIAE

- Trauma from fellatio
- Trauma from severe coughing
- Trauma from severe vomiting
- Prodromal sign of infectious mononucleosis
- Prodromal sign of hemostatic disease

---

green to yellow. Frequently it reappears in another week or so. A careful history taken in confidential surroundings confirms the diagnosis in almost all cases.

Bruising of the palate from severe attacks of vomiting and coughing appears as a broad, linear, red or bluish bruise that follows the junction of the hard and soft palates. Again the history is diagnostic in these cases.

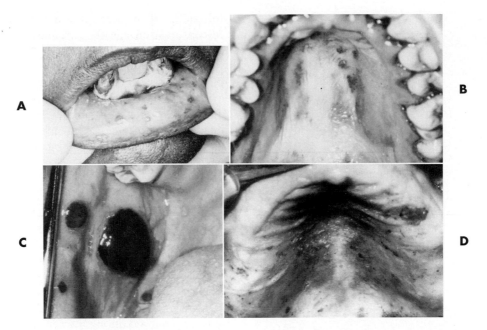

Fig. 12-8. Purpuric macules in hemostatic disease. **A,** Petechial purpuric macules that occurred during a sickle cell crisis. **B,** Petechiae and gingival bleeding occurring in a patient with acute myelogenous leukemia. **C,** Purpuric macules and blood clots in a patient with heroin-induced thrombocytopenic purpura. **D,** Purpuric macules in a patient with leukemia. (**A** courtesy S. Smith, Chicago; **B** courtesy J. Canzona, Chicago; **C** from Kraut RA, Buhler JE: *Oral Surg* 46[5]:637-640, 1978; **D** courtesy M. Lehnert, Minneapolis.)

Prodromal signs of infectious mononucleosis may occur a few days before the patient becomes ill as 6 to 20 petechiae in the soft palate. These petechiae may also occur between the fifth and twentieth days of illness. This feature, along with malaise, enlarged nodes in the neck, and a positive monospot test followed by a positive Paul-Bunnell heterophil test, establishes the diagnosis of the disease.

Because the soft palate sustains a considerable degree of stimulation and mild trauma during swallowing of food, this location is frequently the first to show the petechiae that may herald the onset of hemostatic disease. A complete series of blood tests usually identifies the specific diagnosis. However, the clinician must remember that some individuals bruise easily, so a few scattered petechiae may be present from time to time on the normal palates of these individuals.

Management

The associated hemostatic disorders may be conveniently divided into three groups according to the basic defect: disorders of the vessels, disorders of the platelets, and disorders affecting coagulation. A suitable study of the patient, including a thorough history and clinical examination and the appropriate laboratory tests, identifies the specific underlying systemic defect. Surgery should not be performed until the defect has been identified and treated or at least until the surgical procedure has been

modified on the basis of the clinician's recognition of the defect and its nature.

EARLY HEMATOMA

The hematoma is a pool of effused blood confined within the tissues. When it is superficial, it appears as an elevated, bluish swelling in the mucosa (Fig. 12-9). The early hematoma is fluctuant, rubbery, and distinct in outline, and the overlying mucosa is readily movable. The temperature of the overlying mucosa may be elevated slightly. Digital pressure on the surface may induce a stinging sensation because pressure on the contained pool of blood causes further separation of tissues.

Differential Diagnosis

A history of a traumatic incident (such as accident, surgery, or administration of a local anesthetic) can usually be elicited from the patient and is useful in establishing the diagnosis of early hematoma. Not to be overlooked is the possibility of spontaneous hemorrhage that accompanies the development of a hematoma in patients who have hypertension, blood dyscrasias, or other bleeding diatheses; these may be the first indications of systemic disease.

Early hematoma must be differentiated from all the soft and rubbery bluish lesions that occur in the oral cavity:

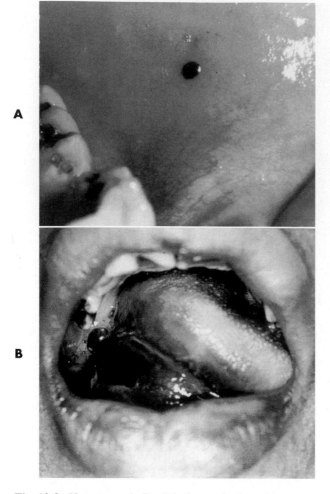

Fig. 12-9. Hematoma. **A,** Small lesion on the buccal mucosa. **B,** Large, dome-shaped hematoma in the right sublingual region caused by damage to the lingual artery during a surgical procedure.

mucocele, ranula, varicosity, hemangioma, lymphangioma, and superficial cyst. The history of a sudden onset after a recent traumatic incident strongly favors a diagnosis of early hematoma. The lesion is tender and fluctuant and cannot be evacuated by digital pressure. Although an early hematoma is usually not painful, palpation generally induces a stinging sensation. There is no thrill or crepitus. The early hematoma is usually a solitary lesion that yields dark blue blood on aspiration.

Management

The hematoma is usually self-limiting in size because the increasing pressure of the blood in the tissue equalizes with the hydrostatic pressure in the injured vessel and thus terminates the extravasation. If a large arteriole is damaged, however, a pressure bandage may be placed over accessible areas to control the hemorrhage and limit the expansion of the hematoma.

Occasionally it may be feasible to evacuate an expanding or painful hematoma with an aspirating syringe and then apply a pressure bandage to prevent its re-

formation. If indicated, the patient may be hospitalized for observation and the offending vessel located surgically and ligated.

An enlarging hematoma in the neck or sublingual area may encroach on the airway, and its management must be evaluated in light of this possibility.[19] Since the hematoma presents an excellent medium for the growth of opportunistic bacteria, the patient must be immediately placed on a suitable regimen of antibiotic medication for several days.

LATE HEMATOMA

A hematoma is usually clotted within 24 hours of hemostasis and then becomes a hard, black, painless mass. It often requires this prolonged period to completely clot because blood continues to leak into the clotting pool from the injured vessels. If the hematoma is superficially located, changes from black to blue to green to yellow may be observed during the following days. It disappears finally when all the hemosiderin from the extravasated blood has been removed from the tissues.

If a hematoma becomes infected, it is painful. Although the clot initially is firm, if the infection is a pyogenic type, the firm clot softens and becomes fluctuant as pus accumulates.

Differential Diagnosis

After a difficult extraction, clinicians frequently see hematomas that have formed adjacent to the extraction site. The submaxillary space is an occasional site for the development of such hematomas, which must be differentiated from an early space infection.

The late hematoma is firm and painless, whereas an early space infection is firm but acutely painful on palpation. In addition, the tissue over the infection has an increased temperature and may be inflamed. Later the infection may become fluctuant and yield pus on aspiration.

Management

If the patient with a large hematoma has not been protected with antibiotics, such prophylactic treatment should be initiated immediately and the patient observed carefully for a few days. A patient who has or appears to be developing a problem with respiration should be hospitalized and appropriate measures instituted to establish and maintain a patent airway.

HEMANGIOMA

The hemangioma is a benign tumor of patent blood vessels that may be congenital or traumatic in origin. A small lesion similar to a telangiectasia, which is a dilatation of a previously existing vessel, may appear. The hemangioma, however, is formed by an increased number of blood vessels. A total of 73% of hemangiomas occur

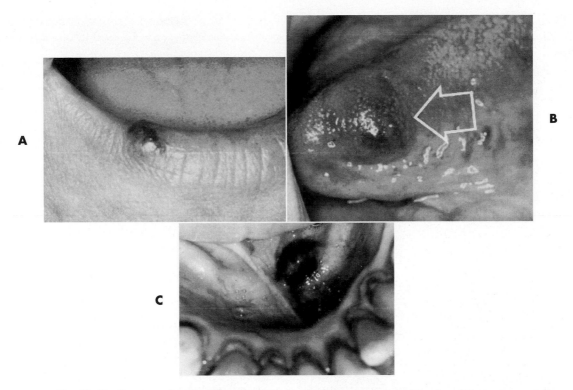

Fig. 12-10. Cavernous hemangioma. **A,** Of the lip. **B,** Of the anterolateral border of the tongue. **C,** Of the floor of the mouth, mimicking a ranula. (Courtesy G. MacDonald, San Jose, Calif.)

within the first year of life.[20] Only hemangiomas that occur superficially are considered in this section. The deeper hemangiomas are rarely detected and do not appear blue.

The cavernous hemangioma is a soft, nonfluctuant, domelike, bluish, and occasionally bosselated nodule that may vary in size from a millimeter or less to several centimeters in diameter (Fig. 12-10). It frequently appears on the lips, buccal mucosa, palate, and other sites in the oral cavity.

Maffucci's syndrome features multiple enchondromas, multiple hemangiomas, and phleboliths. Laskaris and Skouteris[21] reported a case in which the intraoral hemangiomas were the only ones present.

Differential Diagnosis

The hemangioma blanches and may be emptied by the application of digital pressure, which forces the blood from the vascular spaces. This feature accounts for the finding that the lesion is not fluctuant and, in turn, helps differentiate the cavernous hemangioma from the mucocele, ranula, and superficial cyst, which although soft, is fluctuant and cannot be emptied by digital pressure. (See Chapter 3 for a broader discussion of these differences.) A varicosity usually is seen as an elongated enlargement of a superficial vein rather than as a nodule or dome-shaped mass.

Furthermore, a pulse is not detectable within the cavernous hemangioma. This feature distinguishes the he-

mangioma from an arteriovenous shunt or an aneurysm, both which may occur as rubbery, nonfluctuant, domelike, bluish-red nodules with usually discernible throbbing.

In addition to these characteristics, the aspiration of bluish blood with a fine-gauge needle contributes convincing evidence for a working diagnosis of cavernous hemangioma.

Management

Surgical excision and injection of sclerosing agents, solid embolizing materials, or combinations thereof are used for the treatment of a hemangioma. The exact size and extent of the tumor must be determined before any treatment is undertaken, since the visible portion may represent just the tip of the lesion. Angiograms are thus used to detect the lesion's depth.[22] The excision of a moderately large or large hemangioma should not be attempted in the dental office; rather, the patient should be hospitalized and the procedure performed in an operating room, where blood is available for transfusions and where extraoral ligation of cervical arteries may be accomplished more readily.

Cryotherapy has gained acceptance in the treatment of hemangiomas.[23,24,25] Results range from good to excellent.

Sclerosing solutions are injected into the lesion to induce inflammation and the formation of fibrous tissue, which scleroses and shrinks the vascular spaces (Fig. 12-11). Solutions such as sodium tetradecyl sulfate have provided good results.[26-28] Absolute ethanol has also been used.[29]

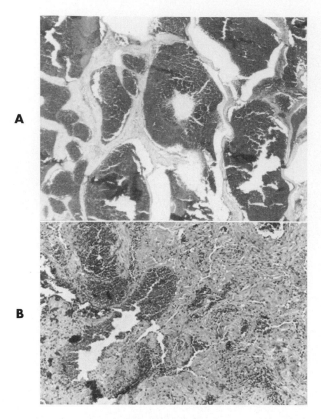

Fig. 12-11. A, Photomicrograph of a cavernous hemangioma shows the many vascular spaces separated by thin connective tissue septa. **B,** Photomicrograph of a cavernous hemangioma that has been sclerosed by an injected agent shows a decreased number of vascular spaces and the increased fibrous tissue component.

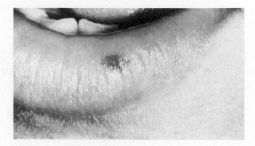

Fig. 12-12. Oral melanotic macule of the lower lip.

This sclerosing technique is useful with slowly flowing lesions in which the sclerosing agent would have more time to act. Sclerosing agents are often used before surgery to reduce the amount of surgery needed and to reduce hemorrhage.[27]

The smaller lesions disappear after injection, whereas the larger lesions require up to 10 biweekly treatments.[26] Lesions usually disappear without scarring, and side effects seldom occur. The injection of a sclerosing agent is frequently all the treatment required. A lesion so treated becomes firm and loses much of its bluish color. If large feeder vessels are present, embolization using materials such as metal coils may significantly reduce arterial blood flow.[30] This may be all the treatment that is required or may be a presurgical benefit.

ORAL MELANOTIC MACULE

The oral melanotic macule is a pigmented entity of the oral mucosa and lips that has been frequently studied during the last 2 decades.[31-34] This lesion is one of the most common pigmentations of the oral cavity of light-skinned individuals. Oral melanotic macule accounts for 0.4% to 0.5% of cases accessioned in oral pathology laboratories.[33,34] The cause is uncertain but may represent post-

traumatic (inflammatory) pigmentation in some cases. A case has been reported in which the entity occurred after external beam radiotherapy.[35] It is an atypical manifestation of physiologic pigmentation, since the histologic appearance is identical to that of melanoplakia.[33]

Features

The oral melanotic macule is usually a solitary lesion that occurs mostly in light-skinned individuals. The lesion is usually well circumscribed and brownish, bluish, or black (Fig. 12-12). The majority are less than 1 cm in diameter; the largest reported lesion is 2 cm in diameter.[32] The macules tend to be larger on the buccal mucosa.[34] The most frequent site is the lower lip, followed by the gingiva, the buccal mucosa, and the hard palate.[31-34]

Mean patient ages are between 31.5 and 44 years.[31-34] Most of the lesions remain constant in size and do not tend to become malignant. Microscopically, increased melanin is seen in the basal cell layer, and the majority also show melanin in the lamina propria, some of which is contained in melanophages. The microscopic appearance is identical to that of melanoplakia.

Differential Diagnosis

Entities that should be included in the differential discussion of oral melanotic macule are melanoplakia, amalgam tattoo, resolving ecchymotic patch, superficial spreading melanoma, nevi, lentigo, and melanocytic hyperplasia.

Melanoplakia is not always distinguishable from the oral melanotic macule, but usually the latter entity is smaller and has a configuration different from that of the melanoplakic patches present in the rest of the mucosa of the patient. The condition commonly occurs in blacks.

The amalgam tattoo in most cases is in a location where it could be associated with a juxtaposed amalgam filling. However, that is not always the case; amalgam tattoos have been seen on mucosa far removed from the alveolar processes.

The resolving ecchymotic patch can be easily differentiated from all the melanin macules. The former entity usually has a browner color and disappears within a few days.

Superficial spreading melanoma is less common than an oral melanotic macule; is seen in patients who are, on the average, 8 years older than those with oral melanotic macules; and slowly spreads by circumferential growth. Gender is not predominant for oral melanoma or the oral melanotic macule, and the palate and maxilla are the predominant sites for melanoma, whereas the palate is a relatively uncommon site for melanotic macules.

Flat nevi and lentigo are rare lesions in the oral cavity but may look clinically identical to the oral melanotic macule. Lesions of melanocytic hyperplasia are very rare but mimic closely the clinical appearance of melanotic macules and junctional nevi.[2,36]

If multiple melanotic patches are present in the oral cavity of a patient, melanoplakia, multiple oral melanotic macules, melanoma, Addison's disease, Albright's syndrome, Peutz-Jeghers syndrome, and postinflammatory pigmentation should be considered.

Management

The oral melanotic macule and an adequate border of normal tissue should be excised as soon as possible in patients with good surgical risk. The excised tissue is submitted for microscopic study because these lesions cannot be differentiated from small, superficial spreading melanomas on a clinical basis. If a static melanin patch is present for a significant period, it is sufficient to observe the lesion every 6 months.

MUCOCELE

The mucocele is one of the most frequent bluish lesions to occur on the lower lip, but it can occur anywhere on the oral mucosa. It is unlikely to be found on the attached gingiva or the anterior hard palate because of the usual absence of minor salivary glands in these regions. The upper lip is another uncommon location for a mucocele.

The mucocele is thought to occur when a duct of a minor salivary gland is severed by trauma and the secretion spilled and pooled in the superficial tissues. It seldom possesses an epithelial lining and therefore is classified as a false cyst. Other mucoceles form as a result of ductal blockage, perhaps by mucous plugs or sialoliths. These types characteristically have an epithelial lining formed by ductal cells.

Features

A mucocele located near the surface appears as a bluish mass (Fig. 12-13) because the thin overlying mucosa permits the pool of mucous fluid to absorb most of the visible wavelengths of light except the blue, which is reflected. A deep mucocele, on the other hand, may be a normal mucosal pink because of the thickness of the covering mucosa. If a mucocele is subjected to chronic irritation, its mucosal covering is inflamed or covered with a thickened layer of keratin.

A mucocele is usually a fluctuant, bluish, soft, and nodular or dome-shaped elevation that is freely movable over the underlying tissue but cannot be moved independent of the

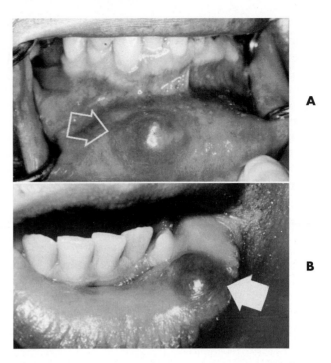

Fig. 12-13. Mucocele *(arrows)*. (**B** courtesy G. MacDonald, San Jose, Calif.)

mucosal layer. It cannot be emptied by digital pressure and on aspiration yields a sticky, viscous, clear fluid. The patient may report that the swelling is somewhat paroxysmal—recurring, rupturing, and draining periodically.

Differential Diagnosis

The differential diagnosis developed for a mucocele must include vascular lesions, superficial nonkeratotic cyst, early mucoepidermoid tumor, and mucinous adenocarcinoma. Both these neoplastic entities may mimic a mucocele in that superficial pools of mucus may be apparent. Consequently the clinician must inspect and palpate the tissue at the base and periphery of the "mucocele" for induration, which might indicate the presence of such tumors. A salivary gland tumor is rare in the lower lip but occurs with a higher frequency in the palate, buccal mucosa, and upper lip.[37]

Management

It is generally advisable to completely remove mucoceles surgically, and the excised tissue should be examined microscopically. This procedure is particularly important because some mucin-producing salivary gland tumors mimic a mucocele clinically. The lesion should be excised in such a way as to sever a minimum number of the ducts of adjacent acini. A good practice is to remove all the glandular units that protrude into the incision because their ducts are likely to have been severed. This practice helps avoid the embarrassing occurrence of numerous iatrogenic satellite mucoceles.

Steroid injection has been an alternative to surgery in the treatment of mucoceles,[38] but there is a danger of overlooking early mucin-producing tumors when such an approach is used.[39] Cryosurgery using liquid nitrogen on cotton swabs has been reported to give good results.[40] Again, careful follow-up is necessary.

Multiple superficial mucoceles are a rare variety that occurs very superficially.[41-44] These multiple lesions are frequently seen on the soft palate but can affect the buccal mucosa, lips, and retromolar pad.[41] They present as clear vesicles (not nodular) on a nonerythematous background. The differential list must include diseases that manifest as vesicles and blebs.[41-44]

RANULA

A ranula is, in effect, a mucocele that occurs on the floor of the mouth—a retention cyst in the sublingual salivary gland (Fig. 12-14). It derives its name from the diminutive form of the Latin word for "frog," *rana;* it is said to resemble a frog's belly. Galloway, Gross, Thompson, and Patterson[45] discuss in detail the various theories regarding etiology.

Features

A pertinent feature to be noted in the history of a ranula is fluctuation in size. The lesion is generally smallest early in the morning before the patient rises and largest just before meals. This fluctuation in size reflects both the increased secretory activity during periods of gustatory stimulation and water absorption from the pooled mucus during inactive periods of sleep.

When superficially located, a ranula is quite bluish (see Fig. 12-14), but a deep ranula appears pinker, reflecting the thicker mucosal covering. It usually occurs unilaterally, is dome shaped, and may vary greatly in size. It is soft and fluctuant and cannot be emptied by digital pressure. It does not pulsate, and on aspiration it yields the sticky, clear fluid characteristic of salivary retention phenomena.

Differential Diagnosis

The differential diagnosis for a ranula is identical to that of a mucocele (see p. 193). It is interesting how closely the vascular lesions depicted in Figs. 12-4, *C,* and 12-10, *C,* resemble a ranula in both location and appearance.

Management

Initially, conservative treatment by marsupialization may be performed by excising the entire roof of the ranula and permitting the area to heal without a dressing. Packing the entire pseudocyst cavity with gauze may minimize recurrence.[46] Such an approach necessitates the careful examination of the lesion's base in case the mucin-producing entity is really a salivary gland tumor. For the same reason, close postoperative surveillance is necessary. The lesion treated by marsupialization may recur in about 25% of cases.[47] A recurring lesion is an indication that ducts

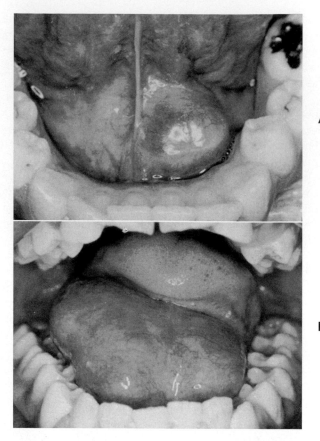

Fig. 12-14. Ranula. **A,** Small, unilateral, dome-shaped, bluish lesion. **B,** Large, bluish ranula occupying the floor of the mouth.

from neighboring sublingual gland units have been severed during operation or occluded by scarring.

Recurrences of the condition may signal the need to adopt a more radical form of treatment, such as the removal of sections of the involved gland or the entire gland. This procedure may result in significant morbidity (e.g., injury to the lingual nerve and to Wharton's duct).[46] If the ranula is large and a considerable degree of postoperative swelling is anticipated, the patient must be hospitalized to care for airway problems that may develop. Removal of the entire gland along with the ranula is the most reliable method.[45,47,48]

A plunging ranula is one that penetrates the mylohyoid muscle with possible enlargement in the upper midline of the neck (Fig. 31-13, *F*).

SUPERFICIAL CYST

The odontogenic and some of the "fissural" cysts that occur just under the epithelial surface and contain straw-colored fluid appear on clinical examination as bluish, nodular swellings. Although they occur in patients with mixed dentition, the most common example is the eruption type of follicular cyst seen in infants.

Actually, several types of odontogenic cysts (radicular, dentigerous, or residual, eruption, and gingival) may ap-

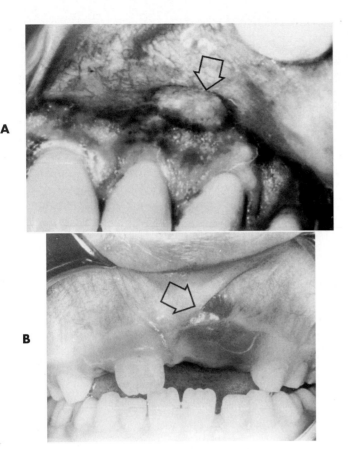

Fig. 12-15. Bluish cysts. **A,** Bluish, translucent, shallow, dome-shaped mass *(arrow),* which proved to be a gingival cyst. **B,** Bluish eruption cyst *(arrow)* involving the left central incisor. The cyst is similar in appearance to an eruption hematoma. (**A** courtesy E. Seklecki, Tucson, Ariz; **B** courtesy A.C.W. Hutchinson Collection, Northwestern University Dental School Library, Chicago.)

pear as nodular, bluish, fluctuant swellings if they are not confined in bone and are located near enough to the surface that the intervening soft tissues can transmit some light to the cyst's mass (Fig. 12-15).

Epidermoid cysts, however, are filled with keratin, so they appear white and are called *Epstein's pearls* when they are small and situated superficially in infants. Superficial keratocysts also appear white for the same reason.

Differential Diagnosis

The superficial cyst must be differentiated from the other soft, bluish lesions. A cavernous hemangioma can be evacuated by digital pressure, whereas a superficial cyst cannot.

A radiograph helps differentiate a superficial bony cyst from a mucocele, since the bony superficial cyst causes demonstrable bone destruction. The mucocele is not apparent on radiographic examination.

A gingival cyst may have the color of adjacent normal gingiva or have a bluish tinge. Most cases occur in the fifth and sixth decade and in the premolar, canine, or incisor areas of the mandible.[49] This cyst generally does

not involve bone, so a radiograph is not helpful in differentiating it from a mucocele. In addition, a mucocele, unlike a gingival cyst, rarely if ever occurs on the gingivae or the alveolar ridges, since minor salivary glands are not normally present in these locations.

If the cyst is not infected, a thin, straw-colored fluid is obtained on aspiration. A clear, viscous, sticky fluid is found in the mucocele.

Eruption cysts in infants and youngsters in the mixed dentition stage are rather common. They characteristically occur in the incisor region, especially in infants.[50] The dome-shaped, fluid-filled swelling is readily seen on the ridge, where the involved tooth is attempting to erupt (see Fig. 12-15). The eruption cyst usually has a light bluish hue and is rubbery.

An eruption hematoma, caused by trauma to the tissue just superficial to the crown of the erupting tooth, closely resembles an eruption cyst. Usually the darker blue color of the eruption hematoma helps the clinician make this distinction.

Also, the lymphangiomas of the alveolar ridges in neonates closely mimic eruption cysts in infants as reported by Levin, Jorgenson, and Jarvey.[51] This special type of lymphangioma occurs on the posterior crests of the maxillary ridges and on the posterior lingual surface of the mandibular ridges. They are dome shaped, blue, and fluid filled. In one study, 15 infants had single lesions; 32 had two lesions each; 2 had three lesions each; and 9 had four lesions each, one in each quadrant. The majority are 3 to 4 mm in diameter. The lesions are also found in black infants; 3.7% of black infants examined have a lesion or lesions. During biopsy, the lesions collapse and the fluid escapes. No teeth are observed deep in the lesion during excision.[51] The fact that eruption cysts in infants usually occur in the incisor region aids in making the distinction between these two entities.

Management

The treatment of intrabony cysts is discussed in Chapters 17 and 19. Eruption cysts usually rupture spontaneously, but if the parents are concerned, simple incision or excision may be performed and followed by microscopic study.

GIANT CELL GRANULOMA

The giant cell granuloma may be central or peripheral. The central variety is discussed in detail in Chapter 19, whereas the peripheral giant cell granuloma (PGCG) is described in Chapter 10 as an exophytic lesion. The exophytic giant cell granuloma, as well as some of the other inflammatory hyperplastic lesions, may be bluish, so it is also included in this chapter.

Differential Diagnosis

The lesions that should be considered in the differential diagnosis of PGCG are other inflammatory hyperplastic lesions, hemangioma, lymphangioma, metastatic tumors of the gingiva, nevi, and nodular melanomas. Other inflammatory hyperplastic lesions need not be differentiated because they represent the same basic pathosis as PGCG.

Most hemangiomas have been present from birth, whereas PGCG is of relatively recent onset. Also, congenital hemangiomas seldom occur on the gingiva; yet the gingiva and alveolar mucosa are the only locations of PGCG.

Oral lymphangiomas are less common than PGCG and rarely occur on the gingiva. In addition, lymphangioma has a much paler color.

Metastatic carcinoma to the gingiva must be considered also. However, in the absence of a history of a primary tumor elsewhere, this entity deserves a low ranking. Evidence of uneven bone destruction under the exophytic lesion prompts the clinician to consider metastatic tumor more likely.

Oral nevi and nodular melanomas occur less frequently than PGCG and in almost all cases are firmer on palpation. Except for the amelanotic varieties, they are usually darker. Finally, a nodular melanoma has a history of rapid growth.

BLACK HAIRY TONGUE

Hairy tongue is a harmless entity that occurs on the dorsum of the tongue in approximately 0.15% of the general population.[52] This condition is the result of an elongation of the filiform papillae, in some cases to such an extent that they resemble hair (Fig. 12-16). This alteration in the papillae results from an increased retention and accumulation of keratin (hyperkeratosis) (see Fig. 12-16). The condition may be provoked by irritation from one or a combination of local factors: (1) food debris remaining on the tongue and becoming impacted between the papillae as a result of inadequate oral hygiene, (2) habitual use of oxidizing or astringent agents in oral preparations, (3) local use of some antibiotics, (4) use of tobacco, and (5) *Candida albicans* infection. Systemic influences such as systemic antibiotic therapy, anemia, and general debilitation play an etiologic role.[52] Zinc deficiency is associated with hairy tongue in sheep.[53]

The hyperplastic, hyperkeratotic papillae are essentially light colored, but the color that they assume is a consequence of local factors. Chromogenic bacteria, mineral and vitamin preparations, drugs, and dark-colored food may be responsible for changing a white hairy tongue

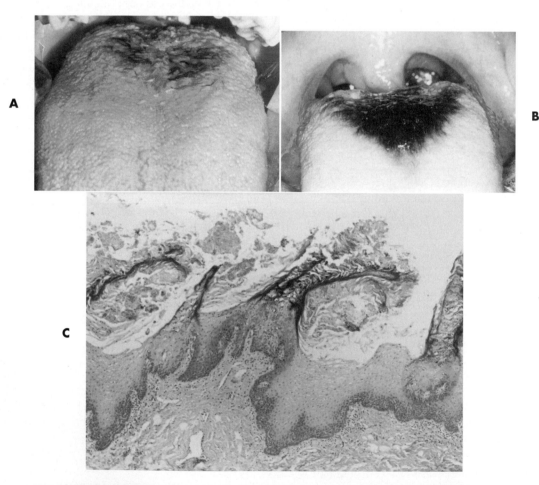

Fig. 12-16. Black hairy tongue. **A** and **B,** Clinical views of patients are shown. **C,** High-magnification photomicrograph shows elongated filiform papillae with increased keratin retention. (**B** courtesy A.C.W. Hutchinson Collection, Northwest University Dental School Library, Chicago.)

from tan to brown and then to black. Pain is usually not a feature, but gagging may be a problem.

Patients with malignant neoplasia are prone to this condition; 22.06% of patients with malignant neoplasms have hairy tongue.[52] There is a slightly increased incidence in elderly patients (0.72%) as well.[52]

Management

An improved tongue-brushing technique after shearing of the elongated papillae with scissors is generally all that is necessary.

LYMPHANGIOMA
Features

A lymphangioma is similar to a cavernous hemangioma. Like the hemangioma, it is usually congenital, but it is less common. Its most frequent intraoral sites are the dorsal surface and lateral borders of the tongue (Fig. 12-17). (Zachariades and Koundouris[54] describe an interesting case on the buccal mucosa.) Its color is less blue than that of a hemangioma, ranging from a normal mucosal pink to bluish, and may be quite translucent. Aspiration yields lymph fluid that is high in lipid content.

The dilated lymphatic channels of a lymphangioma characteristically reach high into the lamina propria and often contact epithelial basement membranes. This feature is often pronounced enough to impart a pebbly appearance to the surface of the lesion. In addition, this feature may hinder the evacuation of the lesion by digital pressure.

Differential Diagnosis

The differential diagnosis of a lymphangioma is identical to a cavernous hemangioma. Aspiration with a fine-gauge needle may be used to differentiate these two lesions.

Management

Even small lesions on the dorsal surface and lateral borders of the tongue are often continually irritated and worry the patient. Surgical excision is the treatment of choice, but a hemangioma must be ruled out before the excisional procedure is undertaken. Excision of a lymphangioma is not as hazardous as that of a hemangioma; still, if the lesion is larger than 2 cm and is located on the tongue, the patient should be hospitalized because of the possibility of extensive postoperative edema and a related airway problem.

"PIGMENTED" FIBROUS HYPERPLASIA

Occasionally a fibrous hyperplasia lesion occurs in a small melanoplakic patch in the oral cavity. It is a small, moderately firm, nodular or polypoid mass bluish in appearance. It is frequently mistaken for a nevus, and its true identity depends on microscopic examination, which demonstrates it to be fibrous hyperplasia with increased melanin deposition in the basal layer of the covering epithelium. The entity then must be included in the differential diagnosis of "nevoidlike" lesions.

MELANOMA

Melanoma is a malignant tumor of nevus cells and is an increasingly common neoplasm of the skin.[55] There has been a 3.16-fold increase in melanoma deaths between 1960 and 1990 in the United States.[56] It is anticipated that 32,000 new melanomas will be found in 1995, 53% of these in male patients.[56] It is also estimated that there will be 7,200 melanoma deaths in 1995, 63% of these in male patients.[56] Cutaneous melanomas are about one fifth as common in blacks as in whites and are less common in moderately pigmented people. People in their 40s and 50s traditionally have had most of these tumors, but the greatest rate of increase is in those under 40 years of age, particularly in women.

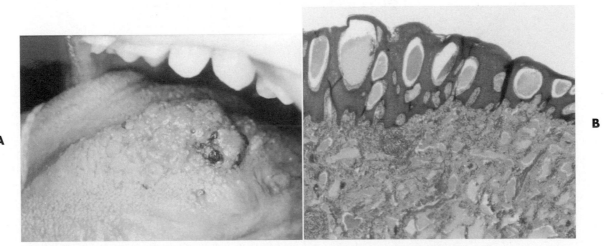

Fig. 12-17. Lymphangioma. **A,** Lesion has a pebbly surface on the dorsum of the tongue. **B,** Numerous lymphatic spaces appear to be in intimate contact with the surface epithelium. (**A** courtesy D. Bonomo, Flossmoor, Ill.)

Although the etiology of melanoma is unknown, it is recognized that over exposure to ultraviolet light is a significant promotive factor. Several risk factors have been recognized[55] and are listed in the box below.

Although many cutaneous melanomas arise from non-lesional nevi, a significant percentage develop from preexisting nevi. Specific changes in preexisting nevi suggest malignant change[55] and are listed in the box at right.

Most primary melanomas of the skin may now be classified as separate lesions on clinical, histologic, and behavioral bases; these include lentigo maligna melanoma, superficial spreading melanoma, nodular melanoma, and acral-lentiginous melanoma.[55] The first three types are listed in ascending order of malignant behavior. The 5-year survival rate for cutaneous melanoma is 84%.[56]

RISK FACTORS FOR CUTANEOUS MELANOMA

- Large number of typical moles
- Atypical moles
- Family history of melanoma
- Prior melanoma
- Freckling
- History of repeated blistering sunburns
- Ease of sunburning
- Inability to tan
- Light hair and blue eyes

Lentigo maligna melanoma has a predilection for the exposed surfaces of older patients. On clinical examination, it is seen as a pigmented macule with an ill-defined margin. During the first phase, it grows slowly in a radial (developing uniformly around a central axis) and superficial manner. This slow-growth phase usually continues for many years, and then behavior becomes more aggressive as the second phase begins. In this stage, invasion becomes advanced and metastasis frequent.[57] Prognosis for the lentigo maligna melanoma is considered to be good, particularly if it is completely excised during the radial-growth phase.

Superficial spreading melanoma is the most common form of melanoma and shows some behavioral characteristics similar to lentigo maligna melanoma. It begins as a pigmented macule that enlarges slowly for several years in a superficial radial-growth pattern (Fig. 12-18). As the name implies, the superficial malignant melanocytes are restricted mostly to the epithelium and the junction. If the

---

SUSPICIOUS CHANGES IN NEVI

- A—asymmetry
- B—border irregularity
- C—color variegation
- D—diameter greater than 0.6 mm

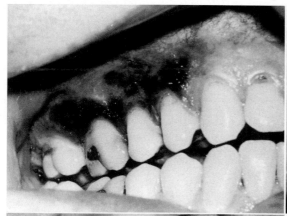
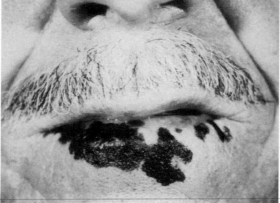
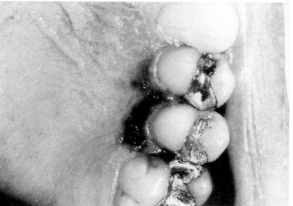

Fig. 12-18. Superficial spreading melanomas. **A** and **B,** Two views of a superficial spreading melanoma on the maxillary ridge of a 45-year-old man. The patient had watched it slowly grow for several months. **B,** Mirror shot showing the spread of the tumor from the labial gingiva through the interproximal area to involve the lingual gingiva. **C,** Superficial spreading melanoma of the lower lip in a 59-year-old man that had been present for 8 years, spreading from two small, pigmented patches. Nodules were now present on the mucosal surface. (**A** and **B** from Robertson GR, Defiebre BK, Firtell DN: Primary malignant melanoma of the mouth, *J Oral Surg* 37:349-352, 1979. **C** from Regezi JA, Hayward JR, Pickens TN: Superficial melanomas of oral mucous membrane, *Oral Surg* 45[5]:730-740, 1978.)

lesion is left untreated, it shifts into the more aggressive, vertical-growth phase and presents as a pigmented nodule or nodules within the larger pigmented patch. Metastasis usually does not occur while the lesion is in the superficial spreading (radial-growth) phase. Therefore if the lesion is completely excised during the superficial phase, the prognosis is much better than that for nodular melanoma.

Nodular melanoma, which arises by itself without a superficial spreading component, grows rapidly, may metastasize early, and has the poorest prognosis. Acral-lentiginous melanoma presents as a darkly pigmented, flat to nodular lesion on the palms or soles and under the nails.[55]

ORAL MELANOMA

Oral melanomas comprise 0.2% to 8% of all melanomas and may, with their cutaneous counterparts, be on the increase.[58] Dismal 5-year cure rates of 5.2% to 20% and median survival times of 18 months have been reported,[58] raising the question of whether oral melanoma behaves differently from cutaneous melanoma. The following reasons have been given for the poorer prognosis for oral melanoma:

1. Excisional surgery is more difficult to achieve.[59]
2. Lesions are diagnosed at a later stage.[59]
3. Modes of metastasis are through hematogenous and lymphatic routes, and these vessels are very abundant in the oral cavity and neck.[60]

Umeda and Shimada[59] report on a treatment protocol that gives much better results (see the section on management).

Although a classification for oral melanoma has not been developed like the one for the cutaneous variety, it seems that superficial spreading melanomas occur in the oral cavity with a nodular (microscopically determined) component in more advanced cases.[57,59-65] It is helpful to identify all melanomas as being in situ or invasive melanoma. Preexisting melanosis occurs in one third of all oral cases.[60] If superficial spreading melanomas are excised during the early stage, the prognosis is better than it is with nodular cases. Only 5% of oral melanomas are amelanotic (lack pigmentation).[58]

Features

Like cutaneous melanoma, the oral variety is slightly more common in male patients[60] and occurs most frequently between the ages of 40 and 70.[59] Some 80% occur on the maxilloalveolar ridge and palate[60] (Figs. 12-18 and 12-19 and Plate J).

The oral melanoma may present as one of four enlarging lesions: a pigmented macule (various shapes, possibly linear); a pigmented nodule; a large, pigmented exophytic lesion perhaps associated with macular pigmentation; or an amelanotic (nonpigmented) variety of any of these three forms (see Figs. 12-18 and 12-19). Melanoma may vary from a mucosal pink through brown and blue to black. It is usually firm on palpation but not as firm as a squamous cell carcinoma. The oral variety may ulcerate but does not possess a rolled, raised border. An erythematous border in the mucosa often surrounds the tumor and represents an inflammatory reaction of the surrounding tissue to the tumor.

The rate of growth in superficial melanoma is slow until the vertical phase is reached. The growth rate for the nodular melanoma, although usually rapid, may be variable. The tumor is usually painless unless ulcerated, infected, or both. Rapid infiltration of the adjacent deep tissues frequently occurs in the nodular type and fixes the superficial tissues to the deeper layers.

Spread is by the lymphatic and hematogenous routes. There is evidently a relationship between tumor thickness and neck metastasis.[59] The most common nodes are submaxillary, and upper jugular contralateral node involvement is common also.[59]

Differential Diagnosis

The early melanoma, which appears clinically as a small, brownish-blue macule, may be readily confused with the entities listed in the box on p. 200.

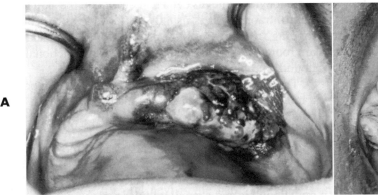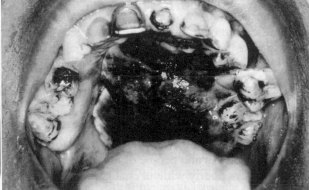

Fig. 12-19. Advanced melanomas of the maxillary ridge and palate. **A,** Melanoma appearing to have a superficial spreading component at the periphery. **B,** Large, advanced melanoma in a 56-year-old woman. (**A** courtesy S. Smith, Chicago.)

25. Gongloff RK: Treatment of intraoral hemangiomas with nitrous oxide cryosurgery, *Oral Surg* 56:20-24, 1983.

26. Minkow B, Laufer D, Gutman D: Treatment of oral hemangiomas with local sclerosing agents, *Int J Oral Surg* 8:18-21, 1979.

27. Chin DC: Treatment of maxillary hemangioma with a sclerosing agent, *Oral Surg* 55:247-249, 1983.

28. Baurmash H, DeChiara S: A conservative approach to the management of orofacial vascular lesions in infants and children: report of cases, *J Oral Maxillofac Surg* 49:1222-1225, 1991.

29. Muto T, Kinehara M, Takahara M, Sato K: Therapeutic embolization of oral hemangiomas with absolute ethanol, *J Oral Maxillofac Surg* 48:85-88, 1990.

30. Perrott DH, Schmidt B, Dowd CF, Kaban LB: Treatment of high-flow arteriovenous malformation by direct puncture and coil embolization, *J Oral Maxillofac Surg* 52:1083-1086, 1994.

31. Weathers DR, Corio RL, Crawford BE, et al: The labial melanotic macule, *Oral Surg* 42:196-205, 1976.

32. Page LR, Corio RL, Crawford BE, et al: The oral melanotic macule, *Oral Surg* 44:219-226, 1977.

33. Buchner A, Hansen LS: Melanotic macule of the oral mucosa: a clinicopathologic study of 105 cases, *Oral Surg* 48:244-249, 1979.

34. Kaugers GE, Heise AP, Riley WT, et al: Oral melanotic macules: a review of 353 cases, *Oral Surg* 76:59-61, 1993.

35. Barrett AW, Porter SR, Scully C, et al: Oral melanotic macules that develop after radiation therapy, *Oral Surg* 77:431-434, 1994.

36. Goode RK, Crawford BE, Callihan MD, et al: Oral melanoacanthoma, *Oral Surg* 56:622-628, 1983.

37. Krolls SO, Hicks JL: Mixed tumors of the lower lip, *Oral Surg* 35:212-217, 1973.

38. Wilcox JW, Hickory JE: Nonsurgical resolution of mucoceles, *J Oral Surg* 36:478, 1978.

39. Abrams AM: Danger of treating mucoceles by steroid injection, *J Oral Surg* 36:583, 1978 (letter to the editor).

40. Toida M, Ishimaru J-I, Hobo N: A simple cryosurgical method for treatment of oral mucous cysts, *Int J Oral Maxillofac Surg* 22:352-355, 1993.

41. McCaul JA, Lamey P-J: Multiple mucoceles treated with gamma-linolenic acid: report of a case, *Br J Oral Maxillofac Surg* 32:392-393, 1994.

42. Tal H, Altini M, Lemmer J: Multiple mucous retention cysts of the oral mucosa, *Oral Surg* 58:692-695, 1984.

43. Evanson JW: Superficial mucoceles: pitfall in clinical and microscopic diagnosis, *Oral Surg* 66:318-322, 1988.

44. Jensen JL: Recurrent intraoral vesicles, *J Am Dent Assoc* 120:569-570, 1990.

45. Galloway RH, Gross PD, Thompson SH, Patterson AL: Pathogenesis and treatment of ranula: report of three cases, *J Oral Maxillofac Surg* 47:299-302, 1989.

46. Baurmash HD: Marsupialization for treatment of oral ranula: a second look at the procedure, *J Oral Maxillofac Surg* 50:1274-1279, 1992.

47. Yoshimura Y, Obara S, Kondoh T, Naitoh S-I: A comparison of three methods used for treatment of ranula, *J Oral Maxillofac Surg* 53:280-282, 1995.

48. Schow SR: Discussion of three methods used for treating ranula, *J Oral Maxillofac Surg* 53:283, 1995.

49. Nxumalo TN, Shear M: Gingival cysts in adults, *J Oral Pathol Med* 21:309-313, 1992.

50. Clark CA: A survey of eruption cysts in the newborn, *Oral Surg* 15:917, 1962.

51. Levin LS, Jorgenson RJ, Jarvey BA: Lymphangiomas of the alveolar ridges in neonates, *Pediatrics* 58:881-884, 1976.

52. Farman AG: Hairy tongue (lingua villosa), *J Oral Med* 32:85-91, 1977.

53. Mann SO, Fell BF, Dalgarno AC: Observations on the bacterial flora and pathology of the tongue of sheep deficient in zinc, *Rev Vet Sci* 17:91-101, 1974.

54. Zachariades N, Koundouris I: Lymphangioma of the oral cavity: report of a case, *J Oral Med* 39:33-34, 1984.

55. Goldsmith LA, Askin FB, Chang AE, et al: Diagnosis and treatment of early melanoma, National Institutes of Health Consensus Statement, NIH Consensus development conference, Jan 27-29, Vol 10, No 1, 1992.

56. American Cancer Society: *Cancer facts and figures: 1995,* American cancer society, Publication No 5008.95, Atlanta, 1995, The Society.

57. Regezi JA, Hayward JR, Pickens TN: Superficial melanomas of oral mucous membrane, *Oral Surg* 455:730-740, 1978.

58. Smyth AG, Ward-Booth RP, Avery BS, To EWH: Malignant melanoma of the oral cavity: an increasing clinical diagnosis? *Br J Oral Maxillofac Surg* 31:230-235, 1993.

59. Umeda M, Shimada K: Primary malignant melanoma of the oral cavity: its histological classification and treatment, *Br J Oral Maxillofac Surg* 32:39-47, 1994.

60. Taylor CO, Lewis JS: Histologically documented transformation of benign oral melanosis into malignant melanoma: a case report, *J Oral Maxillofac Surg* 48:732-734, 1990.

61. van der Waal RIF, Snow GB, Karim ABMF, van der Wall I: Primary malignant melanoma of the oral cavity: a review of eight cases, *Br Dent J* 176:185-188, 1994.

62. Strauss JE, Strauss SI: Oral malignant melanoma: a case report and review of the literature, *J Oral Maxillofac Surg* 52:972-976, 1994.

63. Bennett AJ, Solomon MP, Jarrett W: Superficial spreading melanoma of the buccal mucosa: report of case, *J Oral Surg* 34:1109-1111, 1976.

64. Robertson GR, Defiebre BK, Firtell DN: Primary malignant melanoma of the mouth, *J Oral Surg* 37:349-352, 1979.

65. Rapini RP, Golitz LE, Greer RO, et al: Primary malignant melanoma of the oral cavity, *Cancer* 55:1543-1551, 1985.

66. Yoshida H, Mizukami M, Hirohata H, Hagiwara, T: Response of primary oral malignant melanoma to interferon: report of two cases, *J Oral Maxillofac Surg* 52:506-510, 1994.

67. von Wussow P, Block B, Hartmann F, Deicher H: Intralesional interferon-alpha therapy in advanced malignant melanoma, *Cancer* 61:1071-1074, 1988.

68. Buchner A, Leider AS, Merrell PW, Carpenter WM: Melanocytic nevi of the oral mucosa: a clinicopathologic study of 130 cases from Northern California, *J Oral Pathol Med* 19:197-201, 1990.

69. Watkins KV, Chaudhry AP, Yamane GM, et al: Benign focal melanotic lesions of the oral mucosa, *J Oral Med* 39:91-96, 1984.

70. Chuong R, Goldberg MH: Clinicopathologic conferences. Case 47, Part I. Oral hyperpigmentation, *J Oral Maxillofac Surg* 41:613-615, 1983.

71. Chuong R, Goldberg H: Clinicopathologic conferences. Case 47, Part II. Oral hyperpigmentation associated with Addison's disease, *J Oral Maxillofac Surg* 41:680-682, 1983.

72. ten Bruggenkate CM, Cardoza EL, Maaskant P, et al: Lead poisoning with pigmentation of the oral mucosa: review of the literature and report of a case, *Oral Surg* 39:747-753, 1975.

73. Lockhart PB: Gingival pigmentation as the sole presenting sign of chronic lead poisoning in a mentally retarded adult, *Oral Surg* 52:143-149, 1981.

74. Plack W, Bellizzi R: Generalized argyria secondary to chewing photographic film, *Oral Surg* 49:504-506, 1980.

CHAPTER 13

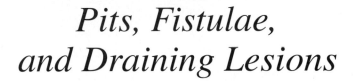

Pits, Fistulae, and Draining Lesions

HENRY M. CHERRICK

NORMAN K. WOOD

Pits, fistulae, and draining lesions of the oral cavity include the following:

PITS
FOVEA PALATINAE
COMMISSURAL LIP PIT
POSTSURGICAL PIT
POSTINFECTION PIT
RARITIES
  Congenital lip pits
  Inverted ductal papilloma
INTRAORAL FISTULAE AND SINUSES
CHRONIC DRAINING ALVEOLAR
  ABSCESS
SUPPURATIVE INFECTION OF THE
  PAROTID AND SUBMANDIBULAR
  GLANDS

DRAINING MUCOCELE AND RANULA
OROANTRAL FISTULA
ORONASAL FISTULA
DRAINING CHRONIC OSTEOMYELITIS
DRAINING CYST
PATENT NASOPALATINE DUCT
RARITIES
  Sinus tract from foreign body
CUTANEOUS FISTULAE AND SINUSES
PUSTULE
SINUS DRAINING A CHRONIC
  DENTOALVEOLAR ABSCESS OR
  CHRONIC OSTEOMYELITIS

EXTRAORAL DRAINING CYST
SPECIFIC SINUSES
THYROGLOSSAL DUCT
SECOND BRANCHIAL SINUS
CONGENITAL AURAL SINUSES
SALIVARY GLAND FISTULA OR SINUS
AURICULOTEMPORAL SYNDROME
OROCUTANEOUS FISTULA
RARITIES
  First branchial arch sinus and fistula

Pits, fistulae, and draining lesions of the cervicofacial complex may present perplexing diagnostic problems, partially because numerous types may occur in the oral cavity and on the skin of the face and neck. The process of differential diagnosis may be facilitated, however, by dividing these lesions into three categories: pits, intraoral fistulae and sinuses, and cutaneous fistulae and sinuses.

The terms *fistula* and *sinus* are used in the present discussion as prescribed by their traditional definitions. A *fistula* (Latin, "reed instrument or pipe") is an abnormal pathway between two anatomic cavities; it has two openings. A *sinus* (Latin, "hollow, bay, or curve") represents the tract of a lesion; it has one opening. The fistula and sinus are designated according to the surface or surfaces on which they open (e.g., oroantral fistula, cutaneous sinus). The clinician is undoubtedly aware that most writers do not strictly adhere to these definitions; furthermore, there is an increasing tendency to use the terms interchangeably in the literature.

PITS

A *pit* is defined as a hollow fovea or indentation. Generally blind tracts lined with epithelium, pits are normal, anatomic landmarks or are congenital, postsurgical, or inflammatory defects.

FOVEA PALATINAE

The fovea palatinae are two indentations formed by a coalescence of several mucous gland ducts near the midline of the palate. These round to oval depressions are always located in soft tissue on the anterior part of the soft palate. They can usually be accentuated when the patient holds the nose and attempts to blow it. The depressions may be probed to a depth of 0.5 to 2 mm and, when manipulated, may secrete a clear, mucinous fluid. On occasion the fovea palatinae are abnormally large and may be confused with fistulae or sinuses (Fig. 13-1).

COMMISSURAL LIP PIT

The commissural lip pit is a relatively common developmental disorder, although there is disagreement concerning its incidence. Everett and Wescott[1] have reported that approximately 0.2% of the population show this anomaly; however, Baker[2] has found that 12% of whites and 20% of blacks in his series demonstrate it.

The commissural lip pit may be bilateral or unilateral. Unilateral pits occur as often on the right as on the left side of the mouth. The pits are located at the angles of the mouth, with the tracts diverging dorsolaterally into the cheek (Fig. 13-2). They range in size from a shallow dimple to a tract measuring 4 mm in length, and the tissue is slightly raised around the opening.

On microscopic examination the tract is lined with stratified squamous epithelium that continues into the vermilion tissue of the lip. Mucous gland ducts may empty into the sinus; as a result, mucus frequently can be milked from the tract.

Differential Diagnosis

Differentiating aspects are discussed in the section on differential diagnosis at the end of the chapter. The commissural lip pit especially must be differentiated from the congenital lip pit, which is seen on the vermilion border of the lower lip but not at the commissures. The congenital lip pit, however, is extremely rare, occurring in approximately 1 of 2 billion births.[3,4]

Management

The commissural lip pit is asymptomatic and requires no treatment.

POSTSURGICAL PIT

The postsurgical pit is the result of wound breakdown secondary to infection or failure to obliterate dead space in wound closure (improper layer closure and inadequate eversion of the wound). The postsurgical pit appears on clinical examination as a dimple or puckering of a portion of or the entire surface of a wound with a comparatively shallow depression that can be probed easily (Fig. 13-3).

Differential Diagnosis

The differentiating aspect is discussed in the section on the differential diagnosis of the postinfection pit.

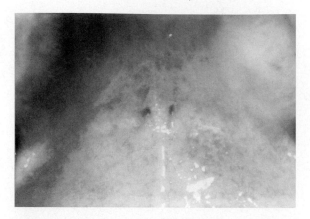

Fig. 13-1. Fovea palatinae on the anterior aspect of the soft palate.

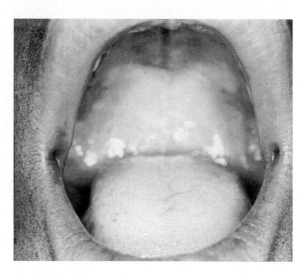

Fig. 13-2. Bilateral commissural lip pits. (Courtesy D. Bonomo, Flossmoor, Ill.)

Management

The management of the postsurgical pit is discussed in the section on the management of the postinfection pit.

POSTINFECTION PIT

The postinfection pit usually results from loss of tissue, often because of necrosis. After the infection has been resolved, a subsequent inversion of the surface tissue into the resultant defect forms a postinfection pit, which clinically resembles the postsurgical pit (Fig. 13-4). Accurate diagnosis may be determined from facts obtained through the patient interview.

Differential Diagnosis

The postsurgical pit or the postinfection pit may appear similar to a stitch abscess, sinus, fistula, or congenital pit; however, they may be distinguished from these entities by a careful history and physical examination, including depth exploration (with lacrimal probes), and by radi-

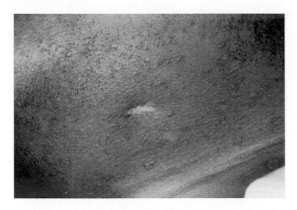

Fig. 13-3. Postsurgical pit after incision and drainage.

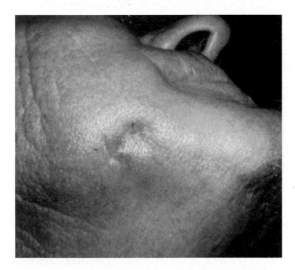

Fig. 13-4. Postinfection pit after the successful treatment of actinomycosis with antibiotic therapy.

ographic examination (performed with lacrimal probes or gutta-percha points inserted into the pits).

Management

Shallow postsurgical and postinfection pits within the oral cavity do not usually require treatment. If they become food traps, however, they should be surgically eliminated. Esthetic and other considerations prompt the same excision and layer closure as for extraoral pits.

RARITIES

The congenital lip pit is extremely rare and consequently is not discussed further here.

INTRAORAL FISTULAE AND SINUSES

CHRONIC DRAINING ALVEOLAR ABSCESS

The dentoalveolar abscess is a common lesion that is a pyogenic infection of the periodontal ligament and

bone[5] and frequently occurs as a draining lesion. The pathogenesis and radiologic appearance are discussed in Chapter 16.

Most dentoalveolar abscesses result from a direct extension of an acute pulpitis or an acute nonsuppurative periodontitis or from an acute exacerbation of a periapical granuloma, cyst, or chronic abscess. Less commonly the dentoalveolar abscess arises from an infection of the alveolar socket after surgical removal of a tooth. In either case the process remains essentially the same: a pyogenic infection of the periodontal ligament and bone.[5]

The surrounding tissue attempts to localize the pyogenic infection by forming an enclosure of granulation tissue, which in turn is surrounded by fibrous connective tissue. This results in a well-circumscribed lesion containing necrotic tissue, disintegrated and viable polymorphonuclear leukocytes, and other inflammatory cells in the periapical region of the tooth or alveolus.

This well-circumscribed, periapical abscess may penetrate the surrounding fibrotic capsule and form a sinus that opens on the mucosa or skin of the face or neck, usually as a result of one or more of the following circumstances:

1. Inability of the body to completely contain or localize the causative organisms
2. Increase in the number of the causative organisms or introduction of a more virulent organism through the carious tooth or by surgical intervention
3. Lowering of the patient's general resistance during the course of formation of the periapical abscess
4. Trauma or surgical intervention, mechanically producing an opening in the fibrous capsule

The enlarging dentoalveolar abscess contains purulent material that is under pressure. The pus proceeds through the bone along the path of least resistance until it reaches the surface, where it temporarily forms a subperiosteal abscess. Eventually it erodes through the periosteum into the soft tissue.

The path of least resistance in the soft tissue is determined by the location of the breakthrough in the bone and the anatomy of the muscles and fascial planes in the area. The expanding abscess may point and discharge onto the nearest external surface in the oral cavity; there are other, more complicated paths of infection, but their discussion is beyond the scope of this chapter. Space infections are discussed in Chapter 31.

Features

In the majority of cases the intraoral sinuses open on the labial and buccal aspects of the alveolus (Fig. 13-5) because the apices of the maxillary and the mandibular teeth are usually located nearer to buccal than to lingual cortical plate. In the maxilla, the roots of the lateral incisors and the palatine roots of the molars frequently lie closer to the palatine cortical plate than to the buccal plate; therefore an infection in these roots often produces a palatine abscess and perhaps a sinus (Fig. 13-6). Also

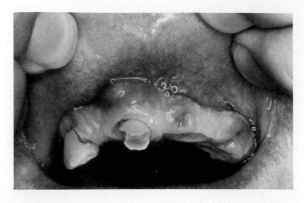

Fig. 13-5. Intraoral sinus from a chronic alveolar abscess of the central incisor. Parulis is evident on the labial aspect.

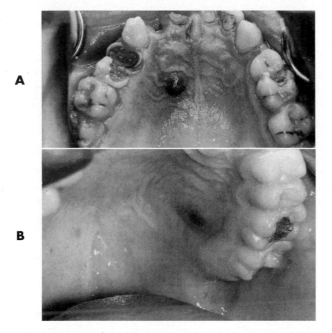

Fig. 13-6. Openings of palatine sinus draining chronically infected, pulpless teeth. **A,** Lateral incisor. **B,** Maxillary first molar.

the mandibular molar roots, particularly of the third molars, are located closer to the lingual plate. In addition, since most of the root tips of these teeth lie below the mylohyoid muscle, the pus drains into the submandibular space and the deeper planes of the neck instead of through an intraoral sinus.

On clinical examination the sinus opening has the appearance of a small ulcer. This opening is commonly found on the buccal alveolus adjacent to the infected tooth. The palatine sinus tract may burrow for a variable distance before it exits through the palatine mucosa. The mucosal opening may be red, may bleed easily, and may be raised (a parulis). This process may run through cycles of healing and recurring drainage, and occasionally multiple sinus scars, patent sinuses, or both may form. Palpation of the surrounding mucosa may cause the expression of pus from the sinus or sinuses.

Pain is a frequent symptom that starts as a dull ache and progresses to an increasingly severe throbbing. A sudden decrease in the pain usually signals the formation of a draining sinus; the pain may disappear completely. The offending tooth has a nonvital pulp and is often tender to percussion.

Dentoalveolar abscesses and sinuses usually appear on radiographic examination as radiolucent areas of bone resorption around a root apex. The radiolucent area is frequently ragged in outline and generally lacks a sclerotic margin, although such a margin may develop. This feature is discussed in detail in Chapter 16.

Differential Diagnosis

The differentiating aspects are discussed in the section on differential diagnosis at the end of the chapter. Rossman, Rossman, and Graber[6] discuss the endodontic-periodontic fistula that originates from necrotic pulp tissue in lateral canals in endodontically treated teeth.

Management

The management of pulpoperiapical sequelae is discussed at length in Chapter 16. Culture and sensitivity tests of the draining fluid usually identify the causative organisms and indicate the antibiotic to use. Occasionally, the infectious organism is *Actinomyces*.[7]

SUPPURATIVE INFECTION OF THE PAROTID AND SUBMANDIBULAR GLANDS

Purulent discharge from Stensen's papillae and the sublingual caruncles indicates the presence of a suppurative infection of the parotid and submandibular salivary glands, respectively (see Fig. 13-7). Thus pus-forming infections of these two major salivary glands are included in this discussion of intraoral draining lesions.

Suppurative infection of the parotid or submandibular salivary glands characteristically occurs in extremely ill or debilitated patients; often, these patients are elderly or are 4 weeks old or younger.[8-10] In the delicate or debilitated newborn of low birth weight, inflammation of the glands usually develops from conditions that produce dehydration.[8] In the older individual, predisposing factors include dehydration, malnutrition, and oral cancer. Surgery, especially an abdominal or orthopedic procedure, is one of the most common predisposing factors for suppurative infection of the salivary glands.[9]

Microorganism contamination is thought to be retrograde, from the oral cavity to the affected gland through the secretory duct, or antegrade, from the bloodstream.[10] *Staphylococcus aureus* is the most frequent infectious agent, but infections of *Streptococcus viridans* and *Escherichia coli* are also common; in addition, many bacteria of the oral flora may induce this infection.

The following predispose to retrograde infection: (1) an increase in the number of microorganisms in the oral flora or introduction of a more virulent type, (2) a lowering of the individual's general resistance, (3) a decrease in salivary secretion, or (4) a decrease in the bactericidal effect of the saliva.[8] The infection commences in the epithelial cells of the large secretory duct and spreads progressively to the smaller ducts and finally to the gland parenchyma. Once infection of the parenchyma has occurred, multiple abscesses may form and then coalesce. If the infection is not eradicated, pus may penetrate the gland capsule and spread into the surrounding tissue, usually along one of the following pathways: inferiorly into the deep fascial planes of the neck, posteriorly into the external auditory canal, or externally on to the skin of the face.[8,9]

Features

Often, pain in the region is the first manifestation of a parotid or submandibular gland infection; this is followed by swelling of the gland, which usually is hot, indurated, and tender to palpation. Redness may be found around the orifices of the duct, and pus may be expressed by pressure on the gland (Fig. 13-7).

The patient may be febrile and quite ill, often out of proportion to what would be expected from such a localized infection. There is usually a concomitant rise in the number of leukocytes in the blood, especially in the neutrophil fraction.

Differential Diagnosis

Contrasting features of similar conditions are discussed in the section on differential diagnosis at the end of the chapter.

Management

The treatment of choice is the immediate institution of type-specific antibiotic therapy, which is indicated by culture and sensitivity tests on the pus expressed from the duct. If there is no improvement within 3 to 4 days, incision and drainage should be undertaken.

DRAINING MUCOCELE AND RANULA

The mucocele and ranula are retention phenomena of the minor salivary glands and the sublingual salivary gland, respectively. These lesions are discussed in Chapter 12 with the bluish lesions. They are included in this chapter because they occasionally occur as chronic draining lesions.

As a mucocele or a ranula increase in size, the overlying epithelium and mucous membrane become stretched and may undergo spontaneous rupture, often as a result of trauma. The exudate is usually clear, viscous, and sticky. The mucocele or ranula decreases in size, but healing rapidly occurs, and the lesion gradually fills and expands again. Repetition of these events can produce a chronic sinus (Fig. 13-8).

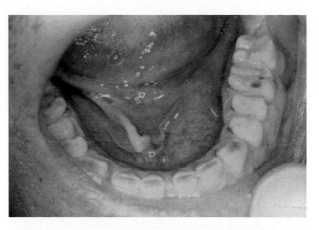

Fig. 13-7. Purulent discharge from Wharton's duct during an acute infection of the submandibular gland.

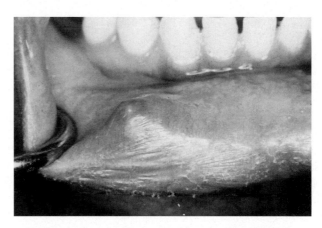

Fig. 13-8. Sinus opening from a chronic draining mucocele.

Differential Diagnosis

The differential diagnosis is discussed in Chapter 12 and at the end of this chapter.

Management

Treatment consists of total enucleation or marsupialization. During surgical correction, other salivary ducts or glands may be injured, so recurrences are fairly common.

OROANTRAL FISTULA

The oroantral fistula (OAF) is a pathologic pathway connecting the oral cavity and the maxillary sinus (Fig. 13-9). In most cases, it is caused by the extraction of a tooth, but it may also be caused by other trauma, tuberculosis,[11] syphilis,[12] or leprosy.[13] Occasionally, it results from tooth-associated pathoses, such as periapical infection or cyst formation.

Usually the apices of the posterior teeth are within millimeters of the cortical floor of the maxillary sinus, or they may project into the maxillary sinus with only a small amount of bony covering. The apex of the mesiobuccal

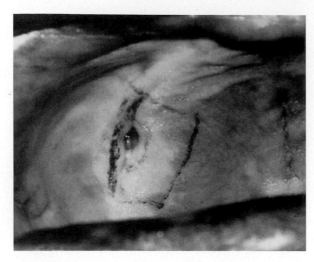

Fig. 13-9. OAF in an edentulous patient. (Courtesy P. Akers, Chicago.)

root of the second molar is closest to the maxillary sinus, with an average distance of 1.63 mm,[14] followed by those of the first molar, third molar, second premolar, first premolar, and canine.

The palatine root apices of the molars are frequently involved in the formation of a fistula.[15] Extraction of the maxillary first molar accounts for 50% of OAFs, with the other 50% almost evenly accounted for by extraction of the second and third molars.[16-18] With extractions of maxillary first molars, 1 in 180 cases result in an oroantral communication.[19]

An OAF generally forms as a result of inadequate blood clot formation in the alveolus after violation of the maxillary sinus. This may be consequential to sinusitis or secondary infection or to the introduction of packs or other hemostatic agents in the socket.

Features

An OAF is frequently seen immediately after extraction of a tooth; however, it may not always be apparent or suspected, especially if the extraction was atraumatic.

The most frequent complaint is the passage of fluids from the oral cavity into the nose, or there may be a foul or salty taste. Facial pain or an associated throbbing frontal headache may develop from an acute maxillary sinusitis exacerbated by any movement of the head. A unilateral nasal discharge may also occur and may be accompanied by a sensation of nasal obstruction or nocturnal coughing resulting from the drainage of exudate into the pharynx. The swallowed exudate may produce morning anorexia. Epistaxis may occur on the affected side. Other, less common symptoms are the eversion of an antral polyp through the fistula, producing the sudden appearance of an exophytic mass on the alveolar crest; the aspiration of air into the mouth through the tooth socket; and the inability to inflate the cheeks or draw on a cigarette.[16]

The OAF provides a direct pathway for oral flora to enter the maxillary sinus and cause sinusitis. The severity depends on several factors. If the diameter of the fistula is quite small, an acute sinusitis is more likely to develop, since sinus exudate cannot escape as freely into the mouth.

Acute maxillary sinusitis may produce swelling and redness overlying the sinus and molar eminence, as well as pain beneath the eye. Palpation over the maxilla increases the pain, and the teeth with roots adjacent to the sinus are often painful or sensitive to percussion. The pain may also be referred to other teeth in the arch and to the ear. Nasal and postnasal discharges, along with a fetid breath and a vague pain or stuffiness in the affected side of the face, are ordinarily present in chronic sinusitis.[12,20]

The maxillary sinus may appear cloudy because of an accumulation of blood, mucus, or purulent exudate on radiologic examination. In some cases a distinct fluid level may be evident.[21]

Differential Diagnosis

The diagnosis is obvious when the fistula is large and a definite communication between the oral cavity and the maxillary sinus can be demonstrated. The diagnosis is more difficult in cases in which the initial opening is small or the inflammation of the sinus mucosa has sealed the fistula. A radiograph may reveal a break in the continuity of the sinus floor, however. Careful probing gives the most dependable results.[19]

Management

An OAF should be repaired as soon as possible after it has occurred because the longer the interval between the genesis of the fistula and closure, the greater the complications.[19] In cases of sinus infection, surgical repair of the fistula must wait until the infection has been eliminated. An intensive course of antibiotic therapy should be instituted for a minimum of 1 week, the duration depending on the extent of the infection. A decongestant should also be used to encourage free drainage of the pus and mucus. Antral lavage is necessary in some cases and may be accomplished through the fistulous opening. Occasionally an antrostomy may be necessary to help drain the sinus.[16,22]

Many elaborate surgical methods have been developed for closing OAFs. The fistula is always excised and the surrounding necrotic tissue curetted. The methods include bone grafts; the use of gold foil grids; absorbable gelatin membranes; and buccal fat pad, buccal, and palatine flap techniques.[23-27] Once the antral infection has been eliminated, closure of the defect is usually successful regardless of the surgical technique used; however, some surgeons prefer to augment the closure by packing the maxillary sinus with gauze and subsequently removing the gauze through a nasal antrostomy. This procedure helps ensure that sinusitis does not develop during the critical stage of closure.

ORONASAL FISTULA

The oronasal fistula is a pathologic, epithelium-lined defect connecting the oral and nasal cavities. The most frequent causes of this type of fistula are congenital cleft palate, trauma, infection, neoplasm, and unsuccessful surgical procedures. The most common traumatic injuries are automobile accidents and gunshot wounds.[28] Although a complete midline cleft of the palate is not a diagnostic problem, occasionally a partial cleft, an unsuccessful repair of a complete cleft, or an anterior cleft resembles an oronasal fistula that results from some other cause (Fig. 13-10).

Occasionally an acute dentoalveolar abscess of a maxillary central incisor burrows through the maxilla or around the anterior aspect of the maxilla into the floor of the nasal cavity.[29] Other, less frequent infectious causes are leprosy, syphilitic gumma, and mycotic infections[13,29] (Fig. 13-11).

Features

When there is an obvious defect in the maxilla, the patient complains of food passing into the nose and often demonstrates nasal speech. Probing of a small defect during radiographic examination usually establishes a definitive diagnosis.

Management

The indicated treatment is usually the surgical removal of the fistula with subsequent flap advancement. When the fistula is too large to close surgically, a prosthetic appliance can be used to cover the defect.

DRAINING CHRONIC OSTEOMYELITIS

Chronic osteomyelitis is discussed in Chapter 16 as a periapical radiolucency, in Chapter 21 as an ill-defined radiolucency, in Chapter 25 as a mixed radiolucent-radiopaque lesion, and in Chapter 28 as a radiopacity. In the present chapter, its draining aspect is featured.

Features

The sinus extends from the medullary bone through the cortical plate to the mucous membrane or skin (Figs. 13-12 and 13-13). The sinus opening may be close to or distant from the offending infection. The mandible is more frequently involved than the maxilla (see Chapter 21). Cases that involve chronic draining are ordinarily painless unless there is an acute or subacute exacerbation. On radiographic examination the involved bone may be radiolucent, mixed radiolucent-radiopaque, or completely radiopaque, depending on the course of the infection. The formation of sequestra and involucra is often noted.

Differential Diagnosis

The differential diagnosis is discussed at the end of the chapter.

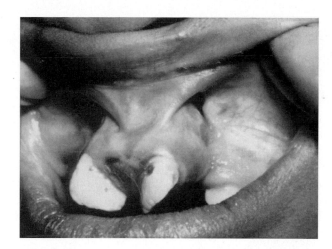

Fig. 13-10. Oronasal fistulae in a patient with a congenital cleft palate. (Courtesy P. Akers, Chicago.)

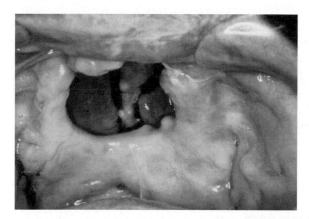

Fig. 13-11. Oronasal fistula as a result of a healed syphilitic gumma.

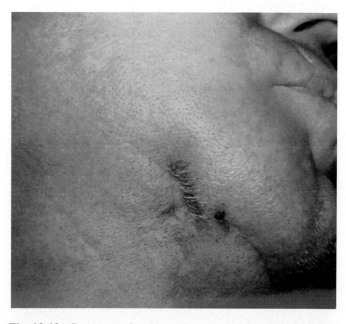

Fig. 13-12. Cutaneous sinus secondary to chronic osteomyelitis at a fracture site.

Management

The management of chronic osteomyelitis is discussed in detail in Chapter 21.

DRAINING CYST

Odontogenic and nonodontogenic cysts of extraosseous and intraosseous origin may perforate and produce sinuses that drain onto the oral mucosa. Secondary infections, or direct extensions of the cysts, generally produce these lesions. Inflammatory cysts (periapical) and other cysts that frequently become large (e.g., dentigerous and odontogenic keratocysts) are the greatest offenders. Dermoid cysts and other soft tissue cysts can also develop sinus tracts.[30]

Features

There is usually pain or swelling of the involved area before sinus formation. Pain ceases when the periosteum and mucosa are perforated, and a purulent discharge ensues. If the sinus is small, the drainage may continue as a chronic case. If the sinus is large, the infection regresses because of the excellent drainage established, and the cyst may disappear completely. When the cyst is large, there is an expansion of the cortical plate. Palpation of the area commonly elicits pain, crepitus, and a purulent or cheesy discharge. A well-delineated radiolucency is visible on radiologic examination.

Differential Diagnosis

The differential diagnosis is discussed at the end of the chapter.

Management

After the infection has been eliminated, the cyst must be treated by enucleation, marsupialization, or decompression. Associated teeth may require root canal therapy or extraction.

PATENT NASOPALATINE DUCT

A completely patent nasopalatine duct or canal is an extremely rare condition, especially in the adult. It arises when the embryologic nasopalatine ducts fail to obliterate. In embryonic life the nasopalatine ducts are paired, epithelium-lined tubes extending from the nasal cavity to the oral cavity within the incisive canal. The nasal orifices of the ducts lie on each side of the nasal septum in the anterior nasal floor. They extend downward in an anterior direction to exit as two slits, one on each side of the palatine papilla, which overlies the incisive foramen.[31-33] Occasionally, examples open posteriorly to the incisive foramen and papilla, and the resultant radiolucency may be cast over the apices of the central incisors.[34]

The nasopalatine duct is lined with ciliated, pseudostratified, columnar epithelium to within 3 or 4 mm of the palatine opening. At this level, there is a transition to cuboidal epithelium and then stratified squamous epithelium.[35-37]

In unusual cases, all or part of the duct persists and remains patent in postnatal life. The completely patent nasopalatine duct is rare; cases in which sections of the duct are patent at the nasal or oral end are more frequent. These are variable-length cul-de-sacs, with the nasal variety being more common. The oral variety of the patent nasopalatine duct may be identified by exposing a radiograph of the region with an orthodontic wire or gutta-percha point inserted into the defect (Fig. 13-14). Central, unilateral, or bilateral canals may be present.[33-41]

Features

The patent nasopalatine duct is usually asymptomatic except when small particles of food or liquid are aspirated into the nose through the duct or infection ensues. This happens most often after the patient has begun wearing

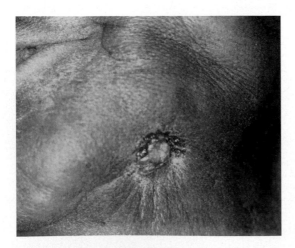

Fig. 13-13. Cutaneous sinus secondary to osteoradionecrosis.

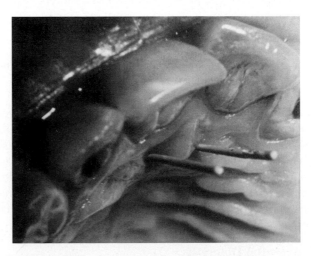

Fig. 13-14. Bilateral patent nasopalatine ducts with gutta-percha cones inserted into the defects. (Courtesy W. Goebel, Edwardsville, Ill.)

dentures, which may force liquid up the canal and into the nose. A salty taste may be a symptom.

Differential Diagnosis

The differential diagnosis is discussed at the end of the chapter. Examples situated in an anterior position may be mistaken for periodontal pockets,[38] and those situated posterior to the papilla may be mistaken for sinus tracts from midline cysts. Also, these may appear as projected periapical radiolucencies over the roots of the central incisors.[34]

Management

Since the nasopalatine duct is usually asymptomatic, it seldom requires treatment.

CUTANEOUS FISTULAE AND SINUSES

PUSTULE

A pustule is a small, superficial elevation of the skin or mucous membrane; it is filled with pus. Pustules are included in this chapter primarily because they become draining lesions for a short time after they rupture, and they are included secondarily because a solitary pustule on the skin overlying the jaws may easily be mistaken for a draining sinus from a chronic alveolar abscess or a chronic osteomyelitis (Fig. 13-15).

Pustules in the skin are common and generally are the result of psoriasis, impetigo, acrodermatitis continua, or superficial bacterial diseases. Intraoral pustules are less common and are the result of superficial foreign bodies or specific diseases such as pustular psoriasis or subcorneal pustular stomatitis. Pustules are classified as primary or secondary (e.g., preceded by a vesicle or papule).

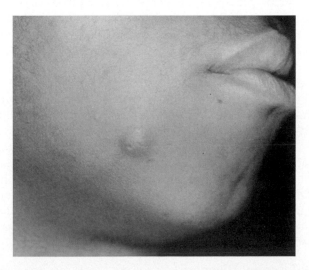

Fig. 13-15. Cutaneous sinus secondary to a periapical infection. This cutaneous lesion resembles a pustule.

Features

On clinical examination the pustule appears as a small, superficial elevation filled with pus and possibly surrounded by a small area of erythema. These lesions are generally asymptomatic but may be tender or painful.

Differential Diagnosis

The differential diagnosis is discussed at the end of the chapter.

Management

A pustule seldom requires definitive treatment.

SINUS DRAINING A CHRONIC DENTOALVEOLAR ABSCESS OR CHRONIC OSTEOMYELITIS

As with intraoral draining lesions, pus from an enlarged dentoalveolar abscess or chronic osteomyelitic lesion burrows along the path of least resistance in hard and soft tissues. This burrowing usually results in the formation of a sinus that empties into the vestibule adjacent to the offending tooth. In some instances, however, the path of least resistance leads to the skin and thus to the formation of cutaneous sinuses (Figs. 13-15 and 13-16).

If the pus exits from bone deep within soft tissue, its spread is governed by structures such as muscles and fascial sheets. Usually the infection spreads through fascial planes to the most available fascial space. A fascial space is a potential space that exists between two or more layers or planes of fasciae and is occupied by loose areolar tissue.

Space infections of the head and neck are usually classified by their anatomic location. Maxillary dentoalveolar infections usually spread to the canine fossa, buccal space, and infratemporal space, whereas mandibular infections spread to the mandibular, submandibular (submaxillary), submental, pterygomandibular, masseteric, parapharyngeal, parotid, and carotid spaces. The infection may spread by direct continuation from the dentoalveolar abscess along the fascial planes or by the lymphatic and blood systems. A further discussion of individual space abscesses of the neck may be found in Chapter 31.

Resolution of the cutaneous sinus usually follows the identification and elimination of the source of infection by endodontic therapy or removal of the involved tooth or teeth.[42-45]

EXTRAORAL DRAINING CYSTS

The phenomenon of intraoral draining cysts is discussed earlier in the chapter. Draining cysts can also occur on the skin of the face and neck (Fig. 13-17). The common cysts that occur in these cutaneous regions are sebaceous, epidermoid, dermoid, thyroglossal, preauricular, and branchial; these cysts are discussed more completely in Chapter 31.

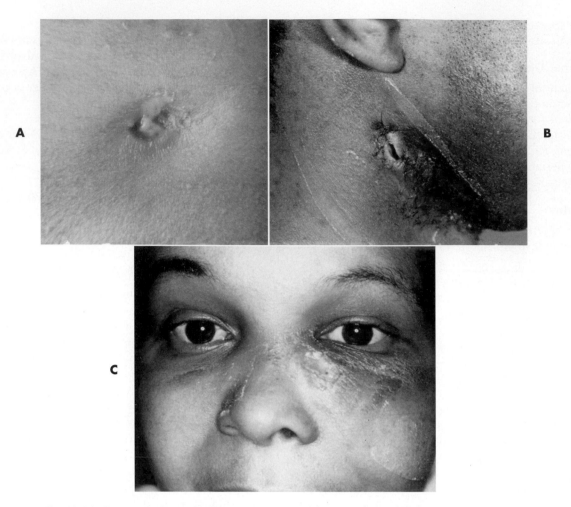

Fig. 13-16. Cutaneous sinuses. **A,** Secondary to a draining dentoalveolar abscess. **B,** Caused by incision and drainage of a submandibular space infection. **C,** Secondary to a canine space infection. (**A** courtesy S. Rosen, Los Angeles.)

SPECIFIC SINUSES
Thyroglossal Duct

The thyroglossal duct is a hollow embryonic tube of epithelial cells marking the descent of the thyroid anlage from the tongue to the normal position of the thyroid gland in the neck. The duct normally becomes a solid stalk and usually degenerates and disappears. The original opening of the thyroglossal duct persists as a vestigial pit, the foramen cecum of the tongue. The literature suggests that the ductal sinus is usually secondary to infection of a thyroglossal duct cyst or incomplete removal in previous operations.

Features

Thyroglossal sinus tracts are commonly seen within the first 2 decades of life, although a duct may begin to drain later in life because of local duct proliferation resulting from irritation. There is no gender predilection.[46-48]

The sinus openings from the thyroglossal duct may occur at any level in the midline of the neck from the foramen cecum to the suprasternal notch, although seldom at these extremes. It is frequently located in the area adjacent to the hyoid bone, being more often observed just below the hyoid than just above (see Fig. 31-13). The sinus opening is mainly in the midline but may be lateral to the midline in a small percentage of cases. On rare occasions, it is far enough from the midline to be confused with a branchial cleft sinus.[49] The cutaneous openings are 1 to 3 mm in diameter with a reddish, inflamed margin. Mucoid (clear) or purulent exudate may be expressed from the opening. The tract may be palpable back to the origin of the problem.

The epithelial lining of the duct is usually squamous epithelium or ciliated, pseudostratified, columnar epithelium. Ducts may show little or no epithelial lining if inflammation has recurred. Rarely, thyroid tissue is entrapped in the duct lining, and neoplastic transformation into papillary thyroid carcinoma occurs.[50] Thyroglossal duct cysts are discussed in Chapter 31.

Differential Diagnosis

The differential diagnosis is discussed at the end of the chapter.

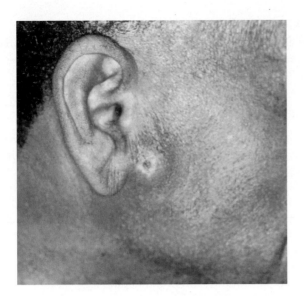

Fig. 13-17. Chronic draining sebaceous cyst.

Management

The indicated treatment is complete surgical excision of all thyroglossal duct epithelium. Because such excision is frequently difficult, the recurrence rate is high.[51]

Second Branchial Sinus (Lateral Cervical Sinus)

A sinus or fistula of the second branchial cleft or pouch is somewhat common; it constitutes the majority of sinuses and fistulas of the lateral neck. This anomaly is thought to occur when the second branchial cleft, the second pharyngeal pouch, or both fail to obliterate in embryonic life. The line of obliteration of the second branchial cleft extends from the lower anterior border of the sternocleidomastoid muscle through the fork of the carotid artery bifurcation and upward toward the tonsillar fossa.[52] Thus there can be three distinct types of branchial tracts:[53] a cutaneous sinus (50%);[54] a pharyngeal mucosal sinus (rarely);[54] and complete fistulae (39%).[54]

Features

The second branchial sinus is gender neutral, and familial tendency is uncertain.[55,56] The sinus or fistula may be unilateral, bilateral, or rarely, near the midline. The sinus or fistula is usually found at birth or within the first year of life. Adults with this anomaly commonly give a history of intermittent drainage since childhood or a spontaneous discharge caused by infection and rupture of a cervical cyst.

Most branchial sinuses or fistulae appear as small dimples or openings in the inferior region of the neck toward the midline, close to the anterior border of the sternocleidomastoid muscle. They sometimes occur in a more superior location along the anterior border of the sternocleidomastoid muscle, and some of these represent a sinus tract associated with a branchial cyst.

Differential Diagnosis

A second branchial sinus may be differentiated from other fistulae or sinuses of the neck by its position.

A thyroglossal duct sinus or fistula is usually found high in the midline, and the very rare first branchial sinus[53] may be found high in the neck, posterior and inferior to the angle of the mandible. The second branchial sinus rarely occurs near the midline or high in the neck.

Suppurative lymphadenitis, most commonly tuberculous adenitis, occurs on occasion as a draining lateral sinus in the neck. This entity can usually be differentiated by the history or by appropriate clinical diagnostic tests. Sometimes, radiographs taken after the injection of radiopaque dye into the sinus or fistula do not help diagnostically.

Management

Once the diagnosis is made, the sinus or fistula must be excised in its entirety, or it recurs.

Congenital Aural Sinuses

Congenital aural sinuses (auricular fistulae, preauricular fistulae, preauricular pits) occur in approximately 1% of the population.[57] They are more common in blacks and Orientals than in whites[58] and are gender neutral, occurring bilaterally in approximately 25% of cases. They are believed to be a non–sex-linked, dominant trait with variable expressivity.[59] Occasionally they are associated with other ear and facial anomalies, but as a rule they occur alone.

Current opinion maintains that they evolved during the embryologic development of the external ear from the six ectoderm-covered mesenchymal nodules (the auditory tubercles) of the first two branchial arches. By the third fetal month, these six nodules have proliferated and merged around the primitive external auditory meatus to form the external ear. The formation of congenital sinuses between the auditory tubercles is likely the result of abnormal development.

Features

Although there are seven possible sites around the ear, 90% are located on the marginal helix, the outer rim of the ear. The vast majority of these occur on the ascending limb of the helix[58] (Fig. 13-18). The openings vary in size from pinpoint to 2 mm, and unless infected, they are not raised. Depth ranges from a slight fossa to 1 cm; they extend internally in an inferoposterior direction anterior to the cartilaginous external auditory meatus (Fig. 13-19). They may be attached to the meatus by a ribbon of fibrous tissue, but they never pierce or open into the meatus.[60] Malformation and partial or complete aplasia of the external ear may accompany these aural sinuses (see Fig. 13-19).

The majority of aural sinuses are asymptomatic, but occlusion of the orifices may result in a cyst. Once the sinuses have been infected, the usual course is chronic, low-grade inflammation with occasional acute inflammatory exacerbations.

Differential Diagnosis

These sinuses may be confused with first branchial cleft anomalies. The two can be differentiated in the following manner: The aural sinuses never open into the external auditory canal and are generally located on the anterosuperior aspect of the external ear, whereas the first branchial cleft anomalies characteristically open into the external auditory canal and produce a purulent discharge with no evidence of middle ear infection. Also the first branchial anomalies usually are fistulae because they have another opening on the skin inferoposterior to the angle of the mandible. These lesions are very rare.[58]

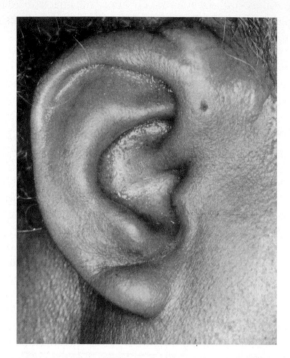

Fig. 13-18. Congenital aural sinus and cyst on the ascending limb of the helix.

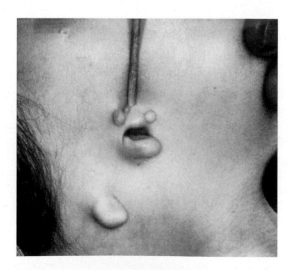

Fig. 13-19. Auricular tags and clinical instrument inserted in a congenital aural sinus located where the ascending limb of the helix would be in the normal external ear.

Management

Treatment is rendered only when the aural sinuses become cystic or infected; in such a case, complete removal of the tract is necessary to prevent recurrent attacks.

SALIVARY GLAND FISTULA OR SINUS

Parotid and submandibular gland fistulae are relatively rare and are caused primarily by accidental trauma, surgery, salivary calculi, malignancy, and infection. Actinomycosis, tuberculosis, syphilis, and cancrum oris have been implicated. For a fistula to be produced, there must usually be damage to the parotid or submandibular duct or one of its large branches. The saliva that escapes from the damaged duct forms a pool within the soft tissue or drains through a fistula in the skin (Figs. 13-20 and 13-21).

The parotid duct lies in the middle third of an area determined by imagining a line drawn across the face from the tragus of the ear to a point midway between the vermilion border of the lip and the ala of the nose. It arises from the merger of numerous smaller branches at the anterior border of the gland. Occasionally, there is an accessory parotid duct that joins the main duct somewhat distal to this border.

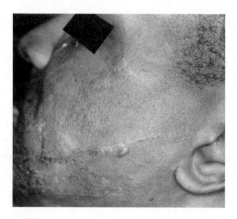

Fig. 13-20. Posttraumatic parotid fistula caused by laceration of the parotid duct.

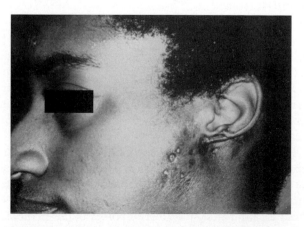

Fig. 13-21. Multiple fistulae resulting from chronic parotitis.

The main parotid duct then crosses superficially to the masseter muscle and turns inward at the anterior border of the muscle, passing through the fat pad of the cheek and forward in an oblique direction to open into the oral cavity opposite the maxillary second molar. When it crosses the outer surface of the masseter muscle, it lies close to the skin and is vulnerable to injury at this site.[61]

A fistula of the submandibular salivary gland complex is rare and is not discussed. Rarely, salivary fistulae develop in the mental region from a plunging ranula of a sublingual gland.[62] Rarely, accessory major glands are present, with the duct opening to the skin.[63]

Differential Diagnosis

The differential diagnosis of salivary gland fistula includes the consideration of fistulae and sinuses that occur as a result of specific and nonspecific infections and foreign bodies in the area of the salivary glands. Definitive diagnosis is accomplished by the history, the probing of the involved duct, and the use of sialography.

Management

If the fistula is the result of trauma, the most common method is apposition of the severed duct ends. Another method is creation of a second mucosal opening by suturing the proximal portion of the duct to the buccal mucosa. Yet another method is formation of an artificial internal fistula using various materials. If these methods are unsuccessful the gland may be removed.

AURICULOTEMPORAL SYNDROME

Auriculotemporal syndrome (Frey's syndrome) is included in this chapter because patients with this disorder have profuse sweating from a small, cutaneous area in the temporal region. Perspiration exuding from such a small area could be confused with an exudate from a draining lesion.

The disorder is caused by damage to the auriculotemporal nerve and reinnervation of the sweat glands by parasympathetic salivary fibers. Surgeries involving the parotid gland, ramus, temporomandibular joint, or condyle are the most common cause.[64,65] Blunt trauma to the side of the face has also been implicated.[66]

Features

Auriculotemporal syndrome becomes evident approximately 5 weeks after damage to the auriculotemporal nerve. The first signs are sweating on the involved side of the face during and after gustatory stimuli. Eventually a feeling of warmth may precede flushing and sweating.[67]

Differential Diagnosis

The definitive diagnosis of auriculotemporal syndrome is made by eliciting a history of trauma or infection in the involved area. The simplest way of identifying the fluid as sweat is to use the Minor starch-iodine test.[67] Other differentiating aspects are discussed in the section on differential diagnosis at the end of the chapter.

Management

Auriculotemporal syndrome is usually considered to be permanent, although an estimated 5% of these patients show regression or disappearance of the disorder.

OROCUTANEOUS FISTULA

Orocutaneous fistula is a troublesome defect because it permits the continual leakage of saliva onto the lower face or neck. It is a common sequela of trauma, oral malignancies, and inflammatory conditions. Cancrum oris, a lesion rarely seen in developed countries, may produce an orocutaneous fistula.

Features

Orocutaneous fistula is usually quite obvious. A traumatic fistula primarily involves soft tissue, but in many neoplastic and infectious conditions the fistula may involve the osseous structures of the jaws.

Traumatic fistula is generally an epithelium-lined communication resulting from an accident or an attempt at surgical repair. It usually does not exhibit the signs of inflammation commonly seen in neoplastic fistulae or fistulae induced by infection.

Neoplastic fistula may be the result of disease that has progressed through soft tissue or bone, beginning in the oral cavity or on the skin surface (Fig. 13-22). Often the fistula is the result of surgical intervention for the neoplastic disease.

Inflammatory fistula is generally not lined with epithelium unless it is of long duration. The fistula may originate in soft tissue or bone (e.g., actinomycosis).

Differential Diagnosis

Establishing a diagnosis of orocutaneous fistula is usually readily accomplished, and the cause is evident.

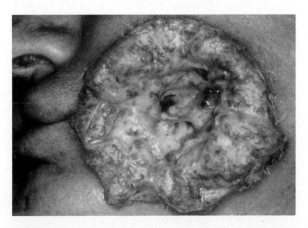

Fig. 13-22. Orocutaneous fistula resulting from a squamous cell carcinoma.

Management

Surgical repair may be successful in most cases of traumatic fistula, but treatment of a fistula caused by malignancy is usually hopeless because of the advanced stage of the tumor. Small, infectious-type fistulae may heal spontaneously after elimination of the infection.

RARITIES

Rare defects such as the first branchial arch sinus and fistula, as well as chronic draining infections of the soft tissue and bone caused by unusual agents such as *Actinomyces,*[68] are included in this category.

DIFFERENTIAL DIAGNOSIS OF PITS, FISTULAE, AND SINUSES

Pits, fistulae, and sinuses may be easily misdiagnosed, if the clinician fails to use a systematic approach. Answers to the following questions should be established during the patient interview:

1. Was the defect present at birth? If not, when did it become apparent?
2. Is fluid draining from it?
3. Is there a bad taste in the mouth?

Pressure should be exerted on the surrounding or associated tissue to determine whether fluid can be expressed from the pit. If fluid is obtained, it should be carefully scrutinized to determine its nature—saliva, pus, blood, or cyst fluid.

In addition, the clinician should attempt to probe the depression to determine whether it is just a shallow pit or indeed a tract. A radiograph of the area should be obtained after insertion of a gutta-percha cone as far as possible to help determine the depth, direction, and termination of the tract. In some cases, shallow pits represent all that remain of quiescent or eradicated tracts.

Routine radiographs help identify lesions of bone as origins of such tracts.

Intraoral Pits, Fistulae, and Sinuses

The following entities must be considered, in this approximate order of frequency:

1. Fovea palatinae
2. Chronic draining dentoalveolar abscess
3. Commissural lip pits
4. Postsurgical and postinfection pit or depression
5. Oroantral fistula
6. Oronasal fistula
7. Draining cyst
8. Draining chronic osteomyelitis
9. Draining mucocele or ranula
10. Suppurative infection of the parotid and submaxillary salivary glands
11. Patent nasopalatine duct

The patent nasopalatine duct is a rare entity. When it is present, the patient may complain of a bad taste. The diagnosis is established by determining the duct's course through the incisive canal by using a gutta-percha point with radiographs.

Suppurative infection of the parotid and submaxillary salivary glands is also quite uncommon. It should be suspected, especially when there is a predisposing dehydration. Expressing pus from the respective duct openings by application of pressure on the glands establishes the diagnosis and differentiates this disorder from infections involving other tissues or viral infections of the glands.

Draining mucocele or ranula is slightly more common. The mucocele is most often located on the lower lip, and the ranula occurs in the floor of the oral cavity. A history of repeated episodes of swelling and draining with regression prompts the clinician to assign a high rank to mucocele and ranula, especially when the fluid is clear, viscous, and sticky.

A chronic osteomyelitis drains through an extraoral sinus opening more frequently than through an intraoral opening. Changes in the basal bone and pus that can be expressed by exerting pressure on a tender or painful expansion of the mandible suggest the assignment of a high rank to osteomyelitis. The probability that chronic osteomyelitis is the likely diagnosis is enhanced if (1) the patient has an uncontrolled systemic disease, such as diabetes; (2) the jawbone has been previously irradiated; or (3) the patient has Paget's disease or other generalized osteosclerotic conditions.

Drainage from a cyst is usually caused by infection. If the cyst is in bone, a radiograph reveals the defect but may not help differentiate between an abscess and a cyst. Such a distinction is academic because an infected cyst may be considered an abscess. Soft tissue cysts within the oral cavity are uncommon.

A large oronasal fistula is easily recognized, so a discussion of its differential features is unnecessary. Small fistulae in the anterior midline could be confused with a patent nasopalatine duct, but these two entities can be distinguished by observing the position of an inserted gutta-percha point on an occlusal radiograph.

Since the majority of oroantral fistulae occur on the ridge in the premolar-molar area, a defect in this region that permits passage of food or drink into the nose is almost certainly an oroantral fistula. Small tracts from infected cysts or abscesses in this region could be confused with purulent drainage of an infected sinus through an oroantral fistula; however, a radiograph made after the insertion of a gutta-percha cone reveals the image of the cone terminating inferior to the antrum when the case is an infected cyst or abscess.

A postsurgical or postinfection defect is seen most often on the alveolus and is diagnosed by learning about the causative experience.

Commissural lip pits always occur in the characteristic location; the probability that other pits or sinus openings could occur in this location is remote.

Chronic draining dentoalveolar abscesses constitute the majority of intraoral draining lesions. If pus can be expressed from the opening by pressing on a tender tooth, the diagnosis is almost certainly chronic abscess. This impression is confirmed if a radiograph exposed after the insertion of a gutta-percha cone shows the image of the cone leading to the tooth roots.

The fovea palatinae are normal anatomic landmarks; however, in some patients, these depressions are so prominent that they may resemble fistulae or sinus openings. The characteristic location is on each side of the midline of the anterior soft palate, and mucus can be expressed from them by pressing on the surrounding soft tissue.

Fistulae and Sinuses of the Face and Neck

The following entities must be considered in the differential diagnosis when a draining lesion is encountered on the skin of the face and neck:

1. Pustule
2. Draining cyst
3. Chronic alveolar abscess or osteomyelitis
4. Salivary gland fistula
5. Orocutaneous fistula
6. Congenital aural sinus
7. Auriculotemporal syndrome
8. Thyroglossal sinus
9. Lateral cervical sinus

Determination of the location, depth, and course of tracts in the neck and face often permits the differentiation of these lesions. Thus injecting radiopaque dye into the defects, along with the use of radiographs, is frequently beneficial as a diagnostic indicator.

Identifying the fluid draining from these lesions may provide a valuable clue for diagnosis. In various cases the fluid may prove to be saliva, cyst fluid, pus, or sweat.

Saliva emanates from orocutaneous and salivary gland fistulae and through the second branchial arch sinus:

1. The second branchial arch sinus can be differentiated from the orocutaneous fistula by the fact that the former is a developmental lesion and is thus usually observed early in life. Also in most cases the former cutaneous defect is more inferior, often positioned just superior to the clavicle at the anterior border of the sternocleidomastoid muscle.
2. The orocutaneous fistula may be differentiated from the salivary fistula in that the defect does not extend from the skin surface to the mucosal surface in the latter. Also the characteristic location of the salivary gland fistula aids in the differentiation.

When the drainage is clear, thin cyst fluid, a tract from a branchial or thyroglossal cyst must be suspected. If the sinus is in the lateral neck, it is most likely draining from a branchial cyst. If it is in or near the midline in the region of the hyoid bone, however, and if it is stressed when the tongue protrudes, the lesion is most likely thyroglossal in origin.

If purulent material emanates from a cutaneous sinus, the entities that must be considered are pustule, infected cyst, chronic alveolar abscess or chronic osteomyelitis, and infected congenital aural sinus:

1. If the lesion is an infected aural sinus, swelling and tenderness are present, as is a small sinus opening on the anterior rim of the external ear. This entity may be confused with a first branchial arch sinus, but the latter is extremely rare (only 24 cases have been reported in the literature).
2. A draining alveolar abscess or chronic osteomyelitis of the mandible may empty onto the skin of the lower face or upper neck. On radiographic examination, bony changes are evident with both entities. If the cause is *Actinomyces* organisms, fine, yellow granules are frequently present in the purulent material (which usually emanates from multiple sinuses).
3. The infected draining cysts most often encountered in these regions are the thyroglossal, branchial, sebaceous, and dermoid.
   a. The sebaceous and dermoid varieties can usually be differentiated from the other two by their more superficial location. The dermoid cyst occurs most often in the midline and is firm, whereas the sebaceous variety may occur anywhere and is not as firm.
   b. The deeper, thyroglossal and branchial types usually can be differentiated by observing that the former are near or in the midline, whereas the latter are situated more laterally.
4. Purulent infections in the lymph nodes and draining space infections must also be considered.

A pustule is the most common of all purulent draining lesions. It is readily recognized by its short course and superficial location and by the presence of multiple skin lesions.

Auriculotemporal syndrome need not be confused with any of the other entities included in this chapter. A history of trauma to the parotid region followed by sweating on gustatory stimulation is practically pathognomonic.

FORDYCE'S GRA
FIBRIN CLOT
SUPERFICIAL AB
SUPERFICIAL NC
   TISSUE
YELLOW HAIRY
ACUTE LYMPHOI
   PHARYNGITIS

Many potentiall
because the cov
fat covered by
Salivary gland
This condition (
and salivary sto
a yellowish ting

FORDYCE'S

Fordyce's granu
small, slightly i
yellow to a disti
form plaquelike
tion of collectio
mucosa. The lol
   The patient
Fordyce's granu
ence may be w
frequently the r
garding cancer.

REFERENCES

1. Everett FG, Wescott WB: Commissural lip pits, *Oral Surg* 14:202-209, 1961.

2. Baker BR: Pits of the lip commissures in Caucasoid males, *Oral Surg* 21:56-60, 1966.

3. Gorlin RJ, Pindborg JJ: *Syndromes of the head and neck,* New York, 1964, McGraw-Hill.

4. Garlick JA, Cal
   multaneous occ
   eral upper lip s
   cyst: a case rep
   genesis, *Oral S*

5. Eisenbud L, K
   scess, *Oral Sur*

6. Rossman LE, F
   endodontic-per
   case, *Oral Surg*

7. Craig RW, A
   Draining fistu
   dodontically tr
   108:851-852, 1

8. Gustafson JR
   29:786-801, 19

9. Krippachne W
   suppurative p:
   Ann Surg 156:

10. Shulman BH:
    of the salivary
    Dis Child 80:4

11. Juniper RP: T
    oroantral fistu
    356, 1973.

12. Shafer WA, H
    of oral pathol
    WB Saunders

13. Lighterman I,
    rosy of the ora
    15:1178-1194

14. Eberhardt JA,
    EL: A compu
    distances betv
    and the apic
    teeth, *Oral Su*

15. Punwutikorn
    Clinically sig
    tions: a study
    Oral Maxillof

16. Killey HC, F
    cases of oroa
    cal flap oper
    1967.

17. Mustian WF
    sinus and its
    J Am Dent As

18. Wowern NV:
    displacement
    sinus: a follo
    29:622-627,

19. Ehrl RA: Or
    ical study of
    cern to seco
    Oral Surg 9:

20. Burket LW:
    treatment, e
    Lippincott.

21. Worth HM:
    radiologic i
    Mosby.

22. Anderson M
    fistula: repor
    863, 1969.

23. Goldman EF
    Treatment c
    closure: repc
    877, 1969.

24. Ziemba RB
    palatal flap
    J Oral Surg

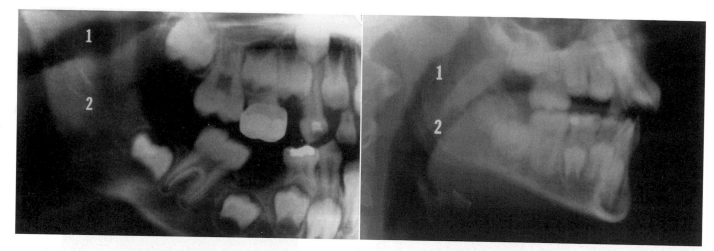

Fig. 15-6. Airway shadow. *1,* Nasopharyngeal airway; *2,* oropharyngeal airway. **A,** Panograph. **B,** Cephalometric view.

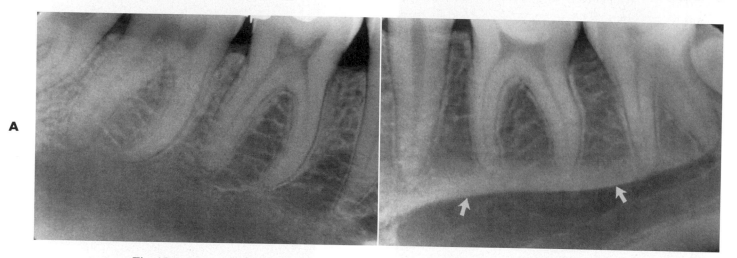

Fig. 15-7. Submandibular fossa. **A,** The fossa appears as a poorly defined radiolucency below the apices of the molars. **B,** The prominent mylohyoid ridge *(arrows)* in this view accentuates the fossa.

MENTAL FOSSA

The image of the mental fossa is similar to the image produced by the submandibular fossa. The mental fossa is situated on the labial aspect of the midline of the mandible just above the mental tubercle. Radiographs of the area often show such a relative radiolucency over the incisor roots that may be mistaken for periapical pathosis (Fig. 15-8).

MIDLINE SYMPHYSIS

The mandibular midline symphysis is present on radiographs at the midline of the mandibles of infants and is represented by a radiolucent line that may be misinterpreted as a fracture (Fig. 15-9). The symphysis usually fuses and ossifies by the age of 1 year and is then no longer apparent. It is not frequently encountered by the dental clinician on radiographs, since few patients have cause to be radiographically examined at this young age.

MEDIAL SIGMOID DEPRESSION

Langlais, Glass, Bricker, and Miles[6] describe a radiolucency that appears below and just anterior to the greatest depth of the sigmoid notch of the mandibular ramus. It may be observed occasionally on a panoramic radiograph (Fig. 15-10). The authors refer to the bony depression that caused this image as the *medial sigmoid depression.* This depression is defined by the temporal crest and the crest of the mandibular neck; its degree of expression, which is quite variable, depends on the robustness (prominence) of these two crests. According to the authors, the medial sigmoid depression is encountered radiographically on approximately 10% of the films examined. However, they point out that the image, regardless of the depression's size, depends on the geometry of the machine used and a particular positioning of the patient. This normal feature of the mandible is important only in that its recognition precludes its misinterpretation as pathosis.

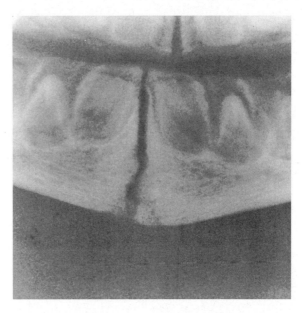

Fig. 15-9. This radiograph of a stillborn child shows the mandibular and the intermaxillary symphysis at birth. These vertical shadows may be erroneously identified as a fracture.

Fig. 15-8. Mental fossa. This radiograph showing a generalized radiolucency in the periapical incisor region illustrates the thinning of the bone resulting from the mental fossa.

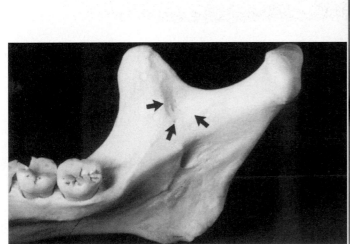

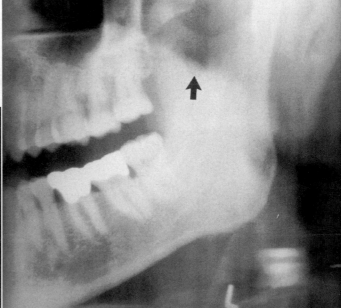

Fig. 15-10. Arrows indicate the presence of the medial sigmoid depression on the medial aspect of the bone (**A**) and the panoramic projection (**B**).

PSEUDOCYST OF THE CONDYLE

Friedlander, Monson, Friedlander, and Esquerra[7] identified and reported the pseudocyst of the condyle, which can appear as a well-defined radiolucency in the anterior aspect of the condyles in panoramic radiographs. These radiolucencies are seen in approximately 1 of 100 patients, are more common in older people, measure at least 0.5 by 0.4 cm, and are surrounded partially (at least 80%) or completely by a discrete sclerotic rim (Fig. 15-11). This image represents a marked cupping of the anterior surface of the condyle.[7] The cupping is produced by the pterygoid fovea and the dense medial and lateral ridges.[7]

ANTERIOR BUCCAL MANDIBULAR DEPRESSION

The anterior buccal mandibular depression has been defined as an anatomic variation occurring just lateral to the mental fossa.[8,9] It is bilateral in the canine region and more common in young children.[8,9] Radiographically, depressions range from an obvious radiolucency to almost imperceptible. Margins are well to poorly defined. A trabecular pattern, which has a pattern similar to the surrounding bone, can always be seen.[8,9]

CORTICAL PLATE MANDIBULAR DEFECTS

In addition to the lingual mandibular bone defect first reported by Stafne in 1942,[10] various cortical plate defects have been reported from time to time in various locations in the mandible. Examples include the following: various locations on lingual of mandibular body,[11,12] lingual surface of the mandibular ramus,[13,14] and the posterior buccal surface of the mandible.[15] It is not always clear whether these entities represent anatomic variations or are the result of pathology. They are included here for completion and are discussed in Chapter 19 with the cystlike radiolucencies not contacting teeth.

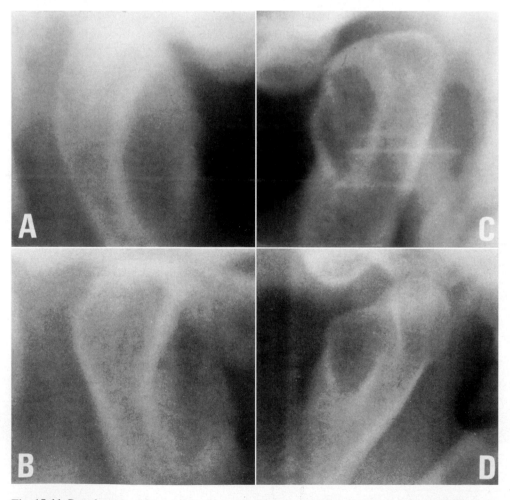

Fig. 15-11 Pseudocysts of the condyle. (From Friedlander AH, Monson ML, Friedlander MD, Esquerra AC: Pseudocysts of the mandibular condyle, *J Oral Maxillofac Surg* 50:821-824, 1992.)

STRUCTURES PECULIAR TO THE MAXILLA

INTERMAXILLARY SUTURE

The intermaxillary suture, between the right and left maxillary bones, can be identified as a thin, vertical radiolucency in the midline between the central incisors (Fig. 15-12). It is usually delineated by two thin, vertical radiopaque lines (cortical bone). It generally fuses later in life and is then no longer represented on the radiograph.

INCISIVE FORAMEN, INCISIVE CANAL, AND SUPERIOR FORAMINA OF INCISIVE CANAL

The incisive foramen (incisive fossa, anterior palatine foramen) frequently shows as a round, oval, diamond-shaped, or heart-shaped radiolucency that is well defined on occlusal films; less often, it appears as a round to ribbon-shaped, poorly defined radiolucency on periapical films, especially of the central incisors. The variation in size of this foramen also parallels its nonuniformity in shape. The position of the foramen on the radiograph ranges from between the roots of the central incisors, close to the alveolar ridge, to the level of the apices (see Fig. 15-12).

This variability in the position of the foramen on radiographs relates to both the angulation of the rays used to expose the film and the position of the foramen itself. The location of the foramen, which is in the midline, may range from the crest of the alveolar ridge to some distance posteriorly.

The incisive canals (nasopalatine or anterior palatine canal) that end at the incisive foramen are occasionally seen on periapical films of the central incisors. Their radiolucency on the film, more apparent than real, is emphasized by the contrast with their relatively sharp, opaque lateral walls, which actually delineate the canals (Fig. 15-13, *B*). The images vary greatly in width and length and may be seen to converge from the nasal fossa toward the foramen, but they usually become indistinct before reaching this terminal.

The images of the superior foramina of the incisive canals are found on periapical films of the maxillary central and lateral incisors and canines, especially if the vertical angle of the radiographic beam is increased sharply (see Fig. 15-13). These foramina are seen on the floor of the nasal fossa, bordering the septum. On the periapical films, their radiolucent images may be projected over the apices of any of the incisor teeth, prompting an impression of periapical pathosis.

NASAL CAVITY (NASAL FOSSA)

The inferior aspect of the nasal cavities is often seen on periapical radiographs of the incisor and canine regions, especially if the vertical angulation is increased. These cavities appear as twin radiolucencies separated by the radiopaque septum and are delimited by radiopaque cortical bone (see Fig. 15-13, *B*). The inferior border of the cavities is often projected above the apices of the incisors and canines.

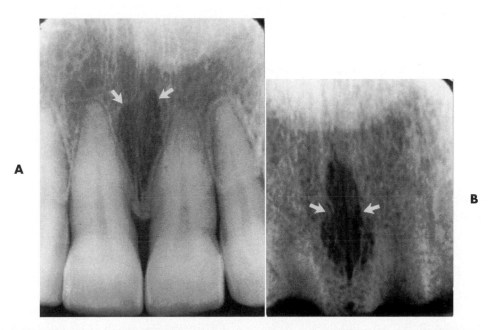

Fig. 15-12. Intermaxillary suture and incisive foramen. The intermaxillary suture can be identified as an indistinct, vertical radiolucent line in the central incisor region in **A.** It is more apparent in **B.** The incisive foramen *(arrows)* represents the oral terminal of the incisive canal. **A,** It is frequently projected onto the central incisor region near the crest of the alveolar process. **B,** The foramen of a nutrient canal is located inferior to the incisive foramen.

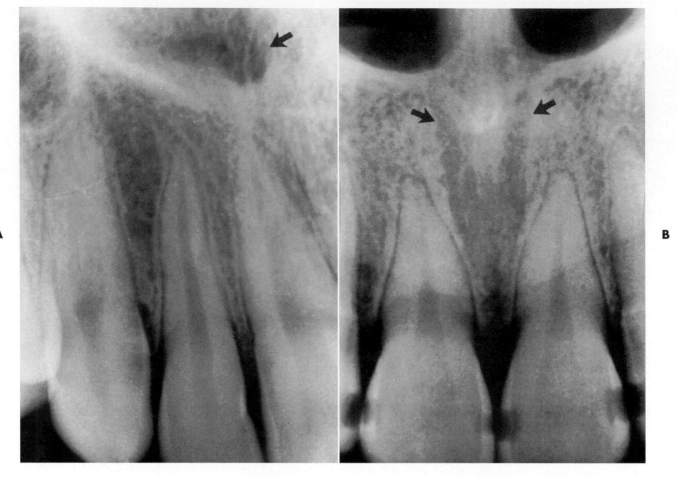

Fig. 15-13. A, Arrow indicates the nasal terminal of the incisive canal. **B,** The paired radiolucencies at the superior border represent the nasal cavities. Arrows indicate the divergent branching of the incisive canals toward their nasal terminals.

NARIS

The image of the nose is sometimes projected over the image of the alveolar bone on anterior periapical films. The density of this soft tissue added to the density of the bone results in a radiographic impression of increased bone density in the area of the superimposition.

Contrariwise, the images of the nares project onto this area of increased density as relative radiolucencies that frequently appear over or on the maxillary incisor region (Fig. 15-14). The nares may then be misinterpreted by the uninitiated diagnostician as evidence of periapical pathosis.

NASOLACRIMAL DUCT OR CANAL

The nasolacrimal duct on each side is usually enclosed in such a thin tube of cortical bone that it is seldom discernible on the usual periapical radiograph (Fig. 15-15, *A*). The orbital extreme of the structure, however, does appear on the maxillary occlusal radiograph, projected onto the posterior hard palate near the first or second molar area as a relatively large, bilateral radiolu-

cency that is well defined by sharp radiopaque borders (Fig. 15-15, *B*).

On the well-centered radiograph the image of each duct is usually at the junction of the radiopaque lines representing the maxillary sinuses and the nasal fossa. These radiopaque lines are situated lateral to and roughly parallel with the midsagittal plane, where the median suture may still be radiographically apparent before fusion.

MAXILLARY SINUS

The maxillary sinus on each side appears as a well-defined radiolucency with thin, sharp radiopaque borders (Fig. 15-16). The radiolucency may be crisscrossed by one or more thin radiopaque lines that represent bony septa appearing to subdivide the sinus. The sinus occurs bilaterally over the molars and premolars and may vary in anteroposterior extent from tuberosity to canine root or even to the lateral incisor root.

Each maxillary sinus may appear to border or overlap the nasal fossa, depending on the angle of exposure. In the adult the inferior aspect of each sinus lies below the

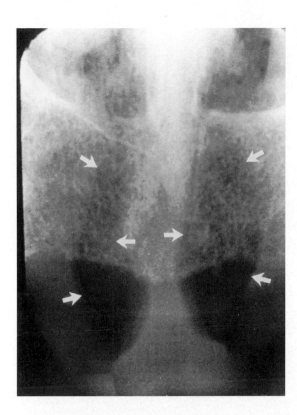

Fig. 15-14. The faint image of the nose and outlines of the nares *(arrows)* are seen in this periapical view of the maxillary incisor region.

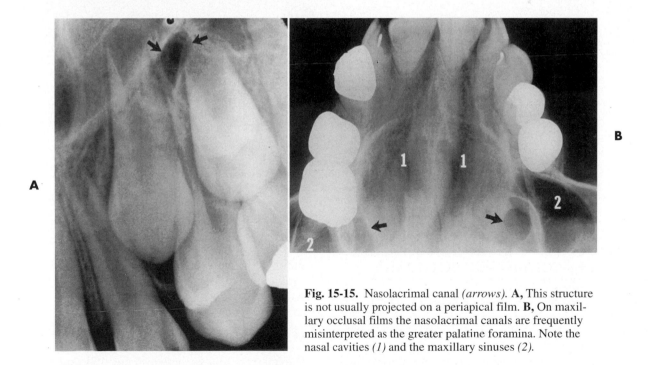

Fig. 15-15. Nasolacrimal canal *(arrows)*. **A,** This structure is not usually projected on a periapical film. **B,** On maxillary occlusal films the nasolacrimal canals are frequently misinterpreted as the greater palatine foramina. Note the nasal cavities *(1)* and the maxillary sinuses *(2)*.

level of the floor of the nasal fossa; frequently, nutrient canals are seen in the sinus wall and, when present, help distinguish this anatomic structure from a cyst or other pathosis. Poyton[16] discusses the radiographic appearance of the maxillary sinus in detail.

GREATER (MAJOR) PALATINE FORAMEN

Occasionally the greater palatine foramen can be identified on each side as a round to oval, ill-defined radiolucency over or between the apices of the maxillary second and third molars.[17]

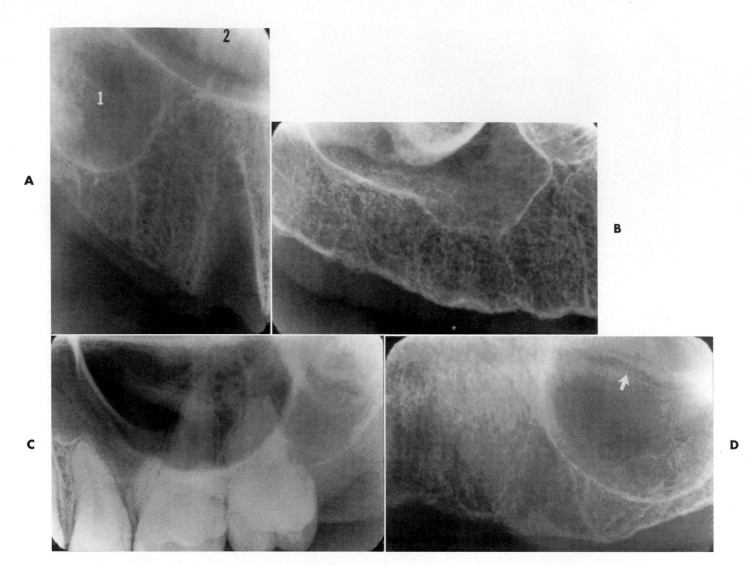

Fig. 15-16. Maxillary sinus. **A,** This periapical view of the canine region shows the maxillary sinus *(1)* the nasal cavity *(2)* and the antral Y. **B,** Maxillary sinus in an edentulous molar region. **C,** Maxillary sinus, showing complex contours and unusual extensions. **D,** Maxillary sinus with a cyst-like configuration. A nutrient canal *(arrow)* in the sinus wall aids in differentiating the sinus from a cyst.

STRUCTURES COMMON TO BOTH JAWS

PULP CHAMBER AND ROOT CANAL

The shadows of pulp chambers and root canals, along with the variations in these anatomic structures, are of great importance in restorative dentistry and in root canal therapy, but a discussion of these features is beyond the scope of this text.

PERIODONTAL LIGAMENT SPACE

Clinicians are well oriented to the radiographic appearance of the smooth radiolucent outline of the periodontal ligament spaces. When the spaces are superimposed over anatomic radiolucencies, however, the resultant radiographic images can simulate a broadening of the spaces and occasionally be mistaken for disease.

MARROW SPACE

The marrow spaces between the trabeculae of spongy bone appear as radiolucent areas that vary greatly in size, shape, and distribution from person to person, as well as throughout the jaws of the same individual (Fig. 15-17). In general, however, the radiographic representations of these structures throughout the maxilla are relatively uniform in size, whereas throughout the mandible the marrow spaces are smaller and more numerous in the anterior portion and tend to be larger in the posterior areas.

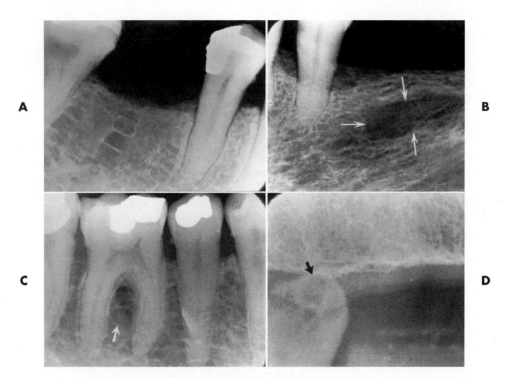

Fig. 15-17. Marrow space. **A,** This pattern occurs adjacent to the mandibular molar roots with some frequency. **B,** Large marrow space *(arrows)* that was mistaken for a lesion. **C,** Large marrow spaces *(arrow)* frequently occur in the bifurcation of the mandibular molars. These variations must be differentiated from periodontal involvement in the bifurcation. **D**, A large marrow space *(arrow)* in the coronoid process was mistaken for a lesion. Note the relatively small marrow spaces in the maxilla compared with those usually occurring in the posterior region of the mandible.

In some persons the trabecular spaces above and below the roots of the molars are so large and the trabeculae so sparse that the combined appearance may resemble and be misinterpreted as cysts, traumatic bone spaces, rarefying osteitis, or other such pathoses. These are referred to as *focal osteoporotic bone marrow defects.*[18,19] In areas where trabeculae are few and marrow spaces are large, the thinly scattered trabeculae are often relatively dense. The size of the marrow spaces is not a particularly reliable criterion for evaluating the status of the jawbone.

NUTRIENT CANAL

The nutrient canals appear as ribbonlike radiolucencies of fairly uniform width that are most often found between the roots of teeth (Figs. 15-12, *B,* and 15-18). These interdental canals, which are most frequently observed on radiographs of the mandibular incisor region, become less numerous in the mandibular premolar area, and the bone supporting the maxillary premolars is the third most likely area in which they are found.

Occasionally a relatively large nutrient canal, carrying the posterosuperior alveolar artery and traversing the lateral wall of the maxillary sinus, is apparent on a maxillary posterior radiograph (see Fig. 15-18, *C*). Although nutrient canals are rarely seen in the anterior region of the maxilla and are seldom recognized below or between the mandibular molars, one is found infrequently in the mandibular posterior region, where the trabeculae are few and the marrow spaces large. In this region a canal or two accentuated by fine radiopaque walls may be apparent.

In all the regions of both jaws, the canals become more marked when the teeth are missing. If the beam of the radiograph is directed parallel to a canal and through its foramen in the cortical bone, the canal appears as a small, round radiolucency (see Fig. 15-18, *C*). These radiolucencies technically are accessory canals and foramina. Occasionally, they are confused with pathologic radiolucencies. Patel and Wuehrmann[20] and Kishi, Nagaoka, Gotoh, et al[21] have studied the radiographic appearance of nutrient canals in the jaws.

DEVELOPING TOOTH CRYPT

Tooth crypts are seen on radiographs of developing dentitions, so they are seldom present in patients over 15 years of age. If the developing tooth is uncalcified, the crypt appears as a roundish homogeneous radiolucency and is mistaken for a cyst by the uninitiated diagnostician (Fig. 15-19). If just the tips of the cusps have calcified, the radiographic appearance is of a well-defined radiolucency containing radiopaque foci.

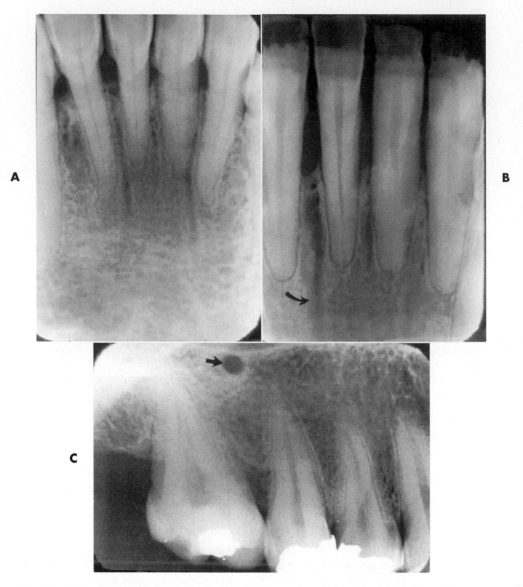

Fig. 15-18. Nutrient canal. **A,** These canals are frequently prominent between the roots of the mandibular incisors, and they terminate as small foramina on the crest of the interseptal bone. **B,** The prominent nutrient canal *(arrow)* in this view could be mistaken for a fracture. **C,** The prominence of this unusually large nutrient canal or accessory foramen *(arrow)* is produced by directing the x-rays parallel to the canal.

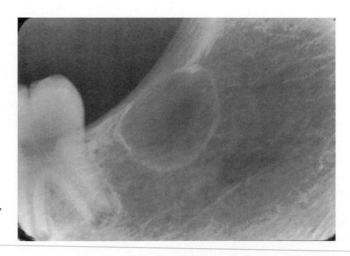

Fig. 15-19. Developing tooth crypt of a third molar. This cystlike radiolucency may be correctly identified by its position in the jaw, its bilateral occurrence, the age of the patient, and serial radiographs.

REFERENCES

1. Hayward BS, Richardson ER, Malhotra SK: The mandibular foramen: its anteroposterior position, *Oral Surg* 44:837-843, 1977.
2. Kaffe I, Ardekian L, Gelerenter I, et al: Location of the mandibular foramen in panoramic radiographs, *Oral Surg* 78:662-669, 1994.
3. Farman AG, Nortje CJ, Grotepas FW: Pathological conditions of the mandible: their effect on the radiographic appearance of the inferior dental (mandibular) canal, *Br J Oral Surg* 15:64-74, 1977.
4. Green RM: The position of the mental foramen: a comparison between southern (Hong Kong) Chinese and other ethnic and racial groups, *Oral Surg* 63:287-290, 1987.
5. Goodday RHB, Precious DS: Duplication of mental nerve in a patient with cleft lip-palate and rubella syndrome, *Oral Surg* 65:157-160, 1988.
6. Langlais RP, Glass BJ, Bricker SL, and Miles DA: Medial sigmoid depression: a panoramic pseudoforamen in the upper ramus, *Oral Surg* 55:635-638, 1983.
7. Friedlander AH, Monson ML, Friedlander MD, Esquerra AC: Pseudocysts of the mandibular condyle, *J Oral Maxillofac Surg* 50:821-824, 1992.
8. Kaffe I, Littner MM, Arensburg B: The anterior buccal mandibular depression: physical and radiologic features, *Oral Surg* 69:647-654, 1990.
9. Arensburg B, Kaffe I, Littner MM: The anterior buccal mandibular depressions: ontogeny and phylogeny, *Am J Phys Anthropol* 78:431-437, 1989.
10. Stafne EC: Bone cavities situated near angle of the mandible, *J Am Dent Assoc* 29:1969-1972, 1942.
11. Langlais RP, Cottone J, Kasle MJ: Anterior and posterior lingual depressions of the mandible, *J Oral Surg* 34:502-509, 1976.
12. Buchner A, Carpenter WM, Merrell PW, Leider AS: Anterior lingual mandibular salivary gland defect, *Oral Surg* 71:131-136, 1991.
13. Mann RW, Keenleyside A: Developmental lingual defects on the mandibular ramus, *Oral Surg* 74:124-126, 1992. (radiology forum)
14. Wolf J: Bone defects in mandibular ramus resembling developmental bone cavity (Stafne), *Proc Finn Dent Soc* 81:215-221, 1985.
15. Kocsis GS, Marcsik A, Mann RW: Idiopathic bone cavity on the posterior buccal surface of the mandible, *Oral Surg* 73:127-130, 1992.
16. Poyton HG: Maxillary sinuses and the oral radiologist, *Dent Radiogr Photogr* 45:43-59, 1972.
17. Grier DC: Radiographic appearance of the greater palatine foramen, *Dent Radiogr Photogr* 43:34-38, 1970.
18. Gordy FM, Crews KM, O'Carrol MK: Focal osteoporotic bone marrow defect in the anterior maxilla, *Oral Surg* 76:537-542, 1993.
19. Makek M, Lello GE: Focal osteoporotic bone marrow defects of the jaws, *J Oral Maxillofac Surg* 44:268-273, 1986.
20. Patel JR, Wuehrmann AH: A radiographic survey of nutrient canals, *Oral Surg* 42:693-701, 1976.
21. Kishi K, Nagaoka T, Gotoh T, et al: Radiographic study of mandibular nutrient canals, *Oral Surg* 54:118-122, 1982.

CHAPTER 16

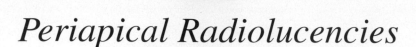

Periapical Radiolucencies

NORMAN K. WOOD
PAUL W. GOAZ
MARIE C. JACOBS

Periapical radiolucencies include the following:

ANATOMIC PSEUDOPERIAPICAL RADIOLUCENCIES
TRUE PERIAPICAL RADIOLUCENT LESIONS
PULPOPERIAPICAL RADIOLUCENCIES
  Periapical granuloma
  Radicular cyst
  Scar
  Chronic and acute dentoalveolar abscesses
  Surgical defect
  Osteomyelitis
  Pulpoperiapical disease and hyperplasia of maxillary sinus lining
DENTIGEROUS CYST
PERIAPICAL CEMENTOOSSEOUS DYSPLASIA (PERIAPICAL CEMENTOMA)

PERIODONTAL DISEASE
TRAUMATIC BONE CYST
NONRADICULAR CYSTS
MALIGNANT TUMORS
RARITIES
  Ameloblastic variants
  Amcloblastoma
  Aneurysmal bone cyst
  Benign nonodontogenic tumors
  Buccal cyst
  Cementifying and ossifying fibromas
  Cementoblastoma—early stage
  Central odontogenic fibroma—WHO type[1,2]
  Cholesterol granuloma[3]
  Cytomegaloviral lesions in human immunodeficiency virus disease
  Gaucher's disease

Giant cell granuloma
Giant cell lesion of hyperparathyroidism
Hyaline ring granuloma[4]
Juvenile ossifying fibroma[5]
Langerhans' cell disease (idiopathic histiocytosis)
Leukemia
Lingual salivary gland depression (anterior)
Mandibular infected buccal cyst
Myofibroma
Odontoma—early stage
Osteoblastoma—early stage
Paradental cyst
Pseudotumor of hemophilia
Solitary and multiple myeloma

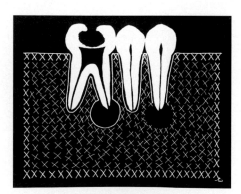

Radiolucent shadows are cast over the periapical regions of teeth in practically all oral radiographic surveys of dentulous patients. Some of these periapical radiolucencies represent innocent anatomic variations, whereas others are caused by benign conditions and require treatment to preserve the associated teeth; still others represent systemic disease conditions that many times become the responsibility and obligation of the dental clinician to recognize and bring to the attention of the patient's physician. The dental clinician should in every case afford whatever cooperation facilitates the most effective treatment.

  Malignancies represent a small group of these periapical shadows, and early detection, recognition, and treatment represent the only hope the patient has of being cured. In Marmary and Kutiner's survey[6] of periapical jawbone lesions, 51% showed radiographic evidence of an inflammatory process in the jawbone. A survey in the United Kingdom showed a very significant increased rate of periapical lesions over 17 years.[7] The high incidence and broad spectrum of conditions causing periapical radiolucencies make it imperative that all dental clinicians acquire a broad and comprehensive working knowledge of the conditions listed or discussed in this chapter.

ANATOMIC PERIAPICAL RADIOLUCENCIES

All periapical radiolucent shadows may be readily divided into two categories: true or false. True periapical radiolucencies represent lesions that truly are in contact with the apex of a tooth: Their shadow cannot be shifted from the periapex by taking additional radiographs at different angles. In contradistinction, false periapical radiolucencies are produced by anatomic cavities or lytic bony lesions that do not contact the apex of a tooth: These radiolucent shadows may be shifted from the periapex by taking additional periapical radiographs at different angles.[8] Different films of the area in question (e.g., a panoramic, occlusal, or Waters' projection) frequently aid in differentiating the normal anatomic shadows from periapical radiolucent lesions.

Furthermore, a complete examination, including the patient history and clinical, laboratory, and pulp tests, aids in this differentiation. If the radiolucencies are anatomic in origin, a comparison with the radiographs of the opposite side frequently reveals an identical situation. Clinicians should be aware not only of the normal location and appearance of the normal ranges, but also of variations of these structures.

The normal structures that may be responsible for radiolucencies and that could be confused with those caused by disease processes are discussed in some detail in Chapter 15. Therefore just a few anatomic structures that may appear at the periapex of periapical films are illustrated here (Figs. 16-1 to 16-3).

PERIAPICAL RADIOLUCENT LESIONS
Pulpoperiapical Radiolucencies

The seven distinct periapical radiolucent lesions that are sequelae of pulpitis follow:
1. Periapical granuloma
2. Radicular cyst
3. Scar
4. Abscess
5. Surgical defect
6. Osteomyelitis
7. Hyperplasia of sinus mucosa

Pathogenesis Each of the listed conditions share a common cause: irritating inflammatory products from an in-

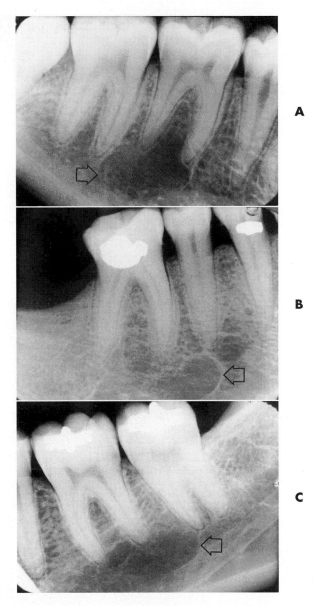

Fig. 16-1. Periapical focal osteoporotic bone marrow defects *(arrows).* **A,** Poorly defined borders. **B** and **C,** Well-defined, smoothly contoured borders.

jured or dead pulp. Microorganisms play an additional role in the infected lesions. The irritating substances set up an inflammation in the periodontal ligament at the periapex that causes lysis of bone and a soft tissue component. This process often expands beyond the periodontal ligament. Various irritants can activate several pathways of inflammation.[9] The egress of antigens from the root canal can initiate a combination of various types of immunologic reactions.[9-11] Rat studies indicate that the pathogenesis of periapical lesions is a multifactoral phenomenon and does not totally depend on the presence of T-cell lymphocytes.[12] Rat studies further indicate that the bone-resorbing activity of these lesions is mostly mediated by the cytokine interleukin-1α; prostaglandin E_2 accounts for the 1% to 15% of the remaining resorptive activity.[13]

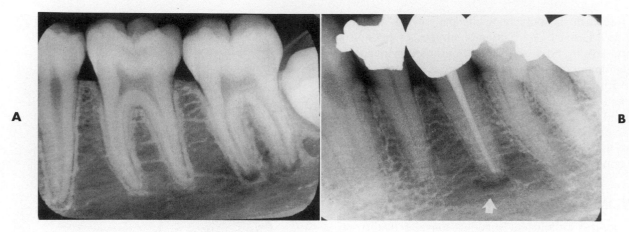

Fig. 16-2. A, Dental papillae (radiolucencies) at the apices of the second molar. **B,** Mental foramen in the periapex of the second molar.

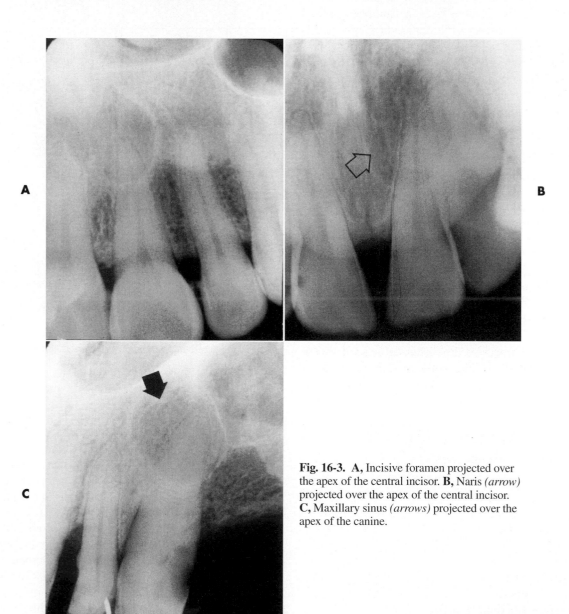

Fig. 16-3. A, Incisive foramen projected over the apex of the central incisor. **B,** Naris *(arrow)* projected over the apex of the central incisor. **C,** Maxillary sinus *(arrows)* projected over the apex of the canine.

```
                  ┌─────────────────────────┐
                  │   Periapical granuloma   │
                  └─────────────────────────┘
                    ↙   ↖    ↗   ↘
        ┌───────────────────┐      ┌───────────────────────────┐
        │   Radicular cyst   │ ───> │   Periapical abscess       │
        │                    │ <─── │   (chronic and acute)      │
        └───────────────────┘      └───────────────────────────┘
```

Fig. 16-4. Potential dynamics of pulpoperiapical lesions.

Generally the periapical granuloma is the first entity to be formed; depending on prevailing conditions, it may change to a radicular cyst or a secondary abscess (Fig. 16-4).

Features   The pulps in almost all cases are nonvital except when one of the roots of a multirooted tooth still retains some vital pulp tissue. Consequently, teeth associated with these lesions characteristically give a negative vitalometer reading. It is helpful to know the signs that would suggest that a certain tooth is nonvital. These are listed in the box at right.

Teeth with a dens in dente have a higher incidence of pulp death and a higher incidence of pulpoperiapical lesions (Fig. 16-5). Burton, Saffos, and Scheffer[14] described various charactcristics of dens in dente, which explains its frequent association with pulpoperiapical lesions. Dens in dente may also lead to pulpoperiapical lesions.[15]

Radiographic considerations

Lamina dura.   The shadow of the lamina dura normally varies greatly from person to person and even from region to region and from tooth to tooth in the same person. The lamina dura at the periapex of the maxillary canines often is impossible to discern even in good radiographs. The thin bone over the apex, as well as the pointed shape of the canine root, is responsible for this phenomenon. This information must be kept in mind when evaluating radiographs for early bony change at the apex of a suspicious tooth. If the lamina dura is consistently faint, the apparent diminution of lamina dura at the apex of the suspect tooth may be within normal limits. Earlier radiographs might be helpful to see if the lamina dura has changed.[16]

Amount of bone destruction.   Generally, 30% to 60% of regional bone destruction must have occurred for a change to be detected on radiographs. (Recently a 5% bone decalcification has been detected using digital subtraction under in vitro conditions.[17]) Consequently an actively growing lesion is slightly larger than it appears on radiographs. Various studies have addressed how much bone or what region of the periapical bone needs to be resorbed before the lesion shows on periapical radiographs.[18-22]

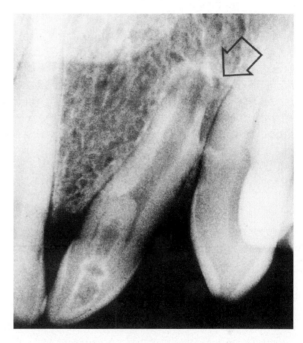

Fig. 16-5. Lateral incisor tooth in a 22-year-old patient with a nonvital pulp, an extensive dens in dente, and a pulpoperiapical radiolucent lesion. Arrow indicates radiolucency. Note the arrested development of the pulp canal with an open apex.

FEATURES SUGGESTIVE OF NONVITAL PULPS

- History of trauma
- History of painful pulpitis
- Dark hue of crown
- Reddish hue of crown
- Crown that is more opaque than its mate
- Large cavity
- Large restoration
- Fracture of crown
- Draining sinus tract
- Dens in dente (see Fig. 16-5)
- Fracture of root
- Absence of root canal shadow
- Open apex when mates are closed

Root resorption. Mild to moderate resorption of the root end commonly occurs and can be seen at the microscopic level. More serious resorption occurs with same frequency and is evident on radiographs as a rough blunting of the root end. In the senior author's experience (NKW), resorption caused by inflammation or infection is characteristically more ragged in outline, whereas resorption resulting from tumor may be more linear or curvilinear.

Periapical granuloma

The periapical granuloma by far represents the most common type of pathologic radiolucency. These lesions represented between 69.7% and 94% of all pulpoperiapical lesions in reports of series.[23-25]

Basically the periapical granuloma is the result of a successful attempt by the periapical tissues to neutralize and confine the irritating toxic products that are escaping from the root canal. The continual discharge of chronic irritating products from the canal into the periapical tissue is, however, sufficient to maintain a low-grade inflammation in these tissues; this inflammatory reaction continues to induce a vascular inflammatory response, which makes up the entity.

The microstructure of the granuloma consists of proliferating endothelial cells, capillaries, young fibroblasts, a minimal amount of collagen, and chronic inflammatory cells (lymphocytes, plasma cells, macrophages) (Fig. 16-6). Occasionally, nests of odontogenic epithelium, Russell bodies, foam cells, and cholesterol clefts are present. Approximately 20% of granulomas have these nests.[25]

Classically, more inflammation is seen in the center of the lesion, where the apex of the tooth is usually located, because at this point the irritating substances from the pulp canal are most concentrated. At the periphery of the lesion, fibrosis (healing) may already have begun, since the irritants are diluted and neutralized some distance from the apex. However, the orderly picture just described may not often be found. Occasionally, cholesterol clefts may form a major portion of the lesion. These would be examples of cholesterol granuloma of the jaws.[26]

Features. On radiographic examination the lesion is a well-circumscribed radiolucency somewhat rounded and surrounding the apex of the tooth (see Fig. 16-6). This periapical radiolucency may have a thin radiopaque (hyperostotic) border. Radiographs of the involved tooth may reveal deep restorations, extensive caries, fractures, or a narrower pulp canal than in the contralateral tooth. All these features would lead the clinician to suspect the presence of pulpoperiapical pathosis. A periapical granuloma cannot be differentiated from a radicular cyst by radiographic appearance alone. It was hoped that digital radiometric analysis would differentiate between granulomas and cysts,[27] but apparently results are disappointing.[28] Cysts tend to be larger than granulomas,[23,27,28] but differentiation on these criteria is not possible because some granulomas are large and some cysts are small. Few granulomas become larger than 2.5 cm in diameter. Any granuloma with a diameter of more than 2.5 cm probably represents a resolving chronic alveolar abscess rather than a primary type of granuloma.

The pulp of the offending tooth tests nonvital. The tooth is completely asymptomatic, including an absence of sensitivity to percussion. Swelling or expansion of the cortical plates over the area of the apex is unusual, since periapical granulomas rarely reach a size to produce such an effect.

Differential diagnosis. A differential diagnosis for a periapical granuloma is included in the corresponding section in the discussion of the radicular cyst.

Management. The management of a periapical granuloma is included in the management section of the discussion of the radicular cyst.

Radicular cyst

The radicular (periapical) cyst is the second most common pulpoperiapical lesion. This lesion has been reported to represent 6% to 17% to 25.9% of all pulpoperiapical lesions in published series of cases.[23-25] It is the most common of all odontogenic cysts. The radicular cyst is classified as an inflammatory cyst because it is thought that inflammatory products initiate the growth of

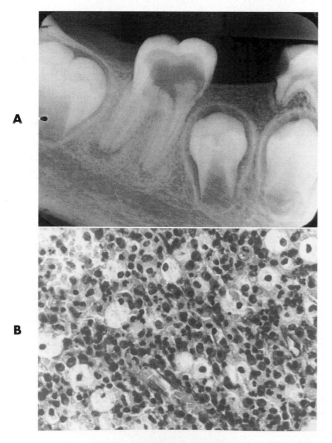

A

B

Fig. 16-6. Periapical granuloma. **A,** The pulp of the first molar was nonvital. **B,** Photomicrograph.

the epithelial component. It is classified as an odonto-genic cyst because of its origin in the Malassez rests' periodontal ligament cells, which are remnants of the Hertwig root sheath; the latter, in turn, is a product of the odontogenic epithelial layers (the inner and outer enamel epithelium).

Almost all radicular cysts probably originate in preexisting periapical granulomas, and their inflammatory reaction may start to proliferate within the granuloma. As the proliferating epithelial nests increase in size, the central cells start to degenerate and liquify because of ischemia to the central cells and because the capillaries in the tissue surrounding the developing cyst are being compressed. This sequence of events leads to the formation of a liquid-filled cavity lined with epithelium (i.e., a cyst). The cyst continues to grow because of a combination of factors. Two cytokines, interleukin-1 and interleukin-6, appear to be synthesized mainly by epithelial cells, which are known for inflammatory and osteolytic activity.[29] The pressure exerted by the enlarging cyst on the alveolar bone induces osteoclastic action and resorption of bone at the periphery of the cyst.

Features. Most radicular cysts involve the apices of the permanent teeth: 58% involve the lateral incisors.[24] These cysts involve deciduous teeth, most commonly the molars.[30] The history and clinical and radiographic features are identical to those of the periapical granuloma (Fig. 16-7). Studies by Lalonde[31] show that such a lesion is more likely to be a radicular cyst if the periapical radiolucency is at least 1.6 cm in diameter. Almost 20% of apices associated with radicular cysts show resorption.[32]

An untreated cyst may slowly enlarge and cause expansion of the cortical plates. In these instances a domelike swelling is observed on the alveolus over the periapical region of the involved tooth. The swelling may develop on the buccal or lingual side of the alveolar process and is covered with normal-appearing mucosa. Initially, it is bony hard to palpation, but later it may demonstrate a crackling sound (crepitus) as the cortical plate becomes thinned. In these cases of a destroyed cortical plate, the swelling is rubbery and fluctuant because of the cyst fluid (see Fig. 16-7, *E*). Large cysts may involve a complete quadrant, with some of the teeth occasionally mobile and some additional pulps nonvital. If it becomes infected, the tooth and swelling develop all the painful symptoms of an abscess.

On microscopic examination the radicular cyst is classically described with a lumen surrounded by an epithelial lining on a connective tissue wall that may vary in thickness from region to region and from cyst to cyst (see Fig. 16-7, *F*). Peripherally it is fibrous, although its inner regions may be composed of granulation tissue where foci of chronic inflammatory cells, foam cells, Russell bodies, and cholesterol clefts may be found. Various types of epithelium may be present; the epithelium varies greatly in form, thickness, and continuity.

Aspiration of a noninfected radicular cyst produces a light, straw-colored fluid, usually containing an abundance of shiny granules (cholesterol crystals).

Differential diagnosis. If a well-defined radiolucency is at the apex of an untreated asymptomatic tooth with a nonvital or diseased pulp and if anatomic structures can be ruled out, the radiolucency is a dental granuloma or a radicular cyst in approximately 90% of cases. Although these two entities cannot be distinguished by radiographic features alone, if the radiolucency is 1.6 cm or more in diameter, or 200 mm^2, it is more likely to be a cyst.[23,31] In practice, it is unnecessary to differentiate between small periapical granulomas and cysts, since both respond well to conservative root canal therapy.

Periapical scars and surgical defects are frequently confused with a periapical granuloma or cyst. In teeth that have received nonsurgical endodontic treatment for granulomas and cysts and are assumed to be well sealed, a persistent, asymptomatic, nonenlarging radiolucency is most likely a periapical scar. Similarly, an asymptomatic radiolucency that persists after root resection is likely a surgical defect. It is unlikely to be any type of residual or more serious pathosis if the tooth remains asymptomatic and the radiolucency does not increase in size.

The periapical cementoosseous dysplasia (PCOD) (cementoma) in its early lytic and fibroblastic stage cannot be distinguished from a periapical granuloma or cyst by radiographic examination (see Fig. 16-16). However the pulp is vital and healthy, whereas the tooth with a granuloma or cyst has a nonvital pulp. PCOD frequently involves the lower teeth (in a ratio of about 9:1), especially the incisors.

Although a traumatic bone cyst in a periapical area may be mistaken for a dental granuloma or cyst (see Fig. 16-19), as with PCOD, the pulps of the associated teeth are usually vital. Also, approximately 90% of traumatic bone cysts occur in the mandible, where they are most frequently seen in the molar, premolar, and incisor regions (in that order). Periapical cysts and granulomas have no predilection for the lower jaw and are more common in the anterior region. An intact periapical lamina dura is seen in the case of a traumatic bone cyst.

When a patient's history indicates a systemic disorder (e.g., hyperparathyroidism, primary malignant tumor, multiple myeloma), the working diagnosis of periapical granuloma or cyst must be broadened to include these more serious entities.

The periapical lesion associated with periodontal disease usually shows moderate to severe crestal bone loss (see Fig. 16-18). According to Brynolf,[33] this is coupled with a pattern of periapical bone loss morphologically distinct from that usually produced by pulpitis in that the radiolucency associated with marginal bone loss is of greatest width around the apex but extends laterally, tapering along the root for a short distance. Occasionally a periodontal fenestration over the apex mimics a true periapical radiolucency (see Fig. 16-18).

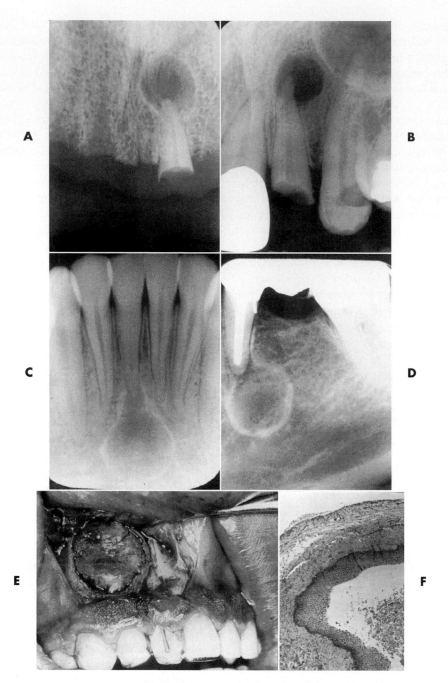

Fig. 16-7. Radicular cyst. **A** to **D,** Smoothly contoured, well-defined margins are evident in periapical radiographs. Hyperostotic borders can be seen in **A, C,** and **D. E,** Erosion of the labial cortex can be seen under the mucoperiosteal flap. **F,** Photomicrograph of a cyst wall shows the epithelial layer that surrounds the lumen.

The mandibular infected buccal cyst (molar area) is located on the buccal aspect of a lower molar tooth, which is usually but not invariably erupted.[34,35] On periapical radiographs the inferior aspect of the shadow of the cyst can be seen crossing the root at variable levels and sometimes includes the periapex. The size varies from 1 cm in diameter to considerably larger. The patient is usually young, the first molar is the most frequently involved, the pulp is usually vital, and the lamina dura around the

apices is intact. These last two characteristics permit differentiation from a periapical granuloma or cyst.

Malignancies always present serious difficulties in early diagnosis.[36] Many of the classic radiographic findings of malignancy are not seen in early lesions.[36] A symmetric or asymmetric bandlike widening of the periodontal ligament shadow is *very* suggestive of malignancy.

Management. Ordinary periapical shadows with a working diagnosis of granuloma or cyst should be treated with nonsurgical endodontics if the treatment plan calls for maintenance of the tooth. Protocol calls for a 1- to 3-month recall with clinical and radiographic examination to ensure that the lesion is not enlarging, whether there is doubt about the cause.[37] The success rate is very high for this type of approach. Studies show approximately 88% partial or complete resolution of radiolucencies.[38,39] One of these studies has observed these results within 12 months.[38] Other studies report success rates of 80% to 84.4%.[40,41]

When the suspicion index warrants, root canal therapy should be supplemented with apicoectomy and microscopic examination of the surgical specimen from the apex.[38,42,43] If extraction is indicated, the periapical area should be judiciously curetted and the specimen sent for microscopic examination.

On occasion, large radicular cysts that have destroyed a considerable amount of bone are encountered. Six approaches may be used for the management of such lesions. These approaches are surgical enucleation; surgical enucleation and restoration of the defect with a graft, preferably autogenous bone; marsupialization; decompression; decompression with delayed enucleation; and creation of a common chamber with the maxillary sinus or the nasal cavity (used occasionally for large maxillary cysts).

Liposky[44] described a technique of decortication and bone replacement for large cysts. Enucleation followed by collapse of a mucoperiosteal flap to eliminate the dead space has been used successfully for large cysts.[45] Nonsurgical endodontic failures can be treated by apicoectomy and biopsy. Freeze-dried bone allograft has been used successfully with this protocol.[46]

Sequential postsurgical radiographs are essential to ensure that the defect is regressing, no matter which method is used. The average healing time for cysts of more than 10 mm in diameter is approximately 2½ years. Incomplete removal of the cyst lining may result in the formation of a residual cyst or, in rare instances, of a more aggressive type of pathosis.

Periapical scar

The periapical scar is composed of dense fibrous tissue and is situated at the periapex of a pulpless tooth in which usually the root canals have been successfully filled. It represents a previous periapical granuloma, cyst, or abscess whose healing has terminated in the formation of dense scar tissue (cicatrix) rather than bone (Fig. 16-8). From 2% to 5% of all periapical radiolucent lesions are estimated to be periapical scars.

On microscopic examination a mature periapical scar shows a few spindle-shaped fibroblasts scattered throughout dense collagen bundles, and the collagen bundles often show an advanced degree of hyalinization. Inflammatory cells are not a feature, and vascularity is meager (see Fig. 16-8, *C*).

In our experience a significant percentage of lesions diagnosed microscopically as periapical granulomas have contained isolated areas of scar tissue, as well as regions of granulation tissue. Such lesions are in reality mixed lesions and probably should be thought of as scarring periapical granulomas or perhaps as a relatively young, less dense scar experiencing intermittent inflammation. A substantial portion of periapical granulomas microscopically examined are found to be such mixed lesions; therefore it would seem that, if the lesions are properly treated by nonsurgical endodontics, their granulomatous portion readily resolves and their reduced area may persist as periapical scar tissue. Serial radiographs of such lesions probably show a decrease in the size of the periapical radiolucency proportional to the amount of granulomatous tissue present at the time endodontic treatment was initiated.

It would seem then that the majority of persisting radiolucencies at the apex of asymptomatic teeth whose canals have apparently been successfully sealed by nonsurgical endodontic procedures are periapical scars. Periapical scars also frequently occur in cases initially treated by periapical curettage or root resection.[47]

Features. The periapical scar causes a well-circumscribed radiolucency that is more or less round and on radiographic examination resembles the periapical granuloma and cyst (see Fig. 16-8). It is frequently smaller than either of these entities. The tooth is asymptomatic, and the associated radiolucency remains constant in size or perhaps shrinks slightly.

The periapical scar occurs most often in the anterior region of the maxilla. Most of the involved teeth have been treated endodontically. Occasionally, such a scar occurs at the periapex of a pulpless tooth that has not been endodontically treated.

Differential diagnosis. The differential diagnosis of these lesions is included in the corresponding section in the discussion of periapical surgical defects.

Management. When the periapical scar is associated with an asymptomatic root canal–filled tooth, it requires no treatment once the clinician has established that the area is not enlarging.[48]

Chronic and acute dentoalveolar abscesses

Abscesses make up about 2% of all pathologic periapical radiolucencies. In the context of this chapter, the periapical or dentoalveolar abscesses are subdivided as follows, according to whether they are radiolucent:

1. Primary or neoteric abscesses are pulpoperiapical inflammatory or infectious conditions associated with teeth that have not developed apparent periapical radiolucent lesions; they are usually described as an acute apical periodontitis or an acute periapical abscess (Fig. 16-9).
2. Secondary or recrudescent abscesses develop in a previously existing asymptomatic periapical radiolucent lesion (e.g., granuloma, cyst, scar, cholesteatoma) (see Fig. 16-9).

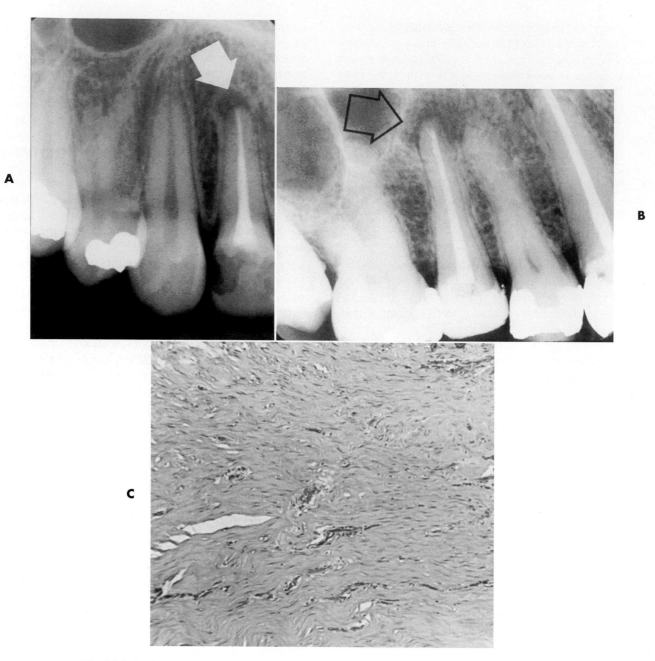

Fig. 16-8. Periapical scars. **A** and **B,** The periapical lesions have become markedly smaller in these two asymptomatic teeth after conservative root canal therapy. **C,** Photomicrograph shows dense fibrous tissue that makes up the periapical scar.

The primary (neoteric) abscess develops in a periapical region that is normal on radiographic examination. The infection is usually acute and exudative, involving the periodontal tissues at the apex of the tooth with a necrotic pulp. The canal contains large numbers of virulent bacteria that rapidly spread to the periapical tissues and cause an acute periodontitis, a very sensitive tooth, and perhaps alveolar swelling. The onset and course of the infection are so sudden that resorption of bone has not yet occurred. Frequently the infection and inflammation in the apical area forces the tooth slightly from its socket, creat-

ing an increased periodontal ligament space around the entire root that is usually apparent on the radiograph (see Fig. 16-9).

The secondary (recrudescent) abscess may be of the chronic or the acute type, depending on the number and virulence of the invading organisms, the resistance of the host, and the type and timing of the treatment instituted. Some 88% of periapical granulomas show microbial growth when homogenized and cultured: 55% of isolates are facultative anaerobes, and 45% are strict anaerobes.[49] Consequently, it is not surprising that granulomas become

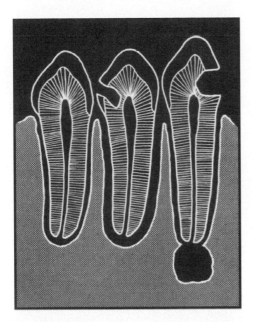

Fig. 16-9. Radiographic changes in pulpoperiapical infection. The middle tooth, illustrating primary acute abscess, displays the absence of a preexisting pulpoperiapical lesion and the widened periodontal ligament space. The tooth on the right represents a pulpoperiapical secondary abscess in which a radiolucent lesion has been present before this acute onset. This latter instance can also show a widening of the periodontal ligament space.

abscesses in some instances. There is general agreement that the microbial flora of the dental abscess is polymicrobial and that anaerobes play a major role in these infections.[50-56] These are mostly carbon dioxide–dependent streptococci, strict anaerobic gram-positive cocci, and strict anaerobic gram-negative bacilli.[56]

At the molecular level, lipopolysaccharides from the outer wall of gram-negative bacteria exert a plethora of biologic effects that result in the amplification of inflammatory reactions.[53] Capsule-associated material from gram-negative bacteria play a major role in tissue breakdown.[57]

Features. The primary lesion in which the infection occurs may be a granuloma, cyst, or rarely a scar; therefore a periapical radiolucency is a feature of the secondary abscess. The radiolucency may vary from small to quite large to involve much of the jaw. The initial periapical lesion may even have caused an expansion of the cortical plate.

If the acute infection is discovered soon after its onset and depending on its duration and acuteness or chronicity, the margins of the radiolucency may vary from well defined with possibly a hyperostotic border to poorly defined in chronic cases (Fig. 16-10). Sometimes the radiolucency is represented as a blurred area of somewhat lessened density than that of surrounding bone. Radiographs of the related tooth frequently show features such as deep restorations, caries, narrowed pulp chambers, or canals, which suggest that the pulp is nonvital. The roots of these teeth may also show resorption at the apex (see Fig. 16-10).

The microscopic picture varies somewhat, depending on the stage of the infection, but basically it consists of a central region of necrosis containing a dense accumulation of polymorphonuclear leukocytes surrounded by an inflamed connective tissue wall of varying thickness. A chronic resolving abscess may have fewer polymorphonuclear leukocytes; less necrosis; and more lymphocytes, plasma cells, macrophages, and granulation tissue (see Fig. 16-10). On the contrary, an acute abscess may contain only necrotic and unidentifiable soft tissue.

The tooth with an acute abscess is painful on percussion, and the patient may complain that it seems "high" to bite on. As a rule it does not respond to electrical pulp tests. The application of ice, however, relieves the pain somewhat, in contrast to the application of heat, which intensifies the pain. The tooth may demonstrate increased mobility.

If permitted to progress without treatment, the abscess may penetrate the cortical plate at the thinnest and closest point to the apex and form a space infection in the adjacent soft tissues. The space abscess is painful, and the surface of the skin or mucosa over the abscess feels warm and rubbery to palpation and demonstrates fluctuance (see Fig. 10-27, *D*). Systemic temperature may be elevated. Aspiration usually produces yellowish pus. Regional lymph nodes may become enlarged and painful.

Serial, total, and differential leukocyte counts are valuable in determining the course and nature of the infection. If circumstances are unfavorable, such as lowered host resistance (diabetes[58]) combined with virulent multiplying organisms and inadequate early treatment, serious complications may ensue. These include osteomyelitis, septicemia, septic emboli, asphyxia from a Ludwig's angina or another space infection that compromises the airway, and cavernous sinus thrombosis—any of which could be fatal.

A chronic infection ensues when the virulence and number of organisms are low and host resistance is high. If untreated, the chronic abscess frequently forms a sinus tract, permitting the pus to drain to the surface. A small proliferation of granulation tissue often forms on the surface and is referred to as a *parulis* (see Fig. 16-10, *C*). When drainage is established, pain is relieved, since the pain-producing pressure of the abscess is reduced.

Differential diagnosis. There is little question that the diagnosis is abscess when a painful fluctuant swelling is present. When the abscess is determined to be of the secondary type, however, the original periapical lesion may be difficult to identify. Such identification is often impossible because the histomorphology has been destroyed by the infection. The clinician must always be alert to the possibility that the apical radiolucency might be a secondarily infected primary tumor or a secondary tumor. However, malignancies seldom become abscessed, although superficial infection and necrosis are common.

In addition, any of the nonodontogenic cysts (e.g., incisive canal, globulomaxillary, median) may become infected

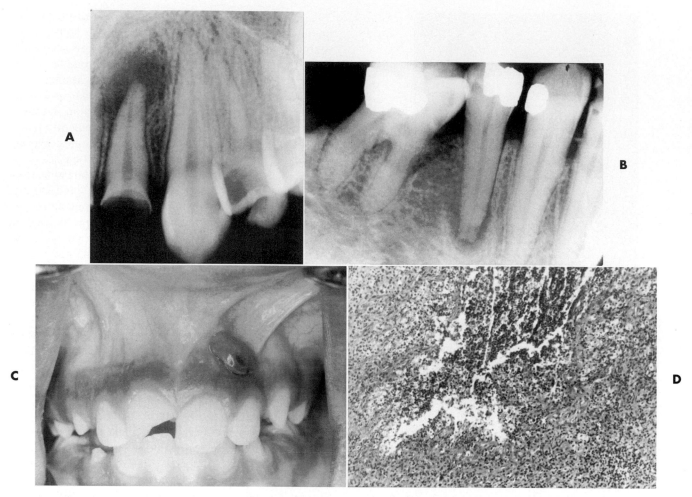

Fig. 16-10. Chronic periapical abscess. **A** and **B,** Ill-defined ragged borders. **C,** Parulis resulting from a chronic draining abscess at the apex of the pulpless left central incisor. **D,** Microscopy of a chronic abscess surrounded by granulation tissue.

and on radiographic examination may be projected over the apices of teeth with vital pulps, simulating an infected radicular cyst. In this case the image would not be very radiolucent.

Not all abscesses involving teeth are of pulpal origin. The periodontal abscess, originating in a deep periodontal pocket, is a common lesion; it can be distinguished from the incited periapical abscess by proper radiographic procedures showing the absence of a periapical radiolucency and usually the presence of an intrabony periodontal pocket. In addition, the pulps of teeth with such periodontal abscesses are usually vital. Endodontal and periodontal situations also occur and require special considerations in diagnosis and treatment.[59,60]

Management. The acute abscess should be treated aggressively to alleviate the patient's pain and to ensure that untoward sequelae do not occur. Immediate drainage should be achieved if possible. This may involve opening into the pulp chamber and passing a file down a root canal, extracting the tooth, or incising and draining soft tissue abscesses in a dependent method. A through and

through drain may be placed in the soft tissue abscess and irrigated frequently.

Oral penicillin is the empirical antibiotic of choice,[50,51,56,61] with metronidazole as an alternative or combination drug.[50,56] Oral penicillin G has been the standard, but amoxicillin may give better results.[50,62] If erythromycin is used in cases of penicillin allergy, erythromycin acistrate appears to provide higher active drug levels in the tissues than erythromycin stearate.[63] Specimens should be taken for culture and sensitivity tests and results used to redesign antibiotic coverage if necessary.

If the tooth is expendable, the correct time to extract is a judgment decision, but in most cases aggressive treatment and early extraction speeds recovery.[64] Systemic diseases that lower resistance to infection must be considered in these cases.

When a chronic draining sinus is present, the exact origin of the abscess can be located by inserting a gutta-percha cone into the extent of the sinus. The image of the cone points to the abscess on the radiograph. The procedure may not only direct attention to the offending tooth, but also demonstrate whether the abscess is of pulpal or periodontal origin. Sinus defects usually close when the infection has been eradicated and the root canals properly obliterated.

Surgical defect

A surgical defect in bone is an area that fails to fill in with osseous tissue after surgery, and it accounts for approximately 3% of all the periapical radiolucencies. It is frequently seen periapically after root resection procedures, especially when both labial and lingual plates have been destroyed. Approximately 45% of all periapical radiolucencies treated surgically require 1 to 10 years for complete resolution, and another 30% take longer than 10 years. In the remaining 25% the surgical defects resulting from root resection procedures do not heal completely. The post–root resection defect represents an area where the cortical plate is entirely lacking. A periapical scar may be present as well.

Features. The periapical radiolucency produced by a surgical defect is usually rounded in appearance, is smoothly contoured, and has well-defined borders (Fig. 16-11). It usually does not measure more than 1 cm in diameter. The radiolucent shadow may be projected directly over the apex or a few millimeters beyond the apex of the resected root of the endodontically treated tooth (see Fig. 16-11). If a time-sequence series of radiographs is available from the time of the resection, the radiolucency usually decreases in size. Frequently, it resolves to a certain size and then remains constant.

The tooth and periapical area are usually completely asymptomatic. A careful clinical examination may reveal the mucosal scar from the previous surgery. The defect may be detected by palpation if it is large enough.

Differential diagnosis. The periapical radiolucency produced by a surgical defect may be confused with any of the periapical lesions included in this chapter. A history of root resection, combined with the radiographic appearance of a resected, asymptomatic, endodontically treated tooth associated with a well-defined periapical radiolucency no larger than 1 cm and a small depression in the mucosa over the apical area, is highly suggestive of surgical defect.

If changing the angle of the beam shifts the radiolucent shadow in the periapical area, this can be taken as additional evidence that the entity is not at the periapex but in the cortical plate. If the shadow is caused by a surgical defect, it should show a reduction in size as it is periodically reexamined, especially during the first 6 months after surgery.

Management. Correct identification and periodic surveillance with radiographs are required for the management of periapical surgical defects.

Osteomyelitis

Occasionally a periapical abscess develops into an acute or chronic osteomyelitis, especially in patients with depressed systemic resistance or with very dense bone. *Os-*

teomyelitis is defined as an infection of bone that involves all three components: periosteum, cortex, and marrow. On this basis the periapical abscess can be considered a localized type of osteomyelitis (see Chapter 21).

Although the terms *osteomyelitis* and *osteitis* are often used interchangeably, the latter describes the more localized condition, and the former describes the more aggressive diffuse condition. This distinction of nomenclature should be made, although the pathologic processes may be fundamentally similar because there are clinical and radiographic differences between the entities and a difference in the regions of the jaw involved. Furthermore, the differences in the architecture, circulation, and character of the marrow between the alveolus and the body of the jawbone are apparently responsible for the usual localized, restricted nature of the osteitis—in contrast to the diffuse, almost unrestricted spread of the infection through the medullary spaces of the jawbone in an osteomyelitis. Differing responses to treatment also aid in the delineation of the two entities: An osteitis may be readily managed, whereas an osteomyelitis often proves difficult to eradicate. In summary, osteitis is restricted to the alveolar process and perhaps the superior aspect of the basal bone of the jaw. Osteomyelitis intimately involves the basal bone. Inasmuch as osteomyelitis is discussed in detail in Chapter 21, only a brief description in relation to periapical radiolucencies is presented here.

Acute osteomyelitis is similar to an acute primary alveolar abscess, since the onset and course may be so rapid that bone resorption has not occurred; thus a radiolucency may not be present. Chronic osteomyelitis, on the other hand, represents a low-grade infection of bone, which if untreated follows a protracted course of bone destruction. Chronic osteomyelitis may demonstrate four distinct radiographic pictures: completely radiolucent, mixed radiolucent and radiopaque, completely radiopaque, and proliferative periostitis. This last can be recognized as a somewhat opaque layering of the periosteum, with bone proliferating peripherally. In this discussion, only the chronic destructive type, causing a periapical radiolucency, is considered.

Features. Osteomyelitis is seldom observed in the maxilla, probably because of the comparatively rich blood supply; when it does occur, however, it may be a more fulminating infection than that in the mandible.

The offending tooth usually contains a nonvital pulp, may be sensitive to percussion, and may have been previously associated with an acute or chronic periapical abscess. There is a somewhat rounded periapical radiolucency that resembles the image seen in a periapical cyst, granuloma, or abscess. Frequently, however, the borders of the radiolucency are poorly defined and ragged (Fig. 16-12). Such an appearance is characteristic of infections in bone and results from the irregular extensions of the inflammation and infection through marrow spaces and channels in the bone.

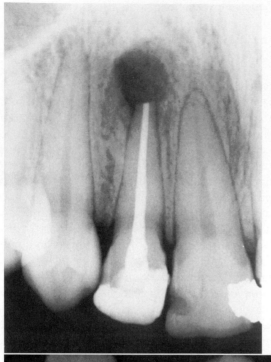

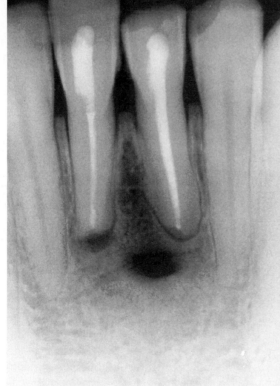

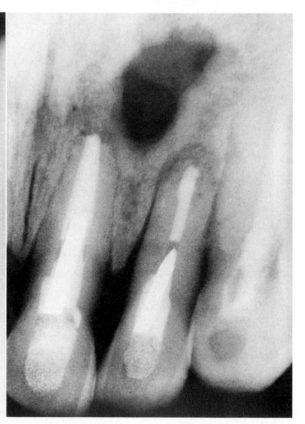

Fig. 16-11. Periapical surgical defects.

The bony course of a draining tract traversing the body of the jawbone may be seen as a radiolucency from the periapical radiolucency through the cortical plate beneath the sinus opening on the mucosa or skin (see Fig. 16-12). The course of this tract is deeper or longer than that seen with a pointed chronic alveolar abscess, since it is traversing the body of the jaw, in contrast to the shorter course characteristic of the draining restricted to the alveolar process.

If a sequestrum (segment of dead bone) is present and large enough, it shows as a radiopacity within a radiolucency. The patient complains of malaise and may have a fever, and there is a concomitant swelling on the bone and mucosa around the osteomyelitis that may vary from

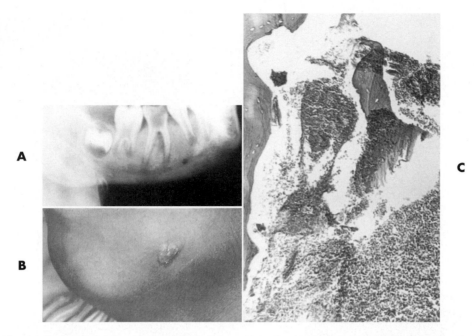

Fig. 16-12. Chronic osteomyelitis. **A,** Radiolucencies around the roots of the first molar. **B,** Sinus draining extraorally. **C,** Nonvital bony trabeculae (empty lacunae), inflammatory infiltrate, and necrotic material. (**A** courtesy R. Moncada, Maywood, Ill.)

slight to moderate. The swelling is firm, painful, and hot to palpation; pressure on the swelling or tooth may cause pus to be discharged from the sinus opening.

The microscopic picture is identical to that produced by a chronic alveolar abscess: necrotic tissue containing polymorphonuclear leukocytes and regions of granulation tissue. More dead bone (spicules with empty lacunae) is seen in osteomyelitis than in a chronic alveolar abscess (see Fig. 16-12). Although such spicules may be found in the radiolucent lesions, they are not large enough to show on the radiographs.

Differential diagnosis. The entities that should be included in the differential diagnosis of osteomyelitis are chronic alveolar abscess, an infected malignant tumor, Paget's disease complicated with osteomyelitis, and eosinophilic granuloma. If the draining sinus involves the body of the jawbone and courses through the marrow, the prognosis for the lesion is less favorable than that for a chronic alveolar abscess.

If the area of bone destruction is large and the region not painful, eosinophilic granuloma must be considered. A biopsy establishes the final diagnosis.

Osteomyelitis superimposed on a malignant tumor of bone is rare but may completely disguise the more serious lesion, which becomes apparent again only after successful treatment of the osteomyelitis. The suspicion that a lesion may be osteomyelitis can be qualified considering the following circumstances:

1. If only the alveolar portion of the jawbone is infected, the diagnosis is alveolar abscess.

2. If the tooth suspected of precipitating the condition is in a fracture line, the diagnosis of chronic osteomyelitis is strengthened. This diagnosis is also supported if an accompanying uncontrolled systemic disease such as diabetes is present.

3. Also, an attending bone disease, such as Paget's disease or previous radiation therapy, along with some pathognomonic symptoms of infection, tends to strengthen the impression of osteomyelitis. Paget's disease is evident when several bones are involved and the classic cotton-wool appearance is apparent.

When considering Paget's disease, the clinician must remember that there is an increased incidence of osteosarcoma in this disease and that the radiographic appearance of the disease and osteogenic sarcoma can be confused with that of chronic sclerosing osteomyelitis.

Management. The management of osteomyelitis is discussed in detail in Chapter 21. Risks and benefits must be carefully considered when attempting to maintain involved teeth. Systemic disease must be ruled out.

Pulpoperiapical disease and hyperplasia of maxillary sinus lining

Pulpoperiapical inflammation or infection and periodontal conditions frequently produce local inflammatory hyperplasia of the adjacent antral soft tissue floor.[64-70] These appear as gray shadows that may be dome shaped in the maxillary sinus floor or a gray radiopacity that appears as a cap over the adjacent troublesome root (Fig. 16-13). Radicular cysts can pouch up into the sinus and may show

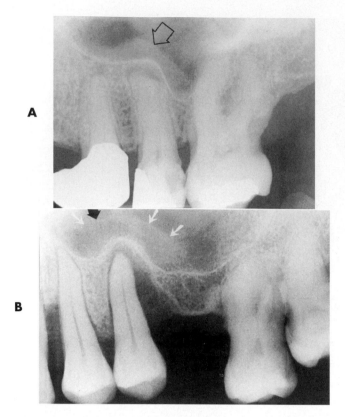

Fig. 16-13. Hyperplasia of the soft tissue membrane of the maxillary sinus floor *(arrows).* **A,** Etiology is a pulpoperiapical infection involving the second premolar tooth. **B,** Etiology is advanced periodontal disease involving the second premolar tooth.

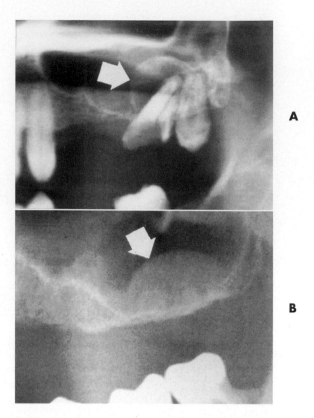

Fig. 16-14. Shadows in the sinus floor. **A,** Radicular cyst at the periapex of the second molar *(arrow).* Note the thin, curved bony rim of the cyst that separates the cyst from sinus. **B,** Benign mucosal cyst on the sinus floor *(arrow).*

a thin, curved radiopaque rim of bone separating the cyst from the sinus cavity (Fig 16-14, *A*). The free margin of the soft tissue shadow is usually smoothly contoured and distinct, although the soft tissue shadow may show varying degrees of grayness. The cortex of the sinus floor just superior to the offending apex may show indistinctness or in some cases may show minimal thickening.[68] Most of these soft tissue shadows disappear after treatment.[69] In one study, 78% disappeared completely after 11 to 20 months of dental treatment.[70] The persistent lesions probably represent lesions of fibrous hyperplasia, especially in cases in which the osteitis has disappeared.

Differential diagnosis. The differential diagnosis list would include benign mucosal cyst (Fig. 16-14, *B*), buccal exostosis, polyps of the maxillary sinus, malignant tumors, and antral exostoses.[71]

Dentigerous Cyst

Although a dentigerous cyst forms adjacent to the crown of an unerupted tooth, sometimes the position of the crown of the involved tooth and the extension of the cyst is such that the pericoronal radiolucency is projected over the apex of a neighboring tooth (Fig. 16-15, *A*). In 55% of such instances, root resorption of the neighboring tooth occurs.[32] On rare occasions, the radiolucency is projected over the apex of the same tooth, especially in cases of a circumferential or lateral dentigerous cyst (Fig. 16-15, *B*). In such situations, it may not be immediately apparent whether the radiolucency is pericoronal or periapical. The confusion is compounded if the tooth over whose apex the image of the dentigerous cyst is cast has a nonvital pulp. Dentigerous cysts are discussed in detail in Chapter 17.

Periapical Cementoosseus Dysplasia

PCOD is the lesion previously known as *periapical cementoma* and is by far the most common fibrocementoosseous lesion. PCOD is a reactive fibroosseous lesion and is thought to arise from elements in the versatile periodontal ligament,[72-75] where mature osteoblasts, cementoblasts, and precursor cells reside. The box on p. 267, left, provides a classification of fibroosseous lesions.[75]

These periapical lesions have the following stages of development, which are apparent on radiographic examination:

1. The early (osteolytic or fibroblastic) stage is radiolucent; the microstructure consists chiefly of a cellular fibroblastic stroma that may contain a few small foci of calcified material (see Figs. 16-16 and 16-17).
2. As these lesions mature, they pass through an intermediate stage, which is indicated by a radiolucent area containing radiopaque foci.

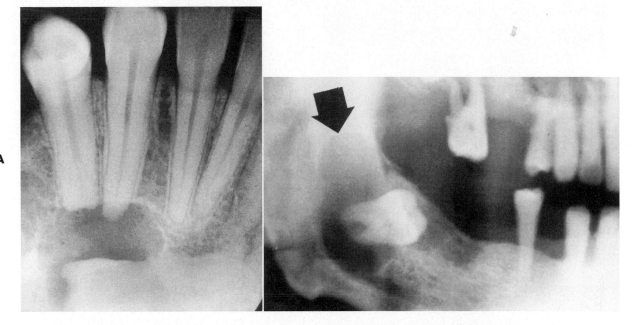

Fig. 16-15. Dentigerous cysts seen as periapical radiolucencies. **A,** The pulps of the canine and first premolar teeth tested vital. **B,** Unusual radiographic shadow of a circumferential dentigerous cyst *(arrow),* which gives the illusion that the cyst is associated with the root rather than the crown. (**B** courtesy R. Latronica, East Amhurst, NY.)

CLASSIFICATION OF FIBROOSSEOUS LESIONS

  I. Fibrous dysplasia
 II. Reactive (dysplastic) lesions arising in the tooth-bearing area.
      These are presumably of periodontal ligament origin. It is convenient to divide them into three types based on their radiologic features, although they seem to represent the same pathologic process.
      Periapical cementoosseous dysplasia
      Focal cementoosseous dysplasia
      Florid cementoosseous dysplasia
III. Fibroosseous neoplasms
      These are widely designated as cementifying fibroma, ossifying fibroma, or cementoossifying fibroma.

Modified from Waldron CA: Fibro-osseous lesions of the jaws, *J Oral Maxillofac Surg* 51:828-835, 1993.

DIFFERENTIAL LIST FOR PCOD

• Anatomic radiolucency
• Pulpoperiapical radiolucency
• Traumatic bone cyst
• Focal cementoosseous dysplasia[74]
• Cementoossifying fibroma
• Cementoblastoma
• Malignancy

---

3. The final stage is referred to as the *mature lesion;* it has become almost completely calcified and appears as a well-defined, solid, homogeneous radiopacity surrounded in most cases by a thin radiolucent border.

The calcified material in periapical lesions may be entirely cementum, may be entirely osseous, or may be a combination.

This chapter deals with the periapical radiolucencies, so only the osteolytic fibroblastic or radiolucent stage of the lesion is discussed.

Features In the early stage of development, PCODs occur as radiolucencies that are usually somewhat rounded, have well-defined borders, and are associated with teeth having vital pulps (Fig. 16-16). Blacks are more commonly affected than whites; 80% of the lesions occur in women, 5.9% in black women.[76] The lesions are seldom seen before the fourth decade of life. Although any tooth may be affected, approximately 90% of PCODs occur in the mandible, where the periapical region of the incisors is the most frequently involved site. The lesions may be solitary or multiple, are completely asymptomatic, and seldom exceed 1 cm in diameter. It is unusual for a PCOD to become large enough to produce a detectable expansion of the cortical plate.

Differential diagnosis The differential diagnosis list for PCOD is located in the box above. Anatomic radiolucencies are often projected over periapices but usually can be separated from the periapex by changing the angle of the x-ray.

The osteolytic or early stage of PCOD could be confused with the pulpoperiapical radiolucencies. The PCOD

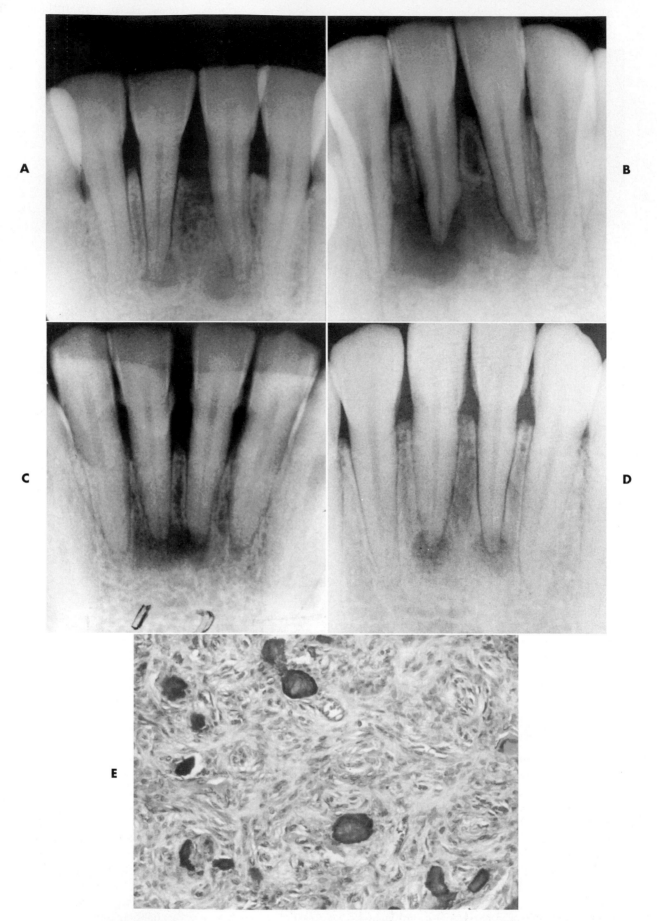

Fig. 16-16. Periapical cementoosseus dysplasia (PCOD) (early stage). **A** to **D,** All incisors were vital, and all patients were over 30 years of age. **E,** Photomicrograph of an early PCOD showing a few small foci of cementum-like material in a fibroblastic field.

is totally asymptomatic, the pulp of the involved tooth is usually vital, and the lesion most frequently affects the mandibular incisors. These features contrast with those of a pulpoperiapical lesion, which is associated with pulp disease or pulp death in a tooth that is frequently (or has been) sensitive to pressure, percussion, or both. The two lesions cannot be differentiated on radiographic examination while the PCOD is in the radiolucent stage. In some instances, although not always, the apex of a tooth with PCOD gives the appearance of having been sharpened in a pencil sharpener (see Fig. 16-16, *C*).

A traumatic bone cyst may be projected over the apex of a tooth with a vital pulp and may be confused with PCOD, but it is usually much larger and is characteristically found in a younger age-group. If its identity is in doubt, however, radiographs taken later reveal the developing calcifying foci within the radiolucency. Differentiating the PCOD from pulpoperiapical pathosis in the intermediate stage is also easier because of the radiopaque areas present at this time within the radiolucent area. The traumatic bone cyst most often involves the mandibular premolar or molar teeth; PCOD has a marked predilection for the lower incisors.

Focal cementoosseous dysplasia is similar to PCOD: It occurs commonly in the premolar or molar region of the mandible (Fig. 16-17). It differs from PCOD in that the margins are so not discrete and the tissue is attached to bone at the margins.[74]

The cementoossifying fibroma occurs at the apices of vital teeth, is more commonly seen in the mandible, goes through maturation stages similar to those of PCOD, and thus could be confused with this latter entity. It differs in the following ways: (1) It occurs in younger people; (2) it occurs most often in the premolar region; (3) it has the potential to be a large lesion; and (4) it requires prompt surgical removal.

The cementoblastoma in its early stage may also be confused with early PCOD, but the former is a rare lesion that occurs almost exclusively at the periapices of the mandibular molars (see Fig. 16-25, *C*). Furthermore, it characteristically extends higher on the root.

Although the rare malignancy at the periapex must always be considered, it should be given a low ranking unless the patient's history or the behavior of the lesion directs otherwise.

Management Observation is all that is required when the working diagnosis of PCOD is ensured.

Periodontal Disease

A discussion of periodontal disease is not within the scope of this text. Nevertheless, periodontal disease must be considered here because it causes a relatively common periapical radiolucency. Such a radiolucency is usually caused by advanced periodontal bone loss involving one tooth more severely than the teeth immediately adjacent. The entire bony support of the involved tooth may be destroyed, and the tooth may appear to be floating in a radiolucency (Fig. 16-18). Sometimes a narrow vertical pocket extends to the apex and appears to be a fairly well-defined periapical

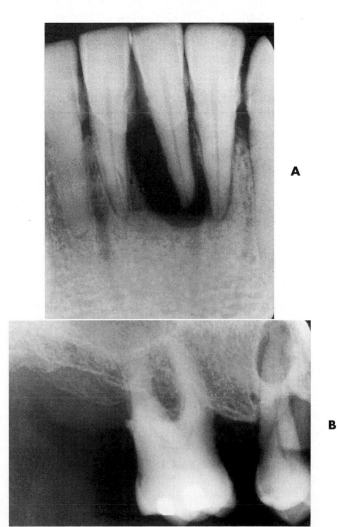

A

B

Fig. 16-18. Periodontal disease. Periapical radiolucencies caused by periodontal disease. The teeth tested vital.

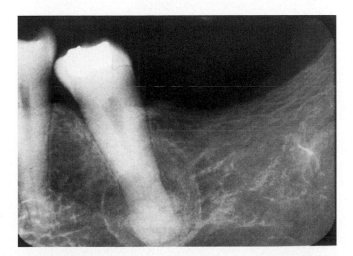

Fig. 16-17. Focal cementoosseous dysplasia (FCOD) and root of the second premolar tooth. Some intralesional calcification is present.

radiolucency, which in one projection seems to be surrounded by bone (see Fig. 16-18). Brynolf[33] describes specific characteristics that may be useful in differentiating between periodontal disease–produced periapical radiolucencies and pulpoperiapical radiolucencies. The diagnosis is best established with a clinical examination of the supporting structures by identifying and probing all periodontal pockets. Pocket depth relative to the root length of associated teeth can be demonstrated by placing gutta-percha points in the pockets to their full depths and then taking radiographs of the area with the points in place.

Teeth with advanced periodontal destruction are usually quite mobile and sensitive to percussion; surprisingly, many remain vital, and the demonstration of such vitality aids the clinician in determining the correct diagnosis. Nevertheless, endodontic and periodontal problems may be concomitant, and cases have been reported of advanced periodontally involved teeth, which had nonvital pulps that almost certainly occurred as a result of the periodontal condition.[77]

Extraction of the tooth may be the indicated treatment. The soft tissue must be curetted from the region of the apex and sent for microscopic examination to establish the final diagnosis and rule out more serious diseases that can cause a similar pattern of bone loss.

Traumatic Bone Cyst

Although the traumatic bone cyst (hemorrhagic bone cyst, extravasation cyst, simple bone cyst, solitary bone cyst, progressive bony cyst, blood cyst) is discussed in detail in Chapter 18, it should also be included in this series, since it may present a difficult diagnostic problem when it occurs as a periapical radiolucency. The traumatic bone cyst is classified as a false cyst of bone because it does not have an epithelial lining. Its cause is unknown.

Features A history of trauma may be elicited. The lesion is usually discovered on routine radiographs and is asymptomatic except when it occasionally reaches a size sufficient to cause expansion of the jaw. In such instances, cortical plates are expanded rather than eroded, and this produces a bony, hard bulge on the jaw. Sometimes the lesion involves half the mandible. The mandible is involved more frequently than the maxilla. The premolar and molar regions are the most common locations, but the symphysis is also frequently involved (Fig. 16-19). Bilateral cases have been reported,[78] and unusual cases have occurred in the ramus and condyle.[79]

Teeth involved with this type of periapical radiolucency are vital, and the lamina dura is intact. Tipping, migration of teeth, and root resorption are not features. Traumatic bone cysts usually occur in patients under 25 years of age.

On radiographic examination a traumatic bone cyst is a well-defined (cystlike) radiolucency above the mandibular canal, is predominantly round to oval, and may be positioned somewhat symmetrically about the periapex of a root (see Fig. 16-19). It usually extends superiorly between the premolar and molar roots, producing a scalloped appearance. The lateral and inferior borders of the elongated variety have smooth, regular contours (see Fig. 16-19).

Aspiration usually is fruitless, but in some cases serosanguineous fluid, a small quantity of blood, or a serumlike fluid may be obtained.[80] At surgery, the clinician may find scanty tissue which on microscopic examination proves to be loose or dense fibrous connective tissue containing some hemosiderin.

Differential diagnosis The traumatic bone cyst that is projected around and between the roots of teeth is most frequently mistaken for a radicular cyst. The pulps of the associated teeth are vital in traumatic bone cysts, however, which makes the distinction between the two entities clear in most cases.

Differentiating between a periapical traumatic bone cyst and relatively large, early stage PCOD may pose a diagnostic problem, since the pulps of the associated teeth in both cases should be vital (barring a concomitant, nonrelated pulpal problem). In distinguishing between these two, the clinician can measure from the size of the lesion: PCOD is seldom

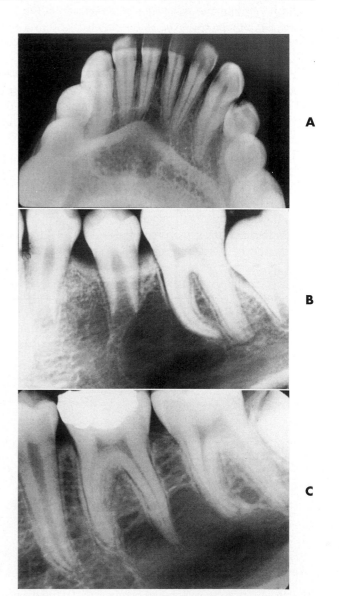

Fig. 16-19. **A** and **B,** traumatic bone cyst. All teeth tested vital. (**B** courtesy M. Kaminski, deceased.)

more than 0.7 cm in diameter, whereas the traumatic bone cyst is usually larger than 1 cm. Also the traumatic bone cyst usually occurs in individuals under 25 years of age, whereas PCOD is seen in patients over 30 years of age. PCOD has a marked predilection for the lower incisors, whereas the traumatic bone cyst is seen mostly in the premolar and molar regions. Periodic radiographs show the maturational changes of the radiolucent PCOD—through the mixed radiolucent-radiopaque stage to the mature radiopaque stage—thus permitting the working diagnosis of PCOD.

A traumatic bone cyst may also be confused with the rare median mandibular cyst. Both entities have similar features. The surrounding teeth have vital pulps. Both can occur in the midline of the lower jaw and may project between the teeth, although the median mandibular cyst frequently causes a separation of the teeth, whereas the traumatic bone cyst does not. Both are usually asymptomatic. Even though expansion of the cortical plates is an unusual finding in either case, such a deformity is even less common in the traumatic bone cyst. Aspiration may produce similar and confusing results.

Management   The treatment of choice is to open the area surgically, establish a diagnosis of traumatic bone cyst, remove the tissue debris present, curette the walls of the bony cavity to induce bleeding, and close the soft tissue flap securely. The patient should be protected with antibiotics, since the clinician has in effect produced an intrabony hematoma. This mode of treatment has proved to be quite successful, with bone filling the defect after the clot has organized. A careful follow-up to confirm healing is advised.[81]

Nonradicular Cysts

On occasion, nonradicular cysts may be projected over the apices of teeth. Therefore their description is appropriate in this chapter.

The most common offenders are the incisive canal cyst, midpalatine cyst, median mandibular cyst (refer to discussion of traumatic bone cyst), and primordial cyst (Fig. 16-20). With the exception of primordial cysts, these occur in specific regions of the jawbones. In general, they must be differentiated from anatomic shadows,

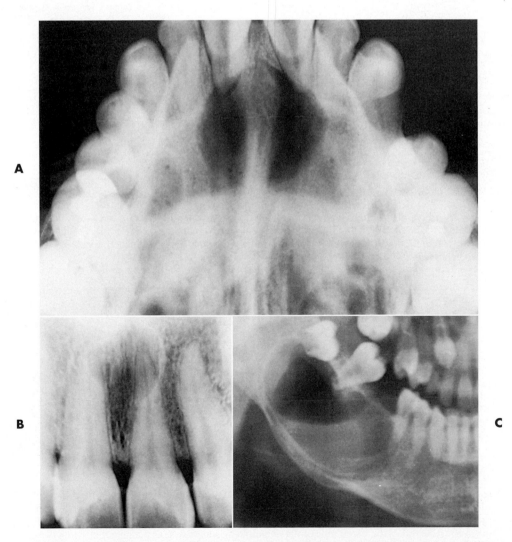

Fig. 16-20. Nonradicular cyst. **A** and **B,** Incisive canal cysts. **C,** Primordial cyst. (Courtesy N. Barakat, Beirut, Lebanon.)

radicular cysts, periapical granulomas, traumatic bone cysts, early PCOD, and other less common entities.

Changing the angle at which the radiograph is taken frequently projects the radiolucent image of the nonodontogenic cyst away from the superimposed apices, and this differentiates the nonodontogenic from the radicular cyst and from the dental granuloma or other pulpoperiapical lesions as well. Also the teeth seemingly associated with these nonradicular cysts are usually vital.

Differential diagnosis If a cystlike radiolucency larger than 2 cm in diameter is present over the apex of a vital maxillary incisor and can be projected away from the apex by changing the horizontal angle at which a second radiograph is taken, the most likely diagnosis for the lesion is incisive canal cyst.

If a cystic area at the periapex of a maxillary first molar on a periapical film is shown on an occlusal film to involve the whole palate and if all the maxillary teeth are vital, the most appropriate diagnosis is midpalatine cyst.

Malignant Tumors

Malignant tumors may be found as a single periapical radiolucency mimicking a more common benign lesion. Biopsy is mandatory for periapical lesions that do not respond to endodontic therapy, are surgical cases, or are otherwise suspect.[42,43] Cases of malignant salivary gland tumors occurring as periapical radiolucencies that were mistaken for pulpoperiapical lesions have been reported.[82,83] Malignant tumors may be primary or secondary. Primary malignancies that cause radiolucent lesions are discussed in detail in Chapter 21. Metastatic tumors of the jaws frequently produce a variable radiographic appearance, and those that resemble benign conditions most often escape early diagnosis. Unfortunately, early malignant lesions at the apices seldom present with features that suggest their identity.[36]

The malignancies that should be considered are squamous cell carcinoma, malignant tumor of the minor salivary glands (Figs. 16-21 through 16-23), metastatic tumors, osteolytic sarcoma, chondrosarcoma, melanoma,

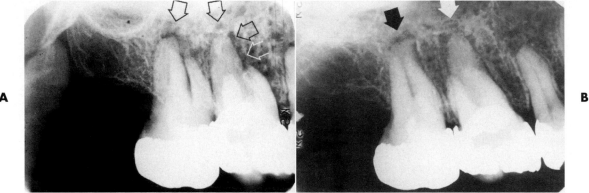

Fig. 16-21. Periapical radiographs. Arrows indicate bony destruction and periapical radiolucencies at the apices of the premolar and molar teeth, all caused by squamous cell carcinoma of the maxillary sinus. Note the bandlike widening of periodontal ligament spaces in the periapices. (Courtesy R. Copeland, Libertyville, Ill.)

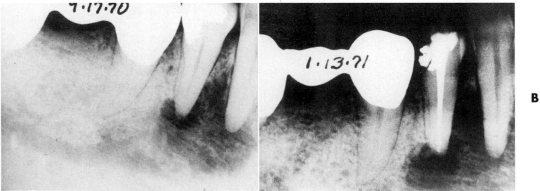

Fig. 16-22. Adenoid cystic carcinoma. **A,** Periapical radiograph showing the existing periapical radiolucency before endodontic treatment. **B,** Periapical radiograph taken 4 months later showing enlargement of the radiolucency. Surgery and microscopic study established the diagnosis. (From Burkes JE: Adenoid cystic carcinoma of the mandible masquerading as periapical inflammation, *J Endodont* 1:76-78, 1975.)

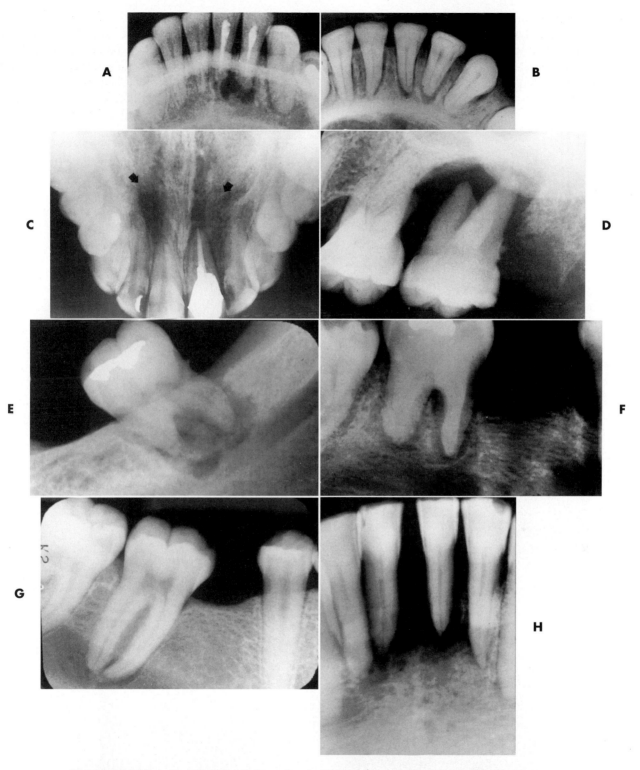

Fig. 16-23. Malignant periapical radiolucencies. **A,** Chondrosarcoma. **B** and **C,** Osteogenic sarcoma. (The bandlike widening of the periodontal ligament spaces around the incisor roots is evident in **B.**) **D,** Adenoid cystic carcinoma on the posterolateral hard palate. **E,** Metastatic carcinoma from the pancreas. **F,** Hemangiosarcoma. The radiolucencies at the apices of the molar and the bandlike widening of the periodontal ligament spaces are evident on all teeth shown. **G,** Metastatic rhabdomyosarcoma at the periapex of a molar. **H,** Metastatic carcinoma at the apices of the central incisors. (**A** courtesy O.H. Stuteville, deceased; **B** and **G** courtesy R. Goepp, Chicago; **C** from Curtis M, Elmore J, Sotereanos G: Osteosarcoma of the jaws: report of a case and review of the literature, *J Oral Surg* 32:125-130, 1974; **F** courtesy D. Skuble, Hinsdale, Ill; **H** courtesy R. Oglesby, Stroudsburg, Pa.)

fibrosarcoma, reticulum cell sarcoma, and multiple myeloma. Other than symmetric and asymmetric band-like widening of periodontal ligaments, the findings in Figs. 16-21 through 16-24 are not pathognomonic for malignancy. Granted, enlarging lesions with ragged, moth-eaten borders are always worrisome (see Chapter 21).

Mesenchymal malignant tumors and metastatic tumors originating within bone are more apt to produce a localized periapical radiolucency than a peripheral squamous cell carcinoma, which almost always originates in the surface and erodes through the alveolar bone to arrive at the apex. However, a squamous cell carcinoma originating within a

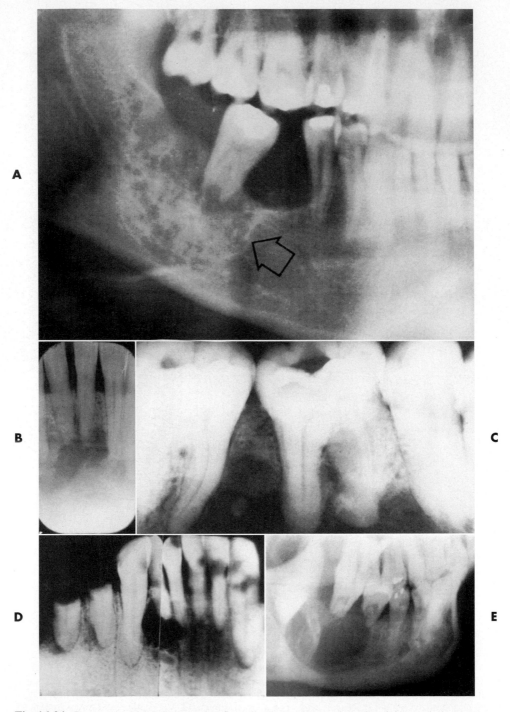

Fig. 16-24. Rare periapical radiolucencies. **A** to **C,** Giant cell granuloma involving teeth that were vital. **D** and **E,** Ameloblastoma. **F** and **G,** Langerhans' cell disease. **F,** Radiolucency at the apex of the lateral incisor and canine in an adult. **G,** Three periapical radiolucent lesions *(arrows)* in a 14-year-old boy. **H,** Periapical lesion in a 62-year-old woman with multiple myeloma. The lesions in myeloma usually have smoother contours than shown. (**A** courtesy N. Barakat, Beirut, Lebanon; **B** and **F** courtesy R. Goepp. Chicago; **C** courtesy J. Ireland, deceased, and J. Dolci, Mundelein, Ill; **D** courtesy P. Akers, Chicago; **E** courtesy O.H. Stuteville, deceased.)

cyst could be seen as a localized periapical radiolucency.

In summary, malignant periapical radiolucencies may produce the following images: (1) a well-defined periapical radiolucency; (2) a poorly defined periapical radiolucency; or (3) a large, ragged, well-defined radiolucent tumor that has destroyed a large segment of the surface bone and has involved the apex of a tooth. Root resorption and bandlike widening of periodontal ligament spaces (see Fig. 16-21 through 16-23) may accompany any of the three images.

Features The signs and symptoms of most malignancies of the oral cavity and jaws have much in common. Although these tumors occur in patients of all ages, they are more common in patients of middle and old age. Pain may be a feature. The involved teeth may retain their vitality. If the tumor is advanced, there may be migration, loosening, tipping, and spreading of teeth. There may also be gingival bleeding. Paresthesia or anesthesia of the soft tissues is sometimes present and is ominous.

Expansion of the jaw is a feature in advanced lesions. At first, this expansion has a smooth surface covered with normal-appearing mucosa unless the tumor is squamous cell carcinoma. Later in the course of the tumor's growth, the mucosa breaks down because of chronic trauma, ulcerates, and then develops into a fulminating necrotic growth of tissue.

Differential diagnosis The advanced lesions are readily recognized as malignancies. The earlier lesions, however, present a problem because they may mimic the benign conditions just discussed; unless other subtle symptoms of malignancy are recognized, the clinician is not alerted to the seriousness of the case.

Management Fortunately, two basic principles are used by clinicians who manage periapical radiolucencies.

First, the tooth and the area in question are observed with periodic clinical and radiographic examination, and the lesion and tooth are treated with conservative

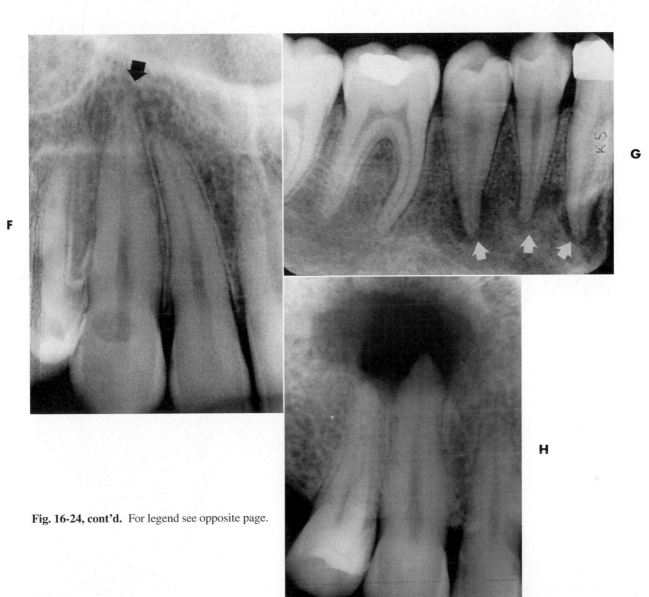

Fig. 16-24, cont'd. For legend see opposite page.

endodontic techniques. Therefore if a small malignant periapical radiolucency has been misdiagnosed and treated as a pulpal sequela, this error soon becomes apparent.

Second, if the clinician chooses to perform a root resection in addition to the root canal filling, the tissue recovered from the periapex is routinely sent for microscopic study. Consequently, the malignancy is diagnosed immediately, and more extensive management may be instituted promptly at the discretion of the local tumor board.

RARITIES

The rare pathologic entities that at times occur as periapical radiolucencies are listed at the beginning of this chapter. Specific points obtained from the patient's history or by clinical, radiographic, or laboratory examination would presumably direct the examiner to the lesion most likely responsible for the patient's periapical radiolucency (Figs. 16-24 to 16-26).

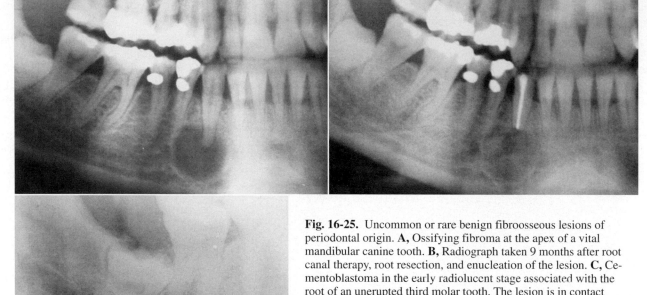

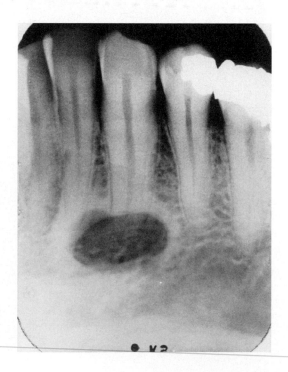

Fig. 16-25. Uncommon or rare benign fibroosseous lesions of periodontal origin. **A,** Ossifying fibroma at the apex of a vital mandibular canine tooth. **B,** Radiograph taken 9 months after root canal therapy, root resection, and enucleation of the lesion. **C,** Cementoblastoma in the early radiolucent stage associated with the root of an unerupted third molar tooth. The lesion is in contact with a considerable length of the root. Periapical cementomas seldom extend to this extent in a cervical direction. (**A** and **B** courtesy N. Barakat, Beirut, Lebanon; **C** courtesy P. Pullen, Palm Beach Gardens, Fla.)

Fig. 16-26. Periapical radiograph showing well-defined radiolucency projected over the apex of the mandibular canine tooth. This radiolucency was produced by an anterior lingual mandibular bone concavity. (From Connor MS: Anterior lingual mandibular bone concavity, *Oral Surg* 48:413-414, 1979.)

REFERENCES

1. Allen CM, Hammond HL, Stimson PG: Central odontogenic fibroma, WHO Type, *Oral Surg* 73:62-66, 1992.

2. Kaffe I, Buchner A: Radiologic features of central odontogenic fibroma, *Oral Surg* 78:811-818, 1994.

3. Hirshberg A, Dayan D, Buchner A, Freedman A: Cholesterol granuloma of the jaws: report of a case, *Int J Oral Maxillofac Surg* 17:230-231, 1988.

4. Chou L, Ficarra G, Hansen LS: Hyaline ring granuloma: a distinct oral entity, *Oral Surg* 70:318-324, 1990.

5. Slootweg PJ, Panders AK, Koopmans R, Nikkels PGJ: Juvenile ossifying fibroma: an analysis of 33 cases with emphasis on histopathological aspects, *J Oral Pathol Med* 23:385-388, 1994.

6. Marmary Y, Kutiner G: A radiographic survey of periapical jawbone lesions, *Oral Surg* 61:405-408, 1986.

7. MacDonald-Janowski DS: The detection of abnormalities in the jaws: a radiological survey, *Br Dent J* 170:215-218, 1991.

8. Richards AG: The buccal object rule, *Dent Radiogr Photogr* 53:37-56, 1980.

9. Torabinejad M: Mediators of acute and chronic periradicular lesions, *Oral Surg* 78:511-521, 1994.

10. Torabinejad M, Kettering JD: Detection of immune complexes in human dental periapical lesions by anticomplement immunofluorescence techniques, *Oral Surg* 48:256-261, 1979.

11. Torabinejad M, Theofilopoulos AN, Ketering JD, et al: Quantitation of circulating immune complexes, immunoglobulins G and M, and C_3 complement component in patients with large periapical lesions, *Oral Surg* 55:168-190, 1983.

12. Wallstrom JB, Torabinejad M, Kettering J, McMillan P: Role of T cells in the pathogenesis of periapical lesions: a preliminary report, *Oral Surg* 76:213-218, 1993.

13. Stashenko P, Wang C-U, Tani-Ishii N, Yu SM: Pathogenesis of induced rat periapical lesions, *Oral Surg* 78:494-502, 1994.

14. Burton DJ, Saffos RO, Scheffer RB: Multiple bilateral dens in dente as a factor in the etiology of multiple periapical lesions, *Oral Surg* 49:496-499, 1980.

15. Stewart RE, Dixon GH, Graber RB: Dens evaginatus (tuberculated cusps): genetic and treatment considerations, *Oral Surg* 46:831-836, 1978.

16. Wood NK: Periapical lesions. In Taylor G, editor: Endodontics, *Dent Clin North Am* 28(4):725-766, 1984.

17. Southard KA, Southard TE: Detection of simulated osteoporosis in human anterior maxillary alveolar bone with digital subtraction, *Oral Surg* 78:655-661, 1994.

18. Bender IB: Roentgenographic and direct observation of experimental lesions in bone. I. *J Am Dent Assoc* 62:152-160, 709-716, 1961.

19. Ramadan AE, Mitchell DF: Roentgenographic study of experimental bone destruction, *Oral Surg* 15:934-943, 1961.

20. Shoha RR, Dowson J, Richards AG: Radiographic interpretation of experimentally produced bony lesions, *Oral Surg* 38:294-303, 1974.

21. Valasek P, Emmering TE: Unpublished data, 1983.

22. Van der Stelt PF: Experimentally produced bone lesions, *Oral Surg* 59:306-312, 1985.

23. Kizil Z, Energin K: An evaluation of radiographic and histopathological findings in periapical lesions, *J Marmara Univ Dent Fac* 1:16-23, 1990.

24. Stockdale CR, Chandler NP: The nature of the periapical lesion: a review of 1108 cases, *J Dent* 16:123-129, 1988.

25. Block RM, Bushell A, Rodridgues H, Langeland K: A histopathologic, histobacteriologic, and radiographic study of periapical endodontic surgical specimens, *Oral Surg* 42:656-678, 1976.

26. Hirschberg A, Dayan D, Buchner A, Freedman A: Cholesterol granuloma of the jaws: report of a case, *Int J Oral Maxillofac Surg* 17:230-231, 1988.

27. Shrout MK, Hall MJ, Hildebolt CE: Differentiation of periapical granulomas and radicular cysts by digital radiometric analysis, *Oral Surg* 76:356-361, 1993.

28. White SC, Sapp JP, Seto BG, Mankovich NJ: Absence of radiometric differentiation between cysts and granulomas, *Oral Surg* 78:650-654, 1994.

29. Bando Y, Henderson B, Meghji S, et al: Immunochemical localization of inflammatory cytokines and vascular adhesion receptors in radicular cysts, *J Oral Pathol Med* 22:221-227, 1993.

30. Lustmann J, Shear M: Radicular cysts arising from deciduous teeth: review of the literature and report of 23 cases, *Int J Oral Surg* 14:153-161, 1985.

31. Lalonde ER: A new rationale for the management of periapical granulomas and cysts: an evaluation of histopathological and radiographic findings, *J Am Dent Assoc* 80:1056-1059, 1970.

32. Struthers R, Shear M: Root resorption by ameloblastoma and cysts of the jaws, *Int J Oral Surg* 5:128-132, 1976.

33. Brynolf I: Radiography of the periapical region as a diagnostic aid. I. Diagnosis of marginal changes, *Dent Radiogr Photogr* 51:21-39, 1978.

34. Stoneman DW, Worth HM: The mandibular infected buccal cyst—molar area, *Dent Radiogr Photogr* 56:1-14, 1983.

35. Camarda AJ, Forest D: Mandibular infected buccal cyst: report of two cases, *J Oral Maxillofac Surg* 47:528-534, 1989.

36. Wannfors K, Hammarström L: Periapical lesions of mandibular bone: difficulties in early diagnosis, *Oral Surg* 70:483-489, 1990.

37. Morse DR, Bhambhani SM: A dentist's dilemma: non-surgical endodontic therapy or periapical surgery for teeth with apparent pulpal pathosis and an associated periapical lesion, *Oral Surg* 70:333-340, 1990.

38. Murphy WK, Kaugers GE, Collett WK, Dods RN: Healing of periapical radiolucencies after non-surgical endodontic therapy, *Oral Surg* 71:620-624, 1991.

39. Barbakow FH, Cleaton-Jones PE, Friedman D: Endodontic treatment of teeth with periapical radiolucent areas in a general dental practice, *Oral Surg* 51:552-559, 1981.

40. Natkin E, Oswald RS, Carnes LI: The relationship of lesion size to diagnosis, incidence, and treatment of periapical cysts and granulomas, *Oral Surg* 57:82-94, 1984.

41. Shah N: Nonsurgical management of periapical lesions, *Oral Surg* 66:365-371, 1988.

42. Schlagel E, Seltzer RJ, Newman JI: Apicoectomy as an adjunct to diagnosis, *NY State Dent J* 39:156-158, 1973.

43. Weisman MI: The importance of biopsy in endodontics, *Oral Surg* 40:153-154, 1975.

44. Liposky RB: Decortication and bone replacement technique for the treatment of a large mandibular cyst, *J Oral Surg* 38:42-45, 1980.

45. Yih WY, Morita V: A modified technique for obliteration of large bony defects after cystectomy, *J Oral Maxillofac Surg* 49:689-692, 1991.

46. Saad AY, Abdellatief E-SM. Healing assessment of osseous defects of periapical lesions associated with failed endodontically treated teeth with use of freeze-dried bone allograft, *Oral Surg* 71:612-617, 1991.

47. Arwill R, Persson G, Thilander H: The microscopic appearance of the periapical tissue in cases classified as "uncertain" or "unsuccessful" after apiectomy, *Odont Rev* 25:27-42, 1974.

48. Peters E, Monopoli M, Woo SB, Sonis S: Assessment of the need for treatment of postendodontic asymptomatic periapical radiolucencies in bone marrow transplant recipients, *Oral Surg* 76:45-48, 1993.

49. Iwu C, MacFarlane TW, MacKenzie D, Stenhouse D: The microbiology of periapical granulomas, *Oral Surg* 69:502-505, 1990.

50. Lewis MAO, MacFarlane TW, McGowan DA: A microbial and clinical review of the acute dentoalveolar abscess, *Br Dent J* 28:359-366, 1990.

51. Holbrook WP: Bacterial infections of oral soft tissues, *Curr Opin Dent* 1:404-410, 1991.

52. Fisher LE, Russell RRB: The isolation and characterization of Milleri group streptococcus from dental periapical abscesses, *J Dent Res* 72:1191-1193, 1993.

53. Seltzer S, Farber PA: Microbiological factors in endodontology, *Oral Surg* 78:634-645, 1994.

54. Sundqvist G: Taxonomy, ecology, and pathogenicity of the root canal flora, *Oral Surg* 78:522-530, 1994.

55. Moenning JE, Nelson CL, Kohler RB: The microbiology and chemotherapy of odontogenic infections, *J Oral Maxillofac Surg* 47:976-988, 1989.

56. Gill Y, Scully C: Orofacial odontogenic infections: review of microbiology and current treatment, *Oral Surg* 70:155-158, 1990.

57. Harris M: Pathological bone destruction and the pathogenesis of the inflammatory odontogenic cyst, *J Jpn Stomatol Soc* 42:847-848, 1993.

58. Veta E, Osaki T, Yoneda K, Yamamoto T: Prevalence of diabetes mellitus in odontogenic infections and oral candidiasis: an analysis of neutrophil suppression, *J Oral Pathol Med* 22:168-174, 1993.

59. Belk CE, Gutmann JL: Perspectives, controversies and directives on pulpal-periodontal relationships, *J Can Dent Assoc* 56:1013-1017, 1990.

60. Christie WH, Holthuis AF: The endo-perio problem in dental practice, *J Can Dent Assoc* 56:1005-1011, 1990.

61. Topazian RG, Peterson LJ: Which antibiotic? *Oral Surg* 73:612-622, 1992 (letter to the editor).

62. Paterson SA, Curzon MEJ, The effect of amoxicillin versus penicillin V in the acutely abscessed primary teeth, *Br Dent J* 174:443-448, 1993.

63. Tuominen RK, Lehtinen R, Peltola J, et al: Penetration of erythromycin into periapical tissues after repeated doses of erythromycin acistrate and erythromycin stearate: a pilot study, *Oral Surg* 71:684-688, 1991.

64. Maloney PL, DoKu HC: Maxillary sinusitis of odontogenic origin, *J Can Dent Assoc* 34:591-603, 1968.

65. Pellegrino SV: Extension of dental abscess to the orbit, *J Am Dent Assoc* 100:873-875, 1980.

66. Mattila K: Roentgenological investigations into the relation between periapical lesions and conditions of the mucous membrane of the maxillary sinus, *Acta Odontol* 23:5-77, 1965.

67. Matilla K, Westerholm N: Rounded shadows in maxillary sinus, *Odont Tidskv* 76:121-136, 1968.

68. Powell RN: Peridontal disease and the maxillary sinus, *Oral Surg* 19:24-27, 1965.

69. Worth HM, Stoneman DW: Radiographic interpretation of antral mucosal changes due to localized dental infection, *J Can Dent Assoc* 38:110-116, 1972.

70. Ericson S, Welander N: Local hyperplasia of maxillary sinus mucosa after elimination of adjacent periapical osteitis, *Odont Rev (Malmo)* 17:153-159, 1966.

71. Ohba T, Langlais RP, Langland OE: Antral exostosis in panoramic radiographs, *Oral Surg* 76:530-533, 1993 (radiology forum).

72. Waldron CA, Giansanti JS: Benign fibroosseous lesions of jaws: a clinical-radiologic-histologic review of sixty-five cases. II. Benign fibro-osseous lesions of periodontal ligament origin, *Oral Surg* 35:340-350, 1973.

73. Waldron CA: Fibro-osseous lesions of the jaws, *J Oral Maxillofac Surg* 43:249-262, 1985.

74. Summerlin D-J, Tomich CE: Focal cemento-osseous dysplasia: a clinicopathologic study of 221 cases, *Oral Surg* 78:611-620, 1994.

75. Waldron CA: Fibro-osseous lesions of the jaws, *J Oral Maxillofac Surg* 51:828-835, 1993.

76. Neville BW, Albenesius RJ: The prevalence of benign fibroosseous lesions of periodontal ligament origin in black women: a radiographic survey, *Oral Surg* 62:340-344, 1986.

77. DiFranco CF, Gargiulo AV: Isolated advanced periodontal defects with pulpal involvement, *Perio Case Rep* 5:1-4, 1983.

78. Patrikiou A, Sepheriadou-Marropoulou T, Zambelis G: Bilateral traumatic bone cyst of the mandible: a case report, *Oral Surg* 51:131-133, 1981.

79. Shigematsu H, Fujita K, Watanabe K: Atypical simple bone cyst of the mandible, *Int J Oral Maxillofac Surg* 23:298-299, 1994.

80. Donkor P, Punnia-Moorthy A: Biochemical analysis of simple bone cyst fluid: report of a case, *Int J Oral Maxillofac Surg* 23:296-297, 1994.

81. Forssell K, Forssell H, Happonen R-P, Neva M: Simple bone cyst: review of the literature and analysis of 23 cases, *Int J Oral Maxillofac Surg* 17:21-24, 1988.

82. Burkes JE: Adenoid cystic carcinoma of the mandible masquerading as periapical inflammation, *J Endodont* 1:76-78, 1975.

83. Gingell JC, Beckerman T, Levy BA, et al: Central mucoepidermoid carcinoma: review of the literature and report of case associated with an apical periodontal cyst, *Oral Surg* 57:436-440, 1984.

CHAPTER 17

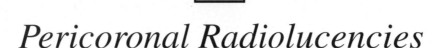

Pericoronal Radiolucencies

NORMAN K. WOOD
IRIS M. KUC

The entities producing pericoronal radiolucencies include the following:

PERICORONAL OR FOLLICULAR SPACE
DENTIGEROUS CYST
UNICYSTIC (MURAL)
   AMELOBLASTOMA
AMELOBLASTOMA
ADENOMATOID ODONTOGENIC TUMOR
CALCIFYING ODONTOGENIC CYST OR
   TUMOR
AMELOBLASTIC FIBROMA
RARITIES
   Ameloblastic variants

Calcifying epithelial odontogenic tumor
Envelopmental primordial cyst
Ewing's sarcoma
Extrafollicular dentigerous cyst
Follicular primordial cyst
Langerhans' cell disease
Malignant teratoma
Odontogenic carcinoma
Odontogenic fibroma
Odontogenic keratocyst
Odontogenic myxoma

Odontoma in pericoronal location (pre-
   mineralized stage)
Ossifying fibroma
Other radiolucencies projected onto images
   of impacted tooth crowns
Paradental cyst
Pseudotumor of hemophilia
Salivary gland tumors (central)
Squamous cell carcinoma
Squamous odontogenic tumor

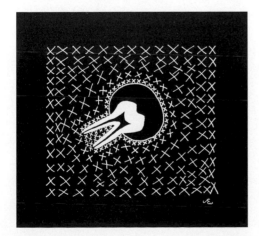

Characteristic features of the entities that commonly produce periocoronal radiolucencies are shown in Table 17-1.

PERICORONAL OR FOLLICULAR SPACE

The crowns of unerupted teeth are normally surrounded by a dental follicle—a soft tissue remnant of the enamel organ that is frequently referred to as the *reduced enamel epithelium.*

The dental follicle is necessary for tooth eruption,[1-4] and increased numbers of monocytes are present in this structure during eruption.[2] Osteoclasts are also present on the coronal surface of the bony crypt.[3] On microscopic examination the dental follicle is shown to be composed of soft myxomatous to dense collagenous fibrous tissue containing nests or cords of odontogenic epithelium (Fig. 17-1). It is important to distinguish between dental follicle and odontogenic tumors microscopically.[5]

Table 17-1 Pericoronal radiolucencies*

	Predominant gender	Peak age (year)	Most frequent jaw involved	Most frequent area of jaw involved	Most frequent tooth involved	Signs or symptoms	Recurrence
Follicular spaces Developing teeth	—	4-12				None	
Impacted teeth	M ~ F	Over 18	Mandible	Posterior	Mandibular third molar	Delayed eruption of tooth	Recurs as cyst or ameloblastoma
Dentigerous cysts	?	Over 18	Mandible	Posterior	Mandibular third molar	Delayed eruption of tooth Swelling, asymmetry	Recurs as cyst or ameloblastoma
Unicystic (mural) ameloblastomas	M ~ F	85% under 30 (average 21)	Mandible	Posterior	Mandibular third molar	Delayed eruption of tooth Swelling, asymmetry	Occasional
Ameloblastoma	M ~ F	Average 38.9	Mandible	Posterior	Mandibular third molar	Delayed eruption of tooth Swelling	Significant
Adenomatoid odontogenic tumors	$\frac{F}{M} = \frac{2}{1}$	10-21 (average 16.5)	Maxilla	Anterior (90%)	Maxillary canine (60%)	Delayed eruption of tooth Swelling, asymmetry	Unusual
Ameloblastic fibromas	M ~ F	70% under 20 (average 14 to 15.5)	Mandible	Posterior	Mandibular molar and premolar	Delayed eruption of tooth Advanced swelling, asymmetry	Unusual

*Entities listed according to frequency of occurrence.
~, Approximately equal.

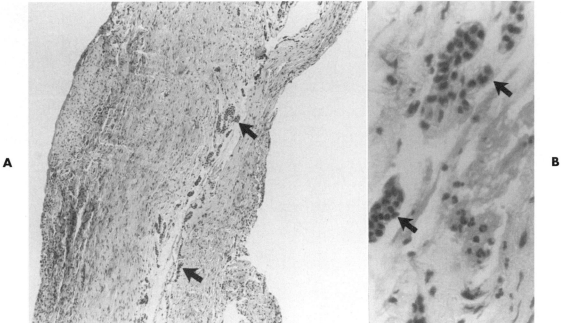

Fig. 17-1. Photomicrographs of a pericoronal follicle. Low (**A**) and high (**B**) magnifications. Nests and cords of odontogenic epithelium *(arrows)* are found throughout the fibrous and myxomatous stroma.

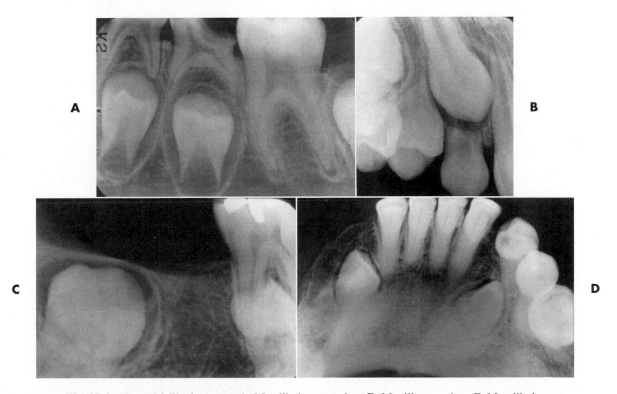

Fig. 17-2. Normal follicular space. **A,** Mandibular premolars. **B,** Maxillary canine. **C,** Mandibular second molar. **D,** Impacted mandibular canines.

The follicle appears on radiographic examination as a homogeneous radiolucent halo. The halo has a thin outer radiopaque border (Fig. 17-2) representing compact bone that is continuous with the lamina dura. This radiolucent halo merges with the periodontal ligament space; the halo varies in breadth because of the varying thicknesses of the follicles and the accumulation of fluid between the capsule of the reduced epithelium and the crown of the tooth.

Teeth that have been impacted for some years frequently show a meager pericoronal space (Fig. 17-3).

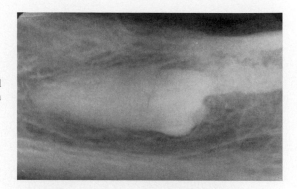

Fig. 17-3. Meager follicular space associated with an impacted premolar. Diminished follicular spaces are frequently seen with impacted teeth of long standing.

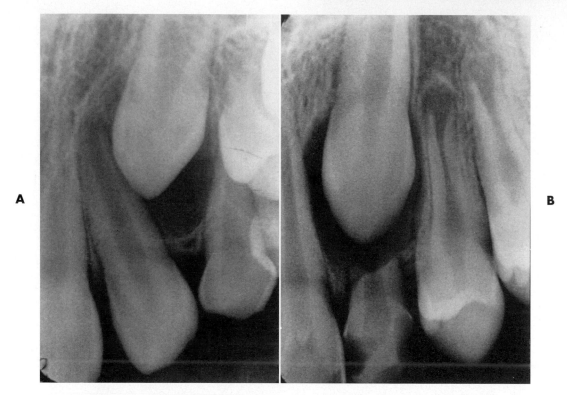

A

B

Fig. 17-4. Follicular spaces surrounding maxillary canines frequently achieve these proportions and are often misdiagnosed as dentigerous cysts.

By contrast, the unerupted maxillary canines frequently have enlarged follicular spaces, especially when their eruption has been delayed (Fig. 17-4). Because cystic and other pathologic changes can take place in such follicles and delay eruption or displace unerupted teeth, it is important to identify any developing pathosis. Unfortunately, these entities are usually painless, and there is no specific criterion that enables the dentist to distinguish between a normal and an abnormal (enlarging) follicle.

Some children have generalized enlargement and hyperplasia of their follicular spaces. Fig. 17-5 illustrates such a case. In this figure, almost all the follicular spaces surrounding the unerupted teeth are abnormally large, but only the largest one, which surrounds the crown of the mandibular left first premolar tooth, represents a lesion (a

dentigerous cyst). The clinicians in charge of this case after surgery on two areas observed the boy closely to ensure that tooth eruption was not delayed. Hyperplastic dental follicles have been reported with rough hypoplastic amelogenesis imperfecta[6] and in Lowe syndrome (Fig. 17-6).[7]

The following guidelines have been used to distinguish between a normal and an abnormal follicle:

1. When an asymptomatic follicular radiolucency becomes approximately 2.5 cm in diameter and the surrounding cortical plate is poorly defined, disease is strongly suggested.[8]
2. If the pericoronal space reaches 2.5 mm in width on the radiograph, this is presumptive evidence that fluid is collecting within the follicle and pathosis is present in 80% of cases.[9]

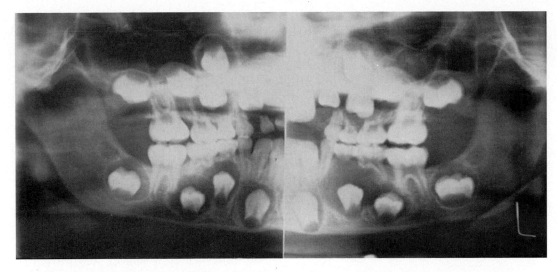

Fig. 17-5. Enlarged follicular spaces within normal limits. Panorex radiograph of an 8-year-old child showing multiple enlarged follicular spaces around unerupted permanent teeth. Surgery and microscopic study demonstrated a dentigerous cyst associated with the crown of the lower left first premolar tooth. Follow-up examinations showed the eruption of the remainder of the teeth without surgical intervention. (Courtesy J. Dolce, and J. Ireland, deceased.)

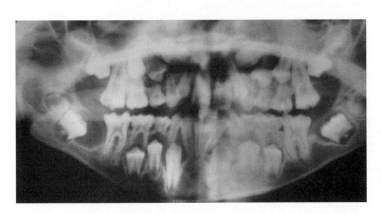

Fig. 17-6. Enlarged dental follicles, dentigerous cyst associated with the right second mandibular molar, and hypoplasia of the crowns of the first permanent molars. The 11½-year-old boy had oculocerebrorenal syndrome. (From Roberts MW, Blakey GH, Jacoway JR, et al: Enlarged dental follicles: a follicular cyst and enamel hyperplasia in a patient with Lowe syndrome, *Oral Surg* 77:264-265, 1994.)

The latter guideline has not proved useful for evaluating the pericoronal spaces of the upper canines, which are usually larger than those surrounding other erupting teeth.

Differential Diagnosis

For a discussion of the differential diagnosis of a pericoronal or follicular space, see the section on differential diagnosis at the end of this chapter.

Management

In the absence of clinical symptoms, it is advisable to radiographically examine equivocally enlarged or enlarging follicles at least every 6 months or until it becomes apparent that eruption is being delayed, the tooth is being displaced, or the tooth erupts. If eruption is delayed, a dentigerous cyst or another pericoronal pathologic condition must be considered, and surgical intervention is indicated. Clinical judgment must be used in each case because it is difficult, if not impossible, to distinguish between a small dentigerous cyst and a large dental follicle unless surgery is performed.[10]

DENTIGEROUS (FOLLICULAR) CYST

After the radicular cyst, the dentigerous cyst is the most common odontogenic cyst.[11,12] Dentigerous cysts are associated with the crowns of unerupted or developing teeth. The etiology of cystic formation is unknown, although a study in rats shows that periapical infection produces dentigerous cysts in the underlying teeth.[13]

Features

The dentigerous cyst is the most common pathologic pericoronal radiolucency. It has a lumen lined with epithelium derived from the enamel organ or from other remnants of the dental lamina. Various types of epithelial linings may be seen (Fig. 17-7); occasionally some are of odontogenic keratocysts, but the orthokeratinized type is more common than the parakeratinized.[14]

The teeth most frequently affected are the mandibular third molars, the maxillary canines, the mandibular premolars, and the maxillary third molars (in that order).

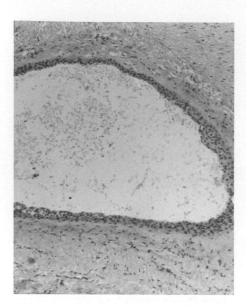

Fig. 17-7. This dentigerous cyst wall is lined with stratified epithelium. The thick wall consists mostly of dense fibrous connective tissue.

The highest incidence occurs during the second and third decades of life.

If multiple dentigerous cysts are found, the patient should be examined for multiple basal cell nevus syndrome or cleidocranial dysplasia. In the latter condition, there are many supernumerary teeth and thus multiple impactions with increased possibilities of dentigerous cyst formation. Dentigerous cysts associated with unerupted supernumerary teeth constitutes 5% to 6% of all dentigerous cysts.[15] Approximately 90% of this type of dentigerous cyst was associated with a maxillary mesiodens.[15]

It has been reported that 2.6% of patients with one or more unerupted teeth have dentigerous cysts,[16] and it has been estimated that dentigerous cystic changes occur in 0.81% of impacted third molars.[17] The cysts vary greatly in size, from less than 2 cm in diameter to massive expansions of the jaws[18] (Fig. 17-8). The expansion may in turn produce gross deformity of the region involved.

Although a slowly expanding cyst may markedly thin the cortical plates, it seldom erodes them. When the cortical plates are eroded, palpation reveals a rubbery, fluctuant, nonemptiable mass (in contrast to the crepitus or crackling quality of the sensation revealed on palpation of the expanded, thin walls of the bony cyst). Dentigerous cysts cause resorption of adjacent tooth roots in 55% of cases.[19] The term *paradental cyst* has been recommended for cysts that occur at the distal or buccal surfaces of the crown of the impacted tooth.[12]

Aspiration often yields a straw-colored, thin liquid. Cholesterol crystals may be seen in the aspirate when the syringe is slowly rotated in front of a strong light.

Because a cyst is usually painless, delayed eruption of a tooth may be the first and only clinical sign suggesting

pericoronal pathosis. Pain usually indicates the presence of infection. A dentigerous cyst rarely expands so rapidly that it presses on a sensory nerve and causes pain. When this occurs, the pain may be referred to any part of the face and is frequently described as a headache. Paresthesia, anesthesia, or mobile teeth are almost never produced.

The eruption cyst is a dentigerous cyst that has developed, or is discovered, when the associated tooth is near the surface. The tooth may be found immediately below the gingiva, producing a domelike swelling on the ridge. The eruption cyst should not be considered a separate entity. It is described in greater detail in Chapter 12.

A pathologic fracture is an inherent danger associated with a large cyst that has destroyed an extensive segment of the jaw. The jaw may become so weakened that it must be splinted before surgery to prevent fracturing during the procedure.

Differential Diagnosis

For a discussion of the differential diagnosis of a dentigerous cyst, see the section on differential diagnosis at the end of this chapter.

Management

Complete enucleation must be accomplished; enucleation reduces the possibility of potentially dangerous cells remaining in the region after surgery to form residual cysts, ameloblastomas, or other lesions.[21] All excised tissue is sent for microscopic study and periodic follow-up ensured. If the microscopic diagnosis is parakeratinizing odontogenic keratocyst, surgery and follow-up are more aggressive because recurrence rates are high.[14] The odontogenic keratocyst is discussed in detail in Chapter 19.

Prophylactic Prevention of Dentigerous Cysts

Researchers debate whether all impacted third molars should be prophylactically removed in the late teens and early twenties to prevent the subsequent development of dentigerous cysts and other lesions. Space permits just a short discussion. Recent studies indicate that pathologic sequelae are low from the retention of third molars: between 7% and 12%.[7,17,22] Furthermore, a certain proportion erupt late.[23] Cases of extensive pathologic conditions developing in long-standing impacted third molars can buttress the case for prophylactic removal.[24] Some researchers call for a more conservative approach to prophylactic removal.[17,22,25] One argument seldom raised for prophylactic removal is the danger of loss of the second molar when impacted third molars are surgically removed later in life because of infection. Such infection often results from a communication between the third molar crown and the periodontal pocket on the distal side of the second molar. The bone removed in surgical removal fails to return at this age, and often the second molar is subsequently lost. This is a more significant

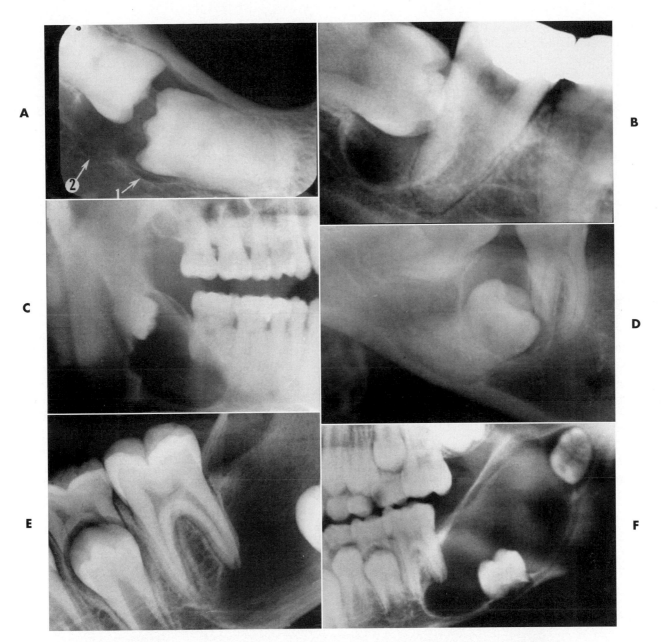

Fig. 17-8. Dentigerous cyst. **A,** Molar impactions showing, a follicular space *(1)* and, a dentigerous cyst *(2)*. Microscopic examination confirmed this impression. **B** and **C,** Dentigerous cysts associated with impacted mandibular third molars. **D,** Dentigerous cyst surrounding an impacted second molar. **E** and **F,** Two views of the same cyst surrounding the crowns of impacted second and third molars. This case illustrates the importance of obtaining adequate radiographs to grossly determine the extent of the lesion. (**C** courtesy D. Skuble, Hinsdale, Ill.)

problem in the maxilla. There are many disease indications for the removal of impacted third molars.

UNICYSTIC (MURAL) AMELOBLASTOMA

The unicystic ameloblastoma that forms in the wall of a dentigerous cyst ranks next to the dentigerous cyst as the most frequently occurring pathologic pericoronal radiolucency. The terms *mural* and *unicystic* are used to identify this type, although unicystic ameloblastoma occurs in other locations and does not necessarily contact teeth.

The mural ameloblastoma represents approximately 5% of all ameloblastomas.[26] The ameloblastoma and mural ameloblastoma are similar in predilections for gender (occurring approximately equally in men and women) and site (mandibular third molar region).[26] However, the mural variety occurs in a younger age group: 21.8 years[24] for the mural ameloblastoma vs. 38.9 years for the ameloblastoma.[20,26] In one study the majority of unicystic ameloblastomas were associated with dentigerous cysts,[27] all of which were found in patients under 30 years of age.[26] Other cyst types associated with mural ameloblastoma are residual, radicular, globulomaxillary, and primordial cysts. Ackermann, Attini, and Shear[20] divide histopathologic features into (1) lining of variable nondescript epithelium with characteristics of early ameloblastic transformation in some areas, (2) intraluminal proliferation of ameloblastoma, and (3) ameloblastomatous invasion of the connective tissue wall. Various studies report that between 15% and 30% of all ameloblastomas form in the wall of a dentigerous cyst.[28-30] Apparently the ameloblastomatous potential of dentigerous cysts declines markedly in patients over 30 years of age.[30]

Features

The unicystic (mural) ameloblastoma is asymptomatic and remains undetected until the pericoronal radiolucency is seen on the routine radiograph (Fig. 17-9). As the lesion slowly enlarges, a slight, nontender swelling becomes apparent on clinical examination. This swelling is the result of an expansion of the cortical plates of the jaw and can be identified by palpation as hard and bony. With enlargement of the tumor, the overlying cortical plates are thinned to the point of destruction, and palpation discloses softer areas, some of which may be fluctu-

ant cystic spaces. Other softer areas are firm but not bony hard and represent solid masses of tumor or fibrous tissue that has extended through the eroded bone.

Radiographically a localized thinning and haziness of the hyperostotic radiopaque rim of the pericoronal radiolucency should prompt the clinician to suspect that a mural ameloblastoma may have penetrated the fibrous capsule of a dentigerous cyst and is initiating the invasion of bone between trabeculae.

Differential Diagnosis

For a discussion of the differential diagnosis of a mural ameloblastoma, see the section on differential diagnosis at the end of this chapter.

Management

Before a surgeon undertakes the treatment of a pericoronal radiolucency, a differential diagnosis that includes the unicystic (mural) ameloblastoma and the full-blown ameloblastoma must be completed. Subsequently, at surgery the "cyst" should be enucleated, and if a mural mass is discovered, the surgeon should flag it with sutures to enable the pathologist to concentrate on it as the area of greatest concern. Such a discrepancy on the surface of the lining may prove to be localized de-

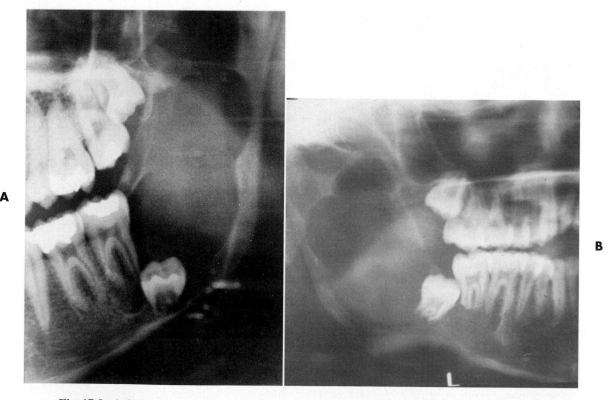

Fig. 17-9. A, Unicystic ameloblastoma in a young adult; it is seen as a pericoronal radiolucency associated with the impacted mandibular third molar tooth. **B,** Orthopantomograph showing another case of a unicystic ameloblastoma seen as a pericoronal radiolucency. Both of these lesions presented challenges in surgical management even though ameloblastoma had not invaded the connective tissue wall. (**A** courtesy D.E. Cooksey, Los Angeles; **B** courtesy E. Casper, Chicago.)

posits of cholesterol, fibrous tissue, granulation tissue, an area showing ameloblastic change, a mural ameloblastoma, another type of odontogenic tumor, salivary gland tumor,[31] or central squamous cell carcinoma (Fig. 17-10). If the pathologist's frozen-section examination establishes the mass as an ameloblastoma that has not penetrated the basement membrane, further surgery is not done. If the neoplasm has penetrated the basement membrane, more bone should be removed by curettement.[20]

The frequency of recurrence after simple enucleation of cysts containing mural ameloblastomas is much lower than that of ameloblastomas treated in a similar manner.[26,27] Further and more extensive surgery for unicystic (mural) ameloblastoma should be done only in the event of recurrence.[27,32-36] In cases of proven capsular infiltration of tumor into bone, more bone should be removed in that region. The clinician should consider all findings before deciding on an approach to treatment. In all cases, careful, periodic follow-up is always indicated.

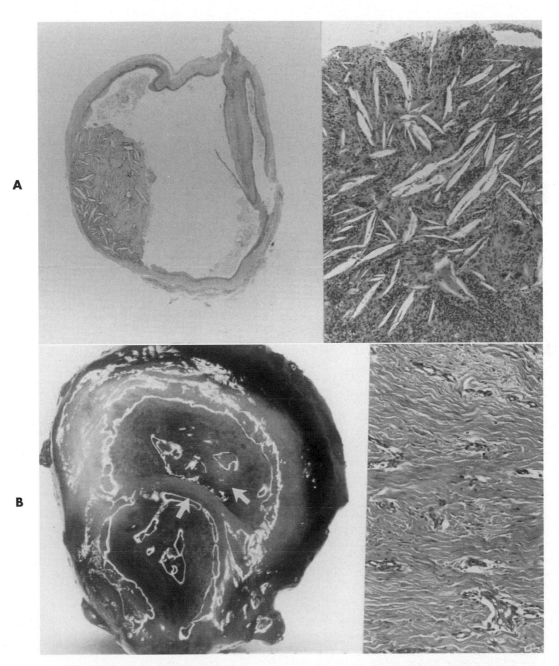

Fig. 17-10. Mural nodules on dentigerous cyst walls. **A,** Mural cholesteatoma found in a dentigerous cyst wall (low and high magnification). **B,** Mural nodules *(arrows)* composed of fibrous tissue.

Continued

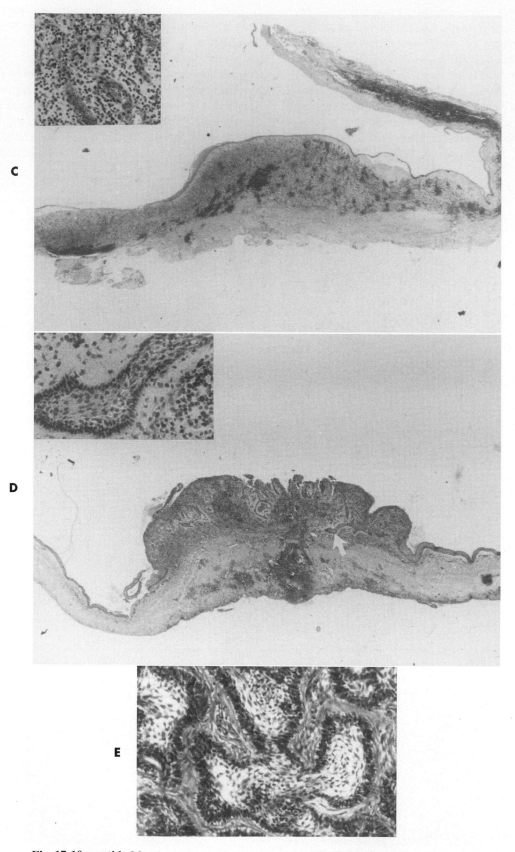

Fig. 17-10, cont'd. Mural nodules on dentigerous cyst walls. **C,** Mural nodule composed of granulation tissue. **D,** Mural nodule containing odontogenic epithelial nests, which are undergoing ameloblastic change. **E,** This mural nodule proved to be a follicular ameloblastoma.

AMELOBLASTOMA

The pericoronal radiolucency under investigation may prove to be an ordinary ameloblastoma at surgery and microscopic study. In other words the radiolucent cavity may be completely filled by ameloblastoma that has infiltrated peripherally into the bony margins. Presumably, such examples represent mural (unicystic) ameloblastomas that have developed into full-blown ameloblastomas. At any rate, these should be recognized as locally aggressive lesions that require extensive surgery. This type of ameloblastoma is discussed as a multilocular radiolucency in Chapter 20.

ADENOMATOID ODONTOGENIC TUMOR (ADENOAMELOBLASTOMA)

The adenomatoid odontogenic tumor (AOT) is uncommon, benign, and noninvasive and makes up approximately 3% of all odontogenic tumors.[10,37] The origin of the AOT is uncertain, but it is thought to arise from residual odontogenic epithelium. Some authorities suggest that instead of classifying the AOT as a benign tumor, it might be better to consider it a hamartoma of residual odontogenic epithelium.[38] Most AOTs are follicular, but some are extrafollicular[39,40]; only the former are discussed here. The AOT must be distinguished from the ameloblastoma because these two lesions differ radically in clinical, radiographic, and microscopic features and behavior. The AOT is a slow-growing tumor that does not infiltrate bone. These tumors are inclined to displace teeth rather than cause root resorption.[39]

The AOT is almost twice as common in women and usually occurs in the second decade of life; the average age at occurrence is 17 years.[39] At least 73% of these tumors occur in association with unerupted teeth or in the walls of dentigerous cysts.[39] Approximately 27% of AOTs are not associated with teeth, and a few cases of extraosseous forms have been reported.[39] Approximately 90% have occurred in the anterior portions of the jaws; they are about 1½ times more frequent in the maxilla than in the mandible.

Unerupted teeth frequently associated with this tumor (in order of frequency) are the maxillary canine, lateral incisor, and mandibular premolar. Small calcifications within the tumor are not seen on radiographs, so the lesion is completely radiolucent and mimics a dentigerous cyst in growth pattern and appearance (Fig. 17-11, *A*). Continued slow growth may expand the cortical plates and produce a clinical swelling and asymmetry, but invasion of the soft tissue does not occur (Fig. 17-11, *D*).

Management

The AOT is best treated by enucleation, since it separates easily and cleanly from its bony defect and does not show a tendency to recur[39] (Fig. 17-11, *E*). The surgical specimen may be solid or cystic, and on gross inspection, elevations of varying size and shape may be found projecting from the lining into the fluid-filled lumen (Fig. 17-11, *F*). Some areas of the cystic wall are thinner and smooth, however, and are in essence segments of a typical dentigerous cyst wall. An examination of frozen sections should be undertaken at surgery to establish a definite diagnosis. This permits the surgeon to remove more tissue if the diagnosis indicates.

CALCIFYING ODONTOGENIC CYST OR TUMOR (CENTRAL)

On first consideration the calcifying odontogenic cyst or tumor should be included with the mixed radiolucent-radiopaque lesions in Chapters 24 and 25. However, a wide variation in the amount of calcified material has been observed in these lesions; this variation ranges from extremely small foci that can be seen only at the microscopic level (Fig. 17-12) to moderate-sized foci that can readily be seen as white flecks in the cystic radiolucency

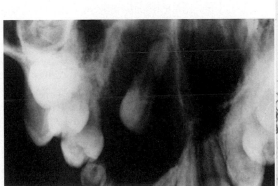
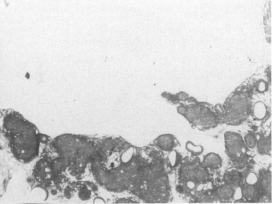

Fig. 17-11. AOT. **A,** Maxillary occlusal radiograph showing a large radiolucency involving and displacing the maxillary right canine. **B,** Low-power photomicrograph showing fingers of tumor tissue projecting into the lumen. (**A** courtesy W. Smith, San Diego.)   *Continued*

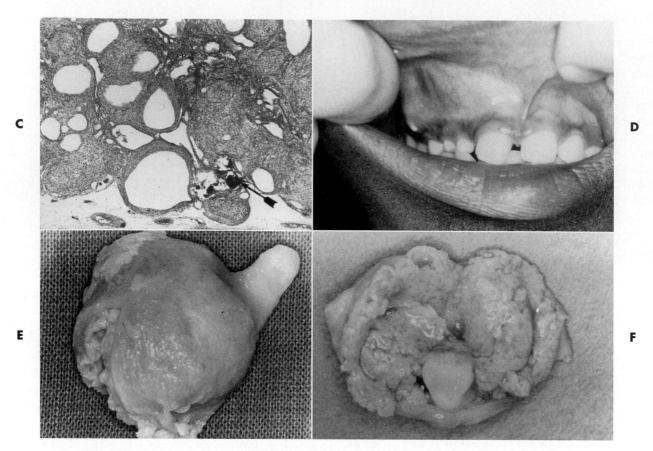

Fig. 17-11, cont'd. AOT. **C,** Higher-power photomicrograph showing the typical picture of pseudo-ducts and pseudoacini. The small areas of calcification *(arrow)* were not large enough to show as radiopaque foci on the radiograph of this lesion. **D,** Expansion of the alveolar process and vestibule in the upper right canine region in a 14-year-old patient. This tumor had eroded the labial plate. **E,** Surgical enucleation. The smooth, regular periphery permitted ready enucleation from the surrounding bone. The root tip of the permanent canine is protruding from the mass. **F,** Bisected specimen from the same patient in **E.** Papillomatous projections are evident from the wall into the lumen of this cystic tumor. (**D** to **F** courtesy W. Smith, San Diego.)

(see Fig. 24-12) to a calcified component so large that it almost completely obliterates the radiolucency. Therefore it is apparent that in the early stage the calcifying odontogenic cyst or tumor appears as a completely radiolucent cystlike lesion. Some of these occur as pericoronal radiolucencies and are thus included here (see Fig. 17-12). The calcifying odontogenic cyst or tumor is discussed in greater detail in Chapter 24 as a mixed radiolucent-radiopaque lesion.

AMELOBLASTIC FIBROMA

The ameloblastic fibroma is a true mixed odontogenic tumor, containing nests and strands of odontogenic and ameloblastic epithelium in a primitive, dental papilla–like connective tissue (Fig. 17-13, *B*). Calcified dental structures are not present. The ameloblastic fibroma should be considered a separate entity, not an immature odontoma.[41]

Features

The ameloblastic fibroma is not as frequently associated with an unerupted tooth as the AOT, although both are usually found in the same age-group (under 20 years of age). The ameloblastic fibroma does not demonstrate a predilection for either gender. More than 70% of these fibromas occur in patients under 20 years; the average age has been reported as 15 years.[42,43] Although this tumor may arise in either jaw, the majority occur in the mandible, and the highest incidence is in the premolar and molar region. This mixed odontogenic tumor grows slowly by expansion of the cortex and usually does not invade bone.

On radiographic examination the ameloblastic fibroma is usually seen as a pericoronal radiolucency but may appear unilocular or multilocular, not associated with an unerupted tooth. It may show cortical expansion (see Fig. 17-13) and may spread the roots of adjacent teeth.[44]

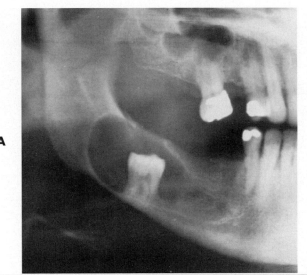

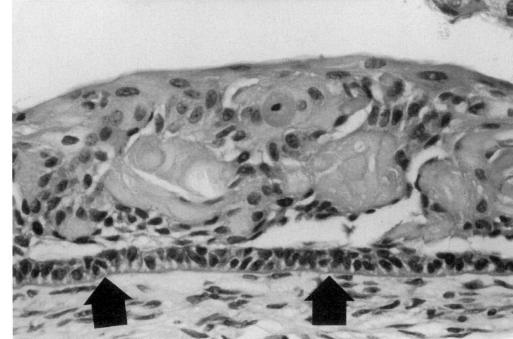

Fig. 17-12. Calcifying odontogenic cyst. **A,** Panorex radiograph shows a pericoronal radiolucency in association with an impacted mandibular molar tooth. The calcified areas in this case are so small that they cannot be seen in the radiograph as radiopaque flecks. **B,** Photomicrograph of an early lesion before calcification, showing the ghost cells with keratinization. Arrows indicate the basal cell layer of the cyst wall.

Management

The treatment indicated for ameloblastic fibroma is enucleation. The tumor readily separates from the bone, and ameloblastic cells generally do not invade the connective tissue capsule. Recurrence rates are around 18%,[45] but they are higher for this tumor than for the AOT. In rare instances, tumors have several recurrences. Consequently, periodic ra-

diographic reexamination of the treated area is a necessary precaution. Ameloblastic fibrosarcomas have been reported.

RARITIES

Almost any pathologic process may occur around the crowns of unerupted teeth (Fig 17-14 through 17-18). An incomplete list of lesions that rarely produce a pericoronal

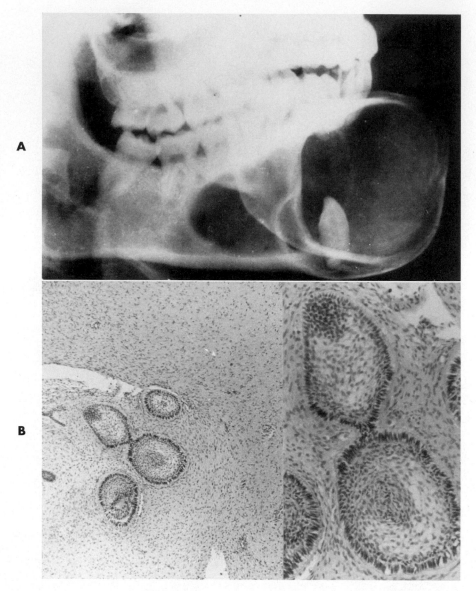

Fig. 17-13. Ameloblastic fibroma. **A,** This large, well-defined radiolucency displacing the mandibular canine and expanding the cortical plates proved to be an ameloblastic fibroma. **B,** Low and high magnification of the histologic features of an ameloblastic fibroma showing ameloblastic nests in a pulplike stroma. (**A** courtesy O.H. Stuteville, deceased.)

radiolucent lesion is located at the beginning of this chapter.

DIFFERENTIAL DIAGNOSIS OF PERICORONAL RADIOLUCENCIES

When the clinician is confronted by a pericoronal radiolucency, the surgical team must be prepared for the anticipated procedure. This is best accomplished by the formulation of a list of possible diagnoses arranged in order of probability, with the most probable lesion heading the list. If all the discernible features of the pathosis under study give ameloblastoma a low level of probability, the need to prepare the surgical team for an extensive procedure (e.g., a resection with bone graft) is obviated.

To illustrate the usefulness of formally developing a differential diagnosis, this chapter closes with an analysis of the circumstances attending a 50-year-old woman with a well-defined pericoronal radiolucency associated with an impacted lower right third molar.

The lesion was discovered on a routine radiographic survey. It was asymptomatic and measured 2 cm in diameter with an intrafollicular space measuring 1 cm. Because normal follicular spaces usually decrease in size with age, it was initially recognized, on the basis of its proportions, not as a simple, enlarged, uncomplicated follicle, but rather as a pathologic process.

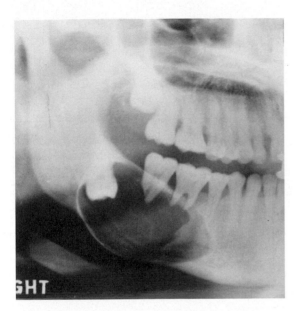

Fig. 17-14. Calcifying epithelial odontogenic tumor (Pindborg tumor) seen as a well-defined pericoronal radiolucency involving the impacted third molar in a 30-year-old woman. (From Smith RA, Roman RS, Hansen LS, et al: *J Oral Surg* 35:160-166, 1977.)

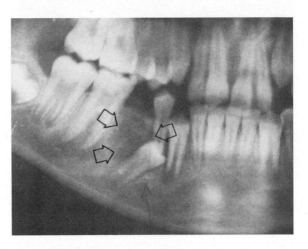

Fig. 17-15. Arrows indicate ragged, ill-defined pericoronal radiolucency involving the impacted mandibular right second premolar tooth. Biopsy specimen in this 15-year-old revealed Ewing's sarcoma. (Courtesy N. Barakat, Beirut, Lebanon.)

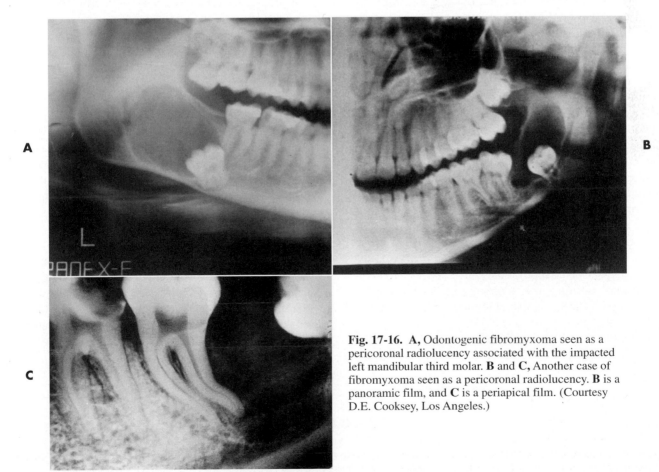

Fig. 17-16. A, Odontogenic fibromyxoma seen as a pericoronal radiolucency associated with the impacted left mandibular third molar. **B** and **C,** Another case of fibromyxoma seen as a pericoronal radiolucency. **B** is a panoramic film, and **C** is a periapical film. (Courtesy D.E. Cooksey, Los Angeles.)

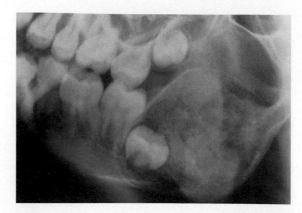

Fig. 17-17. Cementoossifying fibroma. The large radiolucent area appears to contact the crown of the displaced mandibular third molar. The thin radiopaque borders of the lesion are evident. The increased buccolingual thickness of the ramus composed of dense fibrous tissue imparts a hazy semiradiopaque appearance to this lesion that contained minimal foci of calcification.

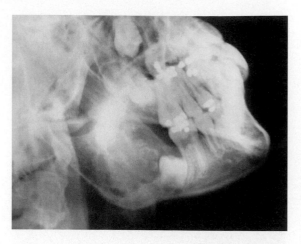

Fig. 17-18. Pseudotumor of hemophilia seen as a pericoronal radiolucency in this lateral oblique radiograph of a young man with a hereditary deficiency of factor VIII. (Courtesy G. Blozis, Columbus, Ohio.

Although the lesion under investigation occurred in the mandibular third molar area, a frequent site of the unicystic (mural) ameloblastoma, this entity was not assigned a prominent rank, since it seldom occurs in persons over 30 years of age.[30]

The odontoma and its ameloblastic variants commonly occur in a supracoronal position in close approximation to the occlusal surface of an unerupted tooth. Therefore in radiographs these lesions in their unmineralized stages could be seen as pericoronal radiolucencies. However, the chances of the lesion in question representing an odontoma or one of its ameloblastic variants is remote because these lesions develop at the same time as the dentition and thus would have already passed into the completely radiopaque stage in a patient who is 50 years old.

The calcifying odontogenic cyst may occur as a pericoronal radiolucency and may be unsuspected until small radiopaque foci appear. Since its management is identical to that of the uncomplicated dentigerous cyst, extensive attempts at ranking are academic rather than practical.

Although the ameloblastic fibroma is 4 times more common in the mandible, the choice of this entity as the working diagnosis is inappropriate, since this mixed odontogenic tumor occurs most frequently in the mandibular premolar–first molar area and seldom is seen in patients over 20 years of age.

Further, none of the lesion's characteristics (e.g., location, age of patient) suggest an AOT, since these entities show a predilection for the anterior region of the jaws of young persons.

Envelopmental primordial cysts and follicular primordial cysts are interesting possibilities. The envelopmental primordial cyst is a true primordial cyst that occurs in close proximity to the crown of an unerupted tooth, and superimposition of the image may cause the cystlike radiolucency to appear as a dentigerous cyst on radiographic examination.[46] The follicular primordial cyst, in counter distinction, surrounds the crown, and the cyst lining is attached to the neck of the tooth in a true dentigerous relationship. To enhance the process of differential diagnosis, different angulations of radiographs shift the image into a different relationship in the case of envelopmental primordial cysts, thus showing that they are not true dentigerous cysts. The follicular primordial cyst image could not be differentiated from that of the dentigerous cyst. The important point is that a high percentage of the primordial cysts are odontogenic keratocysts (high recurrence rate), whereas only a small percentage of true dentigerous cysts are odontogenic keratocysts.

Consequently the working diagnosis—or the condition assigned the highest rank in the differential diagnosis for this radiolucent lesion—was dentigerous cyst. The possibility that any of the other pericoronal radiolucencies might be found at operation was remote; nevertheless, the unicystic (mural) ameloblastoma was a distant second on the formulated list.

REFERENCES

1. Marks SC Jr, Cahill DR, Wise GE: The cytology of the dental follicle and adjacent alveolar bone during tooth eruption in the dog, *Am J Anat* 168:271-289, 1983.

2. Marks SC Jr, Cahill DR: Experimental study in the dog of the non-active role of the tooth in the eruptive process, *Arch Oral Biol* 29:311-322, 1984.

3. Wise GE, Lin F: The molecular biology of initiation of tooth eruption, *J Dent Res* 74:303-306, 1995.

4. Larson EK, Cahill DR, Gorski JP, Marks SC: The effect of removing the true dental follicle on premolar eruption in the dog, *Arch Oral Biol* 39:271-275, 1994.

5. Kim J, Ellis GL: Dental follicle tissue: misinterpretation as odontogenic tumors, *J Oral Maxillofac Surg* 51:762-767, 1993.

6. Peters E, Cohen M, Altini M: Rough hypoplastic amelogenesis imperfecta with follicular hyperplasia, *Oral Surg* 74:487-492, 1992.

7. Roberts MW, Blakey GH, Jacoway JR, et al: Enlarged dental follicles: a follicular cyst and enamel hypoplasia in a patient with Lowe syndrome, *Oral Surg* 77:264-265, 1994.

8. Worth HM: *Principles and practice of oral radiologic interpretation,* Chicago, 1963, Mosby.

9. Stafne EC: *Oral roentgenographic diagnosis,* ed 3, Philadelphia, 1969, WB Saunders.

10. Daley TD, Wysocki GP: The small dentigerous cyst: a diagnostic dilemma, *Oral Surg* 79:77-81, 1995.

11. Daley TD, Wysocki GP, Pringle GA: Relative incidence of odontogenic tumors and oral and jaw cysts in a Canadian population, *Oral Surg* 77:276-280, 1994.

12. Ackermann G, Cohen MA, Altini M: The paradental cyst: a clinicopathologic study of 50 cases, *Oral Surg* 64:308-313, 1987.

13. Bando Y, Nagayama M: Odontogenic cyst induction by periapical infection in rats, *J Oral Pathol Med* 22:323-326, 1993.

14. Crowley TE, Kaugars GE, Gonsolley JC: Odontogenic keratocysts: a clinical and histologic comparison of the parakeratin and orthokeratin variants, *J Oral Maxillofac Surg* 50:22-26, 1992.

15. Lustmann J, Bodner L: Dentigerous cysts associated with supernumerary teeth, *J Oral Maxillofac Surg* 17:100-102, 1988.

16. Mourshed F: A roentgenographic study of dentigerous cysts. I. Incidence in a population sample, *Oral Surg* 18:47-53, 1964.

17. Stanley HR, Alattar M, Collett WK, et al: Pathological sequelae of "neglected" impacted third molars, *J Oral Pathol* 17:113-117, 1988.

18. Kaya Ö, Bocutoglu Ö: A misdiagnosed giant dentigerous cyst involving the maxillary antrum and affecting the orbit: case report, *Aust Dent J* 39:165-167, 1994.

19. Struthers P, Shear M: Root resorption by ameloblastomas and cysts of the jaws, *Int J Oral Surg* 5:128-132, 1976.

20. Ackermann GL, Altini M, Shear M: The unicystic ameloblastoma: a clinicopathological study of 57 cases, *J Oral Pathol* 17:541-546, 1988.

21. Holmlund A, Anneroth G, Lundquist G, Nordenram Å: Ameloblastomas originating from odontogenic cysts, *J Oral Pathol Med* 20:318-321, 1991.

22. Eliasson S, Heimdahl A, Nordenram Å: Pathological changes related to long-term impaction of third molars: a radiographic study, *Int J Oral Maxillofac Surg* 18:210-212, 1989.

23. Ventä I, Murtomaa H, Turtola L, et al: Clinical follow-up study of third molar eruption from ages 20 to 26 years, *Oral Surg* 72:150-153, 1991.

24. Girod SC, Gerlach K-L, Krueger G: Cysts associated with longstanding impacted third molars, *Int J Oral Maxillofac Surg* 22:110-112, 1993.

25. van der Linden W, Cleaton-Jones P, Lownie M: Diseases and lesions associated with third molars: review of 1001 cases, *Oral Surg* 79:142-145, 1995.

26. Shteyer A, Lustmann J, Lewin-Epstein J: The mural ameloblastoma: review of the literature, *J Oral Surg* 36:866-872, 1978.

27. Robinson L, Martinez MG: Unicystic ameloblastoma: a prognostically distinct entity, *Cancer* 40:2278-2285, 1977.

28. Kane JP: Odontogenic tumors: a statistical and morphological study of 88 cases, master's thesis, Washington, DC, 1951, Georgetown University.

29. Mehlisch DR, Dahlin DC, Masson JK: Ameloblastoma: a clinicopathologic report, *J Oral Surg* 30:9-22, 1972.

30. Stanley HR, Diehl DL: Ameloblastoma potential of follicular cysts, *Oral Surg* 20:260-268, 1965.

31. Breitenecker G, Wepner F: A pleomorphic adenoma (so-called mixed tumor) in the wall of a dentigerous cyst, *Oral Surg* 36:63-71, 1973.

32. Rapidis AD, Angelopoulos AP, Skouteris CA, et al: Mural (intracystic) ameloblastoma, *Int J Oral Surg* 11:166-174, 1982.

33. Gardner DG, Corio RL: The relationship of plexiform unicystic ameloblastoma to conventional ameloblastoma, *Oral Surg* 56:54-60, 1983.

34. Gardner DG, Corio RL: Plexiform unicystic ameloblastoma: a variant of ameloblastoma with a low-recurrence rate after enucleation, *Cancer* 53:1730-1735, 1984.

35. Marks R, Block M, Sanusi DI, et al: Unicystic ameloblastoma, *Int J Oral Surg* 12:186-189, 1983.

36. Leider AS, Eversole LR, and Barkin ME: Cystic ameloblastoma, *Oral Surg* 60:624-630, 1985.

37. Regezi JA, Kerr DA, Courtney RM: Odontogenic tumors: an analysis of 706 cases, *J Oral Surg* 36:771-778, 1978.

38. Courtney RM, Kerr DA: The odontogenic adenomatoid tumor, *Oral Surg* 39:424-435, 1975.

39. Philipsen HP, Reichart PA, Zhang KH, et al: Adenomatoid odontogenic tumor: biologic profile based on 499 cases, *J Oral Pathol Med* 20:149-158, 1991.

40. Philipsen HP, Samman N, Ormiston IW, et al: Variants of the adenomatoid odontogenic tumor with a note on tumor origin, *J Oral Pathol Med* 21:348-352, 1992.

41. Slootweg PJ: An analysis of the interrelationship of the mixed odontogenic tumors: ameloblastic fibroma, ameloblastic fibro-odontoma, and the odontomas, *Oral Surg* 51:266-276, 1981.

42. Gorlin RJ, Chaudhry AP, Pindborg JJ: Odontogenic tumors: classification, histopathology and clinical behavior in man and domestic animals, *Cancer* 14:73-101, 1961.

43. Trodahl JN: Ameloblastic fibroma: a survey of cases from the Armed Forces Institute of Pathology, *Oral Surg* 33:547-558, 1972.

44. Hager RC, Taylor CG, Allen PM: Ameloblastic fibroma: report of case, *J Oral Surg* 36:66-69, 1978.

45. Zallen RD, Preskar MH, McClary SA: Ameloblastic fibroma, *J Oral Maxillofac Surg* 40:513-517, 1982.

46. Altini M, Cohen M: The follicular primordial cyst–odontogenic keratocyst, *Int J Oral Surg* 11:175-182, 1982.

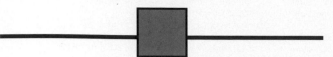

CHAPTER 18

Interradicular Radiolucencies

NORMAN K. WOOD
CHARLES G. BAKER

In this chapter the following interradicular radiolucencies are presented:

ANATOMIC RADIOLUCENCIES
PRIMARY TOOTH CRYPT
MENTAL FORAMEN AND MENTAL
 CANAL
MAXILLARY SINUS
INCISIVE FORAMEN
LATERAL FOSSA
BONE MARROW PATTERN
NUTRIENT CANAL
PATHOLOGIC RADIOLUCENCIES
PERIODONTAL POCKET (BONY)
FURCATION INVOLVEMENT

LATERAL RADICULAR CYST
TRAUMATIC BONE CYST
PRIMORDIAL CYST
OTHER ODONTOGENIC CYSTS
ODONTOGENIC TUMORS
GLOBULOMAXILLARY
 RADIOLUCENCIES
INCISIVE CANAL CYST
MALIGNANCIES
LATERAL (INFLAMMATORY)
 PERIODONTAL CYST

LATERAL (DEVELOPMENTAL)
 PERIODONTAL CYST
BENIGN NONODONTOGENIC TUMORS
 AND TUMORLIKE CONDITIONS
MEDIAN MANDIBULAR CYST
RARITIES
ADENOMATOID ODONTOGENIC TUMOR
BUCCAL CYST
HISTIOCYTOSIS X
OSTEORADIONECROSIS
PARADENTAL CYST

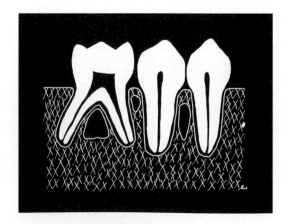

Interradicular radiolucencies, as the name and introductory drawing imply, are radiolucencies that occur between the roots of teeth. The most common are the harmless anatomic radiolucent shadows that may occur in this location and are usually readily recognizable. Logic dictates that the majority of lesions in this location are related to teeth or odontogenesis or are tumors of odontogenic tissue; in practice, this is true. A third group comprises lesions that could develop anywhere in the skeleton but by chance occur occasionally in the alveolar bone between the roots of teeth; neurofibroma is an example of this type of lesion.

ANATOMIC RADIOLUCENCIES

Some of the anatomic radiolucencies seen in films of the jawbone, described in detail in Chapter 15, may occur between the roots of teeth (Fig. 18-1).

Radiolucent primary tooth crypts are normal structures seen as radiolucencies of young children. The in-

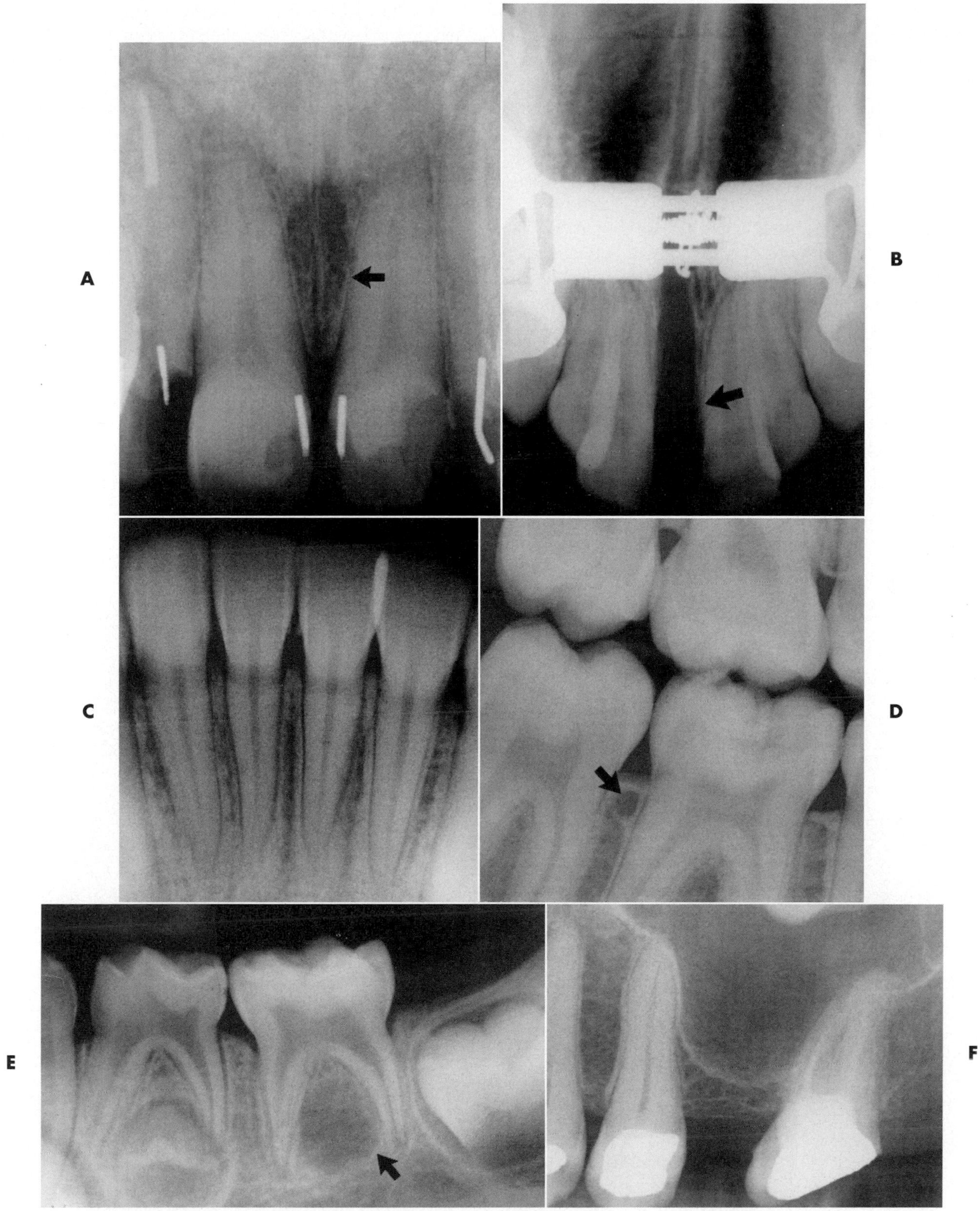

Fig. 18-1. Anatomic interradicular radiolucencies. **A,** Arrow indicates the incisive foramen. Vertical radiolucent line is the midline suture. **B,** Marked widening of the midline suture *(arrow)* is a result of an orthodontic appliance. **C,** Vertical radiolucent lines in several interradicular areas represent nutrient canals. **D,** Near the alveolar crest the arrow shows a "wormhole" radiolucency that is a nutrient canal running parallel to the direction of the x-rays. **E,** Radiolucent tooth crypt of a second premolar tooth *(arrow)* between the roots of the primary deciduous molar tooth. **F,** Radiolucent shadow of a maxillary sinus extending down between the molar and premolar teeth.

terradicular ones represent the developing premolars and are located between or among the roots of the deciduous molar teeth at approximately 2 years of age (see Fig. 18-1).

The mental foramen is seen as a small, roundish radiolucency in the periapices of the mandibular premolar teeth. Occasionally, it occurs between the roots of these teeth, and the bandlike radiolucency of the mental canal is also observed in some cases.

The shadow of the maxillary sinus has many variations. In some individuals, it dips down between the molar roots (see Fig. 18-1). Its configuration usually is bilaterally similar. In unusual circumstances a small buccal outpouching of the sinus wall shows as a cystlike radiolucency between the tooth roots.

The shadow of the incisive foramen is prominent in some individuals and faint in others. When present, it usually projects as a well-defined, contoured radiolucency between the roots of the central incisors in the midline (see Fig. 18-1). Its superior or inferior position is influenced by the degree of vertical angulation at which the radiograph was taken.

The lateral fossa is the vertical depression often present in the labial alveolar plate between the lateral incisor and canine teeth. This narrowing of the alveolus, which produces a definite radiolucency in this region (see Fig. 18-9), is discussed in this chapter with the globulomaxillary shadows. Such a normal narrowing of the alveolus may occur in other interradicular sites also.

Bone marrow patterns in the mandible are prominent in some individuals and nondescript in others. In the former instance, variously shaped radiolucent patterns are dispersed throughout the alveolar and basal bone; some occur interradicularly and are recognizable by the characteristic patterns seen throughout the mandibular films (see Fig. 18-3).

Nutrient canals are obvious in the mandibular periapical radiographs of some individuals. In radiographs of dentate persons, they are seen as vertical, narrow, bandlike radiolucencies running between the teeth (see Fig. 18-1) and sometimes to the apices of the teeth. Occasionally, when the x-ray beam is directed to the long axis of the particular canal (see Fig. 18-1), a nutrient canal is seen as a small "wormhole."

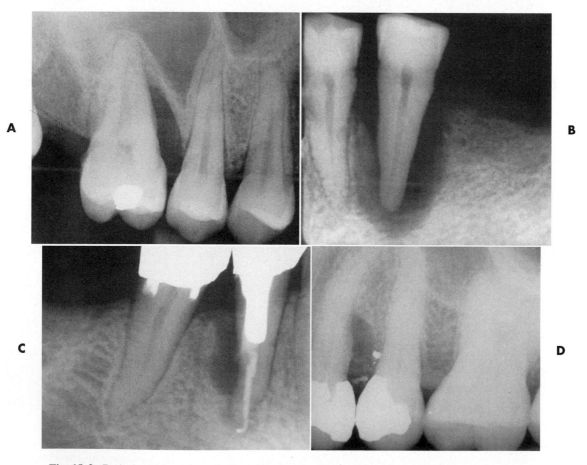

Fig. 18-2. Periodontal bone loss. **A,** Deep intrabony pocket on the mesial side of the first molar. **B,** Extensive periodontal bone loss associated with a premolar tooth. **C,** Root fracture with distal bone destruction. **D,** Periodontal bone destruction distal to the root of the first premolar tooth that is a reaction to amalgam.

PERIODONTAL POCKETS

Periodontal bone loss of the horizontal variety produces familiar changes on periapical films. In cases of intrabony pockets or vertical bone loss that occurs locally on the mesial or distal aspect of a tooth, the resultant radiolucency is interradicular but closer to the involved tooth contacting its surface (Fig. 18-2, *A*). The relatively straightforward diagnosis in such cases is established by placing a periodontal probe into the defect. In cases of severe bone loss the radiolucency surrounds the root (Fig. 18-2, *B*).

FURCATION INVOLVEMENT

Advanced periodontal disease frequently produces furcation involvement. The defect is easily detected, particularly in films of mandibular molars, since the bifurcation is devoid of bone and shows as a radiolucency (Fig. 18-3). Usually a periodontal probe can be maneuvered into bifurcation defects from the buccal or the lingual aspect. Two entities may mimic this condition: (1) a bone marrow space in the bifurcation (see Fig. 18-3) and (2) endodontic involvement with rarefying osteitis in the bifurcation area as a result of an accessory canal connecting the floor of the pulp chamber to the bifurcation. A

significant number of molar teeth have this particular accessory canal.[1] In these two cases the clinician is usually unable to enter the bifurcation with a probe. In the case of the bone marrow pattern the lamina dura remains unchanged over the bone in the bifurcation area but is absent in periodontal disease and in the pulp-related rarefying osteitis. In the case of the rarefying osteitis of endodontic origin, the pulp gives abnormal readings to pulp testing. Occasionally, tooth fractures also produce rarefying osteitis in the furcation region (see Fig. 18-3).

LATERAL RADICULAR CYST

The radicular cyst is discussed in detail as a periapical radiolucency in Chapter 16. Associated teeth have nonvital pulps, and lateral radicular cysts may occur when a sizable accessory canal opens to the lateral root surface (Fig. 18-4). An early small cyst is restricted to a small area of the interradicular bone adjacent to the root surface. In larger cysts the thickness of interseptal bone is destroyed, and it may be more difficult to make the diagnosis or identify the offending tooth. When the cyst becomes infected, pain and swelling occur, and the offending tooth or both teeth may become sensitive to percussion.

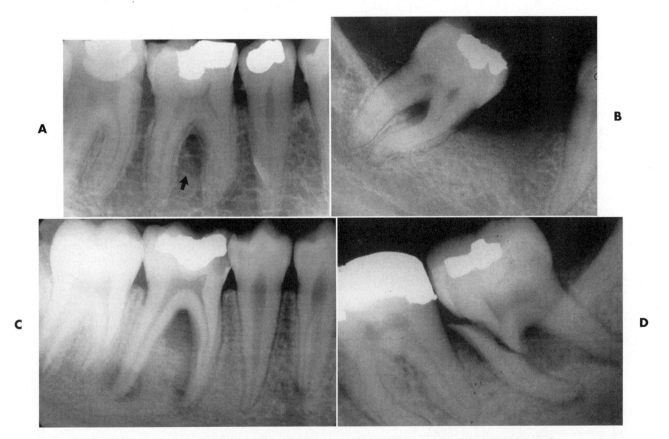

Fig. 18-3. Furcation involvement. **A,** Prominent bone marrow pattern *(arrow).* **B,** Periodontal involvement of a molar bifurcation. **C,** Bone destruction in a bifurcation associated with the first molar caused by pulp disease. **D,** Bone destruction in a bifurcation of the second molar caused by a tooth fracture.

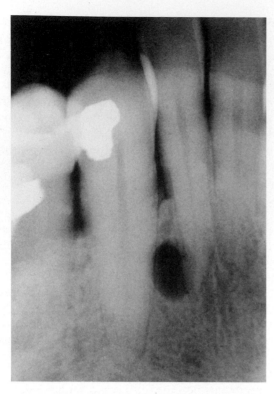

Fig. 18-4. Lateral radicular cyst involved with a nonvital canine tooth with a lateral canal.

TRAUMATIC BONE CYST

The traumatic bone cyst as a periapical radiolucency is discussed in detail in Chapter 16. Characteristically this cyst primarily involves the bone inferior to the apices of the mandibular premolars and first molar and may extend superiorly into the area between the roots of these teeth (Fig. 18-5). In unusual cases, when the primary involvement is in the interradicular bone, there may be very little classic destruction of the bone just inferior to the apices. These interradicular radiolucencies are more oval or slit-like and are not as round as the lateral radicular cyst or the lateral periodontal cyst. The traumatic bone cyst occurs primarily in the tooth-bearing region of mandibles in people under 30 years of age.

PRIMORDIAL CYST

Discussed in Chapter 19 as cystlike radiolucencies not contacting teeth, primordial cysts may occur interradicularly in a region where a tooth may have failed to develop.

OTHER ODONTOGENIC CYSTS

Almost any of the other odontogenic cysts can involve the interradicular region occasionally. The dentigerous cyst is an example, but its pericoronal location usually aids in its recognition (Fig. 18-6).

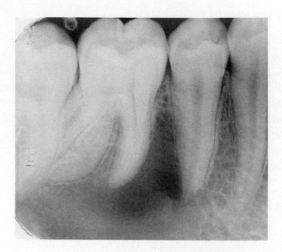

Fig. 18-5. Traumatic bone cyst in a young patient with extensive interradicular involvement between the molar and second premolar roots.

ODONTOGENIC TUMORS

Odontomas are the most common odontogenic tumors by far and usually involve at least a portion of the alveolar bone. Consequently, they frequently occur as interradicular lesions (Fig. 18-7). They are seldom seen in their completely radiolucent stage because young children's jaws are seldom radiographed. Nevertheless, small odontomas in the radiolucent stage are cystlike with a well-defined border, and foci of mineralization soon begin to appear within the radiolucency in subsequent radiographs.

Ameloblastomas are discussed in Chapter 19 as cystlike radiolucencies and in Chapter 20 as multilocular radiolucencies. They can originate in the interradicular bone, so in the early stage, they can mimic many of the other lesions discussed in this chapter (Fig. 18-8).

GLOBULOMAXILLARY RADIOLUCENCIES
Globulomaxillary Cyst

Thoma[2] identified the globulomaxillary cyst and speculated that it occurred in nests of epithelium in the fusion line between the maxillary process and the globular process of the frontonasal process in embryonic life. Lately, this embryonic fusion process has been reaffirmed.[3] However, most authorities now believe that the vast majority of, if not all, cysts that occur in this region are odontogenic in origin.[4-9] If globulomaxillary cysts do occur, they must be rare. Various odontogenic cysts, as well as other types of pathologic conditions, occur in this location.[6,8,9] Certainly a significant number of lateral radicular cysts occurring between the maxillary lateral incisor and canine teeth have been misdiagnosed as globulomaxillary cysts. A more careful workup would have demonstrated that one of the teeth had a nonvital pulp resulting from a dental or traumatic cause.

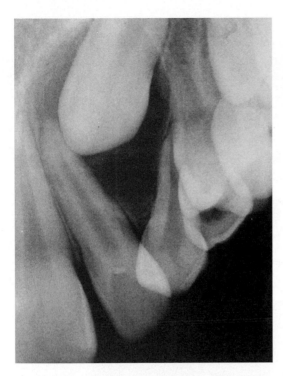

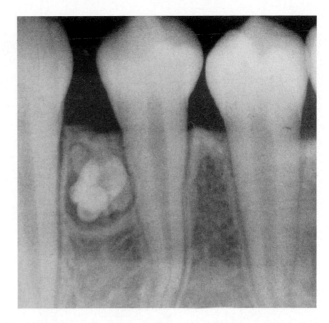

Fig. 18-7. Complex odontoma in an interradicular position. In its premineralization stages, this would have appeared as a radiolucency.

Fig. 18-6. Dentigerous cyst associated with the crown of a permanent canine tooth, which appears as an interradicular radiolucency.

The classic radiographic picture is of a more or less inverted pear- or tear-shaped, well-defined radiolucency between the separated roots of the lateral incisor and canine (see Fig. 18-10). Furthermore, a careful examination of the radiograph discloses that the lamina dura around the roots of both teeth is intact.

Features

The globulomaxillary cyst (if it occurs at all) is asymptomatic and is discovered on routine radiographic examination. As it becomes larger and expands the cortical plate buccally, the patient may complain of swelling or pain, especially if it becomes secondarily infected. The astute examiner notices that the contact point between the lateral incisor and canine has shifted toward the incisal edges of these teeth because of rotation of the crowns by the spreading roots. The mucosa over the buccal swelling is normal in appearance, and palpation of the surface produces crepitus if the cortical plate is still intact but fluctuance if it is not. Aspiration often yields typical amber-colored cyst fluid.

Differential Diagnosis

When an inverted tear-shaped radiolucency is found on the radiographs of a patient, the clinician must be especially careful not to make an impulsive diagnosis. Each case must be evaluated separately and thoroughly. An odontogenic cyst, a giant cell granuloma, an adenomatoid odontogenic tumor, surgical defects, myxomas, an-

terior bony clefts, and especially anatomic variations have masqueraded as a globulomaxillary cyst (Figs. 18-9 and 18-10).

If an amber-colored fluid is found on aspiration, the clinician can be reasonably sure that the lesion is a cyst, although there is a remote chance that the lesion is a cystic ameloblastoma.

Having determined a working diagnosis of cyst, the clinician must establish whether it is a radicular lateral periodontal or a globulomaxillary cyst. This distinction must be made before treatment is initiated because the root canals of the involved teeth have to be treated and filled before surgery if the pulps are nonvital. Pulp vitality tests aid in establishing whether the radiolucency is pulpoperiapical.

The most common cause of a radiolucency between the maxillary canine and lateral incisor tooth is a normal anatomic depression in the labial plate of the lateral fossa in this region (see Fig. 18-9). This trough can be readily identified by visual inspection and by palpation. In contrast, almost all pathologic bony lesions do not produce depressions but expand the jaws as soon as growth is sufficient to do so. The second most common cause of radiolucencies is pulpoperiapical lesions, perhaps positioned laterally because of the presence of lateral canals. Various authors have published papers on globulomaxillary radiolucencies.[5,9-11]

Management

The management of this cyst is identical to that described for other bony cysts; nonvital pulps must be addressed as well.

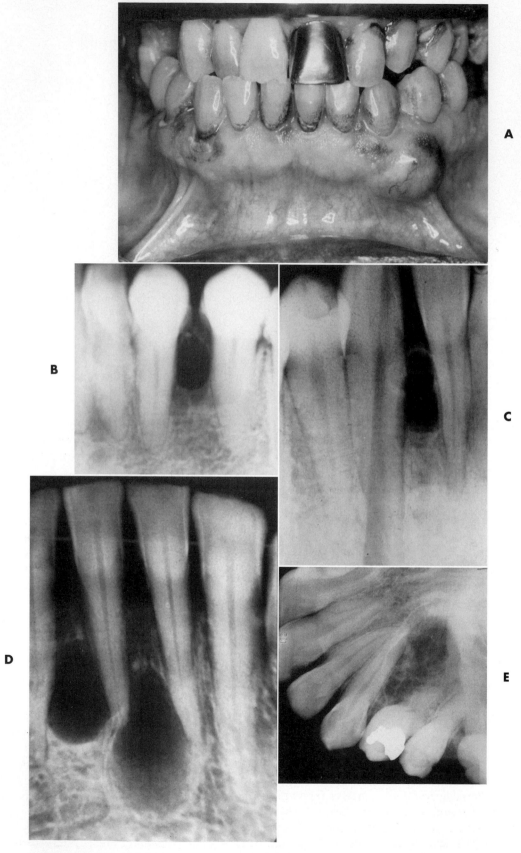

Fig. 18-8. Interradicular ameloblastomas. **A** and **B** are from the same patient. (**C** courtesy M. Wolfe, Chicago; **D** courtesy K. Tsiklakis, Athens, Greece.)

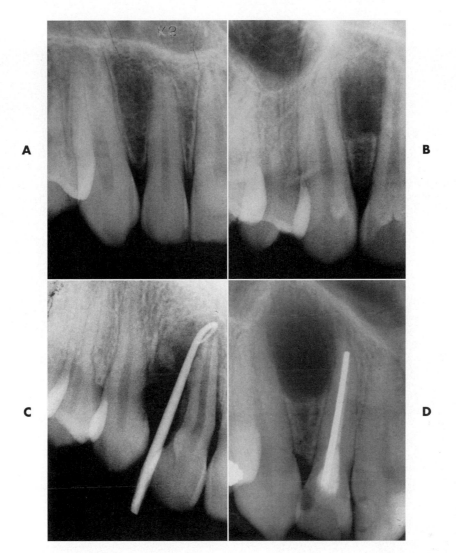

Fig. 18-9. Globulomaxillary radiolucencies. **A,** Shadow of a lateral fossa. **B,** Lateral rarefying osteitis in a nonvital lateral incisor with dens in dente. **C,** Chronic alveolar abscess. Lateral incisor is nonvital. **D,** Lateral radicular cyst from the lateral canal of a lateral incisor, after treatment.

INCISIVE CANAL CYST

Cysts of the incisive canal and of the palatine papilla are subclassifications of nasopalatine cysts originating in nests of epithelium that remain after the disintegration of the nasopalatine duct, an early epithelial fetal structure present within the incisive canal (Fig. 18-11).

This bilateral epithelium-lined duct structure runs superiorly through the incisive canal area to become Jacobson's organ, which is bilaterally positioned on the lateral aspects of the nasal septum. These lateral structures disintegrate in later fetal life, but nests of epithelium remain and are sometimes stimulated to produce cysts of the incisive canal and palatine papilla.

Features

The nasopalatine duct cyst is the most common nonodontogenic cyst[12] and occurs in 1 of every 100 persons. The overall age at diagnosis is 42.5 years. There is a slight male predilection.[13] Symptoms were present in at least 70% of cases; the mean radiographic diameter was 17.1 mm, but in 70% of cases, it was 22 mm or less.[13] A cyst of the palatine papilla is located in soft tissue, so it usually does not produce a radiolucency.

The incisive canal cyst is evident as a cystlike radiolucency on occlusal and periapical radiographs of the maxillary central incisor area (see Fig. 18-11). Frequently, its image is projected over the apices of the central incisors, and it must be differentiated from a radicular cyst. Often the anterior nasal spine is seen over the superior portion of the cyst as a radiopaque shadow, thus producing a heart-shaped radiolucency (see Fig. 18-11).

On occasion, the cyst forms in a superior aspect of one of the incisive canals at a point where the canals are discernibly separate, in which case it is positioned slightly to

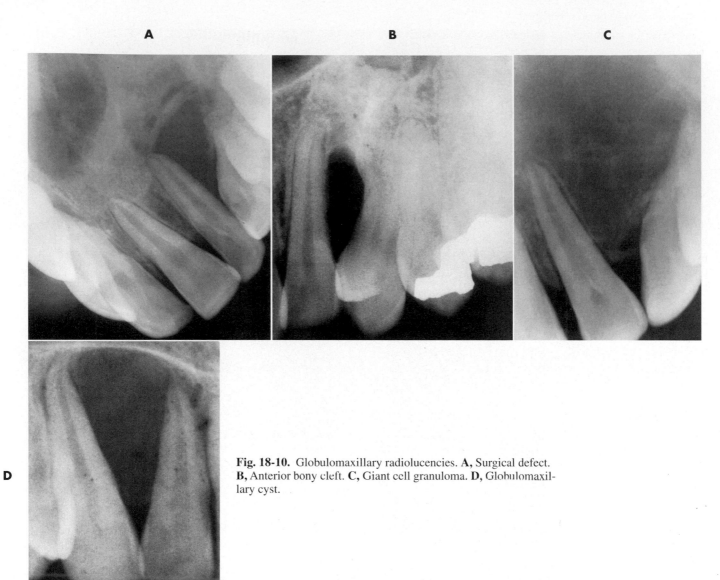

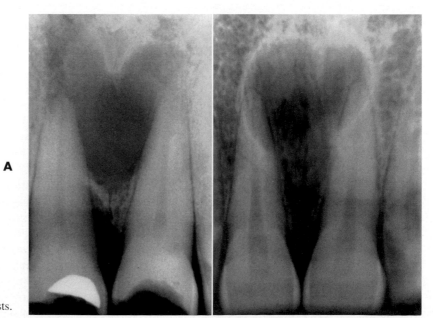

Fig. 18-10. Globulomaxillary radiolucencies. **A,** Surgical defect. **B,** Anterior bony cleft. **C,** Giant cell granuloma. **D,** Globulomaxillary cyst.

Fig. 18-11. Incisive canal cysts.

one side of the midline and the displacement is perceptible on radiographs. Sometimes, two separate cysts develop simultaneously in the left and right branches of the canal and cause paired cystlike radiolucencies. The appearance of separate cysts, however, may be an illusion resulting from a cyst at the juncture of canals extending superiorly into the separate branches of the incisive canal.

A cyst of the palatine papilla may be evident on clinical examination as a nodular fluctuant mass involving the area of the papilla, but it is not demonstrable on radiographs, since it is primarily of soft tissue and extends into the soft tissue more readily than into bone; bony destruction in the incisive foramen therefore does not usually result. On occasion, however, an incisive canal cyst at the oral limits of the bony canal bulges out of the canal into the soft tissue papilla. It produces a nodular swelling that appears on clinical examination as a cyst of the palatine papilla but that can also be correctly recognized from the obvious bony destruction apparent on the radiograph. A cyst in the canal may also erode the bone posterior to the canal, bulge into the mucosa posterior to the papilla, and create the clinical impression of a midpalatine cyst. Other cysts may bulge into the nasal cavity and extend so far posteriorly as to appear to be midline cysts of the palate.

The microscopic structure of the incisive canal cyst is similar to that of other cysts, although the epithelium lining the lumen is occasionally of the respiratory type and mucous glands are frequently present in the cyst wall.

Differential Diagnosis

Several types of cysts may occur in the anterior maxillary region and be projected over the apices of the incisors. Also, the incisive canal and foramen may normally vary greatly in size. Consequently the clinician may have some difficulty distinguishing between a large incisive foramen and a small asymptomatic incisive canal cyst on the basis of radiographic evidence alone. Some clinicians follow the rule of thumb that radiolucencies of the incisive canal measuring less than 0.6 cm in diameter should not be considered cystic in the absence of other symptoms.

A diagnostic problem frequently arises when a cystlike radiolucency is projected over the apex of a maxillary central incisor. The clinician must distinguish whether this is an incisive canal cyst or a radicular cyst (see Fig. 18-11).

Management

Enucleation is the treatment of choice for incisive canal cysts. The recurrence rate is approximately 2%.[13] Since this cyst lacks aggressive behavior, observation is justified in selected cases.[13]

MALIGNANCIES

Malignancies can begin in the interseptal bone and usually present as radiolucencies with poorly marginated

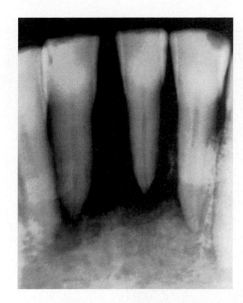

Fig. 18-12. Metastatic carcinoma.

borders (Fig. 18-12). Furthermore, malignancies that involve the periodontal ligament early in their development characteristically produce a bandlike widening of the image of the periodontal ligament. These features are described in detail in Chapter 21.

LATERAL (INFLAMMATORY) PERIODONTAL CYST

Lateral (inflammatory) periodontal cysts occur in the periodontal ligament, usually near the alveolar crest. They are thought to arise as the result of periodontal disease and can affect any tooth. (Some may be lateral radicular cysts resulting from lateral canals.) Pocket contents may be the irritant that stimulates adjacent rests of Malassez in the periodontal ligament. Fig. 18-13 illustrates a case in a periapical film. These cysts must be distinguished from lateral (developmental) periodontal cysts.[14,15]

LATERAL (DEVELOPMENTAL) PERIODONTAL CYST

The lateral (developmental) periodontal cyst is an unusual odontogenic cyst whose cause is unclear. Theories of the formation and development of the cyst hold that it is or results from (1) an early dentigerous cyst left in place after eruption of the tooth, (2) a primordial cyst, (3) the rests of Malassez in the periodontal ligament, (4) reduced enamel epithelium,[16] and (5) remnants of the dental lamina.[17,18]

These cysts occur in an interradicular position and have a high predilection for the mandibular canine and premolar region (Fig. 18-14), although some series report as many in the maxilla.[16] The adjacent teeth have vital pulps. On radiographic examination, these small to

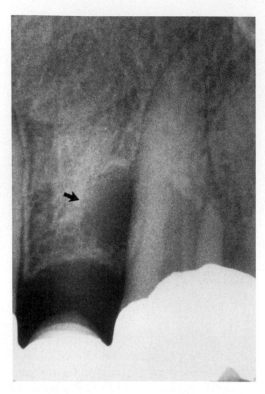

Fig. 18-13. Lateral (inflammatory) periodontal cyst *(arrow).*

medium cysts are round to oval and usually have a well-marginated, often hyperostotic border. Some authors include the botryoid odontogenic cyst as an example of the lateral periodontal cyst.[19] Microscopy shows a thin, nonkeratinized epithelial lining one to five cells thick.[17]

Entities among those to be considered in the differential diagnosis are the lateral radicular cyst, lateral (inflammatory) periodontal cyst, odontogenic keratocysts, radiolucent odontogenic tumors, and benign mesenchymal tumors.

Management

Management involves enucleation and microscopic study of the specimen. Care should be taken to preserve teeth if possible.

BENIGN NONODONTOGENIC TUMORS AND TUMORLIKE CONDITIONS

Any benign tumor of the tissues found within bone may occur and characteristically appear as a smoothly contoured, well-defined radiolucency much like a cyst (Fig. 18-15). These tumors or tumorlike conditions are uncommon in the jawbone and occur less commonly in the interradicular region.

MEDIAN MANDIBULAR CYST

The median mandibular cyst occurs in the symphyseal region of the lower jaw. It is uncommon, and its origin is in dispute. Some authorities contend that it is a true fissural

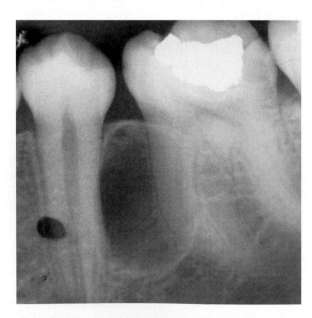

Fig. 18-14. Lateral (developmental) periodontal cyst.

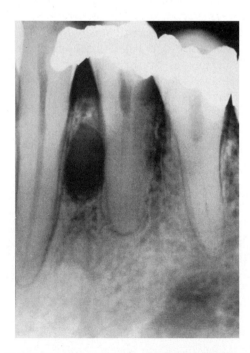

Fig. 18-15. Neurilemoma. (From Morgan G. Morgan P: Neurilemmoma-neurofibroma, *Oral Surg* 25:182-189, 1968.)

cyst originating from epithelium trapped in the fusion or from merging of the paired mandibular processes during the fourth week of embryonic life; others suggest that it probably represents a primordial cyst that formed in a supernumerary tooth bud, and others favor a theory of nests of odontogenic epithelium from the dental lamina.[20] Still others raise the possibility that it may be a lateral periodontal cyst developing on the medial aspect of the central incisors.[21] Nanavati and Gandhi[22] detail five criteria that they thought should be fulfilled before identifying a lesion as a median mandibular cyst. Rapidis and Langdon[23] are of the opinion that this is not a true clinical entity. If the central incisors adjacent to a median mandibular cyst are nonvital, it is reasonable to conclude that the particular example is a radicular cyst in most cases.

RARITIES

Rare entities that can occur interradicularly are the adenomatoid odontogenic tumor, buccal cyst, Langerhans' cell disease, osteoradionecrosis, and paradental cyst (Fig. 18-16). Other, more common entities such as giant cell granulomas may rarely appear primarily as interradicular radiolucencies (Fig. 18-17).

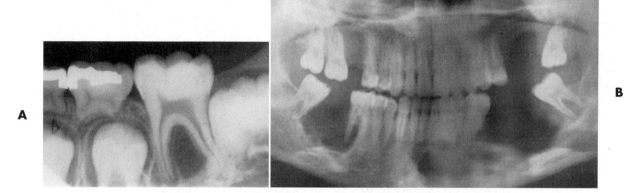

Fig. 18-16. A, Buccal cyst. **B,** Eosinophilic granulomas in all four quadrants.

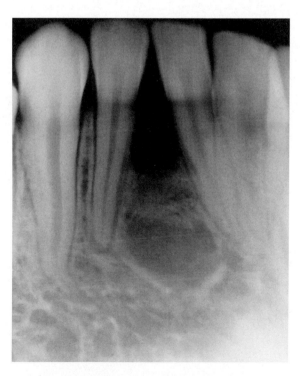

Fig. 18-17. Giant cell granuloma between the central incisors.

REFERENCES

1. Vertucci FJ, Anthony RL: A scanning electron microscopic investigation of accessory foramina in the furcation and pulp chamber floor of molar teeth, *Oral Surg* 62:319-326, 1986.
2. Thoma K: Facial cleft or fissural cyst, *Int J Orthod Oral Surg* 23:83-89, 1937.
3. D'Silva NJ, Anderson L: Globulomaxillary cyst revisited, *Oral Surg* 76:182-184, 1993.
4. Christ TF: The globulomaxillary cyst: an embryonic misconception, *Oral Surg* 30:515-526, 1970.
5. Wysocki GP: The differential diagnosis of globulomaxillary radiolucencies, *Oral Surg* 51:281-286, 1981.
6. Wysocki GP, Goldblatt LI: The socalled "globulomaxillary cyst" is extinct, *Oral Surg* 76:185-186, 1993.
7. Hollingshead MB, Schneider LC: A histologic and embryologic analysis of so-called globulomaxillary cysts, *Int J Oral Surg* 9:281-286, 1980.
8. Vedtofte P, Holmstrup P: Inflammatory paradental cysts in the globulomaxillary region, *J Oral Pathol Med* 18:125-127, 1989.
9. Taicher S, Azaz B: Lesions resembling globulomaxillary cysts, *Oral Surg* 44:25-29, 1977.
10. Zegarelli DJ, Zegarelli EV: Radiolucent lesions in the globulomaxillary region, *J Oral Surg* 31:767-771, 1973.
11. Dunlap CL, Barker BF: Myospherulosis of the jaws, *Oral Surg* 50:238-243, 1980.
12. Daley TD, Wysocki GP, Pringle GA: Relative incidence of odontogenic tumors and oral and jaw cysts in a Canadian population, *Oral Surg* 77:276-280, 1994.
13. Swanson KS, Kaugers GE, Gunsolley JC: Nasopalatine duct cyst: an analysis of 334 cases, *J Oral Maxillofac Surg* 49:268-271, 1991.
14. Killey HC, Kay LW, Seward GR: *Benign cystic lesions of the jaws: their diagnosis and treatment,* Edinburgh, 1977, Churchill Livingstone.
15. Eliasson S, Isacsson G, Köndell PA: Lateral periodontal cysts: clinical, radiographical and histopathological findings, *Int J Oral Maxillofac Surg* 18:191-193, 1989.
16. Altini M, Shear M: The lateral periodontal cyst: an update, *J Oral Pathol Med* 21:245-250, 1992.
17. Rasmusson LG, Magnusson BC, Borrman H: The lateral periodontal cyst: a histopathological and radiographic study of 32 cases, *Br J Oral Maxillofac Surg* 29:54-57, 1991.
18. Wysocki GP, Brannon RB, Gardner DG, et al: Histogenesis of the lateral periodontal cyst and the gingival cyst of the adult, *Oral Surg* 50:327-334, 1980.
19. Phelan JA, Kritchman D, Fusco-Ramer M, et al: Recurrent botryoid odontogenic cyst (lateral periodontal cyst), *Oral Surg* 66:345-348, 1988.
20. Tenaca JI, Giunta JL, Norris LH: The median mandibular cyst and its endodontic significance, *Oral Surg* 60:316-321, 1985.
21. DiFiore PM, Hartwell GR: Median mandibular lateral periodontal cyst, *Oral Surg* 63:545-550, 1987.
22. Nanavati SD, Gandhi PP: Median mandibular cyst, *J Oral Surg* 37:422-425, 1979.
23. Rapidis AD, Langdon JD: Median cysts of the jaws: not a true clinical entity, *Int J Oral Surg* 11:360-363, 1982.

CHAPTER 19

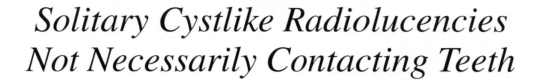

Solitary Cystlike Radiolucencies Not Necessarily Contacting Teeth

NORMAN K. WOOD

PAUL W. GOAZ

In this chapter the cystlike radiolucencies that usually do not involve the teeth are presented:

ANATOMIC PATTERNS
Marrow spaces
Maxillary sinus
Early stage of tooth crypts
Median sigmoid depression
POSTEXTRACTION SOCKET
RESIDUAL CYST
TRAUMATIC BONE CYST
LINGUAL MANDIBULAR BONE DEFECT
ODONTOGENIC KERATOCYST
PRIMORDIAL CYST
AMELOBLASTOMA—UNICYSTIC
FOCAL OSTEOPOROTIC DEFECT OF THE
    JAWS
SURGICAL DEFECT
GIANT CELL GRANULOMA
GIANT CELL LESION
    (HYPERPARATHYROIDISM)
FOCAL CEMENTOOSSEOUS DYSPLASIA
INCISIVE CANAL CYST
MIDPALATINE CYST

CEMENTIFYING AND OSSIFYING
    FIBROMA (EARLY STAGE)
BENIGN NONODONTOGENIC TUMORS
RARITIES
    Adenomatoid odontogenic tumors
    Ameloblastic variants
    Aneurysmal bone cyst
    Aneurysms in bone
    Arteriovenous malformation in bone
    Artifact
    Calcifying odontogenic cyst
    Central calcifying epithelial odontogenic
        tumor
    Central calcifying odontogenic cyst or
        tumor[1,2]
    Central hemangioma of bone
    Central odontogenic fibroma[3]
    Central odontogenic myxoma[4]
    Central salivary gland tumor[5]
    Central squamous cell carcinoma in cyst
        lining

Cholesterol granuloma[6]
Dentinoma (immature)
Desmoplastic fibroma
Hemangioma of bone
Langerhans' cell disease
Hydatid cyst
Lipoma (intraosseous)
Low-grade metastatic carcinoma
Metastatic carcinoma
Minor salivary gland tumor in bone
Myospherulosis (paraffinoma)
Odontogenic fibroma
Odontoma (early stage)
Oral pulse granuloma
Osteoblastoma (early stage)
Postoperative cyst of maxillary sinus
Postoperative maxillary cyst
Plasmacytoma
Pseudotumor of hemophilia[7]
Pulse granuloma
Squamous odontogenic tumor

The term *cystlike radiolucency* describes a dark radiographic image that is approximately circular in outline and usually smoothly contoured with well-defined borders. On occasion the radiolucency may be somewhat elongated, especially in the horizontal plane, and therefore may appear more elliptic. A thin hyperostotic border of bone may be present.

This group includes the imposing spectrum of entities from normal anatomic spaces to cysts of various types, benign tumors, ameloblastomas, dangerous intrabony hemangiomas, and malignancies (e.g., slow-growing metastatic tumors, squamous cell carcinomas within cysts). Consequently a careful differential diagnosis is mandatory before treatment.

The radicular, lateral, and dentigerous cysts are discussed not here but in other chapters. Some lesions included in this chapter (e.g., traumatic bone cysts, early cementoosseous dysplasias) occur as periapical radiolucencies

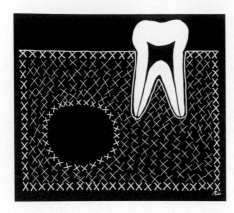

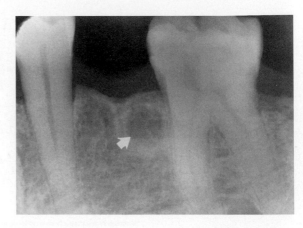

Fig. 19-1. Cystlike marrow space or focal osteoporotic bone marrow defect *(arrow).*

and are included in Chapter 16, but since these entities also occur with some frequency independent of the roots of teeth, they satisfy the criterion for inclusion in this chapter.

Cysts, giant cell granulomas, giant cell lesions of hyperparathyroidism, ameloblastomas, aneurysmal bone cysts, myxomas, metastatic carcinomas, and hemangiomas may have more than one radiographic appearance, so these lesions are also included in other chapters.

Finally, lesions such as metastatic carcinoma are not discussed here but are merely listed in the rarities section because they do not commonly cause a cystlike radiolucency. They are dealt with in other chapters, however, in which their more common appearances are discussed. The charactcristic features of the common solitary cystlike radiolucencies are shown in Table 19-1.

ANATOMIC PATTERNS

The anatomic radiolucencies found in radiographs of the jawbones are discussed in Chapter 15. Consequently, consideration of them is restricted here to a brief comment on the four entities: marrow spaces, maxillary sinus, early tooth crypts, and the median sigmoid depression.

Marrow Spaces

There is great variation among the patterns of marrow spaces from person to person and from one jaw to the other in the same person. When marrow spaces occur as larger-than-normal, somewhat rounded radiolucencies with borders that appear to be hyperostotic and not contacting teeth, these may be mistaken for any of the cystlike radiolucencies included in this chapter (Fig. 19-1). Larger examples may be termed *focal osteoporotic bone marrow defects.*[8-11]

Such unusual marrow space patterns occur more frequently in the mandible and are seldom seen on radiographs of the maxilla. When the clinician encounters what is interpreted as an uncommon marrow space pattern, a comparison with the spaces in the same area on the opposite side of the jaw usually shows a similar picture if indeed the clinician is dealing with an anomalous condition. This finding, coupled with an absence of local or systemic symptoms, is usually sufficient to permit the correct diagnosis.

However, contralateral areas may be subject to entirely different occlusal forces that significantly affect the trabecular patterns. Furthermore, some abnormal changes in the size of the marrow spaces occur with certain systemic disorders, and these changes are usually bilateral. Consequently, comparison of contralateral patterns might be misleading.

Nevertheless, if in doubt about the diagnosis, the clinician should reexamine the radiographs at regular intervals to ascertain that the radiolucent image is not enlarging. If symptoms exist, the region should be investigated surgically and a biopsy taken.

Maxillary Sinus

Frequently a cystlike outpouching of the maxillary sinus occurs on a radiograph of an edentulous upper jaw, and this normal variation presents a difficulty in differentiation from a pathologic process (Fig. 19-2). Radiographs of the area taken from different angles (Clark technique) often show a connection between such an outpouching and the larger maxillary sinus cavity and resolve the question of identity. Large nutrient canals in the walls of the sinus also contribute to a tentative identification (see Fig. 19-2, *A* and *B*).

Although the maxillary sinuses are frequently asymmetric, comparing their configurations may be helpful in the correct interpretation of a cystlike projection. Again, as is true of the changes in marrow space patterns in response to altered function, the sinus may expand, and its shape may be altered when stresses are reduced as a result of the loss of maxillary posterior teeth on the corresponding side.

Finally, if the clinician cannot satisfy doubts about the nature of the structure in question, periodic radiographs demonstrate whether the radiolucency is changing. As a last resort, aspiration of air from the cavity identifies it as the maxillary sinus.

Early Stage of Tooth Crypts

The radiographic picture of a tooth crypt in the early stages of development before calcification is round,

Table 19-1   Solitary cystlike radiolucencies

Entity	Predominant gender	Usual age (years)	Predominant jaw	Predominant region	Other radiographic appearances	Additional features
Marrow spaces (focal osteoporotic defects)	M = F	All	Mandible	Molar	Routine / Multilocular / Multiple cystlike	Asymptomatic; similar patterns contralaterally
Postextraction sockets	M = F	Over 20	Mandible	Molar	Osteosclerosis	Radiolucency does not enlarge; history of extraction; asymptomatic
Residual cysts	$\frac{M}{F} = \frac{3}{2}$	Over 20 (average 52)	Maxilla 57%	Molar	Multilocular	Asymptomatic; preextraction radiograph showing tooth with associated cyst
Traumatic bone cysts	M > F Slight	Under 30	Uncommon in maxilla	Premolar and molar / Incisor	Periapical radiolucency	Teeth vital; asymptomatic; possible history of trauma; usually no aspirate
Lingual mandibular bone defects	F > M	All ages	Mandible only	Third molar	Semicircular, oval	Teeth vital
Odontogenic keratocysts	M = 56.9%	Peak: 10-30 (average 28)	Mandible 65%	Third molar	Scalloped borders / Multilocular	Occasionaly radiolucency appears hazy; high recurrence rate
Primordial cysts	M ~ F	10-30	Mandible	Third molar	Multilocular	Permanent tooth fails to develop
Ameloblastomas	M ~ F	20-50 (average 40)	Mandible 80%	Posterior 70%	Ill-defined ragged borders / Multilocular	Erode cortical plates; may cause paresthesia
Surgical defects	M = F	Over 10	Equal	Anterior	Ragged and irregularly shaped borders	History of previous surgery; radiolucency does not enlarge
Central giant cell granulomas or lesions	$\frac{F}{M} = \frac{2.4}{1}$	Under 30 (average 26)	Mandible 70%	Anterior to second molars	Multilocular	History of previous trauma (?); serum chemistry levels normal
Giant cell lesions (secondary hyperparathyroidism)	$\frac{F}{M} = \frac{2}{1}$	50-80	Mandible	None	Multilocular / Indistinct borders	History of kidney disease; serum calcium levels normal to ↓; serum phosphate levels ↑; serum alkaline phosphatase levels ↑
Giant cell lesions (primary hyperparathyroidism)	$\frac{F}{M} = \frac{7}{1}$	30-60	Mandible	None	Multilocular / Indistinct borders	Polydipsia; polyuria; serum calcium levels ↑; serum phosphate levels ↑; serum alkaline phosphatase levels ↑
Incisive canal cysts	$\frac{M}{F} = \frac{3}{1}$		Maxilla only	Incisive canal	Heart shaped	Teeth vital; salty taste
Midpalatine cysts			Maxilla only	Palatine midline / Posterior to papilla	None	Uncommon
Early cemento-ossifying fibromas	M ~ F	26.4 (average)	Mandible 70%	Premolar and molar	Radiolucent-radiopaque	Teeth vital
Benign nonodontogenic tumors			Mandible	Molar / Ramus	Radiopaque / Elongated	Teeth vital

~, Approximately equal.

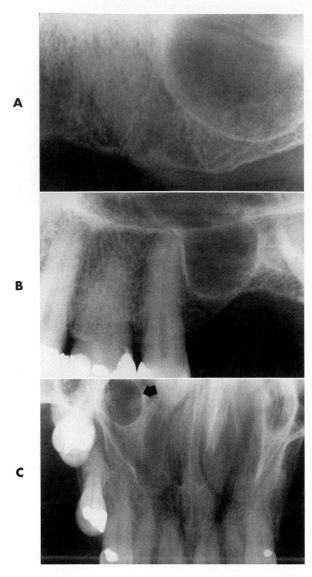

Fig. 19-2. A, Cystlike maxillary sinus. **B,** Cystlike outpouching of the maxillary sinus. **C,** Large nasolacrimal duct *(arrow).*

smooth, and well defined, and the crypt has a radiopaque rim identical to that of a cyst (Fig. 19-3). These entities are readily recognized, but sometimes a single tooth may have delayed development compared with its mate and with the corresponding tooth in the opposite quadrant. It may present a diagnostic problem mimicking a primordial cyst.

The clinician can differentiate between the two entities (delayed calcification or primordial cyst) by periodic radiographs for approximately 6 months.* If the radiolucent area is a retarded developing tooth, radiopaque foci representing the initiation of mineralization at the cusp tips are soon found. If no calcification is detected within 6 months

---

*The alert clinician should consider, however, that occasionally teeth are unusually slow in developing. Cunat and Collard[12] described premolars that developed 5 to 8 years later than normal.

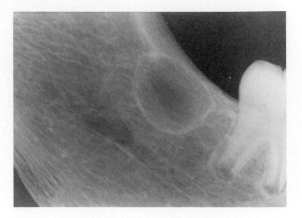

Fig. 19-3. Early molar crypt.

to 1 year, the discontinuity in the bone is most likely a primordial cyst that began within the odontogenic epithelium of the tooth bud before calcification was initiated.

Median Sigmoid Depression

The median sigmoid depression is an anatomic radiolucent shadow recognized and described by Langlais, Glass, Bricker, et al.[13] The radiolucent foramen-like shadow is produced by an osseous depression in some mandibles in the medial portion of the ramus just below the sigmoid notch area.[13] The radiolucency may be unilateral or bilateral. Langlais, Glass, Bricker, et al[13] reported that this radiolucency was seen in 10% of panoramic radiographs of patients, with 6% occurring unilaterally and 4% bilaterally.

POSTEXTRACTION SOCKET

Sometimes the socket resembles a cystlike radiolucency after an extraction and presents a problem in developing a working diagnosis (Fig. 19-4). A recent extraction may be verified clinically by a depressed area on the ridge. Sockets at extraction sites sometimes remain uncalcified for years as unchanging cystlike radiolucencies, but a check of other edentulous areas usually reveals similar-appearing sockets. If the clinical impression is reasonably certain, periodic radiographic examination of the area may be indicated. If serious doubts exist, surgical exploration of the area and possible biopsy are indicated.

RESIDUAL CYST

A *residual cyst,* as the name implies, is a radicular, lateral, dentigerous, or another cyst that has remained after its associated tooth has been lost. In practice, determining whether the cyst was present at the time of extraction or developed later in the residual rests of Malassez (residual odontogenic epithelial nests from Hertwig's root sheath) is not possible unless a radiograph showing that it was present before the extraction can be obtained. It has been postulated that low-grade inflammation of the parent cyst

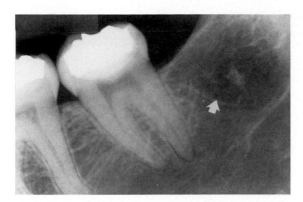

Fig. 19-4. Extraction site *(arrow)* 3 years after a tooth's removal.

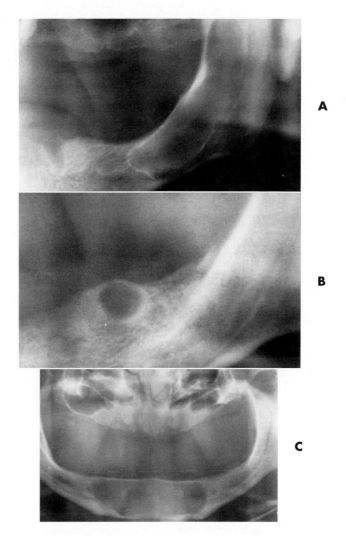

Fig. 19-5. A and **B,** Residual cysts. **C,** Midline cyst of the mandible, type unidentified (could be a residual, primordial, or true midline cyst). (Courtesy F. Prock, Joliet, Ill.)

(or nest of epithelium) might predispose it to the formation of residual cysts.[14]

No radiographic features permit differentiation between this type of cyst and any of the other lesions included in this chapter.

Features

The residual cyst occurs in the alveolar process and body of the jawbones in edentulous areas but may also be found in the lower ramus. Patients over 20 years of age have the highest incidence of residual cysts, the average age being 52 years. The ratio of men to women is 3:2, and the maxilla is more commonly involved than the mandible.[15] The residual cyst appears as a rounded to elliptic radiolucency with well-defined borders (Figs. 19-5 and 19-6). It seldom reaches more than 0.5 cm in diameter but may be large enough to cause jaw expansion and asymmetry. Its symptoms, clinical characteristics, and histopathologic features are identical to those of the other odontogenic cysts discussed in Chapters 16 and 17. Surprisingly, nearly half are symptomatic.[14,16] The microscopic picture is nonremarkable, although cases that contain a piece of legume have been reported.[17] Squamous cell carcinoma has been observed arising from these cysts as well.[18]

Differential Diagnosis

All the entities included in this chapter must be considered when a residual cystlike radiolucency is found; however, the cystlike anatomic patterns, primordial cyst, keratocyst, and traumatic bone cyst are the entities most likely to cause confusion. Postsurgical cysts of the maxillary sinus occur with significant frequency 10 to 30 years after surgical intervention in the maxillary sinus. Such an entity must be differentiated from residual radicular cysts of the posterior maxilla.[19] Differential diagnoses for these entities are given in detail in the section on keratocysts.

Management

The treatment of a residual cyst is identical to that of any other intrabony odontogenic cyst except that the offending teeth have already been lost. Circumstances such as the patient's age and systemic condition and the size of the cyst may prompt the use of one of the following methods in preference to the others:

1. Complete enucleation of the cyst wall with its epithelium and primary closure of the mucoperiosteal flap
2. Complete enucleation of the cyst tissue with the placement of a surgical pack, which is slowly withdrawn as the defect fills
3. Complete excision and replacement with autogenous particulate bone or a single segment of bone fixed in place
4. Marsupialization
5. Decompression
6. Decompression combined with delayed enucleation
7. Enucleation and collapsing of mucoperiosteal flap[20] (Some advocate suction drainage for large cysts when only enucleation is used.[21] All excised tissue is sent for microscopic study.)

Just before surgical intervention, aspiration of the area with at least an 18-gauge needle is a precaution that prevents

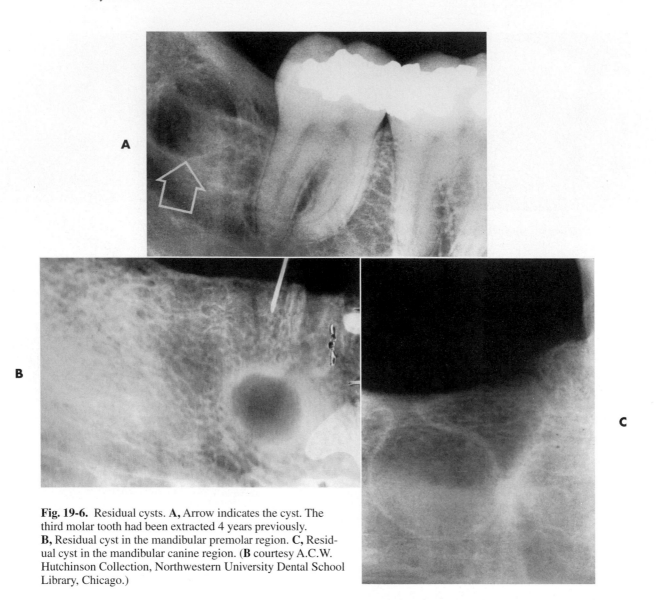

Fig. 19-6. Residual cysts. **A,** Arrow indicates the cyst. The third molar tooth had been extracted 4 years previously. **B,** Residual cyst in the mandibular premolar region. **C,** Residual cyst in the mandibular canine region. (**B** courtesy A.C.W. Hutchinson Collection, Northwestern University Dental School Library, Chicago.)

the surprise of a more serious lesion than anticipated (e.g., solid tumor, intrabony hemangioma, or aneurysmal bone cyst). It has been postulated that if inflammation is not a feature, these cysts tend to undergo slow resolution.[14]

TRAUMATIC BONE CYST

The traumatic bone cyst (TBC) includes the idiopathic bone cavity, hemorrhagic bone cyst, extravasation cyst, simple bone cyst, solitary bone cyst, progressive bony cyst, and blood cyst. It occurs in other bones as well as the jaws and is classified as a false cyst because it does not have an epithelial lining.

TBCs occurring at the apices of teeth are included in Chapter 16 as periapical radiolucencies. They are discussed in detail in this chapter as solitary cystlike radiolucencies not necessarily contacting teeth.

The cause of TBCs is unknown, although a number of patients give a history of prior trauma. The lesions are mostly asymptomatic and are thus detected on routine ra-

diographs. Classically the TBC is located above the mandibular canal and is usually round to oval with contoured, well-defined borders (Figs. 19-7 and 19-8). Often the superior border extends between the roots of the teeth, giving a scalloped appearance (see Fig. 19-7, *A*). Lesions usually do not measure more than 3 cm in diameter, but examples have expanded almost the entire ramus and body[22] (see Fig. 19-7, *C*). Multiple (bilateral) lesions have been reported,[23] but the majority are solitary. Most occur in the mandible,[24-26] with the most common site being the premolar and molar region followed by the lower ramus and the midline. The TBC seldom occurs in the maxilla,[24,26] especially in the anterior region.[24] Atypical locations, such as the condyle, ramus, and area below the mandibular canal, have been reported.[27,28] The majority occur in patients under 30 years of age, there is a slight male predominance, and approximately 95% of lesions contain fluid or are empty.[24] Aspiration is usually fruitless but in some instances yields a serumlike fluid.[29] Reports of these cavities being filled with air or other gases are likely erroneous.[30]

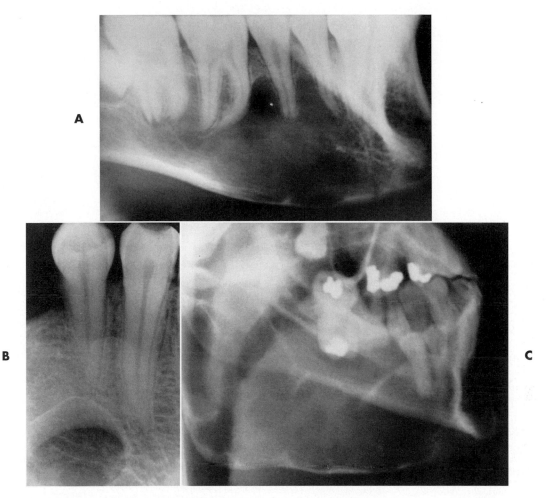

Fig. 19-7. Traumatic bone cyst. The pseudomultilocular appearance and cortical expansion of the large lesion in **C** are evident. (**A** and **C** courtesy M. Kaminski, deceased, and S. Atsaves, Chicago; **B** courtesy R. Goepp, Chicago.)

Saito, Hoshina, Nagime, et al[31] have reported on an older group and a younger group of TBCs. The findings from the younger group correspond to those of the lesions previously discussed. The older group showed a definite female predominance (80%), maxillary predominance, a frequent association with radiopaque lesions, a loss of the lamina dura, and the presence of periapical cementoosseous dysplasia or hypercementosis.[31]

This lesion must be surgically explored to ensure the correct diagnosis, and the subsequent curettement, which produces hemorrhage into the cavity, usually ensures a successful regression of the defect as it is slowly obliterated by bone. The healing period should be closely observed radiographically.[32]

LINGUAL MANDIBULAR BONE DEFECT (STAFNE'S CYST)

The lingual mandibular bone defect (LMBD) of the mandible (known also as *static bone cyst* or *defect, latent bone cyst* or *defect,* and *developmental submandibular gland defect of the mandible*) is an invagination in the me-

dial surface of the mandible, usually in the third molar–angle area (see Fig. 19-9, *A* and *B*). The defect is generally believed to be caused by the mandible developing around the lobe of the submandibular salivary gland during embryonic life. A case of a defect that contained a lymph node rather than salivary tissue has been reported.[33]

Features

The invagination producing the LMBD is lined by cortex, so it projects as a radiolucency surrounded by a smooth, dense radiopaque rim (Figs. 19-9 and 19-10). Shape is round to ovoid to semicircular; the image is usually unilocular but may be bilocular. Lesions are characteristically unilateral but occasionally may be bilateral (see Fig. 19-9). Size may vary from 1 to 3 cm, and the usual location is inferior to the mandibular canal in the third molar region. LMBDs occur in about 0.3% of adults and predominately in male patients. In some series, all patients were male.[34-36] Although most cases are seen as static lesions in adults, cases have been found in adolescents.[37] Lesions have also demonstrated growth.[37-38] The LMBD is classically asymptomatic, and pain is rarely reported.[39] Researching

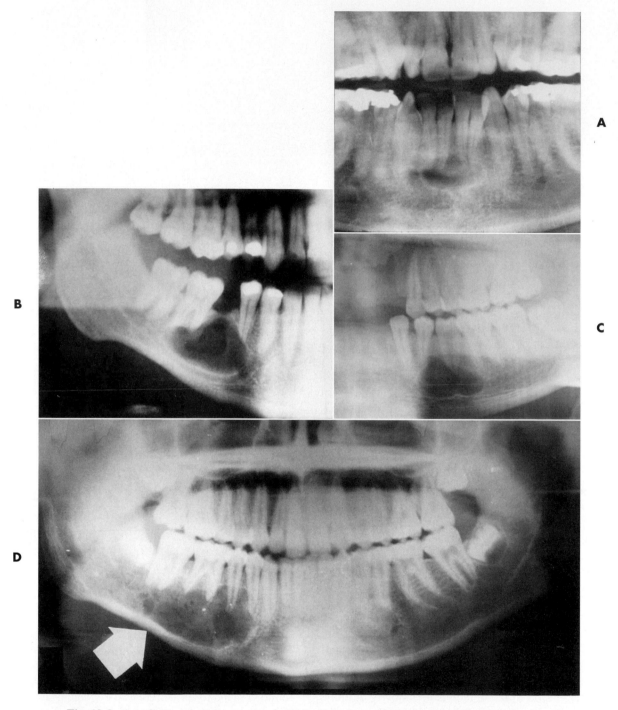

Fig. 19-8. A to **C,** Traumatic bone cysts. **A,** Lesion is in the symphysis region, where it has projected over the apices of the incisor teeth. **B,** Lesion is in the first molar region. **C,** Lesion is in the premolar region. **D,** Central cavernous hemangioma of bone resembles a traumatic bone cyst *(arrow)*. Note the "wormhole" appearance sometimes seen in bony hemangiomas. (**A** courtesy P. Akers, Evanston, Ill; **B** courtesy M. Lehnert, Minneapolis; **C** courtesy W. Heaton, Chicago; **D** from Zalesin HM, Rotskoff K, Silverman H: *J Oral Surg* 33:877-884, 1975.)

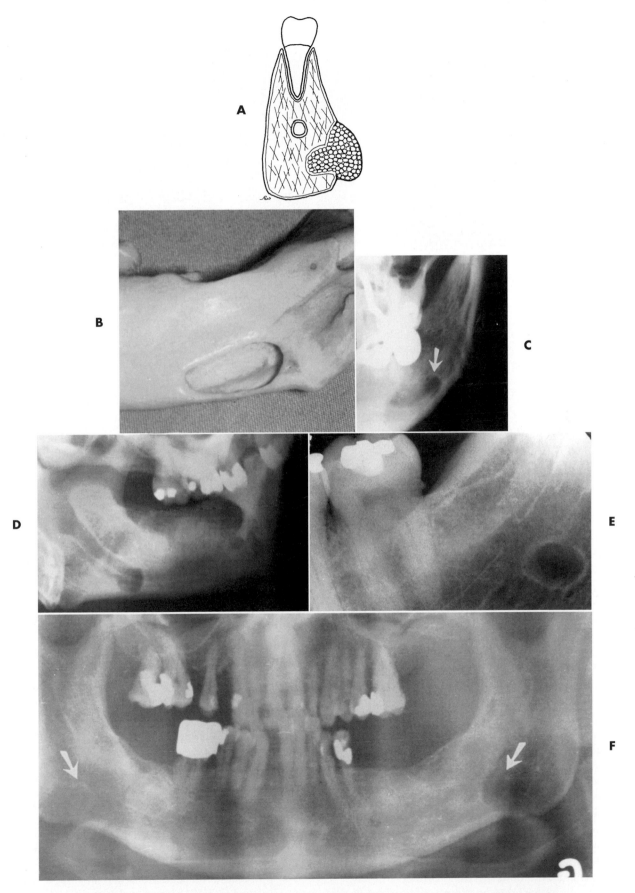

Fig. 19-9. Lingual mandibular bone defects. **A,** Diagram of a cross section of the mandible with the submandibular gland within the defect. **B,** Defect in the mandibular bone. **C to F,** Radiographs of several cases. **F,** Bilateral defects. Arrows in **C** and **F** indicate the defects. (**B** and **C** courtesy O.H. Stuteville, deceased; **E** courtesy N. Barakat, Beirut, Lebanon.)

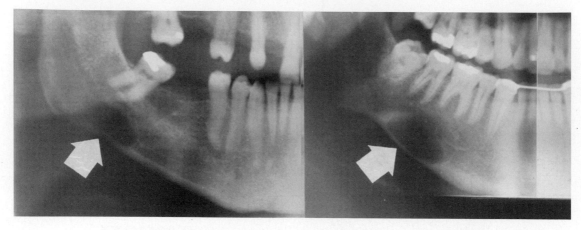

Fig. 19-10. Arrows indicate LMBDs.

skeletal mandibles, Mann has reported a case in which the mylohyoid growth terminated in an LMBD.[40]

Occasionally, these defects are located in the anterior portion of the mandible.[41-45] These are referred to as *anterior lingual mandibular bone defects* and are, at least in some cases, associated with the sublingual gland.[42-45] Some of these radiographic radiolucent shadows are cast over the roots of anterior teeth. Recently, cortical defects have been reported to occur on the lingual aspect of ramus[46] and on the posterior buccal surface of the mandible.[47]

Differential Diagnosis

The position and appearance of this radiolucency are all but diagnostic. Occasionally, when the LMBD is small and situated in a more superior position in a region where teeth are present or have only recently been extracted, it may be mistaken for a radicular or residual cyst. Confusion more frequently occurs with the anterior variety because the entity is often cast over the apices of the teeth (see Fig. 16-26).

Some clinicians use the following procedure to strengthen their impression of developmental bone defect:

1. A curved needle, of approximately 16 gauge for rigidity, is advanced into the tissue intraorally or extraorally until the medial surface of the mandible is encountered.
2. Consequently the lingual surface of the mandible can be explored by walking the needle along the surface of the bone.
3. If a recess is found on the medial wall, the diagnosis of developmental bone defect is certain, provided that all the other findings concur.

Also sialography may show the distribution of dye in the radiolucency, since a portion of the submandibular salivary gland usually lies within this bony pocket.

Management

Recognition of this entity is all that is necessary. These defects should no longer be surgically explored unless the clinician has reason to suspect a more serious diagnosis. Salivary gland tumors have been reported to occur within these defects.

ODONTOGENIC KERATOCYST

The odontogenic keratocyst (OKC) has been recognized and classified as distinct from other types of bony cysts on the basis of its clinical behavior and its distinct and unique microscopic structure. The OKC cuts across the usual classification of cysts because its diagnosis depends entirely on its microscopic features and is independent of its location. It represents 5% to 11% of jaw cysts.[48,49] The primordial cyst and the multiple jaw cysts of basal cell nevus syndrome are predominantly OKCs. In Shafer's series,[50] 45% of primordial cysts were OKCs. Also, a reported 7.8% of all jaw cysts, 8.5% of all dentigerous cysts, and 0.9% of all radicular cysts are OKCs.[51]

On radiographic examination the OKC cannot be distinguished from other intrabony cysts. It is often unicystic (Fig. 19-11, *A*) but sometimes has scalloped borders (Fig. 19-11, *B*), and it often occurs with a multilocular appearance.

In this chapter the discussion of OKCs is limited to those that do not contact teeth. These represent about 28% of these cysts.

Features

The symptoms produced by the OKC are identical to those of the other bony cysts. The cyst may occur in all age-groups, but its peak incidence falls in the second and third decades and shows a gradual decline through the later years. A total of 56.9% occur in male patients; 65% are found in the mandible.[52,53]

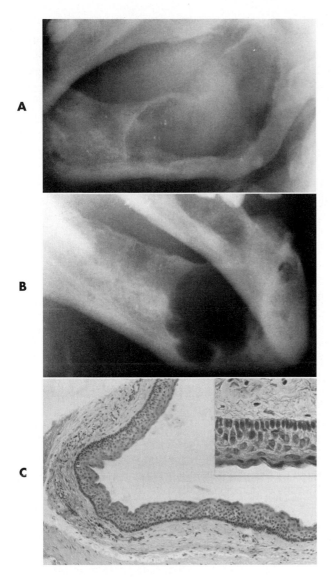

Fig. 19-11. OKC. **A,** Hazy appearance. **B,** Scalloped margins. **C,** Characteristic histopathologic study.

Although multiple OKCs of the jaws have been reported, only some are accompanied by basal cell nevus syndrome. Occasionally the cyst expands the cortical plates and perforates. When palpated, it demonstrates a firmer fluctuance than the usual bony cyst that has perforated the bony plates because the lumen of the OKC is filled with keratin that has a somewhat doughy consistency.

For this reason the clinician should use a large-bore needle when attempting to aspirate these cysts to recover the thick, cheesy, yellow substance that fills the lumen. The OKC differs from other bony cysts in that it has a high recurrence rate (12% to 51%), which increases with years of follow-up.[49,52,54,56] Forssell, Forssell, and Kahnberg[55] found a 43% recurrence rate with few recurrences after the 3-year postoperative period. Occasional recurrences are found 37 to 40 years after surgery.[55,57] Higher recurrence rates are seen in multilocular

cases,[55,56] syndrome cysts, infection fistulation, perforated bony walls, and cysts enucleated in several pieces.[55]

Two types of OKCs exist: a parakeratinizing and an orthokeratinizing. The parakeratinizing type is aggressive, whereas the orthokeratinizing type is similar in behavior to other jaw cysts.[58-61] On microscopic examination the parakeratinized odontogenic keratocyst presents a characteristic picture. The lumen is frequently filled with keratin produced by an epithelial lining whose appearance is distinct from that of the usual stratified squamous keratinizing epithelium and is peculiar to this type of cyst (see Fig. 19-11). The wall is frequently thin and has a similarly thin epithelial lining deficient in rete ridges. The basal cells are columnar or cuboidal and are arranged in a well-defined, palisading row. The prickle cells may be vacuolated, are usually sparse, and are sometimes altogether absent in certain regions. The stratum corneum may be atypical in appearance, with the keratinized cells retaining their nuclei; consequently the keratinization is predominantly of the parakeratotic type. A buddinglike proliferation from the basal layer is frequently seen in OKCs, and microcysts may be present in the walls.

Wright[61] described the orthokeratinized variant of the odontogenic keratocyst: "On microscopic examination this distinct clinicopathologic entity has a thin uniform epithelial lining with orthokeratinization and a granular cell layer just beneath the keratinized layer." The basal cells are usually cuboidal or flattened. Wright[61] described the clinical features as follows: (1) appears as a single cyst, (2) has a predilection for male patients, (3) is most common in the second to fifth decades, (4) appears most often as a dentigerous cyst in the posterior mandible, and (5) shows little aggressiveness on clinical examination.

Differential Diagnosis

Because of its unusually high recurrence rate, the OKC must be distinguished from all other cystlike radiolucencies listed in this chapter.

For example, a cystlike radiolucency measuring 1 cm in diameter is found on a radiograph of an edentulous third molar region of the mandible in a 21-year-old white man. The entity is completely asymptomatic, and there are no related clinical signs. On the radiograph the mandibular canal appears to be displaced inferiorly by the lesion. The differential diagnosis for this radiolucency is discussed in the two sections that follow.

Less likely diagnoses An assessment of the circumstances surrounding the discovery of a cystlike radiolucency undoubtedly lessens the probability that any of the entities in this group warrants further consideration in the differential diagnosis. Nevertheless, since they do have some features in common with the lesion under investigation, the clinician is compelled to include them in the list of possibilities, since they represent unlikely choices.

Benign nonodontogenic tumors of the mandible are uncommon and therefore would be assigned a low ranking in the list of possibilities.

The cementifying or ossifying fibroma is not a common lesion.

Although a developmental bone defect might occur in the third molar region, it would almost never be found superior to the mandibular canal and would not cause displacement of the canal—except (rarely) when an expanding soft tissue tumor in the submaxillary space protrudes into it, causing it to enlarge.

Fissural cysts do not occur in the third molar region.

The giant cell granuloma is usually found in more anterior regions of the jaws.

The giant cell lesion of hyperparathyroidism can often be ruled out by studies of the serum chemistry.

Although the third molar region is a likely location for an ameloblastoma, the young age of the patient and the less frequent occurrence of this odontogenic tumor characterize this possibility as less likely.

The possibility that the radiolucency is a third molar tooth crypt is not likely because the calcification of this tooth is usually initiated in the eighth year and the tooth is fully formed by age 21. Also the contralateral third molar area can be used for a comparison if delayed calcification is suspected. Radiographs taken 6 months later confirm the presence of the calcifying crown, but taking radiographs again in 6 months' time is not a suitable practice if the clinician strongly suspects that the lesion represents a serious pathologic condition.

Comparing the bone trabeculation in the remainder of the jaws aids in determining whether the entity is a cystlike local osteoporotic bone marrow defect, since a single marrow space of this size and shape without similar areas elsewhere in the jawbone would be quite unusual.

More likely diagnoses The clinician's attention is now directed to the following more likely entities, which are similar in several respects and are appropriate for inclusion in the working diagnosis (ranked in descending order of frequency):

Residual cyst
TBC
Primordial cyst
OKC—primordial type
Ameloblastoma

All these entities show a predilection for the third molar area and, except for the ameloblastoma (which usually occurs in an older age-group), for patients in their early to middle twenties. The patient's medical history may produce some clues that aid in arranging the entities in a differential diagnosis, but more often than not, it adds to the confusion.

Although the mandibular third molar region is a characteristic site for the ameloblastoma, this tumor should not be given a high ranking in this 21-year-old patient because the radiolucency is not pericoronal. Paresthesia would switch suspicion toward ameloblastoma.

Aspiration may be helpful in developing a working diagnosis. If the procedure produces an amber-colored fluid, a primordial cyst, residual cyst, or cystic ameloblastoma would be suggested. Conversely, if a thick, yellow, cheesy material is collected, a primordial type of keratocyst would be inferred. If aspiration proved to be nonproductive, the area could then be a TBC or one of the solid entities listed at the beginning of the chapter.

If the clinician can determine that the third molar failed to develop in the affected quadrant, the primordial cyst should be considered as the most likely diagnosis. A patient who has had several posterior teeth extracted during a period of years can seldom be relied on to give sufficiently accurate information regarding whether a third molar ever developed, especially if the other molars are present. Also, if the first permanent molar was extracted relatively soon after its eruption, the patient often becomes confused and reports that a deciduous tooth was lost. Furthermore, the second molar frequently erupts into the position of the first molar, and the third molar drifts into the position of the second molar.

The rarer odontogenic myxoma also must be considered in such a circumstance because this lesion is compatible with the history of a tooth that failed to develop and may be seen as a cystlike radiolucency.

If the patient informs the clinician that a tooth was extracted from the area and a cyst was associated with the tooth, the impression that the radiolucent area is a residual cyst is reinforced, unless there is otherwise conflicting evidence. A previous radiograph showing a tooth present and associated with a cyst, whether radicular, lateral, or follicular, adds credence to the choice of residual cyst.

The following findings are highly suggestive of the diagnosis of OKC: (1) a cystlike radiolucency in the third molar region or mandibular ramus; (2) a diameter of more than 3 cm; (3) a unilocular cystlike radiolucency with scalloped margins; (4) a multilocular cyst; and (5) odorless, creamy or caseous contents.[62]

Management

Aggressive treatment, including enucleation, curettement (mechanical, physical, or chemical), and resection for large cysts with or without loss of continuity of the jaw, is indicated.[63] Adjacent mucosa should be removed in some cases. Great care should be taken to completely remove the cyst lining, and if remnants are left behind, more bone should be curetted at this location.[64] Radical surgery, including resection with or without continuity defects and disarticulation, should be reserved for cysts that demonstrate neoplastic change or for lesions that are not surgically accessible by a conservative approach.[64] An alternative approach, which gives good results, has been recommended for these aggressive lesions: enucleation, liquid nitrogen cryosurgery, and immediate bone grafting.[65] Long-term clinical and radiographic follow-up is mandatory because this lesion behaves more like a tumor than a cyst.

PRIMORDIAL CYST

A primordial cyst is less common than the OKC and is thought to develop as early cystic degeneration in the tooth germ before mineralization has been initiated. The involved tooth bud may be of the regular permanent dentition or a supernumerary tooth. The radiographic picture is nonspecific, showing only a cystlike radiolucency where a tooth has not developed.

Features

The primordial cyst shows no gender predilection and occurs most frequently in patients between the ages of 10 and 30 years. The mandibular molar region, especially the third molar and the area just distal to it, represents the most frequent site of development (Fig. 19-12). These cysts demonstrate all the usual features of cysts and seldom cause cortical expansion. On microscopic examination, they are usually found to be odontogenic keratocysts. On aspiration the clinician frequently obtains a thick, yellowish, granular fluid composed primarily of exfoliated cells and keratin.

Differential Diagnosis

The differential diagnosis of this lesion is discussed in the section on keratocysts.

Management

A significant percentage of primordial cysts appear on microscopic examination as OKCs and thus frequently mimic the behavior of benign tumors.[66] The treatment of OKC is discussed on pp. 319-320.

AMELOBLASTOMA

The ameloblastoma is an odontogenic tumor usually described as locally malignant; it arises from odontogenic epithelium and sometimes from odontogenic cysts.[67] It represents approximately 11% to 13% of odontogenic tumors.[47,68] The unilocular type may be pericoronal or not necessarily contacting teeth (Fig. 19-13). The unilocular ameloblastoma is discussed in detail in Chapter 17 as a pericoronal radiolucency. In this chapter, it is discussed as a cystlike radiolucency not contacting teeth.

Features

The early ameloblastoma is asymptomatic, but as it expands, perforates the cortical plates, or both, it becomes discernible and palpable on clinical examination. A particular ameloblastoma feels firm if it is of the solid type. The cystic type is soft and fluctuant, and straw-colored fluid can be aspirated in some cases. (Also see the section in Chapter 17.)

Differential Diagnosis

To avoid surprise at surgery, the surgeon must consider that every cystlike radiolucency of the jawbones could be an ameloblastoma. The differential diagnosis of the lesion is discussed with that of the OKC (see pp. 319-320).

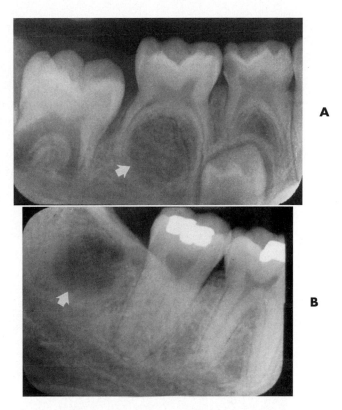

Fig. 19-12. Arrows indicate primordial cysts. The permanent tooth failed to develop in each case.

Management

The unicystic ameloblastoma is a different entity with a much lower recurrence rate than the ordinary ameloblastoma. Its management is discussed in Chapter 17. The multilocular ameloblastoma is described in Chapter 20.

FOCAL OSTEOPOROTIC BONE MARROW DEFECT OF THE JAWS

Focal osteoporotic bone marrow defects of the jaws are relatively common and have been frequently reported.[8-11,68-69] The cause is unknown, but altered healing reactions or marrow hyperplasia may play a role.

Features

Focal osteoporotic bone marrow defects are common in the mandible and uncommon in the maxilla, especially the anterior region.[8,9] From 72% to 91% occur in the premolar and molar region of the mandible.[11,69] There is a strong predilection for female patients, some are bilateral, and almost 25% occur in areas of previous extraction.[11] Radiographic appearance varies from cystlike to multilocular to irregular, and borders are usually well defined but can be vague in some cases.[8,9,11] These defects are seldom symptomatic (pain in less than 15% of cases[11]) and rarely show cortical plate expansion.[8,10] Many are cast over or near the apices of

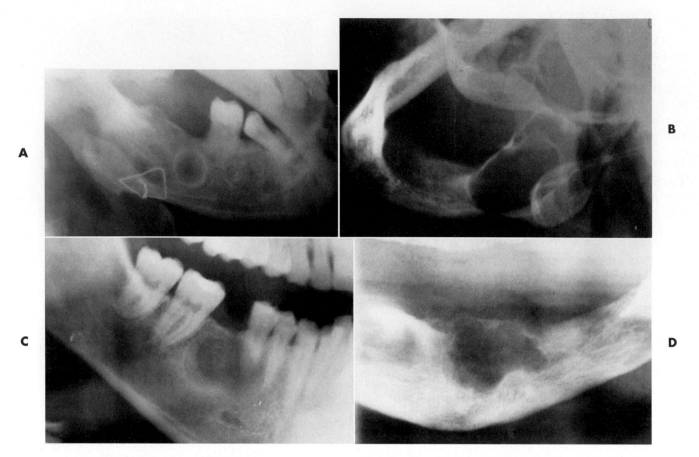

Fig. 19-13. Ameloblastoma. **A** to **C,** Three cystlike ameloblastomas. **D,** Less cystlike shape and some multilocular formation on the left border. (**A** courtesy O.H. Stuteville, deceased; **B** and **C** courtesy D. Skuble, Hinsdale, Ill; **D** courtesy M. Lehnert, Minneapolis.)

teeth (see Fig. 16-1), but lamina duras are intact, and teeth test vital.

Microscopically the defect is filled with hematopoietic marrow[10,11] with a variable fatty component. Approximately 25% of cases in one series were primarily fat.[11]

Differential Diagnosis

A wide range of lesions must be considered, including dental granulomas, rarefying osteitis, odontogenic cysts, TBCs,[8] osteomyelitis, odontogenic tumors, benign and malignant tumors of bone, manifestations of leukemia, Langerhans' cell disease, and advanced anemias.

Management

According to Barker, Jensen, and Howell,[11] a radiolucent shadow with distinct or ill-defined margins in the posterior aspect of the body of the mandible of a middle-aged woman suggests an osteoporotic bone marrow defect. If conflicting evidence is not present in the form of worrisome signs or symptoms, such an area should be radiographed at intervals to ensure that change is not occurring. If malignancy is suspected, surgical exploration and biopsy are carried out.

SURGICAL DEFECT

Defects of a transitory or permanent nature result from bone surgery. The majority of these defects possess well-defined borders; when they are round or ovoid, they have a cystlike appearance on radiographs (Fig. 19-14).

Usually a radiolucency may be suspected as a surgical defect when the clinician learns of prior surgery. Occasionally a surgical defect is permanent, usually because relatively large areas of cortical bone, along with the periosteum and marrow, have been lost; consequently, there is a deficiency of the bone-forming elements. When a patient with such a deformity is seen by a different clinician some years after the surgery, the radiolucency may present a dilemma. The clinician must determine whether it is a surgical defect, a recurrence of the original condition, or a new lesion. If a series of postsurgical radiographs have been taken during the intervening years and are available to the new clinician, whether the area is decreasing, remaining constant, or enlarging will be apparent.

If the area has remained constant, is decreasing slightly in size, or is increasing in radiodensity, it is most likely a surgical defect. If it is increasing in size, however, it must be considered a recurrence of the original

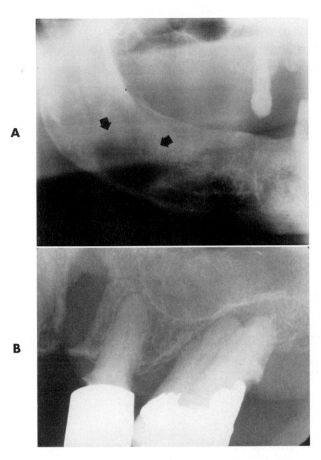

Fig. 19-14. Surgical defect. **A,** Defect *(arrows)* 20 years after cystectomy. **B,** Defect one year after a traumatic extraction.

pathologic process or possibly a new lesion. For example, if a dentigerous cyst was removed some years before, an ameloblastoma may have developed from remnants of the epithelial lining.

If the clinician encounters an asymptomatic radiolucency in an area of the jaw that according to the patient's history was the site of previous surgery and if the original diagnosis can be obtained, the clinician has enough information to consider whether the image is more likely to be a quiescent defect or a recurrence of disease.

If postsurgical radiographs of the area are not available, the size and shape of the asymptomatic radiolucency should be monitored every 6 months. An original diagnosis of a benign condition (i.e., a cyst) does not relieve the clinician of the obligation to periodically reexamine the presumed surgical defect until its benign status has been convincingly demonstrated. Such a demonstration is established by the appearance of a constant or diminishing size in subsequent radiographs. If an increase in size is evident on successive radiographs, the area must be investigated to determine the cause of the change.

Palpation of the jawbone may reveal a depression on the medial or lateral surface in a position corresponding to the location of the radiolucency. Such a finding contributes to the diagnosis of the defect.

CENTRAL GIANT CELL GRANULOMA OR LESION

The central giant cell granuloma of the jaws has often been compared with the giant cell tumor of long bones. It has been proposed that these two entities represent a continuum of a single disease process that is modified by the age of the patient, the site of occurrence, and other factors.[71-72] This would give credence to the theory that the aggressive examples of giant cell granulomas of the jaws may be appropriately designated as *nonmalignant giant cell tumors.*[73] The cause is unknown.

The central giant cell granuloma may occur initially as a solitary, cystlike radiolucency (Fig. 19-15); as it grows larger, it frequently becomes a soap-bubble type of multilocular radiolucency (see Chapter 20). Some 71% have been reported as being unilocular and 17.5% as multilocular.[74]

Features

The central giant cell granuloma occurs most frequently in female patients under 30 years of age, and approximately two of three lesions are found in the mandible.[72,74,75] The portion of the jaws anterior to the molars is the usual site of involvement. Paresthesia is common.

The lesion is painless and grows slowly by expanding and thinning the cortical plates but seldom perforates into the soft tissue. Consequently the clinician usually finds a hard expansion demonstrating some flexibility. If the cortical plates are perforated, however, the swelling is moderately soft on palpation (see Fig. 19-15). This is to be expected because on microscopic examination the lesion consists of multinucleated giant cells scattered throughout a vascular granulomatous tissue stroma that contains a minimum of collagen (see Fig. 19-15).

Hemosiderin is often scattered throughout the tissue and, with the high vascularity, may impart a bluish cast to a lesion that has extended peripherally through the cortical plates and lies just beneath a thin mucosal surface. The covering mucosa appears normal unless traumatized. An expanding lesion may cause some migration of teeth, and root resorption has been reported 43%.[72] Some lesions are more aggressive clinically, radiographically, and microscopically, and they tend to recur. Therefore a spectrum ranging from nonaggressive to aggressive is seen.[72,73,76] More irregularly shaped giant cells and a greater proportion of small giant cells occur in nonaggressive lesions compared with aggressive ones. Also, osteoid is more often seen within the lesional tissue of aggressive lesions.[72] Aggressive lesions usually occur at a younger age, are larger when found, and recur more frequently.[73]

Differential Diagnosis

All the cystlike lesions discussed in this chapter must be considered in the differential diagnosis of giant cell granuloma. The clinical characteristics of the lesion in question

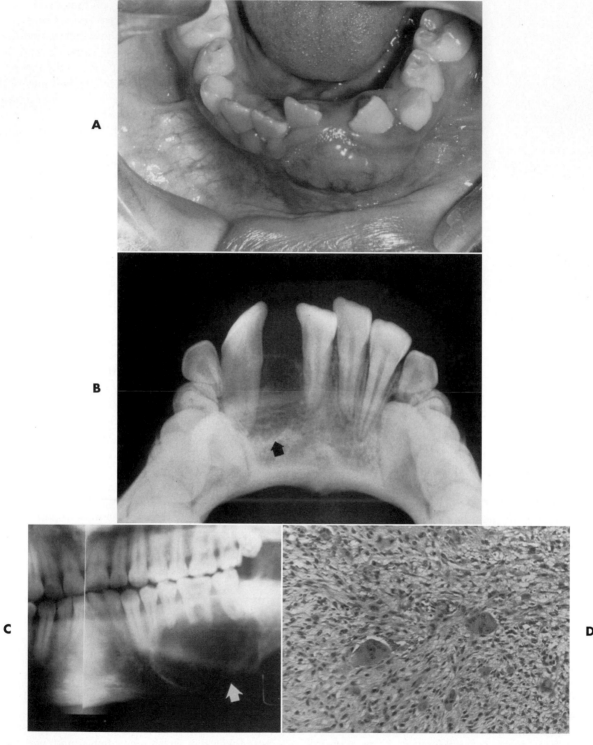

Fig. 19-15. Central giant cell granuloma. **A,** Clinical appearance of an anterior alveolar swelling in a 9-year-old boy. **B,** Radiograph of the lesion. **C,** Another cystlike central giant cell granuloma. **D,** Photomicrograph showing giant cells in the fibrovascular stroma. (**C** courtesy J. Ireland, deceased, and J. Dolci, Mundelein, Ill.).

should be compared with those listed for each entity at the end of the chapter.

When a diagnosis of giant cell granuloma is reported by the pathologist, the results of serum chemistry tests must be studied to exclude the possibility of a giant cell lesion of hyperparathyroidism. In multilesional cases, cherubism and Noonan's syndrome must be considered.[77]

Management

Curettement is the treatment of choice. Recurrence rates between 12% and 49% have been reported[72,78,79] and dictate close long-term follow-up. Reports of successful treatment with intralesional injections of corticosteroids and also with subcutaneous injections of human calcitonin have been published.[80,81] Hyperparathyroidism must be considered as well, especially if the lesion recurs, and serum chemistry tests affirm or negate this consideration. Serum calcium, phosphorus, and alkaline phosphatase tests are indicated to investigate the possibility of hyperparathyroidism. This step is necessary, since the giant cell granuloma cannot be differentiated from giant cell lesion on the basis of a clinical, radiographic, or microscopic examination.

GIANT CELL LESION (HYPERPARATHYROIDISM)

Hyperparathyroidism is discussed in detail in Chapter 23. The giant cell lesion of hyperparathyroidism occurs as a unilocular or multilocular radiolucency (see Chapter 20) and is found in patients with primary, secondary, or tertiary hyperparathyroidism. If the jaws show rarefaction (a possible finding in advanced hyperparathyroidism), the giant cell lesion appears to have poorly demarcated borders because of the rarefied surrounding bone (Fig. 19-16). Establishing its identity depends on serum chemistry tests and demonstration of the concomitant parathyroid, kidney, or other systemic disorder.

Secondary Hyperparathyroidism

Secondary hyperparathyroidism is more common than the primary type. One causative pathologic condition is impaired kidney function[82] from disease (e.g., an ascending infection), which induces a shift in the ionic balance of the blood that ultimately causes a lowered level of serum calcium. The mechanism of this shift is not yet fully understood.

The reduced serum calcium level then leads to parathyroid hyperplasia and an increased production of parathyroid hormone, which in turn causes bone to resorb and return calcium to the blood to maintain serum calcium at normal levels. In moderate to severe cases, enough mineral is removed from the bones that the bones become rarefied and are discernible on radiographic examination (i.e., osteitis fibrosa cystica generalisata, discussed in Chapter 23). The same phenomenon is observed in patients receiving dialysis.

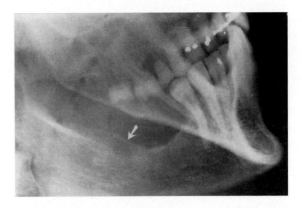

Fig. 19-16. Giant cell lesion of hyperparathyroidism *(arrow)*. The poorly defined borders of the tumor were caused by the generalized rarefaction of the jawbone. (Courtesy O.H. Stuteville, deceased.)

In severe cases of hyperparathyroidism, the cortical plates are especially thinned, and the lamina dura around the roots of the teeth may not be apparent on radiographs. Central giant cell lesions (brown tumors) are prone to occur and are found frequently in the jaws (see Fig. 19-16). They mimic the central giant cell granuloma in clinical, radiographic, and histologic features. The giant cell lesion of hyperparathyroidism may demonstrate a high recurrence rate if the systemic problem is not controlled.

Primary Hyperparathyroidism

Primary hyperparathyroidism detectable on clinical examination is less common than the secondary type and is caused by a functioning adenoma (less often by an adenocarcinoma) of one of the parathyroid glands. The increased level of parathyroid hormone stimulates bone resorption and consequently increases the level of serum calcium, concomitantly inducing an increased excretion of phosphate by the kidney. The skeletal changes and giant cell lesions are identical to those of the secondary type.

Differential Diagnosis

Primary and secondary hyperparathyroidism may be differentiated on the basis of history and laboratory findings.

Patients with primary hyperparathyroidism are usually in a younger age-group, between 30 and 60 years, and may report polydipsia and polyuria because of the increased diuresis. Women are 7 times more likely than men to have this condition. Serum values in advanced primary hyperparathyroidism are increased calcium levels, decreased phosphorus levels, and increased levels of alkaline phosphatase (which is characteristically elevated during increased bony resorption or apposition).

A patient with secondary hyperparathyroidism has the same symptoms and usually a history of kidney disease and is likely to have a decreased renal output. An older age-group (50 to 80 years) is involved, and women are only twice as often afflicted as men. Laboratory tests reveal an inverted relationship of the serum calcium and phosphorus levels compared with those found in primary disease (i.e., the serum calcium levels are normal or decreased, whereas the serum phosphate and alkaline phosphate levels are increased).

Management

If the primary medical problem is corrected, the giant cell lesions often regress without surgery, and the rarefaction disappears. Surgical excision of the parathyroid gland with its adenoma is the treatment for the primary type and is successful. The treatment of the kidney defect in the secondary type is usually more complicated.

FOCAL CEMENTOOSSEOUS DYSPLASIA

Focal cementoosseous dysplasia (FCOD) may be the counterpart of periapical cementoosseous dysplasia that occurs mostly in edentulous, tooth-bearing areas posteriorly in the mandible. (All of these reactive cementoosseous lesions of the periodontal ligament origin are thought to form a continuum).[83] This lesion is asymptomatic, focal, and either radiolucent, radiopaque, or mixed radiolucent-radiopaque with well to poorly defined borders.[83] It shows a marked predilection for blacks.[83,84] Some radiolucent lesions of this entity are basically round with poor or good margination. These may be examples of early lesions, whereas the mature lesion is almost totally radiopaque, often with some vestige of radiolucent rimming. The mixed and radiopaque pictures are discussed in Chapters 24 and 27. Most of these lesions would have once been referred to as *cementomas.*

INCISIVE CANAL CYST

The incisive canal cyst is discussed in detail in Chapter 18 as an interradicular radiolucency. In edentulous anterior maxillas, it can occur as a cystlike radiolucency that does not contact the shadows of teeth (Fig. 19-17).

MIDPALATINE CYST

The midpalatine cyst is an uncommon bony cyst that develops in the midline of the palate posterior to the palatine papilla. It originates in residual embryonic epithelial nests in the fusion line of the lateral palatine shelves. On radiographic examination a unilocular radiolucency is seen in the midline of the palate (Fig. 19-18). Large cysts may destroy the bony palate.

Features

The patient with a midpalatine cyst may complain of a painless bulging that is increasing in size in the roof of the mouth. If the cyst is not traumatized or secondarily infected, the dome-shaped mass is nontender and covered with normal mucosa, which perhaps appears more glossy than usual. The mass is situated over the midline of the palate posterior to the incisive papilla.

Because the bone inferior to the cyst is so thin, the cortical plate is rapidly perforated as the cyst grows; consequently the swelling is soft and fluctuant but cannot be emptied by digital pressure unless a sinus is present. Aspiration produces an amber-colored fluid.

The microscopic picture is identical to that of other cysts. The epithelial lining may be of the respiratory type (with goblet cells and cilia).

Differential Diagnosis

Although many lesions occur on the palate with some frequency, it seems reasonable to limit the differential diagnosis to soft lesions: midpalatine cyst, incisive canal cyst, radicular cyst, palatine space abscess, lipoma, plexiform neurofibroma, mucocele, papillary cyst adenoma, and mucoepidermoid tumor (low grade).

Occasionally an early low-grade mucoepidermoid tumor appears on clinical examination as a mucocele when much mucus is produced by the mucous cells, which are the predominant cell type in the low-grade variety. However, minor salivary gland tumors and retention phenomena are seldom seen in the midline of the hard palate, since there is a paucity of minor salivary glands in this region. These tumors may be seen most frequently in the lateral aspect of the posterior palate in the region of the anterior palatine foramen. Furthermore, although the low-grade mucoepidermoid tumor and the mucocele might demonstrate fluctuance and cannot be emptied by digital pressure—characteristics similar to those of cysts—unlike cysts, they do not yield a typical amber-colored fluid on aspiration but a viscous, clear, sticky liquid (concentrated mucus). Mucoepidermoid carcinoma, papillary cyst adenoma, and mucocele are assigned a low rank in the differential diagnosis for a soft midpalatine swelling.

The plexiform neurofibroma is the only peripheral nerve tumor that is soft and fluctuant. It is the usual type that occurs in von Recklinghausen's disease, so it is a likely choice if the patient has this disease. Also, it can be readily differentiated from a cyst, since it cannot be aspirated.

A lipoma is uncommon in the oral cavity, and like the neurofibroma, it can be readily distinguished from cysts by aspiration.

A palatine space abscess is painful, can be somewhat soft and fluctuant, and yields pus on aspiration. It is generally associated with the palatine roots of nonvital posterior teeth or a vital or nonvital tooth with a lateral periodontal abscess on the lingual aspect of a palatine root. Consequently a palatine space abscess seldom is located in the posterior midline but is found adjacent to the tooth that gave rise to the infection (see Fig. 19-18)—in contrast to an abscess resulting from a secondarily infected midpalatine cyst, which is more symmetrically situated in the midline. The midline palatine space abscess illustrated in Fig. 19-18, *B,* is an exception because it has

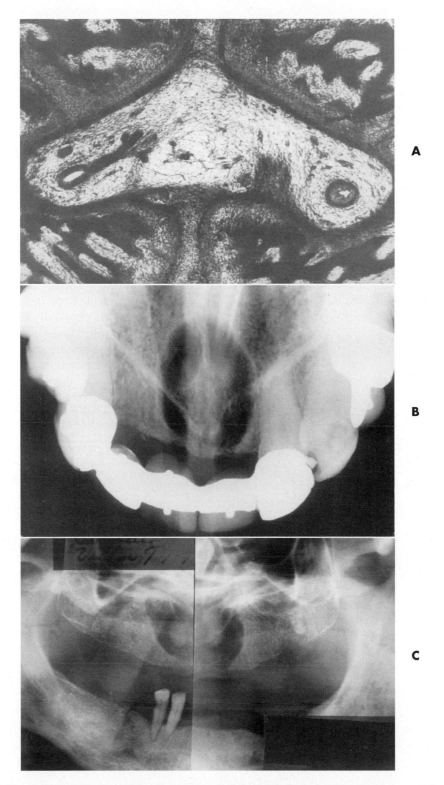

Fig. 19-17. A, Transverse section of a 15-week-old human embryo showing the incisive canal (inverted V-shaped structure). **B,** Occlusal radiograph of incisive canal cyst where some anterior teeth are missing. **C,** Large incisive canal cyst in a Panorex radiograph of an edentulous maxilla.

originated from a lateral incisor tooth and is symmetrically positioned in the midline.

A radicular cyst involving a canine or a premolar rarely perforates the denser cortical bone of the lingual plate; rather, this type of cyst extends through the thinner buccal plate into the buccal vestibule. Further, vitality tests and periapical radiographs aid in the differentiation of the midpalatine cyst from the odontogenic palatine space abscess.

The incisive canal cyst is easily differentiated from the midpalatine cyst in most cases because it occurs in the canal above the palatine papilla, whereas the midpalatine cyst occurs in the midline of the palate posterior to the papilla. When an incisive canal cyst or a midpalatine cyst expands and destroys the posterior limits of the incisive canal, distinguishing with certainty between the two is usually impossible (see Fig. 19-18).

Management

Enucleation is usually all that is necessary, but some curettement may be necessary if infection has played a role.

EARLY STAGE OF CEMENTOOSSIFYING FIBROMAS

Cementoossifying fibromas (benign fibroosseous lesions of periodontal ligament origin) are classified as neoplastic fibroosseous lesions that arise from elements of the periodontal ligament.[85-88] The early stage is osteolytic, in which the surrounding bone is resorbed and replaced by a fibrovascular type of soft tissue containing osteoblasts and cementoblasts. A mixture of small deposits of bone and cementum may be seen in some lesions, whereas just cementum or bone may be seen in others. At this stage, these lesions may appear as solitary cystlike radiolucencies not in contact with teeth (Fig. 19-19). The margins are contoured and distinct.

Features

When small, cementoossifying fibromas are asymptomatic but frequently may grow sufficiently large to expand the jawbone. Approximately 70% occur in the mandible and are primarily found in the premolar and molar region.[87] The average age of patients with ossifying fibroma is 30 years, and the genders are approximately equally affected, with a slight female preference in some studies.[87] The age range in one study was 3 to 63 years.[87] In contrast to periapical cementoosseous dysplasia, these lesions classically occur as solitary entities.

During the initial radiolucent stage, the lesion usually changes progressively from a predominantly fibroblastic lesion to an increasingly calcified structure. During maturation, microscopic examination discloses a number of small droplets of cementum, spicules of bone, cemento-

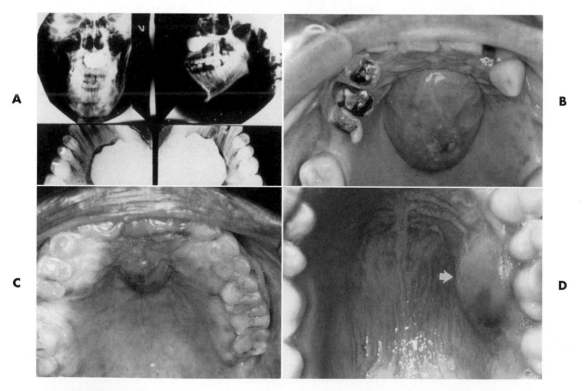

Fig. 19-18.   A, Radiographs of a midpalatine cyst injected with radiopaque dye. **B,** Clinical appearance of a midpalatine abscess. **C,** Palatine swelling from an incisive canal cyst that destroyed the posterior bony boundary of the canal and simulated a midpalatine cyst. **D,** Palatine space abscess *(arrow)* from a pulpless premolar. **(A** courtesy D. Skuble, Hinsdale, Ill.)

blasts, and osteoblasts in a fibrous vascular stroma. As these entities continue to mature, the calcified components become larger, coalesce, and are then apparent on radiographs as radiopaque foci within a well-described radiolucency. Still later, in the mature stage, most of the lesion consists of calcified tissue and appears on radiographs as a well-defined radiopacity usually surrounded by a uniform radiolucent zone that represents a noncalcified area of fibrous tissue at the periphery.

Differential Diagnosis

A period of at least 6 years is required for the lesion to pass from the radiolucent to the radiopaque stage. Usually, this pathosis shows varying degrees of soft tissue density with a few small radiopaque foci present; accordingly, it is usually included in the differential diagnosis of radiolucent areas with radiopaque foci, discussed in Chapter 24. When the lesion (infrequently) is completely radiolucent and not in contact with teeth, it is assigned a low ranking in the differential discussion of such cystlike radiolucencies. Cementoossifying fibromas differ from the more common periapical and focal cementoosseous dysplasias in that they occur in younger patients, most often in the premolar and molar region of the mandible, and if left untreated, attain a much larger size, frequently causing expansion of the jaws.

"Atypical" fibroosseous lesions may closely resemble cementoossifying fibromas but in actuality are more aggressive lesions such as juvenile ossifying fibroma or low-grade osteosarcoma.[89]

Management

To make the correct diagnosis, a surgical approach is necessary so that biopsy material can be obtained. Excision and curettement of the lesion are all that is required, since this lesion seldom recurs.[87,88] "Atypical" lesions may be more aggressive and require more aggressive surgery. This is dictated by the clinical behavior of each lesion.[89]

BENIGN NONODONTOGENIC TUMORS

Specific benign nonodontogenic tumors are rarely observed within the jawbones. If they are considered as a group, however, their composite incidence is high enough to warrant their exemption from the category of rarities. Tumors that have occurred with some frequency within the jaws as cystlike radiolucencies not necessarily in contact with teeth are lipoma, salivary gland adenoma, amputation neuroma, neurofibroma,[90] schwannoma, leiomyoma,[91] fibroma, and myxoma. Because their growth is slow, they present as well-defined radiolucencies of varying shape (Fig. 19-20). Polak, Polak, Brocheriou, and Vigneul[90]

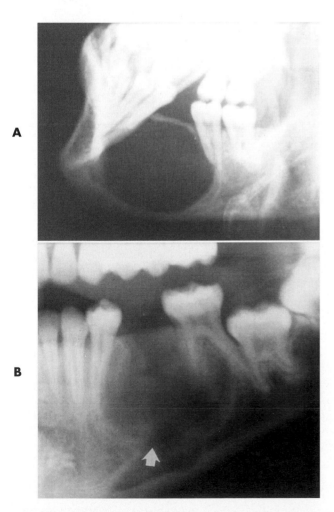

Fig. 19-19. Immature cementoossifying fibroma. The arrow in **B** indicates the lesion. (**A** courtesy S. Atsaves, Chicago; **B,** courtesy R. Goepp, Chicago.)

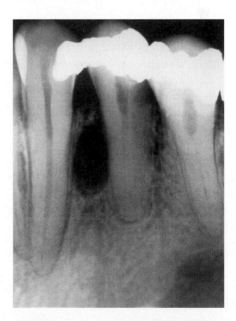

Fig. 19-20. Neurilemoma showing a cystlike radiolucency between the mandibular canine and premolar. (From Morgan G, Morgan P: Neurilemmoma-neurofibroma, *Oral Surg* 25:182-189, 1968.)

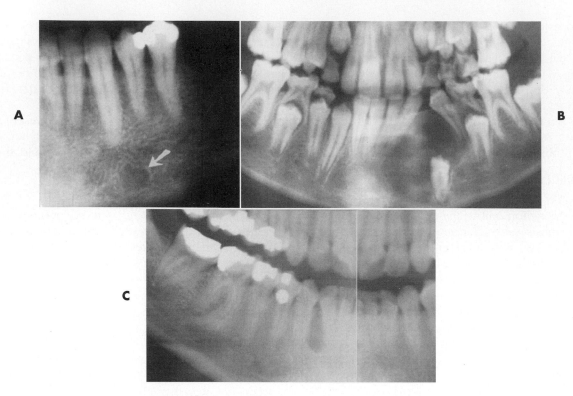

Fig. 19-21. Rarities. **A,** Cystlike metastatic bronchogenic carcinoma *(arrow).* **B,** Pericoronal radiolucency involving an impacted canine that proved to be a myxoma. **C,** Myxoma between the canine and lateral incisor. (**B** and **E** courtesy N. Barakat, Beirut, Lebanon; **C** and **D** courtesy R. Kallal, Chicago.) *Continued*

report a case of a solitary neurofibroma of the mandible and review 29 other cases of neurofibromas in the literature.

Features

Most benign nonodontogenic tumors are asymptomatic, except for the peripheral nerve tumors that develop with major sensory nerves. The patient then usually reports pain, paresthesia, or anesthesia in a region. The patient with an amputation neuroma almost invariably describes a previous traumatic incident: a tooth extraction, a jaw fracture, or major jaw surgery.

If benign tumors of the jaw go untreated, they slowly grow and expand the cortical plates, which because of the slow growth of the tumor frequently remain intact. Aspiration is nonproductive for the benign nonodontogenic tumors just discussed.

Differential Diagnosis

Benign nonodontgenic tumors of the jawbone should be assigned a low ranking in the differential diagnosis of solitary cystlike radiolucencies.

A neurofibroma involving the mandibular canal is sometimes found as an elongated broadening of the canal. When this picture is observed, the possibility that it represents a peripheral nervous tissue tumor should be considered. Arteriovenous pathosis also must be considered in such a case.

When the patient gives a history of major surgery or fracture in a region that has a painful cystlike radiolucency, an amputation neuroma must be considered a possibility.

If the patient has neurofibromatosis, the likelihood that a cystlike radiolucency of the jawbones is a peripheral nerve tumor is much greater than for the general population.

Management

Conservative excision, including enucleation and curettement if necessary—after a presurgical aspiration test has proved nonproductive—is the treatment of choice for these lesions. If the tumor involves the mandibular canal and its contents, the patient should be warned about the likelihood of a postoperative paresthesia or anesthesia of the lip and, if the radiolucency is large, of the possibility of jaw fracture during surgery.

RARITIES

The rare entities, which may appear as cystlike radiolucencies not necessarily in contact with teeth, are listed at the beginning of the chapter. Some are illustrated in Fig. 19-21.

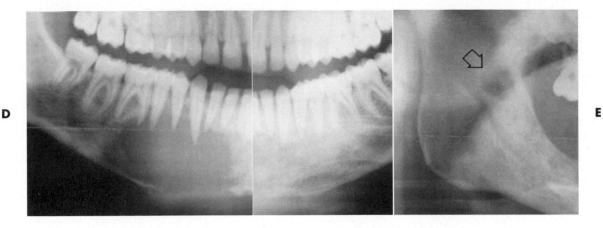

Fig. 19-21, cont'd. Rarities. **D,** Cystlike aneurysmal bone cyst. **E,** Langerhans' cell disease (eosinophilic granuloma) *(arrow).*

REFERENCES

1. Buchner A: The central (intraosseous) calcifying odontogenic cyst: an analysis of 215 cases, *J Oral Maxillofac Surg* 49:330-339, 1991.
2. Hong SP, Ellis GL, Hartman KS: Calcifying odontogenic cyst: a review of ninety-two cases with reevaluation of their nature as cysts or neoplasms, the nature of ghost cells, and subclassification, *Oral Surg* 72:56-64, 1991.
3. Kaffe I, Buchner A: Radiologic features of central odontogenic fibroma, *Oral Surg* 78:811-818, 1994.
4. Peltola J, Magnusson B, Happonen R-P, Borrman H: Odontogenic myxoma: a radiographic study of 21 tumors, *Br J Oral Maxillofac Surg* 32:298-302, 1994.
5. Brookstone MS, Huvos AG: Central salivary gland tumors of the maxilla and mandible: a clinicopathologic study of 11 cases with an analysis of the literature, *J Oral Maxillofac Surg* 50:229-236, 1992.
6. Hirshberg A, Dayan D, Buchner A, Freedman A: Cholesterol granuloma of the jaws, *Int J Oral Maxillofac Surg* 17:230-231, 1988.
7. Machado de Sousa SO, Luiz de Piratininga J, Pinto Jr DS, Soares de Aravjo N: Hemophilic pseudotumor of the jaws: report of two cases, *Oral Surg* 79:216-219, 1995.
8. Gordy FM, Crews KM, O'Carroll MK: Focal osteoporotic bone marrow defect in the anterior maxilla, *Oral Surg* 76:537-542, 1993.
9. Schneider LC, Mesa ML, Fraenkel D: Osteoporotic bone marrow defect: radiographic features and pathogenic factors, *Oral Surg* 65:127-129, 1988.
10. Makek M, Lello GE: Focal osteoporotic bone marrow defects of the jaws, *J Oral Maxillofac Surg* 44:268-273, 1986.
11. Barker BF, Jensen JL, Howell FV: Focal osteoporotic bone marrow defects of the jaws: an analysis of 197 new cases, *Oral Surg* 38:404-413, 1974.

12. Cunat JJ, Collard J: Late developing premolars: report of two cases, *J Am Dent Assoc* 87:183-185, 1973.
13. Langlais RP, Glass BJ, Bricker SL, et al: Medial sigmoid depression: a panoramic pseudoforamen in the upper ramus, *Oral Surg* 55:635-638, 1983.
14. High AS, Hirschmann PN: Age changes in residual radicular cysts, *J Oral Pathol* 15:524-528, 1986.
15. Cabrini RL, Barros RE, Albano H: Cysts of the jaws: a statistical analysis, *J Oral Surg* 28:485-489, 1970.
16. High AS, Hirschmann PN: Symptomatic residual radicular cysts, *J Oral Pathol* 17:70-72, 1988.
17. Marcussen LN, Peters E, Carmel D, et al: Legume-associated residual cyst, *J Oral Pathol Med* 22:141-144, 1993.
18. van der Wal KGH, de Visscher JGAM, Eggink HF: Squamous cell carcinoma arising in a residual cyst: a case report, *Int J Oral Maxillofac Surg* 22:350-352, 1993.
19. Kaneshiro S, Nakajima T, Yoshikawa Y, et al: The postoperative maxillary cyst: report of 71 cases, *J Oral Surg* 39:191-198, 1981.
20. Yung W, Morita V: A modified technique for obliteration of large bony defect after cystectomy, *J Oral Maxillofac Surg* 49:689-692, 1991.
21. Hjørting-Hansen E, Schou S, Worsaae N: Suction drainage in the post surgical treatment of jaw cysts, *J Oral Maxillofac Surg* 51:630-633, 1993.
22. Narang R, Jarrett JH: Large traumatic bone cyst of the mandible, *J Oral Surg* 38:617-618, 1980.
23. Patrickios A, Sepheriadou-Mavrapoulou TH, Zambelis G: Bilateral traumatic bone cyst of the mandible: a case report, *Oral Surg* 51:131-133, 1981.
24. Kuroi M: Simple bone cyst of the jaw: review of the literature and report of case, *J Oral Surg* 38:456-459, 1980.
25. Kaugers GE, Cale AE: Traumatic bone cyst, *Oral Surg* 63:318-324, 1987.

26. Winer RA, Doku HC: Traumatic bone cyst in the maxilla, *Oral Surg* 46:367-370, 1978.
27. Shigematsu H, Fujita K, Watanabe K: Atypical simple bone cyst of the mandible: a case report, *Int J Oral Maxillofac Surg* 23:298-299, 1994.
28. Friedrichsen SW: Longterm progression of a traumatic bone cyst: a case report, *Oral Surg* 76:421-424, 1993.
29. Donkor P, Punnia-Moorthy A: Biochemical analysis of simple bone cyst fluid: report of a case, *Int J Oral Maxillofac Surg* 23:296-297, 1994.
30. Yoshikazu S, Tanimoto K, Wada T: Simple bone cyst: evaluation of contents with conventional radiography and computed tomography, *Oral Surg* 77:296-301, 1994.
31. Saito Y, Hoshina Y, Nagamine T, et al: Simple bone cyst: a clinical and histopathologic study of fifteen cases, *Oral Surg* 74:487-491, 1992.
32. Forssell K, Forssell H, Happonen P, Neva M: Simple bone cyst: review of the literature and analysis of 23 cases, *Int J Oral Maxillofac Surg* 17:21-24, 1988.
33. Pogrel MA, Sanders K, Hansen LS: Idiopathic lingual mandibular bone depression, *Int J Oral Maxillofac Surg* 15:93-97, 1986.
34. Correll RW, Jensen JL, Rhyne RR: Lingual cortical mandibular defects, *Oral Surg* 50:287-291, 1980.
35. Karmoil M, Walsh RF: Incidence of static bone defect of the mandible, *Oral Surg* 26:225-228, 1968.
36. Oikarinen VJ, Julku M: An orthopantographic study of developmental bone defects, *Int J Oral Surg* 3:71-76, 1974.
37. Hansson L: Development of a lingual mandibular bone cavity in an 11-year-old boy, *Oral Surg* 49:376-378, 1980.
38. Wolf J, Mattila K, Ankkuriniemi O: Development of a Stafne mandibular bone cavity: report of a case, *Oral Surg* 61:519-521, 1986.
39. Shibata H, Yoshizawa N, Shibata T: Developmental lingual bone defect of the mandible: report of a case, *Int J Oral Maxillofac Surg* 20:328-329, 1991.

40. Mann RW: Three-dimensional representations of lingual cortical defects (Stafne's) using silicone impressions, *J Oral Pathol Med* 21:381-384, 1992.

41. Connor MS: Anterior lingual mandibular bone concavity: report of a case, *Oral Surg* 48:413-414, 1979.

42. Layne EL, Morgan AF, Morton TH: Anterior lingual mandibular bone concavity: report of case, *J Oral Surg* 39:599-600, 1981.

43. Hayashi Y, Kimura Y, Nagumo M: Anterior lingual mandibular bone cavity, *Oral Surg* 57:139-142, 1984.

44. Buchner A, Carpenter WM, Merrell PW, Leider AS: Anterior lingual mandibular salivary gland defect, *Oral Surg* 71:131-136, 1991.

45. Grellner TJ, Frost DE, Brannon RB: Lingual mandibular bone defect: report of three cases, *J Oral Maxillofac Surg* 48:288-296, 1990.

46. Mann RW, Keenleyside A: Developmental lingual defects on the mandibular ramus, *Oral Surg* 74:124-126, 1992 (radiology forum).

47. Kocsis GS, Marcsik A, Mann RW: Idiopathic bone cavity on the posterior buccal surface of the mandible, *Oral Surg* 73:127-130, 1992.

48. Daley TD, Wysocki GP, Pringle GA, Relative incidence of odontogenic tumors and oral and jaw cysts in a Canadian population, *Oral Surg* 77:276-280, 1994.

49. Shear M: Developmental odontogenic cysts: an update, *J Oral Pathol Med* 23:1-11, 1994.

50. Shafer WG: Presentation to American College of Stomatologic Surgeons, Maywood, Ill, 1978.

51. Payne TF: An analysis of the clinical and histopathologic parameters of the odontogenic keratocyst, *Oral Surg* 33:538-546, 1972.

52. Brannon RB: The odontogenic keratocyst: a clinicopathologic study of 312 cases. I. Clinical features, *Oral Surg* 42:54-72, 1976.

53. Brannon RB: The odontogenic keratocyst: a clinicopathologic study of 312 cases. II. Histologic features, *Oral Surg* 43:233-255, 1977.

54. Vedtofte P, Praetorius F: Recurrence of OKC in relation to clinical and histological features: a 20 year follow-up of 72 patients, *Int J Oral Surg* 8:412-420, 1979.

55. Zachariades N, Papanicolaou S, Triantafyllou D: Odontogenic keratocysts: review of the literature and report of sixteen cases, *J Oral Maxillofac Surg* 43:177-182, 1985.

56. Forssell K, Forssell H, Kahnberg KE: Recurrences of keratocysts: a long-term follow-up study, *Int J Oral Maxillofac Surg* 17:25-28, 1988.

57. Oikarinen VJ: Keratocyst recurrences at intervals of more than 10 years: case reports, *Br J Oral Maxillofac Surg* 28:47-49, 1990.

58. Crowley TE, Kaugers GE, Gunsolley JC: Odontogenic keratocysts: a clinical and histologic comparison of the parakeratin and orthokeratin variants, *J Oral Maxillofac Surg* 50:22-26, 1992.

59. Vuhahula E, Nikai H, Ijuhin N, et al: Jaw cysts with orthokeratinization: analysis of 12 cases, *J Oral Pathol Med* 22:35-40, 1993.

60. Williams TP: Discussion—odontogenic keratocysts: clinicopathologic study of 87 cases, *J Oral Maxillofac Surg* 48:599-600, 1990.

61. Wright JM: The odontogenic keratocyst: orthokeratinized variant, *Oral Surg* 51:609-618, 1981.

62. Forssell K, Sorvari TE, Oksala E: A clinical and radiographic study of odontogenic keratocysts in jaws, *Proc Finn Dent Soc* 70:121-134, 1974.

63. Williams TP, Conner FA: Surgical management of the odontogenic keratocyst: aggressive approach, *J Oral Maxillofac Surg* 52:964-966, 1994.

64. Meiselman F: Surgical management of the odontogenic keratocyst, *J Oral Maxillofac Surg* 52:960-963, 1994.

65. Salmassy DA, Pogrel MA: Liquid nitrogen cryosurgery and immediate bone grafting in the management of aggressive primary jaw lesions, *J Oral Maxillofac Surg* 53:784-790, 1995.

66. Partridge M, Towers JF: The primordial cyst (odontogenic keratocyst): its tumour-like characteristics and behaviour, *Br J Oral Maxillofac Surg* 25:271-279, 1987.

67. Holmlund A, Anneroth G, Lundquist G, Nordenram Å: Ameloblastomas originating from odontogenic cysts, *J Oral Pathol Med* 20:318-321, 1991.

68. Regezi JA, Kerr DA, Courtney RM: Odontogenic tumors: analysis of 706 cases, *J Oral Surg* 36:771-778, 1978.

69. Lipani CS, Natiella JR, Greene GW Jr: The hematopoietic defect of the jaws: a report of 16 cases, *J Oral Pathol* 11:411-416, 1982.

70. Standish S, Shafer W: Focal osteoporotic bone marrow defects of the jaws, *J Oral Surg* 20:123-128, 1962.

71. Auclair PL, Cuenin P, Kratochuil FJ, et al: A clinical and histomorphologic comparison of the central giant cell granuloma and the giant cell tumor, *Oral Surg* 66:197-208, 1988.

72. Whitaker SB, Waldron CA: Central giant cell lesions of the jaws: a clinical, radiologic, and histopathologic study, *Oral Path* 75:199-208, 1993.

73. Chuong R, Kaban LB, Kozakewich H, Perez-Atayde A: Central giant cell lesions of the jaws: a clinicopathologic study, *J Oral Maxillofac Surg* 44:708-713, 1986.

74. Raibley SO, Shafer WG: Unpublished data, 1979.

75. Sidhu MS, Parkash H, Sidhu SS: Central giant cell granuloma of jaws: review of 19 cases, *Br J Oral Maxillofac Surg* 33:43-46, 1995.

76. Ficarra G, Kaban LB, Hansen LS: Giant cell lesions of the jaws: a clinicopathologic and cytometric study, *Oral Surg* 64:44-49, 1987.

77. Betts NJ, Stewart JCB, Fonseca RJ, Scott RF: Multiple central giant cell lesions with a Noonan-like phenotype, *Oral Surg* 76:601-607, 1993.

78. Cherrick HM: Presentation to the American Association of Oral and Maxillofacial Surgeons, Las Vegas, Sept 1983.

79. Eisenbud L, Stern M, Rothberg M, Sachs SA: Central giant cell granuloma of the jaws: experiences in the management of thirty-seven cases, *J Oral Maxillofac Surg* 46:376-384, 1988.

80. Kermer C, Millesi W, Watzke IM: Local injection of corticosteroids for central giant cell granuloma: a case report, *Int J Oral Maxillofac Surg* 23:366-368, 1994.

81. Harris M: Central giant cell granulomas of the jaws regress with calcitonin therapy, *Br J Oral Maxillofac Surg* 31:89-90, 1993.

82. Rao P, Solomon M, Auramides A, et al: Brown giant cell tumors associated with second hyperparathyroidism of chronic renal failure, *J Oral Surg* 36:154-159, 1978.

83. Waldron CA: Fibro-osseous lesions of the jaws, *J Oral Maxillofac Surg* 51:828-835, 1993.

84. Summerlin DJ, Tomich CE: Focal cementoosseous dysplasia: a clinicopathologic study of 221 cases, *Oral Surg* 78:611-620, 1994.

85. Waldron CA, Giansanti JS: Benign fibro-osseous lesions of the jaws: a clinical-radiologic-histologic review of sixty-five cases. I. Fibrous dysplasia of the jaws, *Oral Surg* 35:190-201, 1973.

86. Waldron CA, Giansanti JS: Benign fibro-osseous lesions of the jaws: a clinical-radiologic-histologic review of sixty-five cases. II. Benign fibro-osseous lesions of periodontal ligament origin, *Oral Surg* 35:340-350, 1973.

87. Sciubba JJ, Yoonai F: Ossifying fibroma of the mandible and maxilla: review of 18 cases, *J Oral Pathol Med* 18:315-321, 1981.

88. Zachariades N, Vairaktaris E, Papanicolaou S, et al: Ossifying fibroma of the jaws: review of the literature and report of 16 cases, *Int J Oral Surg* 13:1-6, 1984.

89. Koury ME, Regezi JA, Perrott DH, Kaban LB: "Atypical" fibro-osseous lesions: diagnostic challenges and treatment concepts, *Int J Oral Maxillofac Surg* 24:162-169, 1995.

90. Polak M, Polak G, Brocheriou C, Vigneul J: Solitary neurofibroma of the mandible: case report and review of the literature, *J Oral Maxillofac Surg* 47:65-68, 1989.

91. Burkers EJ: Vascular leiomyoma of the mandible: report of a case, *J Oral Maxillofac Surg* 53:65-66, 1995.

CHAPTER 20

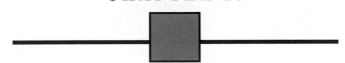

Multilocular Radiolucencies

NORMAN K. WOOD
PAUL W. GOAZ
ROGER H. KALLAL

Multilocular radiolucencies of the oral cavity include the following:

ANATOMIC PATTERNS
MULTILOCULAR CYST
AMELOBLASTOMA
CENTRAL GIANT CELL GRANULOMA
GIANT CELL LESION OF
   HYPERPARATHYROIDISM
CHERUBISM
ODONTOGENIC MYXOMA
ODONTOGENIC KERATOCYST
ANEURYSMAL BONE CYST
METASTATIC TUMORS TO THE JAWS
VASCULAR MALFORMATIONS AND
   CENTRAL HEMANGIOMA OF BONE

RARITIES
Ameloblastic variants
Arteriovenous malformations
Burkitt's lymphoma
Calcifying epithelial odontogenic tumor
Cementoossifying fibroma[1]
Central calcifying odontogenic cyst[2]
Central giant cell tumor
Central salivary gland tumors[3]
Central odontogenic and nonodontogenic
   fibromas[4,5]
Chondroma
Chondrosarcoma

Fibromatosis
Fibroodontogenic dysplasia[6]
Fibrous dysplasia
Hemangiopericytoma
Immature odontoma
Langerhans' cell disease (eosinophilic
   granuloma)
Leiomyoma
Lingual mandibular bone defect
Neurilemoma
Neuroectodermal tumor of infancy
Osteomyelitis
Pseudotumor of hemophilia[7]
Squamous odontogenic tumor

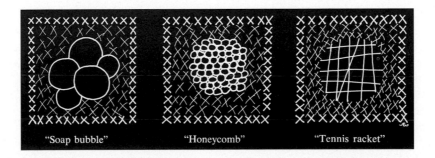

"Soap bubble"   "Honeycomb"   "Tennis racket"

Multilocular radiolucencies are produced by multiple, adjacent, frequently coalescing, and overlapping pathologic compartments in bone. They may occur in the maxilla but are found more commonly in the mandible.

Whereas all the entities included in this chapter appear as multilocular lesions, they may also occur as single, cystlike radiolucencies or even as poorly-defined radiolucencies. The presentation of these lesions in the outline at the beginning of this chapter and in Chapter 19 is according to incidence (to whatever extent such order is known or ordering is possible).

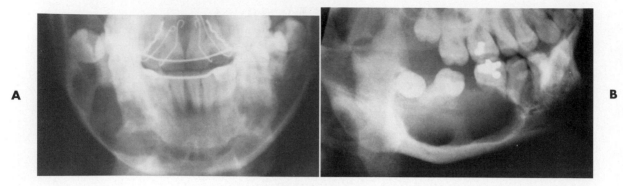

Fig. 20-1. Pseudomultilocular radiolucencies. Both lesions proved at surgery to be unilocular. **A,** Traumatic bone cyst. **B,** Ameloblastoma. (Courtesy M. Kaminski, deceased, and S. Atsaves, Chicago.)

Unilocular lesions that have perforated the cortical plate in one or more areas may cause radiographic images that resemble those from multilocular entities (Fig. 20-1). The true multilocular lesion contains two or more pathologic chambers partially separated by septa of bone, which are usually discernible on radiographic examination. On occasion, the septa may be so thin and their images so indistinct as to cause the multilocular lesion to appear unilocular on radiographic examination.

The terms *soap bubble, honeycomb,* and *tennis racket* are frequently used to describe the various radiographic images of multilocular lesions. *Soap bubble* is reserved for lesions consisting of several circular compartments that vary in size and usually appear to overlap somewhat. *Honeycomb* applies to lesions whose compartments are small and tend to be uniform in size. The *tennis racket* designation is descriptive of lesions composed of angular rather than rounded compartments that result from the development of more or less straight septa. Therefore these compartments tend to be triangular, rectangular, or square. (Refer to the introductory figure for this chapter.)

In this chapter, *multilocular* is used only as a radiographic, not a microscopic, description. Many lesions demonstrate microscopic projections, but these tiny bosses are usually not large enough to be evident on radiographic examination. When studying radiographs of the lesions described in this chapter, the clinician should know that the radiolucent areas making up the images are not empty spaces, as they appear; rather, they are compartments filled usually with neoplastic tissue or at least with cystic fluid or blood.

The following presentation includes descriptions of the primary and distinctive features of each lesion, illustrations of the development of a differential diagnosis, and discussion of the contributing circumstances and considerations that support a suggested course of treatment.

ANATOMIC PATTERNS

To prevent their being mistaken for multilocular lesions, two normal radiolucent structures of the perioral regions

and their radiographic variations are described in this section: the maxillary sinus and bone marrow spaces.

The maxillary sinus usually has several compartments that project into the surrounding maxilla and zygoma and give the radiographic appearance of septa dividing the sinus into lobes.

When many such lobes or compartments are present, the soap-bubble image may result (Fig. 20-2). The anatomic location of the variable extensions of the sinus and the relative location of adjacent structures on radiographs taken from different angles, coupled with the absence of symptoms, are usually sufficient to identify these areas as pouches from the maxillary sinus.

Bone marrow spaces and trabecular patterns appear frequently as multilocular radiolucencies, especially in the mandible (Fig. 20-3). When these spaces and patterns resemble pathologic multilocular radiolucencies, a comparison with the pattern of trabeculation in the remainder of the jawbone usually shows a similar image, so the examiner can conclude with reasonable certainty that the region is a normal variation.

When a trabecular pattern appears only as an isolated area, the correct diagnosis is more difficult to make. In the absence of additional manifestations of disease, however, a satisfactory technique is to observe the area semiannually with radiographs to be certain that no growth occurs and that it is a benign variation of the normal trabecular pattern.

MULTILOCULAR CYST

The multilocular cyst is the most frequently encountered pathologic multilocular radiolucency in the jaws. It is always of the soap-bubble variety, occurs most frequently in the mandible (usually in the premolar and molar region), and varies greatly in size (Fig. 20-4).

Theoretically, any cyst that occurs in the jaws could develop multiple compartments, but the radicular and fissural cysts are usually unilocular lesions, whereas in particular the odontogenic keratocyst, the primordial cyst,

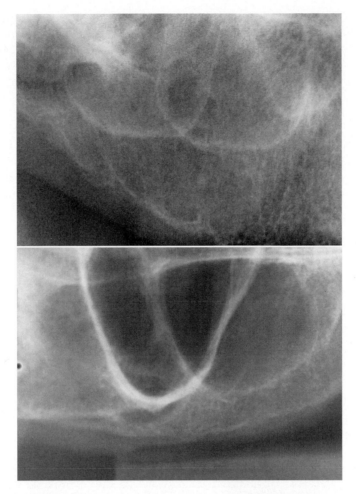

Fig. 20-2. Maxillary sinus showing multilocular patterns.

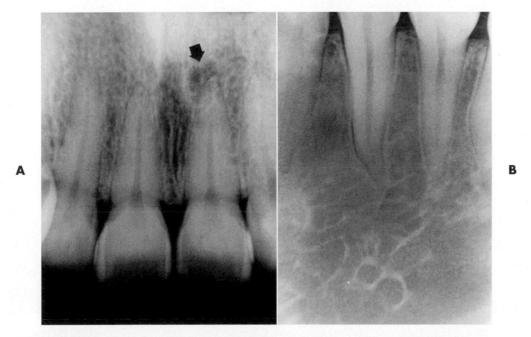

Fig. 20-3. Marrow spaces showing soap-bubble patterns. The arrow in **A** identifies a multilocular bone marrow space at the apices of the central incisor root.

the dentigerous cyst, and the residual cyst occur with some frequency as multilocular cysts.

Features

The multilocular cyst is a true cyst of the jaws and may be found in any age-group but is more frequent in persons over 15 years of age. The small cyst is usually asymptomatic and generally noticed on routine radiographic examination (see Fig. 20-4). It increases in size slowly and may cause displacement of adjacent teeth and occasionally root resorption, but it rarely gives rise to a paresthesia unless it is secondarily infected. If undetected, the cyst may expand the cortical plates as it enlarges and may become apparent on clinical examination as a smooth, bony-hard swelling. If the overlying bone becomes quite thin, a crackling sound (crepitus) may be produced by palpation. Later, if the covering plate is destroyed, the cyst appears as a soft to rubbery, fluctuant mass with perhaps a bluish color.

Aspiration usually yields a thin, straw-colored fluid unless the mass is a keratocyst, which yields a thick, granular, yellow fluid that requires a large-bore needle for successful aspiration. Microscopic study reveals a lumen lined with epithelium and surrounded by a cyst wall varying in thickness and in fibrous tissue content. The botryoid odontogenic cyst is a particular multilocular cyst that gives a "grape bunch" multilocular radiolucent appearance[8-11] (see Fig. 20-4, *B*). It is thought to be a variant of lateral (developmental) periodontal cyst.[12-15]

Differential Diagnosis

All the lesions in this chapter must be considered in the differential diagnosis of multilocular cyst. These are

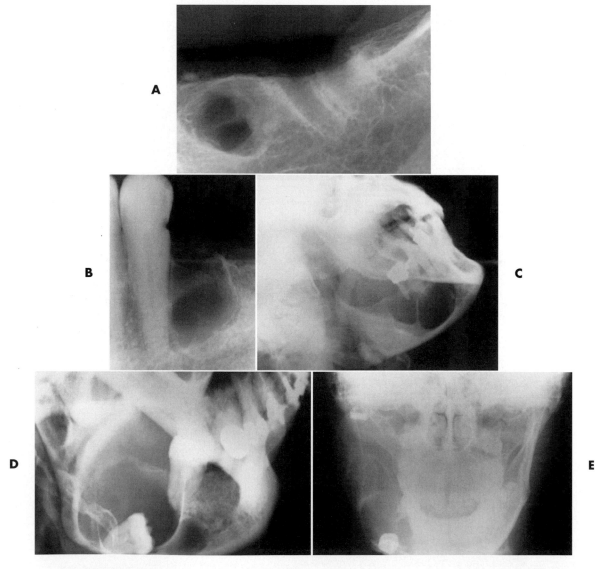

Fig. 20-4. Multilocular cysts. **A,** Residual cyst. **B,** Botryoid cyst. **C,** Radicular cyst. **D** and **E,** Dentigerous cysts. (**A** courtesy M. Smulson, Maywood, Ill; **C** courtesy R. Kallal, Flossmoor, Ill; **D** and **E** courtesy O.H. Stuteville, deceased.)

given in the differential diagnosis section at the end of this chapter and in Table 20-1.

Management

The treatment of cysts is discussed in detail in Chapters 16 and 17. Many factors must be considered before a method of treatment is selected for the multilocular cyst. Enucleation and curettement through bony septa is the treatment of choice for multilocular cysts. Ensuring that all compartments have been eradicated is especially difficult if the more conservative methods are used. However, a conservative approach may be preferable in some cases.

Because the central hemangioma represents a threat of uncontrolled hemorrhage when it is unexpectedly encountered at surgery and because it might be confused with another entity detailed in this chapter, aspiration of any lesion is in order. This test is best used just before initiation of the surgical procedure because of the possibility of contaminating the lesion during aspiration.

AMELOBLASTOMA

The ameloblastoma represents approximately 11% to 13% of all odontogenic tumors.[16,17] They are usually described as locally invasive. It may cast a unilocular cystlike radiolucency or a multilocular image. The multilocular image may be of the soap-bubble or the honeycomb variety (Fig. 20-5). The ameloblastoma is discussed in detail in Chapters 17 and 18 as a unicystic radiolucency. Bone resorption may be mainly mediated by interleukin-1α and interleukin-6: these are synthesized mainly in the stellate reticulum–like cells.[18]

Features

The ameloblastoma grows slowly and silently without clinical signs in the early stages.[19] Later, it can cause migration, tipping, and mob.ility of teeth; root resorption; and paresthesia of the lip. In one series, 81% showed root resorption compared with 55% showing dentigerous cysts.[20] In the advanced stages, this neoplasm may expand cortical plates but frequently erodes them and invades the soft tissue. At this point the ameloblastoma presents clinically as a smooth-surfaced local expansion

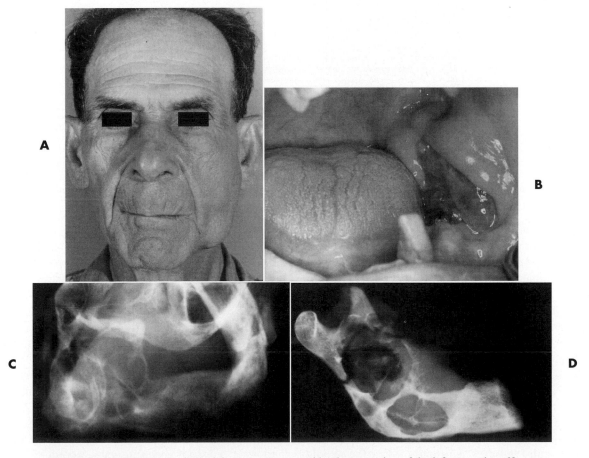

Fig. 20-5. Ameloblastoma. **A,** Facial asymmetry caused by the expansion of the left ramus in a 68-year-old man. **B,** Intraoral swelling in the third molar region of the same patient. The ulcerated surface was caused by trauma from a maxillary molar. **C,** Left lateral oblique radiograph in the patient in **C. D,** Radiograph of the surgical specimen showing the soap-bubble pattern.   *Continued*

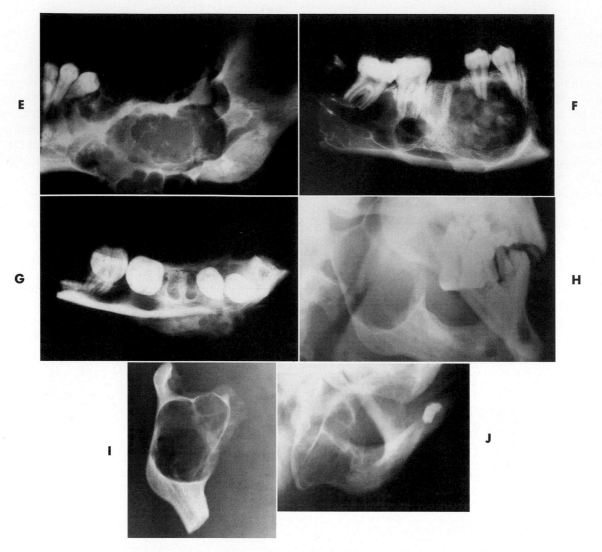

Fig. 20-5, cont'd. Ameloblastoma. **E** to **J,** Radiographs of other ameloblastomas. (Honeycomb patterns are apparent in **E** and **G,** soap-bubble patterns are evident in **H** and **I,** and the angular multilocular pattern is shown in **J.**) (**E** courtesy P. Akers, Chicago; **F** to **J** courtesy O.H. Stuteville, deceased.)

of the jaw producing asymmetry. Lesions may be composed of solid tumor, cystic areas, or both.

The majority (83.5%[21] to 88%[22]) occur in the mandible, where 61% of total tumors involve the third molar region and ascending ramus.[22] It is generally considered to be gender neutral, although it may be slightly more common in men.[23] Incidence peaks between 20 and 50 years, with an average age of 40 years.[24]

Radiographically, these multilocular lesions may appear in a soap-bubble, honeycomb, or tennis-racket pattern (see Fig. 20-5). In places, cortices are spared and expanded, and in other regions, they are destroyed; root resorption is a common finding (see Fig. 20-5).

Although maxillary ameloblastomas are less common, they are potentially lethal,[19] especially when the maxillary sinus is involved or tumor cells invade through bone into the soft tissue. From 71%[25] to 85%[26] occur distal to the canine. Recurrence rates (33%[26] to 53.3%[27]) are higher than those for mandibular tumors, and when con-

servative surgery is used, there is a recurrence rate of 82.5%.[27] A 50% recurrence rate has been reported when the maxillary sinus is involved.[26]

The maxilla lacks the thick, compact plates that tend to limit mandibular ameloblastomas. Maxillary tumors are close to the nasal cavity with its sinuses, orbital contents, pharyngeal tissues, and vital structures at the base of the skull. This contributes to invasion and makes complete resection of the tumor more difficult.

Microscopically, there are at least five histologic types of true ameloblastoma: follicular, plexiform, acanthomatous, desmoplastic, and granular cell (Fig. 20-6). Vickers and Gorlin[28] delineate the histologic criteria for the ameloblastoma. A difference in aggressiveness or tendency to recur does not appear to vary according to histopathologic type. Recently, it has been shown that the desmoplastic ameloblastoma has a greater tendency to occur in the anterior regions of the jaws and characteristically shows a mixed radiolucent-radiopaque pattern radiographically

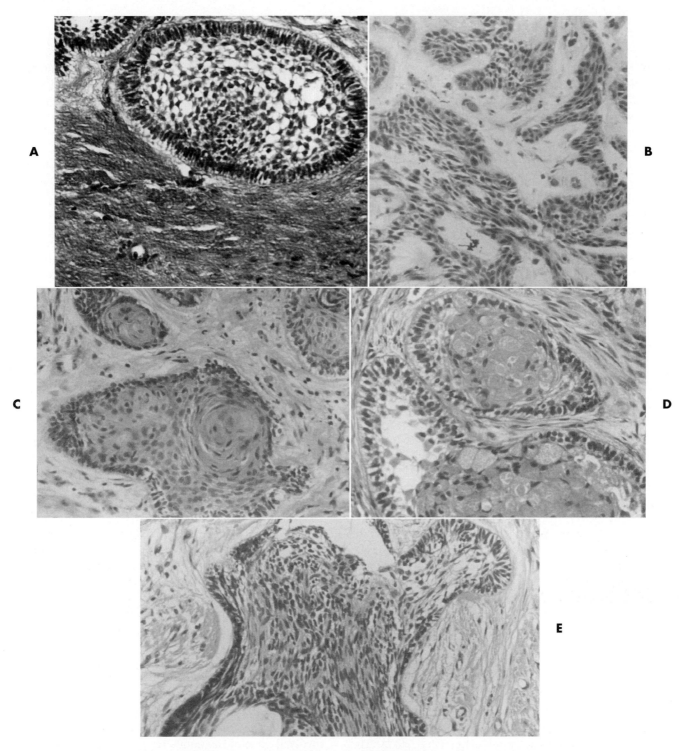

Fig. 20-6. Microscopic types of ameloblastoma. **A,** Alveolar (follicular). **B,** Plexiform. **C,** Acanthomatous. **D,** Granular cell. **E,** Desmoplastic. (**A** courtesy E. Peters, Edmonton, Alberta, Canada.)

(see Fig. 25-18) much like fibroosseous lesions.[22,29,30] One study reports that this variant had a predilection for the maxilla.[29] Slootweg and Müller[31] describe in detail the malignant variants of ameloblastoma and discuss the efficacy of the terms *malignant ameloblastoma* and *ameloblastic carcinoma.* Extraosseous ameloblastomas are rare lesions that occur mostly on the gingiva. They are found in older individuals and follow a nonaggressive course.[32]

Differential Diagnosis

For a discussion of the differential diagnosis of ameloblastoma, see the section on differential diagnosis at the end of this chapter, Table 20-1, and the section on the differential diagnosis of ameloblastoma in Chapters 17 and 18.

Management

The relatively radical surgical treatment of ordinary multilocular ameloblastomas is predicated on the high frequency of recurrence, which results from the small fingers of tumor that extend beyond the apparent margins. It has been reported that ameloblastoma extends 2.3 to 8.0 mm beyond its radiographic margins.[33] Oral surgeons have recommended resecting margins 1 cm[33] to 2 cm into normal bone.[34]

Mehlisch, Dahlin, and Masson[35] aptly describe the successful treatment of an ameloblastoma as that which achieves an acceptable prognosis and causes minimal disfigurement.[35] Their criteria are based on a compromise between variables such as the age and general health of the patient and the size, location, and duration of the tumor. The complete spectrum of approaches, ranging from conservative curettement to wide-block resection, has been practiced over the years. Wide-block resection, with placement of a bone graft, has produced the lowest recurrence rate. Less radical treatment appears to be effective for tumors that are located in the anterior part of the jaw and that measure less than 5 cm in diameter. Ameloblastomas occurring in the anterior region of either jaw have the lowest recurrence rates.

Once the diagnosis of ameloblastoma has been established by biopsy, the first stage of treatment calls for an accurate assessment of extent of tumor by imaging.[19,36] The second stage calls for total excision based on the findings in the first stage.[19] The treatment of choice appears to be resection of the tumor with a 1- to 2-cm margin of normal bone and soft tissue as confirmed by frozen section.[36] The age of the patient and size of the neoplasm may indicate more conservative surgery. The older patient may not be able to tolerate the radical surgery, and life expectancy may modify the concern for recurrence. If the tumor is small and confined to bone, surgery may be less radical.[36] Lifetime follow-up is required.[36]

CENTRAL GIANT CELL GRANULOMA

The central giant cell granuloma may occur initially as a solitary, cystlike radiolucency, but as it grows larger, it frequently develops an architecture that causes a soap-bubble type of multilocular radiolucency (Fig. 20-7). Although trauma was thought to be the causative factor, now many pathologists believe that this is not true; the cause is still in doubt. The central giant cell granuloma is discussed in detail in Chapter 19.

Differential Diagnosis

For a discussion of the differential diagnosis of central giant cell granuloma, see the section on differential diagnosis at the end of this chapter, Table 20-1, and the section on the differential diagnosis of giant cell granuloma in Chapter 19.

GIANT CELL LESION OF HYPERPARATHYROIDISM

The clinical, radiographic, and histologic characteristics of the giant cell lesion of hyperparathyroidism are identical to those of the giant cell granuloma. It occurs as a unilocular or multilocular radiolucency (Fig. 20-8) and is found in patients with primary, secondary, or tertiary hyperparathyroidism. Establishing its identity depends on demonstrating the concomitant parathyroid hormone or kidney disorder. This giant cell lesion is discussed in detail in Chapter 19. Hyperparathyroidism is discussed in detail in Chapter 23.

Differential Diagnosis

For a discussion of the differential diagnosis of the giant cell lesion of hyperparathyroidism, see the section on differential diagnosis at the end of the chapter, Table 20-1, and the section on the differential diagnosis of giant cell lesion in Chapter 19.

CHERUBISM

Although cases without familial involvement have been reported,[37,38] cherubism (familial intraosseous swelling of the jaws) is usually inherited as an autosomal dominant trait. Penetrance is 100% pronounced in male patients.[38] The disease presents with two or more separate, multilocular-appearing lesions (Fig. 20-9). Sometimes the interlocular bone becomes so indistinct that the multilocular appearance is lost.

Features

Cherubism occurs in patients between the ages of 2 and 20 years. It usually commences bilaterally in the rami of the mandible and becomes apparent as painless swellings of the face in these areas. Occasionally the whole mandible is involved. Other bones (e.g., the walls of the maxillary sinus, orbital floor, and tuberosity regions) may also be affected, and the resultant enlargement in these areas produces the cherublike expression by tilting the eyeballs superiorly (see Fig. 20-9). The lesion grows slowly, expanding but not perforating the cortex. Paresthesia is not a feature.

At approximately 8 or 9 years of age, growth of the pathologic region may plateau. At puberty, the lesion may begin to regress. Usually the bony architecture returns to normal by age 30, except for a few instances in which the involved bone of the ramus retains an appearance that resembles ground glass on radiographic examination. Some patients may demonstrate a persistent swelling for years.

A few posterior teeth may be missing in this disease because of the early developing, expanding masses; these expansions destroy the buds and the incipient follicles.

On posteroanterior views the teeth associated with the lesion often seem to be hanging in air. On microscopic examination the lesion is composed of fibroblasts in a highly vascular stroma. The few multinucleated giant cells occur in clusters (see Fig. 20-9). A perivascular eosinophilic cuffing is often present.

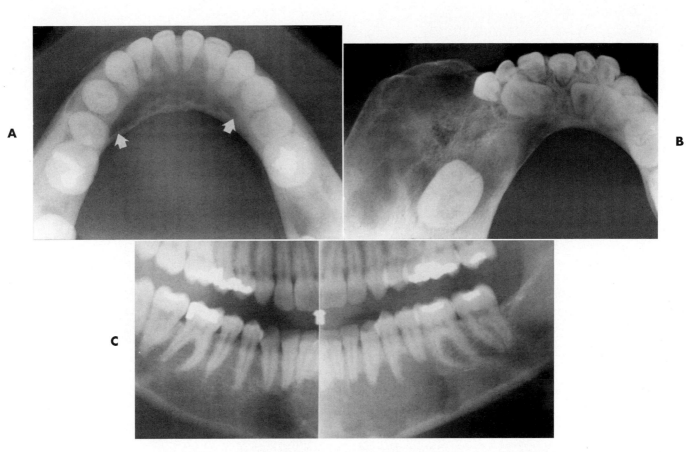

Fig. 20-7. Giant cell granuloma. **A,** Arrows indicate the lateral limits of the soap-bubble lesion. **B,** Large soap-bubble lesion producing marked expansion in the mandible of a 5-year-old boy. See Fig. 19-15, *D,* for the histopathologic features of the lesion.**C,** Lesion in a middle-aged woman. (**A** and **B** courtesy R. Goepp, Chicago; **C** courtesy V. Barresi, DeKalb, Ill.)

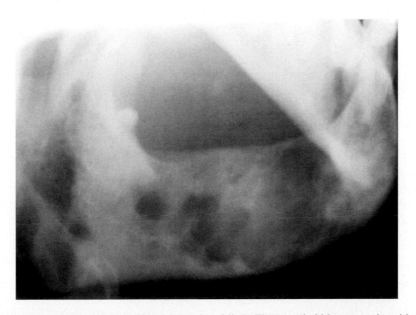

Fig. 20-8. Brown giant cell lesion of hyperparathyroidism. The soap-bubble pattern is evident. (From Rotblat S, Laskin D: Radiolucent lesions of the mandible: differential diagnosis and report of case, *J Oral Surg* 27:820-825, 1969.)

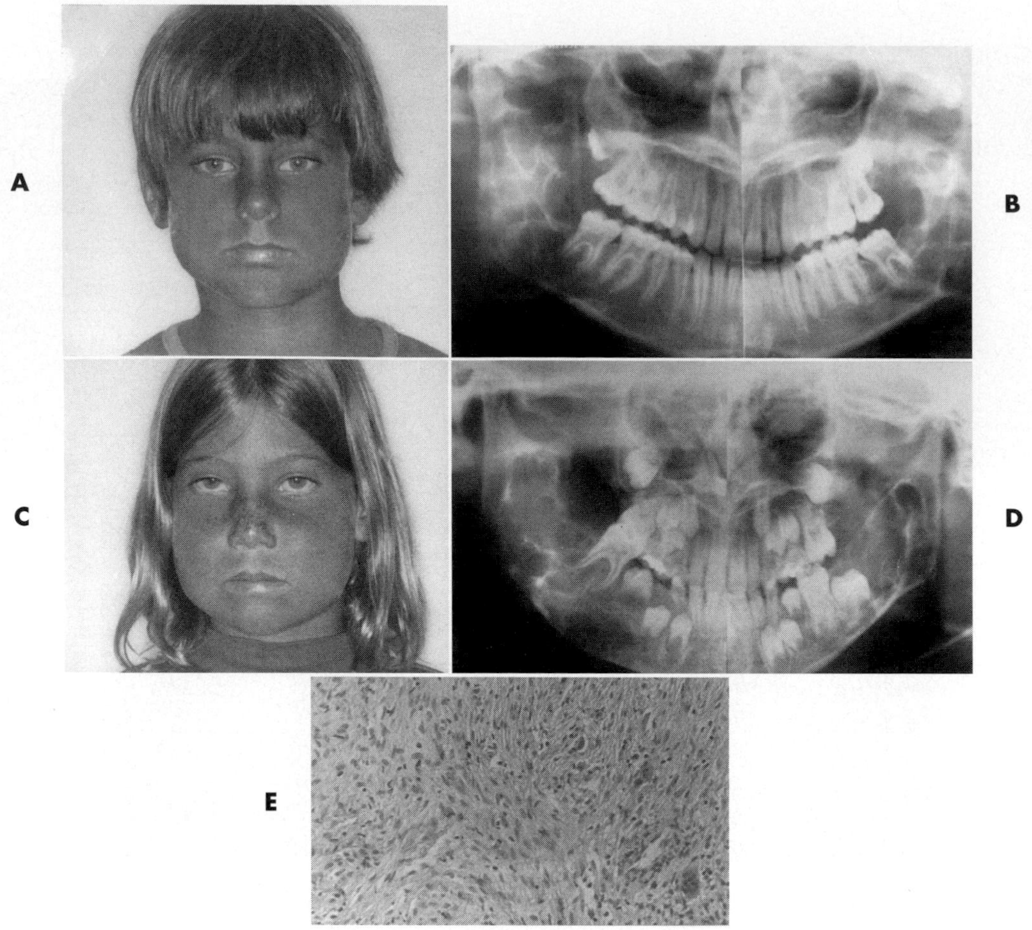

Fig. 20-9. Cherubism. **A,** Clinical appearance of bilateral expansion of the rami in a 12-year-old boy. **B,** Panograph revealing the bilateral soap-bubble expansions of the rami. The maxilla was not involved in this case. **C** and **D,** Seven-year-old sister of the patient in **B.** The maxilla and mandible are involved. The superior tilt of the eyeballs gives the cherubic appearance. **E,** Microscopy of cherubism. (**A** to **D** courtesy J. Hebert, Houston.)

Differential Diagnosis

The multiple lesions occurring bilaterally in the ramus—coupled with the cherubic appearance, the specific age-group, and a history of familial involvement—should readily guide the clinician to the correct impression. This disease is the only entity in this chapter with characteristics specific enough to enable the clinician to feel confident of the working diagnosis. Nevertheless, because nonfamilial cases and unilateral lesions have been reported, the clinician should also consider a list of possible diagnoses. Multiple multilocular lesions with giant cells are seen in hyperparathyroidism and in some cases of Noonan's syndrome,[39] so these must be excluded as well. Other similar, uncommon lesions are multiple or diffuse fibromatous lesions, multiple odontogenic fibromas, and fibroodontogenic dysplasia.[6] The last lesion is polyostotic and familial.[6] For more differential information concerning the differential diagnosis of cherubism, see Table 20-1 and the section on differential diagnosis at the end of the chapter.

Management

The correct identification of the condition and periodic clinical and radiographic examinations are required. If the clinical picture is confusing, an incisional biopsy usually provides the correct diagnosis.

Orthodontic care may be necessary to ensure proper alignment of the teeth, and occasionally, surgical contouring of the lesion is necessary to improve esthetics, especially in cases of rapid growth.[40] Usually by the patient's fourth decade, most evidence of the disease has disappeared, although unusual cases show activity through age 60.[41]

ODONTOGENIC MYXOMA

The odontogenic myxoma is an infiltrative benign tumor of bone that occurs almost exclusively in the jawbones and comprises 3% to 6%[16,17,24] of odontogenic tumors. This neoplasm is mesenchymal, and the myxomatous component is gelatinous in nature. Odontogenic epithelium may occur occasionally in the stroma.

Features

The chief complaint is of a slowly enlarging, painless expansion of the jaw with possible spreading, loosening and migration of teeth. Root resorption is occasionally seen.[42,43] Lip numbness (rare) and pain (occasional) are symptoms.

The majority occur between the ages of 10 and 50 years.[42,43] The average age ranges between 25 and 35 years, and there may be a slight female preference.[42,43] Most are situated in the tooth-bearing areas, and the approximate ratio of maxillary to mandibular lesions has been reported as 3:4.[44] Myxomas of the jawbones tend to be larger in children.[45]

Radiographically the odontogenic myxoma may produce several patterns: unicystic, multilocular, pericoronal (less often), and radiolucent-radiopaque (rare)[42] (Fig. 20-10). Fine intralesional trabeculation occurs in most of the multilocular examples, as well as some of the unicystic types, as a soap-bubble, honeycomb, or tennis-racket pattern. The unilocular types and multilocular types occur with approximately equal frequency.[42] The unilocular variety tend to be small and are mostly located in the anterior region and the multilocular type in the posterior region (see Fig. 20-10). Margins may be poorly or well defined, and border sclerosis have been observed in some cases.[42] The tumor may be scalloped between the roots of the teeth[42] (see Fig. 20-10). The odontogenic myxoma expands the cortical plates, showing as a smooth enlargement of the alveolar and basal bone (see Fig 20-10). Sometimes, it perforates the cortical plate and produces a bosselated surface. The expanding tumor is soft on palpation when the plates are destroyed and gives an impression of fluctuance. Aspiration is nonproductive.

Differential Diagnosis

Again, even though a lesion of this type may be suspected when the clinician encounters a typical multilocular radiolucency, all the lesions discussed in this chapter should be included in the differential diagnosis. If there is a honeycomb or tennis-racket picture, however, the myxoma, along with the ameloblastoma and the intrabony hemangioma, must be especially considered. The honeycomb variant of the myxoma usually shows fine trabeculations within the small lobules, which are not present in the ameloblastoma.

Since the myxoma occurs as a solitary lesion, usually in a slightly older age-group, confusing this lesion with the multiple lesions of cherubism should be obviated.

The giant cell granuloma occurs most commonly in the anterior regions of the jaws, whereas the myxoma is seen most frequently in the ramus and premolar and molar area of the mandible.

Management

Recurrences of the odontogenic myxoma are quite common and have been reported in 25% of treated patients.

Apparently, this behavior is a consequence of the tumor's tendency to spill into the surrounding marrow spaces. To minimize recurrences, resection of the tumor with a generous amount of surrounding bone is necessary in extensive lesions. Teeth in the region often must be included in the section. Many cases are successfully managed, however, with enucleation and curettement. The tumor does not respond to radiation.

ODONTOGENIC KERATOCYST

The odontogenic keratocyst is discussed in detail as a cystlike radiolucency in Chapter 19. It is included in this chapter because it occurs with considerable frequency as a multilocular radiolucency (Fig. 20-11), so it is considered in the differential diagnosis of the lesions included in this chapter. Management is discussed in Chapter 19.

ANEURYSMAL BONE CYST

The aneurysmal bone cyst (ABC) is characterized as a false cyst because it does not have an epithelial lining. It occurs as a unilocular or multilocular radiolucency and, when it is large, frequently balloons out of the cortex (Fig. 20-12). It has been reported most frequently in the long bones, the vertebrae, and occasionally the jaws. Etiology and pathogenesis are unclear.[46] Some pathologists believe that it forms a continuum with the traumatic bone cyst and the central giant cell granuloma. The exaggerated proliferative vascular reaction is thought to be similar to that of the central giant cell reparative granuloma, which it resembles in many respects; however, the developing ABC apparently is continually effused with circulating blood from the injured vessels, whereas granulomas are not.

An extensive study was undertaken to test the hypothesis that the ABC is a secondary phenomenon that occurs in a primary lesion of bone.[20] Areas similar to ABC were found in 28% of the giant cell granulomas, 10% of fibrous dysplasias, one of seven cases of Paget's disease, 14% of fibrosarcomas, and 11% of osteosarcomas. It was postulated that the initiating process of the ABC is the microcyst that forms as a result of intercellular edema in a primary lesion with loose, unsupported stroma.[20]

Features

The ABC is a slow-growing lesion that affects the mandible more often than the maxilla (3:1) but is seldom encountered in the perioral regions.[46] It frequently involves persons under 20 years of age.[20,46] Some 93% occur in the first three decades of life, the molar regions are the most common sites,[20] and there may be a history of rapid growth.[20,46] Because it grows slowly, it may expand and thin the cortical plates, but it usually does not destroy them. It may be slightly tender, and teeth may be missing or displaced, but root resorption is seldom seen.[46] The lesion

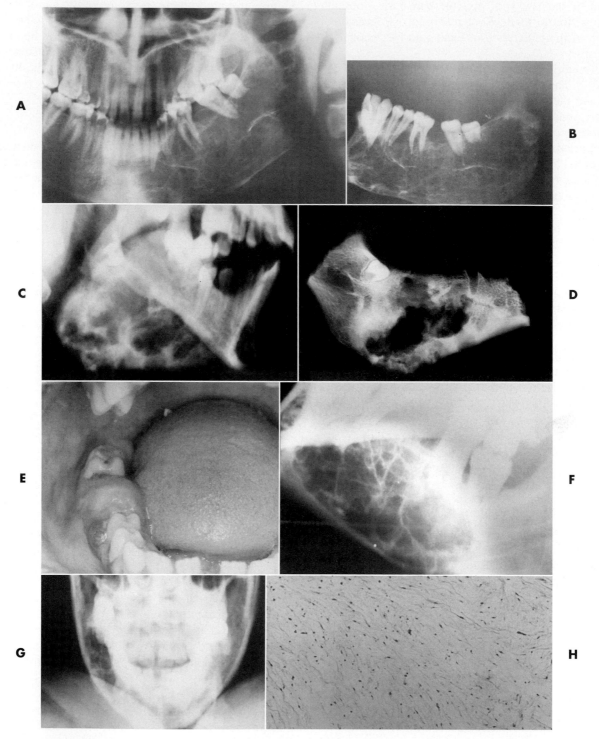

Fig. 20-10. Odontogenic myxoma. **A** and **B,** Orthopantomograph and radiograph of a surgical specimen. **C,** Lateral oblique radiograph of another patient. **D,** Radiograph of the surgical specimen in **A** and **B. E,** Myxoma producing a smoothly contoured oral swelling. **F** and **G,** Radiographs of the lesion shown in **E. H,** Photomicrograph of a myxoma. (**A** and **B** courtesy N. Barakat, Beirut, Lebanon; **C** and **D** courtesy O.H. Stuteville, deceased; **F** courtesy R. Kallal, Flossmoor, Ill; **G** courtesy D. Bonomo, Flossmoor, Ill.)

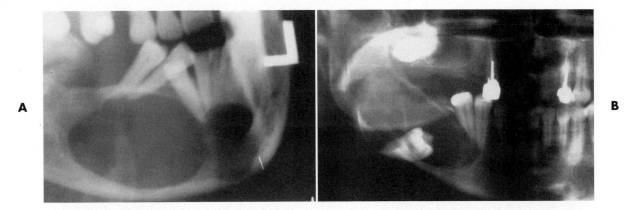

Fig. 20-11. Multilocular odontogenic keratocysts. (**A** courtesy C. Baker, Edmonton, Alberta, Canada; **B** courtesy G. Petrikowski, Edmonton, Alberta, Canada.)

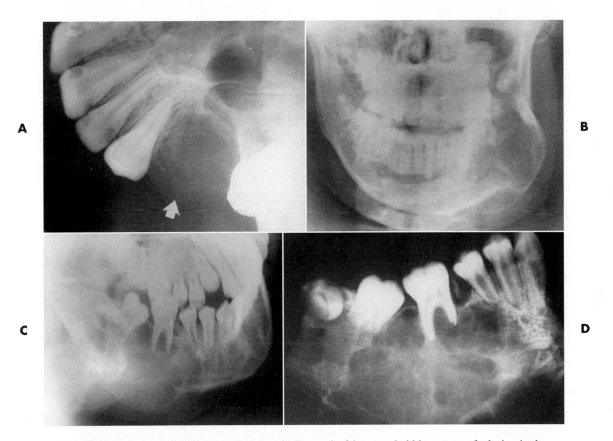

Fig. 20-12. Aneurysmal bone cysts. **A,** Arrow indicates the faint soap-bubble pattern of a lesion in the premolar region. **B** and **C,** Posteroanterior and lateral oblique radiographs of another lesion. **D,** Radiograph of the surgical specimen (from a 12-year-old girl) of lesion shown in **B** and **C.** (**A** courtesy R. Goepp, Chicago; **B** to **D** from Hoppe W: *Oral Surg* 25:1-5, 1968.)   *Continued*

does not appear to show a predilection for either gender.[47,48] Paresthesia is not a feature. ABCs are solitary lesions, but one case of bilateral lesions has been reported.[49] ABCs may occur with other lesions such as fibrous dysplasia, cementoossifying fibroma, and giant cell granuloma.[50]

Grossly the lesion is soft and reddish-brown; because of its rich blood supply, it resembles a sponge filled with blood. On microscopic examination it contains giant cells scattered through a fibrous stroma that contains cavernous, thin-walled blood spaces (see Fig. 20-12). Bone spicules and osteoid may be present.

Differential Diagnosis

The differential diagnosis of aneurysmal bone cyst is discussed in the section on differential diagnosis at the end of this chapter and is included in Table 20-1.

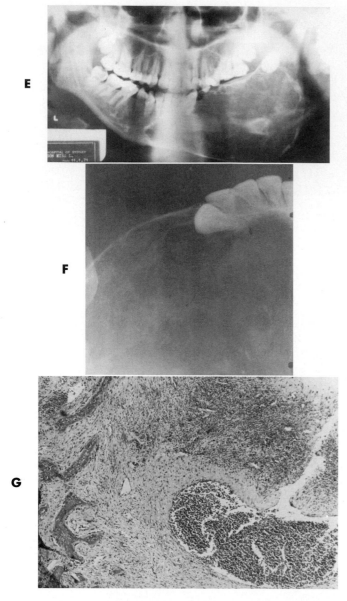

Fig. 20-12, cont'd. Aneurysmal bone cysts. **E** and **F,** Panograph and occlusal radiograph of a large lesion in a 20-year-old woman. The soap-bubble pattern and retention of a thin cortex are characteristic of this benign condition. **G,** Photomicrograph showing a large vascular space. Multinucleated giant cells are frequently present. (**E** and **F** from Oliver LP: *Oral Surg* 35:67-76, 1973.)

Management

Aspiration of the involved area of the bone is recommended to obviate a dangerous, unexpected surgical entrance into an intrabony hemangioma or arteriovenous shunt. Usually a copious amount of blood can be aspirated from an ABC, but not the syringefuls that are readily obtained from hemangiomas or shunts. Surgical curettement is the treatment of choice.[46] Large lesions may require surgical resection and immediate reconstruction.[51] Routine follow-up is necessary because recurrences have been reported.

METASTATIC TUMORS TO THE JAWS

Secondary malignancies to the jawbones represent approximately 1% to 3% of all metastasis, and frequency is more than 2.5 to 5 times the number occurring in oral soft tissue.[52,53] The malignant tumors that most commonly metastasize to the jaw bones in women are those from the breast, adrenal gland, colorectal area, genital organs, and thyroid gland.[52] In men the most common examples are from the lung, prostate, kidney, bone, and adrenal gland.[53] Metastatic jaw tumors arise from parent tumors in other organs and sites, but these are rare.

Malignant cells from distant sites usually are carried via arterial blood. Some pathologists believe, however, that malignant cells travel from their primary site to the jaws via the prevertebral veins of Batson.

Although metastatic jaw tumors are included in this chapter, a multilocular pattern (Fig. 20-13) is not the only one produced by a secondary tumor. Intrabony metastatic jaw tumors may cause several other radiographic appearances:

1. *A solitary, well-defined cystlike radiolucency.* Tumors giving this picture are usually of the slow-growing, well-differentiated type, or the patient is being successfully treated with cytotoxic drugs (see Chapter 19).

2. *A solitary, poorly defined radiolucency.* This picture is usually caused by a localized, rapidly growing tumor (see Chapter 21).

3. *Multiple, separate, poorly defined radiolucencies.* This appearance usually occurs where several foci of malignant nests are present and growing separately from each other (see Chapter 22).

4. *Multiple, punched-out radiolucencies (multiple myeloma–like radiolucencies).* This appearance is characteristic when several nests of slow-growing tumor cells are located close to each other in the bone (see Chapter 22).

5. *Radiopaque patterns with any of the foregoing radiolucent appearances.* The tumors in these cases have induced osteoblastic activity or produced osteosclerosis in the bone (see Chapter 25).

6. *An irregular salt-and-pepper appearance.* This image usually involves a large segment of the jaws and indicates that the tumor is widely disseminated in multiple nests in the bone. These nests appear as small radiolucencies (pepper). They induce sclerotic areas about themselves and thus sprinkle the overall image with small radiopaque foci (salt) (see Chapter 25).

7. *A relatively dense, solitary radiopaque area.* Sometimes a prostatic or a mammary tumor demonstrates osteoblastic activity; the bone thus produced shows as a rather radiopaque area and may resemble condensing osteitis (see Chapter 28).

Features

The mandible is more frequently the site of secondary tumors than the maxilla, and the premolar and molar area is

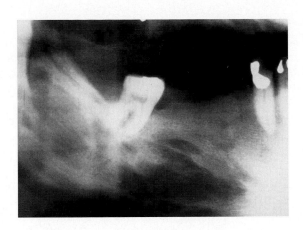

Fig. 20-13. Metastatic renal adenocarcinoma.

the most commonly affected region.[53] Approximately 70% of cases occur in the mandible.[52-54] There may be a slight predilection for female patients,[53-56] but not all reports support this.[52] The oral neoplasm is the first sign of malignancy in about 30% of cases. Most of these are diagnosed in the fifth to seventh decade.[53]

The patient with a secondary tumor of the jaw may seek treatment for pain resulting from a local jaw metastasis or from the parent tumor itself (if it has not been successfully treated). Symptoms induced by the parent tumor usually reflect the altered physiologic condition of the affected organ.

For example, a large bronchogenic carcinoma in the lung may produce symptoms that include chronic cough, hemoptysis, dyspnea, orthopnea, tachycardia, and an overall cachectic appearance. Consequently, if a bony lesion is found in the jaws of such a patient, the clinician should consider the increased possibility of a metastatic tumor. However, in certain cases the metastatic lesion is the first discovered. In such cases the primary tumor is said to be occult, and if the secondary tumor is poorly differentiated on histologic examination, the primary tumor may be difficult to identify and locate.

The local symptoms produced by a metastatic tumor of the jaws are similar to those produced by a primary malignant jaw tumor. These range from nonexistent in an early lesion to marked in an advanced lesion that has caused substantial bone destruction. Advanced tumors often involve the inferior dental canal and cause a paresthesia or anesthesia of the lower lip on the affected side.[57] As the lesion becomes more extensive, pathologic fractures are possible.

An enlarging lesion may erode rapidly through the cortical plates, usually without expanding them, and then invade the surrounding soft tissues, which consequently become fixed to the jawbone. The phenomenon of normally movable soft tissue fixed to bone is an ominous sign and indicates a sclerosing fibrosis or a malignant invasion. If fibrosis, invasion, or both occur in a region where muscles are present, function is impaired. For ex-

ample, a tumor that has perforated the bone and invaded one of the muscles of mastication causes restriction of mandibular opening or perhaps deviation to the affected side. Similarly, if the tongue is fixed in one region by the tumor, its movements may be curtailed, and speech may also be affected.

Pain is not a frequent complaint, but occasionally it is present later, when the tumor encroaches on sensory nerves within bone. The pain is usually of short duration, however, because the tumor rapidly destroys the affected nerve.

The tumor usually erodes rather than expands the adjacent cortical plates. Consequently detectable expansion is not bony hard but firm on palpation. This firmness is caused by the nests, cords, and sheets of closely packed tumor cells that are surrounded by a relatively broad and dense boundary of fibrous tissue. The exophytic mass is frequently nodular and smoothly contoured with a normal-appearing mucosal surface.

The microscopic structure of a metastatic tumor may vary greatly from that of the parent tumor, or both tumors may have an identical microstructure. In addition, a secondary tumor may appear to be more or less malignant than the primary tumor.

Differential Diagnosis

Although the clinician must consider all the multilocular lesions, if the patient has a history of a primary malignancy elsewhere in the body, the possibility of metastatic tumor must be assigned a high rank in the differential diagnosis. For additional features, see Table 20-1.

Management

Once the diagnosis of a metastatic tumor has been made and the primary tumor identified, the case should be managed by a tumor board. The course of action of the tumor board is dictated by the following factors:

1. If the primary tumor was successfully treated some time previously and the present jaw lesion is the only detectable metastatic tumor after a complete examination (including a radiographic skeletal survey and total body bone scans[58]) and if the patient's general medical condition permits, the metastatic lesion should be treated aggressively.

2. Depending on the type and location of the jaw lesion and the way that the primary tumor responded to treatment, surgery, radiation, antitumor medication, or combinations of these techniques might be used. However, the secondary tumor may react differently than the primary tumor to similar treatment.

3. If the primary tumor has shown gross recurrence and there is wide metastases, the jaw lesion should be managed conservatively. Palliative measures may be instituted to provide as much comfort as possible (e.g., a nerve block of alcohol to arrest pain).

VASCULAR MALFORMATIONS AND CENTRAL HEMANGIOMA OF BONE

Vascular malformation (VM) in bone occurs more frequently than the central hemangioma (CH) of bone. Some 35% of VMs occur in bone, whereas CHs of bone are rare.[59] The CH of bone is a benign tumor that rarely occurs in the jaws; it occurs more frequently in the skull and vertebrae. It may be congenital or traumatic in origin and may be difficult to differentiate from VM. The VM and CH are grouped together in this discussion.

These lesions of bone have been referred to as *the great imitators* because they can produce so many different radiographic images. Worth and Stoneman[60] have prepared an excellent and thorough review of the various radiographic appearances. In about 50% of cases a multilocular appearance can be detected (Fig. 20-14).

Another form these lesions can take reveals coarse, linear trabeculae that appear to radiate from an approximate center of the lesion. Small, angular locules of varying shape are seen; however, the general outline is round. A third appearance that may be observed is a cystlike radiolucency with an empty cavity and sometimes a hyperostotic border.

The radiographic margins of these images may be well or poorly defined. Resorption of roots of the involved teeth occurs with some frequency, and calcifications (phleboliths) appearing as radiopaque rings are occasionally seen (see Fig. 29-11).

Features

The usual complaint of a patient with a VM or CH is of a slow-growing asymmetry of the jaw or localized gingival bleeding. Numbness and tenderness or pain may also be described. This solitary tumor is found approximately twice as often in female patients, and about 65% occur in the mandible. Although the tumors affect patients of all ages, the majority have been discovered in patients between the ages of 10 and 20 years. Some tumors demonstrate pulsation and bruits. Paresthesia is occasionally a feature.

As the slow-growing tumor expands the cortical plates, the examiner may observe that the swelling is bony hard and possesses a smooth or bosselated surface covered with a normal-appearing mucosa. Microscopic study reveals that the tumor comprises many thin-walled vascular spaces, some quite cavernous, separated by bony septa (see Fig. 20-14).

Local hemorrhage may be evident around the cervices of the teeth encountered by the enlarging lesion. These teeth may also demonstrate a pumping action; that is, if the examiner depresses the crown of the tooth in an apical direction, the tooth rapidly assumes its former position when the pressure is removed. Extraction of teeth associated with VM or CH lesions may cause a severe bleeding emergency.[61]

Aspiration of an intrabony hemangioma readily yields a copious amount of blood, and caution is necessary. A recommended approach is to introduce the needle through the mucosa some distance from the point where the bone is to be perforated rather than to intro-

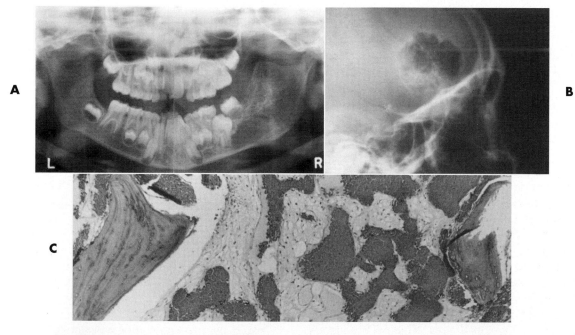

Fig. 20-14. Intrabony hemangioma. **A,** Panograph showing multilocular expansion of the right ramus and the malposition of the developing right mandibular molars. **B,** Multilocular lesion in the frontal bone. **C,** Histologic study showing many vascular spaces between the radiating spicules of bone. (**A** from Gamez-Araujo JJ, Toth BB, Luna A, et al: *Oral Surg* 37:230-238, 1974; **B** courtesy E. Palacios, Maywood, Ill.)

duce the needle directly over the hemangioma. The bleeding that results from the former method usually is more easily arrested, since the mucosa over the point where the bone was penetrated is still intact and the channel through the mucosa can be more effectively compressed.

Differential Diagnosis

Vascular malformations, including the CH, are dangerous lesions of the jaw because rapid exsanguination often follows tooth extraction and jaw fracture.

Because of this lethal potential, when a bony radiolucent lesion is encountered in the jaws, a CH or arteriovenous aneurysm must always be considered, especially since such a tumor often demonstrates a variety of radiographic appearances. Because the multilocular appearance is not pathognomonic for a CH, however, the features listed in Table 20-1 must also be considered in the development of a differential diagnosis.

Specifically the clinician should form a strong impression of CH when encountering a pumping tooth (a tooth that can be pushed apically and then rebounds to its original position) or localized gingival bleeding around a loose tooth coupled with radiographic evidence of bony change in the region. This impression may be further strengthened when large quantities of blood are easily aspirated from the area.

Management

After reaching a working diagnosis of vascular malformation or intrabony hemangioma, the surgeon must urge a complete examination of the patient and the institution of immediate treatment because death may accompany a traumatic incident to the jaws. Angiograms aid greatly in identifying a hemangioma or arteriovenous aneurysm.

Courses of radiation have successfully eliminated manifestations of the tumor and have even induced regression of the bony defects. If the treatment is surgery, a block resection of the lesion (including a safe margin of uninvolved bone) must be performed. Before surgery, the external carotid artery must be ligated, but even this may not control the bleeding during surgery, since unusual vessel aberrations sometimes accompany these tumors.

A promising surgical approach involves ligating the external carotid artery and using muscle fragments, Gelfoam, and metallic pellets (which lodge in the hemangioma) to reduce the size of the vascular channels.[62,63] Recently, absolute alcohol injections[64] and coil embolization[65] have been recommended.

RARITIES

Several other lesions in bone can cause multilocular radiolucencies. These are listed on the first page of this chapter. Figs. 20-15 to 20-20 illustrate some of the entities.

Text continued on p. 354.

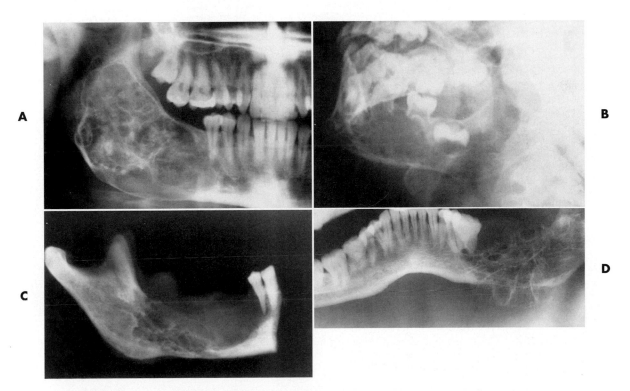

Fig. 20-15. Rare multilocular radiolucencies. **A,** Ameloblastic odontoma. **B,** Intrabony fibroma. **C,** Malignant ameloblastoma. **D,** Intrabony fibroma. (**A** and **C** courtesy O.H. Stuteville, deceased; **B** courtesy N. Barakat, Beirut, Lebanon; **D** from Martis C, Karakasis D: Central fibroma of the mandible: report of a case, *J Oral Surg* 30:758-759, 1972.)   *Continued*

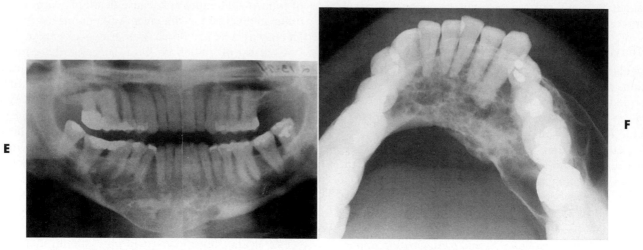

Fig. 20-15, cont'd. Rare multilocular radiolucencies. **E** and **F,** Panographic and occlusal views, respectively, of intrabony central mucoepidermoid carcinoma of the mandible. (**E** and **F** courtesy A. Morof, and W. Schoenheider, Maywood, Ill.)

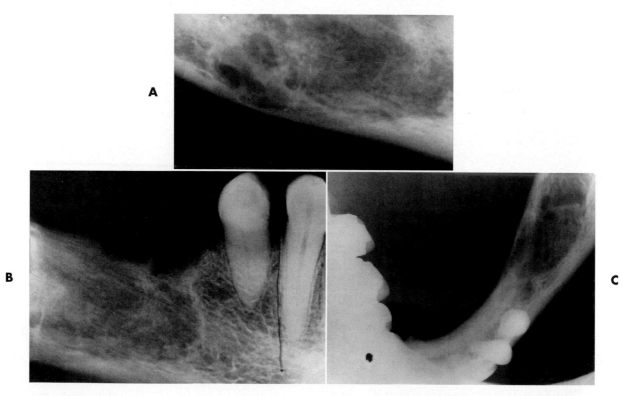

Fig. 20-16. Calcifying epithelial odontogenic tumor of the left mandible. Various views of the same case showing a multilocular pattern. **A** and **B,** Periapical radiographs. **C,** Occlusal radiograph. (Courtesy D. Waite, Lee's Summit, Mo.)

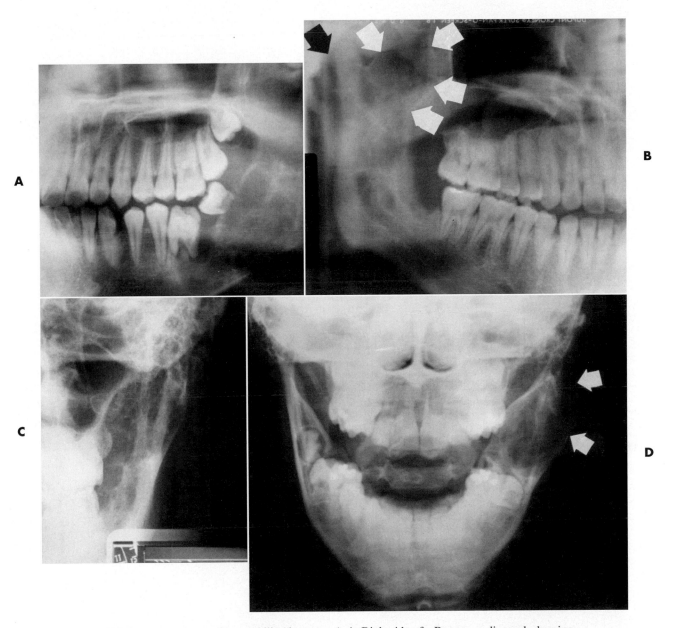

Fig. 20-17. Pseudotumor of hemophilia (three cases). **A,** Right side of a Panorex radiograph showing the multilocular lesion in a 16-year-old boy with severe hemophilia. **B** and **C,** Another case of pseudotumor in the left ramus of a 23-year-old patient with hemophilia. Panorex radiograph (**B**) shows the multilocular expansion of the ramus, coronoid process, and condyle. Cropped posteroanterior radiograph of the affected ramus (**C**) shows the mediolateral dimension of the multilocular expansion. **D,** Another case in an 11-year-old boy with severe hemophilia. Arrows in **B** and **D** identify the lesions. (**A** from Mulkey TF: *J Oral Surg* 35:561-568, 1977; **B** and **C** courtesy T. Mulkey, Inglewood, Calif; **D** courtesy G. Blozis, Columbus, Ohio.)

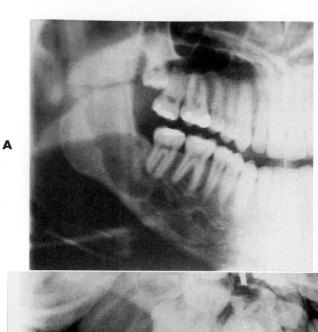

A

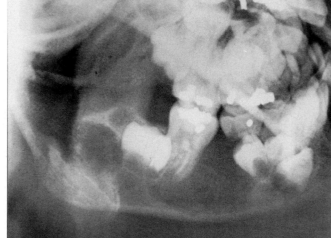

B

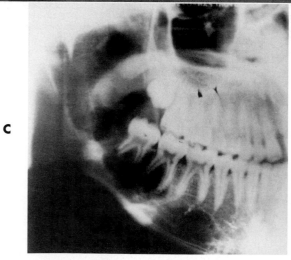

C

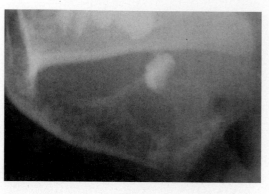

Fig. 20-19. Unilateral case of Burkitt's lymphoma in a young girl. Lateral oblique radiographs showing a rarefied and multilocular pattern of bone loss. (Courtesy D.R. Sawyer, Chicago, and A.L. Nwoku, Lagos, Nigeria.)

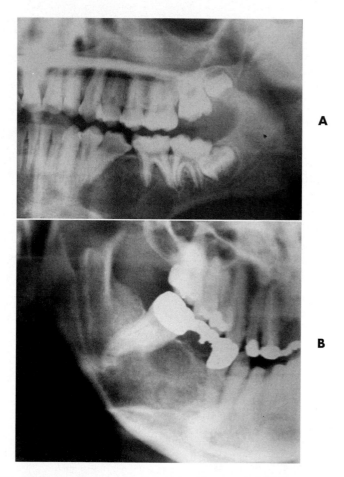

A

B

Fig. 20-18. **A,** Arteriovenous malformation in a 25-year-old man. **B,** Arteriovenous malformation in a 10-year-old patient. **C,** Intra-bony neurilemoma. (**A** from Kelly DE, Terry BC, Small EW: Arteriovenous malformation of the mandible: report of case, *J Oral Surg* 35:387-393, 1977; **B** and **C** courtesy M. Lehnert, Minneapolis.)

Fig. 20-20. Ossifying and cementifying fibroma. **A,** Multilocular-appearing lesion in the premolar and first molar region of the mandible in a 13-year-old boy. **B,** Another multilocular-appearing lesion in the premolar and molar region of a 28-year-old woman. (**A** courtesy W. Heaton, Chicago.)

Table 20-1   Features of lesions producing multilocular radiolucencies

Lesion	Predominant gender	Usual age (years)	Predominant jaw	Predominant region	Predominant multilocular type	Other radiographic appearances	Additional features
Multilocular cysts	M = F	Over 16	Mandible Maxilla—rare	Posterior	Soap bubble	Unilocular cystlike	
Ameloblastomas	M ~ F	20-50 (average 40)	Mandible 80%	Posterior 70%	Soap bubble or honeycomb (Maxilla—unilocular)	Unilocular a. Cystlike b. Ill defined	Paresthesia in some cases
Central giant cell granulomas	$\frac{F}{M} = \frac{2.4}{1}$	Under 30 (average 26)	Mandible 70%	Anterior to second molars	Soap bubble	Unilocular a. Cystlike b. Borders indistinct	Serum chemistry levels normal; 20% cross midline
Giant cell lesion of hyperparathyroidism (secondary)	$\frac{F}{M} = \frac{2}{1}$	50-80	Mandible	None	Soap bubble	Unilocular a. Cystlike b. Borders indistinct	Occasionally multiple; kidney disease; serum calcium level ↓; serum phosphorus level ↑; serum alkaline phosphatase level ↑
Giant cell lesion of hyperparathyroidism (primary)	$\frac{F}{M} = \frac{7}{1}$	30-60	Mandible	None	Soap bubble	Unilocular a. Cystlike b. Borders indistinct	Occasionally multiple; polydipsia; polyuria; serum calcium level ↑; serum phosphorus level ↓; serum alkaline phosphatase level ↑
Cherubism	M > F	2-20	Mandible Maxilla and zygoma	Ramus and molar Sinus and orbital floor	Soap bubble	Unilocular	Multiple; familial history of lesion
Odontogenic myxomas	M = F	10-50 (average 25-35)	Maxilla/mandible = ¾	Ramus, premolar, and molar	Soap bubble Honeycomb Tennis racket	Unilocular a. Cystlike b. Borders indistinct c. Pericoronal	Pain and paresthesia occasionally
ABC	M ~ F	Under 20 70%	Maxilla/mandible = ⅓	Ramus and molar	Soap bubble	Unilocular	Tender
Metastatic tumors to jaws	M = F	50-80	Mandible 95%	Premolar and molar	Honeycomb	Many (see discussion in chapter)	History and symptoms of primary tumor in addition to local lesion
CH of bone	$\frac{F}{M} = \frac{2}{1}$	10-20	Mandible 65%	Body and ramus	Honeycomb	Tennis racket Unilocular a. Cystlike b. Borders indistinct	Local gingival bleeding; pumping action of tooth

~, Approximately equal.

DIFFERENTIAL DIAGNOSIS OF MULTILOCULAR RADIOLUCENCIES

As determined from the previous discussions of multilocular radiolucencies, it is fruitless to attempt to diagnose these lesions using radiographs alone. The clinician can, however, develop a sound differential diagnosis when confronted by a multilocular radiolucency. Table 20-1 lists features of these lesions.

If the suspect region is in the maxillary molar segment of the jaw, a multilobed maxillary sinus must be considered the most likely diagnosis, especially if the pattern is bilateral and the region asymptomatic.

If the multilocular region is in the mandible, the diagnosis most likely is a soap-bubble type of marrow pattern, especially if such a pattern is prominent throughout the mandible.

If the multilocular lesion is situated anteriorly in the jaws of a patient under 30 years of age, it is more likely to be a giant cell granuloma than an ameloblastoma.

If the lesion is situated in the posterior of the mandible in a patient over 30 years of age, it is probably an ameloblastoma, especially if there is an accompanying paresthesia of the lip. If no paresthesia is present, the lesion is more likely a multilocular cyst.

If the patient complains of polydipsia and polyuria or has a history of kidney disease with abnormal serum calcium, phosphorus, and alkaline phosphatase levels, the lesion is most likely a giant cell lesion of hyperparathyroidism.

If the lesions occur in a child and are multiple and if there is a family history of such lesions, the diagnosis is almost certainly cherubism.

A history of primary malignant tumor elsewhere gives metastatic carcinoma a high rank.

Myxoma and CH show several common features: Both frequently have a honeycomb or a tennis-racket appearance, both are usually found in patients between 10 and 30 years of age, and both are usually found in the ramus and premolar and molar regions. Copious amounts of blood obtained by aspiration, the syndrome of the pumping tooth, or cervical hemorrhage are highly suggestive of intrabony hemangioma.

Finally, the clinician must be aware of the various rarities and be ready to elevate one of these within the list of possibilities when the particular circumstances dictate.

REFERENCES

1. Sciubba JJ, Younai F: Ossifying fibroma of the mandible and maxilla: review of 18 cases, *J Oral Pathol Med* 18:315-321, 1989.
2. Buchner A: The central (intraosseous) calcifying odontogenic cyst: an analysis of 215 cases, *J Oral Maxillfac Surg* 49:330-339, 1991.
3. Brookstone MS, Huvos AG: Central salivary gland tumors of the maxilla and mandible: a clinicopathologic study of 11 cases with an analysis of the literature, *J Oral Maxillofac Surg* 50:229-236, 1992.
4. Kaffe I, Buchner A: Radiologic features of central odontogenic fibroma, *Oral Surg* 78:811-818, 1994.
5. Allen CM, Hammond HL, Stimson PG: Central odontogenic fibroma, WHO type, *Oral Surg* 73:62-66, 1992.
6. Dominguez FV, Pezza V, Keszler A: Fibroodontogenic dysplasia: report of two familial cases, *J Oral Maxillofac Surg* 53:1115-1120, 1995.
7. Machado de Sousa SO, Luiz de Piratininga J, Pinto DS Jr, Soares de Araújo N: Hemophilic pseudotumor of the jaws: report of two cases, *Oral Surg* 79:216-219, 1995.
8. Weathers DR, Waldron CA: Unusual multilocular cysts of the jaws (botryoid cysts), *Oral Surg* 36:235-241, 1973.
9. Kaugers GE: Botryoid odontogenic cyst, *Oral Surg* 62:555-559, 1986.
10. Greer RO, Johnson M: Botryoid odontogenic cyst: clinicopathologic analysis of ten cases with three recurrences, *J Oral Maxillofac Surg* 46:574-579, 1988.
11. Eliasson S, Isacsson G, Köndell PA: Lateral periodontal cysts: clinical, radiographical and histopathological findings, *Int J Oral Maxillofac Surg* 18:191-193, 1989.
12. Redman RS, Whitestone BW, Winnie CE, et al: Botryoid odontogenic cyst: report of a case with histologic evidence of multicentric origin, *Int J Oral Maxillofac Surg* 19:144-146, 1990.
13. Rasmusson LG, Magnusson BC, Borrman H: The lateral periodontal cyst: a histopathological and radiographic study of 32 cases, *Br J Oral Maxillofac Surg* 29:54-57, 1991.
14. Altini M, Shear M: The lateral periodontal cyst: an update, *J Oral Pathol Med* 21:245-250, 1992.
15. Shear M: Developmental odontogenic cysts: an update, *J Oral Pathol Med* 23:1-11, 1994.
16. Regezi JA, Kerr DA, Courtney RM: Odontogenic tumors: analysis of 706 cases, *J Oral Surg* 36:771-778, 1978.
17. Daley TD, Wysocki GP, Pringle GA: Relative incidence of odontogenic tumors and oral and jaw cysts in a Canadian population, *Oral Surg* 77:276-280, 1994.
18. Pripatnanont P, Meghji, S: Immunocytochemical localization of osteolytic cytokines in ameloblastomas, *J Dent Res* 74:579, 1995 (abstract 1431).
19. Nastri AL, Wiesenfeld D, Radden BG, et al: Maxillary ameloblastoma: a retrospective study of 13 cases, *Br J Oral Maxillofac Surg* 33:28-32, 1995.
20. Struthers PJ, Shear M: Aneurysmal bone cyst of the jaws. I. Clinicopathologic features, *Int J Oral Surg* 13:85-91, 1984.
21. Regezi JA, Kerr DA, Courtney RM: Odontogenic tumors: analysis of 706 cases, *J Oral Surg* 36:771-778, 1978.
22. Waldron CA, El-Mofty SK: A histopathologic study of 116 ameloblastomas with special reference to the desmoplastic variant, *Oral Surg* 63:441-451, 1987.
23. Kameyama Y, Takehana S, Mizohata M, et al: A clinicopathologic study of ameloblastomas, *Int J Oral Maxillofac Surg* 16:706-712, 1987.
24. Minderjahn A: Incidence and clinical differentiation of odontogenic tumors, *J Maxillofac Surg* 7:142-150, 1979.
25. Sehdev MK, Huvos AG, Strong EW: Ameloblastoma of maxilla and mandible, *Cancer* 33:324-333, 1974.
26. Tsaknis PJ, Nelson JF: The maxillary ameloblastoma: an analysis of 24 cases, *J Oral Surg* 38:336-342, 1980.
27. Cherrick HM: Presentation to American Association of Oral and Maxillofacial Surgeons, Las Vegas, Sept 1983.
28. Vickers RA, Gorlin RJ: Ameloblastoma: delineation of early histopathologic features of neoplasia, *Cancer* 26:699-710, 1970.
29. Kaffe I, Buchner A, Taicher S: Radiographic features of desmoplastic variant of ameloblastoma, *Oral Surg* 76:525-529, 1993.
30. Ng KH, Siar CH: Desmoplastic variant of ameloblastoma in Malaysians, *Br J Oral Maxillofac Surg* 31:299-303, 1993.
31. Slootweg PJ, Müller H: Malignant ameloblastoma or ameloblastic carcinoma, *Oral Surg* 57:168-176, 1984.

32. Buchner A, Sciubba JJ: Peripheral epithelial odontogenic tumors: a review, *Oral Surg* 63:688-697, 1987.

33. Marx RE, Smith BH, Smith BR, et al: Swelling of the retromolar region and cheek associated with limited opening, *J Oral Maxillofac Surg* 51:304-309, 1993.

34. MacIntosh RB: Aggressive surgical management of ameloblastoma, *Clin Oral Maxillofac Surg* 3:73, 1991.

35. Mehlisch DR, Dahlin DC, Masson JK: Ameloblastoma: a clinicopathologic report, *J Oral Surg* 30:9-22, 1972.

36. Williams TP: Management of ameloblastoma: a changing perspective, *J Oral Maxillofac Surg* 51:1064-1070, 1993.

37. DeTomasi DC, Hann JR, Stewart HM: Cherubism: report of a nonfamilial case, *J Am Dent Assoc* 111:455-457, 1985.

38. Kaugers GE, Niamtu J, Svirsky JA: Cherubism: diagnosis, treatment, and comparison with central giant cell granulomas and giant cell tumors, *Oral Surg* 73:369-374, 1992.

39. Betts JN, Stewart JCB, Fonseca RJ, Scott RF: Multiple central giant cell lesions with a Noonan-like phenotype, *Oral Surg* 76:601-607, 1993.

40. Kuepper RC, Harrigan WF: Treatment of mandibular cherubism, *J Oral Surg* 36:638-642, 1978.

41. Waldron CA: Personal communication, 1976.

42. Peltola J, Magnusson B, Happonen R-P, Borrman H: Odontogenic myxoma: a radiographic study of 21 tumors, *Br J Oral Maxillofac Surg* 32:298-302, 1994.

43. Harder F: Myxomas of the jaws, *Int J Oral Surg* 7:148-155, 1978.

44. Farman AG, Nortje CJ, Grotepass FW, et al: Myxofibroma of the jaws, *Br J Oral Surg* 15:3-18, 1977.

45. Keszler A, Dominguez FV, Giannunzio G: Myxoma in childhood: an analysis of 10 cases, *J Oral Maxillofac Surg* 53:518-521, 1995.

46. Hosein M, Motamedi K, Yazdi E: Aneurysmal bone cyst of the jaws: analysis of 11 cases, *J Oral Maxillofac Surg* 52:471-475, 1994.

47. Reyneke J: Aneurysmal bone cyst of the maxilla, *Oral Surg* 45:441-447, 1978.

48. Steidler NE, Cook RM, Reade PC: Aneurysmal bone cysts of the jaws: a case report and review of the literature, *Br J Oral Surg* 16:254-261, 1979.

49. Salmo NAM, Shukur ST, Abulkhail A: Bilateral bone cysts of the maxilla, *J Oral Surg* 39:137-139, 1981.

50. Kershisnik M, Batsakis JG: Pathologic consultation: aneurysmal bone cysts of the jaws, *Ann Otol Rhinol Laryngol* 103:164-165, 1994.

51. Karabouta I, Tsodoulos S, Trigonidis G: Extensive aneurysmal bone cyst of the mandible: surgical resection and immediate reconstruction, *Oral Surg* 71:148-150, 1991.

52. Summerlin D-J, Tomich CE, Abdelsayed RA: Metastatic disease to the jaws. Paper presented to the annual meeting of the American Academy of Oral Pathology, Santa Fe, NM, May 13-18, 1994.

53. Hishberg A, Leibovich P, Buchner A: Metastatic tumors to the jawbones: an analysis of 390 cases, *J Oral Pathol Med* 23:337-341, 1994.

54. Aniceto GS, Peñín AG, Pages R DeLaM, Moreno JJM: Tumors metastatic to the mandible: analysis of nine cases and review of the literature, *J Oral Maxillofac Surg* 48:246-251, 1990.

55. Nishimura Y, Yakata H, Kawaskai T, et al: Metastatic tumors of the mouth and jaws: a review of the Japanese literature, *J Maxillofac Surg* 10:253-258, 1982.

56. Cleveland D, Madani F: Tumors metastatic to the jaws and oral cavity: analysis of 43 cases and review of the recent literature. Paper presented to the American Academy of Oral Pathology, San Francisco, May 9-13, 1992.

57. Cousin GCS, Ilankovan: Mental nerve anesthesia as a result of mandibular metastases of prostatic adenocarcinoma, *Br Dent J* 177:382-384, 1994.

58. Laga EA, Toth BB, Podoloff DA, Keene HJ: Clinical correlation of oral-dental findings with radiographs and total body bone scans, *Oral Surg* 75:253-263, 1993.

59. Kaban LB, Mulliken JB: Vascular anomalies of the maxillofacial region, *J Oral Maxillofac Surg* 44:203-213, 1986.

60. Worth HM, Stoneman DW: Radiology of vascular abnormalities in and about the jaws, *Dent Radiogr Photogr* 52:1-23, 1979.

61. Engel JD, Supancic JS, Davis LF: A case report: arteriovenous malformation of the mandible—life threatening complications during tooth extraction, *J Am Dent Assoc* 126:237-242, 1995.

62. Sadowsky D, Rosenberg RD, Kaufman J, et al: Central hemangioma of the mandible: literature review, case report, and discussion, *Oral Surg* 52:471-477, 1981.

63. Frame JW, Putnam G, Wake MJC, Rolfe EB: Therapeutic arterial embolisation of vascular lesions in the maxillofacial region, *Br J Oral Maxillofac Surg* 25:181-194, 1989.

64. Muto T, Kinehara M, Takahara M, Sato K: Therapeutic embolization of oral hemangiomas with absolute alcohol, *J Oral Maxillofac Surg* 48:85-88, 1990.

65. Perrott DH, Schmidt B, Dowd CF, Kaban LB: Treatment of a high-flow arteriovenous malformation by direct puncture and coil embolization, *J Oral Maxillofac Surg* 53:1083-1086, 1994.

CHAPTER 21

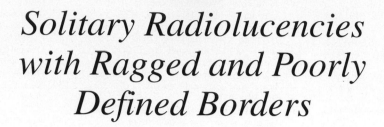

Solitary Radiolucencies with Ragged and Poorly Defined Borders

NORMAN K. WOOD

PAUL W. GOAZ

ORION H. STUTEVILLE

Solitary radiolucencies of the jaws with ragged and poorly defined borders include the following:

CHRONIC OSTEITIS
CHRONIC OSTEOMYELITIS
HEMATOPOIETIC BONE MARROW
   DEFECT
SQUAMOUS CELL CARCINOMA
FIBROUS DYSPLASIA—EARLY LESION
METASTATIC TUMORS TO THE JAWS
MALIGNANT MINOR SALIVARY GLAND
   TUMORS
OSTEOGENIC SARCOMA—OSTEOLYTIC
   TYPE
CHONDROSARCOMA
RARITIES
   Ameloblastic carcinoma
   Ameloblastoma
   Aneurysmal bone cyst
   Angiosarcoma
   Benign tumor in the rarefied jaw

Burkitt's lymphoma
Desmoplastic fibroma
Ewing's sarcoma
Fibromatosis
Fibrosarcoma
Intrabony hemangioma
Langerhans' cell disease (idiopathic histio-
   cytosis)
Liposarcoma
Lymphosarcoma
Malignant ameloblastoma
Malignant fibrous histiocytoma
Malignant lymphoma of bone
Massive osteolysis (phantom bone disease)
Medulloblastoma
Melanoma
Myeloma (solitary, plasmacytoma)
Myosarcoma

Myospherulosis (paraffinoma)
Neuroblastoma
Neuroectodermal tumor of infancy
Neurosarcoma
Odontogenic fibroma
Odontogenic sarcoma
Osteoblastoma
Phosphorus necrosis
Primary intraosseous carcinoma
Reticulum cell sarcoma
Sarcoidosis
Scleroderma
Spindle cell carcinoma
Surgical defect
Tuberculosis
Vascular malformations

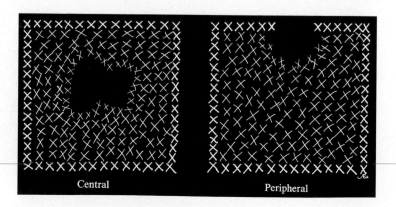

Central   Peripheral

Most solitary radiolucencies with ragged and indistinct borders* are produced by three basic types of pathologic processes: inflammation or infection of bone, fibrous dysplasia (early stage), and osteolytic malignancy of bone. Because of the potentially serious nature of the lesion, every ill-defined radiolucency should be considered malignant until proved otherwise.

Some clinicians depend too heavily on blood chemistry values (such as concentration of plasma calcium, phosphorus, and alkaline phosphatase) for the differentiation of osteolytic lesions. These lesions must cause a substantial amount of bony activity, either mineral absorption or mineral deposition, before significant changes in the blood chemistry values occur. In addition, since pathologic bony activity does not progress at a constant rate, the biochemical values fluctuate with shifts in activity of the pathologic processes. Thus specific altered values of blood chemistry are pathognomonic only periodically and in only a few diseases.

Such instances are identified here when they complement the discussion of a particular entity.

CHRONIC OSTEITIS

Chronic osteitis (chronic alveolar abscess) is a local mild inflammation or infection in bone† that usually occurs around the roots of a tooth. It is commonly a sequela of pulpitis and is perhaps identical to the chronic alveolar abscess discussed as a periapical radiolucency in Chapter 16. It is included in this chapter because it often has ragged, poorly defined borders (Fig. 21-1). As described in Chapter 16, where the features of the chronic alveolar abscess are discussed, the inciting tooth is pulpless and usually tender to percussion. A sinus may be present and may pass through the alveolar bone to open onto the mucosa generally near the level of the apex.

Differential Diagnosis

The presence of an intraalveolar draining sinus is not conclusive evidence that a radiolucent area is a chronic osteitis, an abscess, or osteomyelitis.

Such a lesion could represent an infected malignant tumor in the periapical area. Because of the low incidence of such tumors, however, and because a small malignant lesion is unlikely to become infected, this entity is assigned a low rank in the differential diagnosis of a draining periapical radiolucent lesion.

Management

Although the management of the chronic alveolar abscess is detailed in Chapter 16, it is important to reiterate at least three precepts pertaining to the treatment of radiolucent lesions of the jaws. Compliance with these rules enables the clinician to establish a valid initial diagnosis or at least provides the opportunity to reevaluate the initial impression and treatment. Such confirmation may obviate the disastrous delay that could result if a small periapical malignancy were misdiagnosed as a periapical sequela of pulpitis, treated as such, and then neglected. The three circumstances and the attending considerations follow:

1. If the clinician chooses to treat a periapical radiolucency nonsurgically by obliterating the root canals of the associated tooth, follow-up radiographs are taken to substantiate the initial impression that the bony lesion was pulpoperiapical.
2. If the clinician believes that curettement with or without root resection is needed to complement the canal obliteration, the periapical tissue must be subjected to microscopic examination.
3. If the clinician chooses to extract the tooth, the periapical lesion should also be removed and studied microscopically. Since small malignancies in the area of the roots are uncommon, however, surgical removal and biopsy of every periapical radiolucency are not justified except in extraction cases.

This philosophy ensures the best management of benign-appearing periapical radiolucencies, which include chronic osteitis (chronic alveolar abscess).

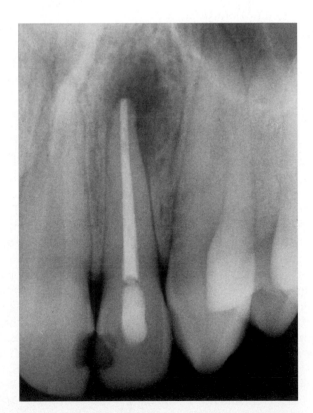

Fig. 21-1. Chronic alveolar abscess at the apex of a lateral incisor preceded the root canal filling, which had been recently completed.

---

*The terms *ragged* and *moth eaten* are also used to connote destructive lesions without smoothly contoured borders. The descriptive phrase *poorly defined* conveys the notion that the borders are fuzzy, indistinct, or difficult to delineate.
†The dry socket is a type of chronic or acute osteitis, but it is excluded from this discussion because it seldom if ever is a diagnostic problem.

CHRONIC OSTEOMYELITIS

Osteomyelitis is an inflammation of the bone caused by pathogenic microorganisms. The disease process is empirically considered osteitis when just the alveolar bone is affected. If the basal bone of the jaws is involved, the process is considered osteomyelitis. The types of osteomyelitis are listed below.

Types of Osteomyelitis

1. Acute osteomyelitis
2. Chronic osteomyelitis
3. Proliferative periostitis
4. Sclerosing osteomyelitis
   a. Local
   b. Diffuse

Chronic osteomyelitis may result from a partial regression of acute osteomyelitis, or it may arise by itself and follow an extended course. A month's duration is arbitrarily used to distinguish between acute and chronic types.[1] Osteomyelitis is uncommon today and seldom occurs in healthy persons, since predisposing factors play important roles in this disease:

1. Hypoxic conditions of the bone related to reduced microvasculature. (This occurs in diabetes, sickle cell anemia, collagen vasular disorders, Paget's disease, osteopetrosis,[1] and florid cementoosseous dysplasia.)
2. Immunodeficiency states such as those seen in acquired immunodeficiency syndrome; leukemia; malnutrition; and prolonged, high-dosage corticosteroid administration
3. Other low-defense-response diseases such as neutropenia and chemotherapy. (A local insult to the jaw such as trauma, surgery, or odontogenic infection may trigger osteomyelitis[1] in these preconditioned individuals. Occasionally, such insults can produce osteomyelitis in normal hosts, but the majority of cases occur in predisposed patients.)

In established cases, this infectious process creates an effective barrier to viable bone and vascularization. The microorganisms are able to initiate thrombosis, and the coagulum produced provides an excellent culture medium for further growth of pathogens.[1] This also functions as an isolating barrier from the host's immune response,[1] from all the benefits of a blood supply already compromised, and from antibiotics. Blood flow generally is increased early in the disease, whereas later in the chronic state, there is a persistent reduction.[2]

Osteomyelitis of the jaws is usually polymicrobial mostly of odontogenic origin.[1] The following bacteria are frequently identified: streptococci, *Bacteroides, Peptostreptococcus,* and other opportunists.[1] As the chronic state is reached, other microorganisms, such as *Actinomyces,*[3-6] *Eikenella,*[3] *Arachnia,*[4] *Coccidioides, Mycobacterium tuberculosis,* and *Klebsiella*[1] may play a major role.

Chronic osteomyelitis may produce at least five different radiographic images: a radiolucency with ragged borders (this chapter), a radiolucency containing one or more radiopaque foci (see Chapter 25), a salt-and-pepper appearance (see Chapter 25), a dense radiopacity (see Chapter 28), and cortical redundancy (see Chapter 28). The patient history, clinical and laboratory features, and processes fundamental to the development of all four types of bony change are basically the same.

Osteoradionecrosis is a condition of bone that has some similarities to osteomyelitis. This disease, which is covered in detail in Chapter 25, seldom occurs as a completely radiolucent lesion. Usually, there is a radiolucency with large radiopaque foci or perhaps a salt-and-pepper appearance.

Microscopic examination of the radiolucent lesions of chronic osteomyelitis shows small spicules of dead bone with empty lacunae scattered throughout necrotic tissue. The radiolucent areas contain varying numbers of lymphocytes, plasma cells, macrophages, and polymorphonuclear leukocytes (see Fig. 16-12). The small sequestra of bone that are microscopically apparent are not large enough to be seen on radiographs.

Features

Although osteomyelitis may occur at any age, it is uncommon in the first three decades except for proliferative periostitis or except when a serious predisposing condition is present. There is a marked predominance for the mandible because of the denser cortical bone and a greater frequency of fractures. In addition, the maxilla enjoys a more generous collateral blood supply, especially in the anterior region. There is also a predilection for male patients, partly because of denser bone and a greater incidence of trauma.

Clinical examination shows signs of infection, which may include inflammation, tenderness, pain, swelling, intraoral and extraoral draining sinus tracts (see Fig. 16-12), regional lymphadenopathy, fever, leukocytosis, and an increased sedimentation rate. Denuded bone may protude from open mucosal or cutaneous ulcers, and small fragments (sequestra) of bone may be shed through these ulcers. The drainage in chronic osteomyelitis is characteristically intermittent and modest in volume.

Radiographically an early acute osteomyelitis does not show bony changes because of the rapid onset. In contrast, one of the images of chronic osteomyelitis is an irregular-shaped radiolucency with ragged, poorly defined borders (Fig. 21-2). The lesion may arise in a recent surgical site or in a fracture line where nonunion may be present. In such a case the lesion often appears as a somewhat linear radiolucency with ragged borders possibly varying in width as it follows the fracture line through the bone (see Fig. 21-2). Often the surrounding bony borders are denser than the adjacent normal bone, reflecting a

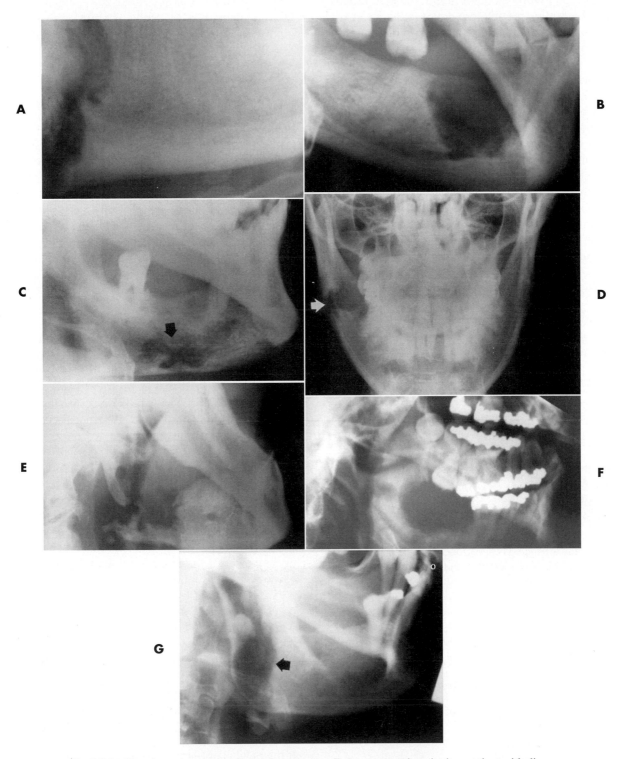

Fig. 21-2. Chronic osteomyelitis. **A,** In a fracture line. **B,** In an extraction site in a patient with diabetes. (See Fig. 16-19, *B,* for an illustration of a draining sinus, and Fig. 16-19, *C,* for the histopathologic appearance of chronic osteomyelitis.) **C** to **E,** Additional examples of osteomyelitis. The arrow in **D** indicates the lesion. **F,** Actinomycotic osteomyelitis. **G,** Airway shadow *(arrow)* simulating a radiolucent pathosis with ragged borders. (**C,** through **E** courtesy O.H. Stuteville, deceased; **F,** courtesy E. Palacios, Maywood, Ill.)

degree of sclerosis induced by the chronic infection. Bone scintigraphy with technetium 99m–labeled diphosphonates is helpful in giving more detail to the lesions.[1,7] Positron emission tomography using radioisotopes of physiologically active compounds, such as glucose, ammonia, and fluoride, is even more useful in helping determine the various margins of metabolic activity.[1]

Osteomyelitis of the mandible most frequently occurs in the body because compound fractures occur more often in this segment.

Intraoral contamination of the fracture site often occurs in compound fractures and increases the likelihood of the development of osteomyelitis. Fractures of the ramus, condyle, and coronoid process seldom become infected; they are rarely compounded in the broken mucosa or skin because of the thick coverage of these segments of the lower jaw by muscles and other tissues. Furthermore, odontogenic infection does not commonly reach these areas because such abscesses occur primarily in the tooth-bearing areas of the jaws.

Differential Diagnosis

The differential diagnosis of osteomyelitis is discussed in the section on differential diagnosis at the end of the chapter.

Management

It is important to work with the patient's physician to bring any predisposing systemic condition under control. The box lists guidelines for the treatment of osteomyelitis.

TREATMENT GUIDELINE FOR ACUTE AND CHRONIC OSTEOMYELITIS

1. Disrupt the infectious foci.
2. Debride any foreign bodies, necrotic tissue, or sequestra.
3. Culture and identify specific pathogens for definitive antibiotic treatment.
4. Drain and irrigate the region.
5. Begin empiric antibiotics based on Gram's stain.
6. Stabilize calcified tissue regionally.
7. Consider adjunctive treatments to enhance microvascular reperfusion (usually reserved for refractory only forms):
   a. Trephination (may be accomplished during debridement)
   b. Decortication (may be accomplished during debridement)
   c. Vascular flaps (muscle)
   d. Hyperbaric oxygen therapy
8. Reconstruct as necessary after resolution of the infection.

From Hudson JW: Osteomyelitis of the jaws: a fifty year perspective, *J Oral Maxillofac Surg* 51:1294-1301, 1993. Adapted from Marx RE: *Oral and Maxillofacial Surgery Clinics of North America: infections of the head and neck*, Philadelphia, PA, 1992, WB Saunders.

Penicillin is still the empiric antibiotic of choice, but other drugs, such as metronidazole, clindamycin, ticarcillin, clavulanic acid, cephalosporins, carbapenem, vancomycin, and fluoroquinolones,[1] are used for refractory microorganisms. Hyperbaric oxygen therapy is useful in refractory cases.

HEMATOPOIETIC BONE MARROW DEFECT

Hematopoietic bone marrow defect has been described as a periapical radiolucency in Chapter 16 and as a cystlike radiolucency in Chapter 19. On occasion, it can appear as a radiolucent lesion with ragged, poorly defined borders (see Fig. 16-1, *A*); as such, it requires differentiation from the other lesions in this chapter. Usually the suspicion index is so low with these lesions that the clinician chooses to radiograph the lesion in 3 to 6 months' time to ensure that it is not enlarging. Nevertheless, in cases of suspected metastatic disease, such a lesion can be worrisome.

SQUAMOUS CELL CARCINOMA

Squamous cell carcinoma (SCC) (epidermoid carcinoma) is described as a red lesion in Chapter 5, a white lesion in Chapter 8, a red and white lesion in Chapter 9, an exophytic lesion in Chapter 10, and an ulcer in Chapter 11. This discussion primarily concerns its bone-destroying image.

Since SCC is the most common malignant lesion in the oral cavity, it is also the most common malignancy to produce radiolucent lesions in the jawbones. Not all intraoral SCCs invade and destroy bone, however. SCCs of the tongue, floor of the mouth, buccal mucosa, lips, soft palate, and oropharynx do not invade bone unless they are permitted to reach a large size and develop unusual extensions. The carcinomas that originate on or near the crest of the mandibular ridge, the maxillary molar ridges, or the posterior hard palate are the tumors most likely to cause bony destruction.

SCCs that destroy bone can be divided into two basic types according to origin: the peripheral or mucosal type, which is the more common, and the central type (within bone), which is rare. Since clinicians and pathologists have become increasingly aware of the central type, however, more of these tumors are being recognized and reported; they are thought to originate in nests of epithelium within the jawbone or the epithelial lining of cysts.

Features

If the SCC is of the peripheral type, the patient may complain of a worsening oral ulcer or red, white, or pink mass that bleeds easily; may be somewhat tender; and is situated over bone of the alveolus or jaw or on the hard palate (Fig. 21-3). The patient usually has poor oral hygiene and admits to the heavy use of tobacco, alcohol, or both. Other frequent complaints are foul odor and taste, paresthesia or anesthesia of the lip, and crepitus and pain on movement of the jaw if a pathologic jaw fracture is present (Fig. 21-4).

If the lesion is of the central type, the patient commonly complains of pain, paresthesia, and swelling of the jaw; the last occurs in the advanced stages of the disease (Fig. 21-5, *E*).

Radiographs of bone invaded by the peripheral type of SCC show lytic defects with either of two forms:

1. A roughly semicircular or saucer-shaped erosion into the bony surface with ragged, ill-defined bor-

ders that illustrate the varying, uneven osteolytic invasion (see Fig. 21-3)

2. A mandibular lesion with advanced horizontal resorption of the ridge and basal bone in the involved area and only a thin, fairly well-defined inferior border of the mandible remaining (see Fig. 21-5)

Small sequestra of bone may be present as ragged radiopacities in either type of radiolucent lesion (see Fig. 25-2).

Teeth involved with either type of lesion become loose, migrate, or show root resorption.

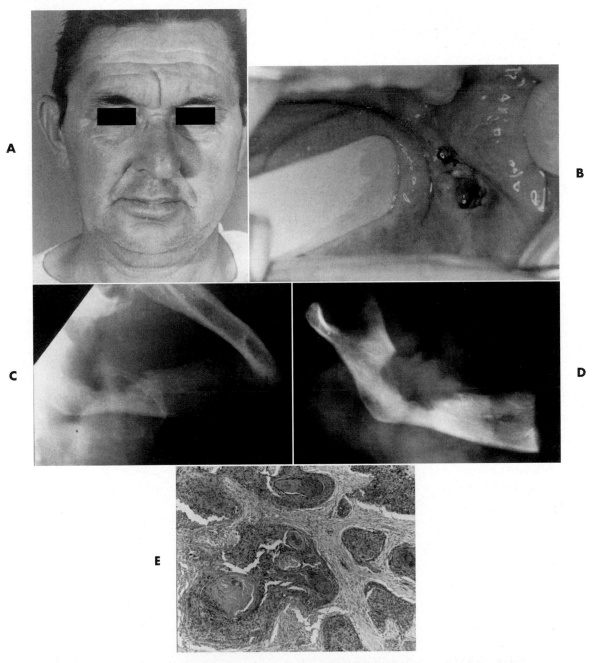

Fig. 21-3. SCC. **A,** Expansion of the face over the left molar region in a 58-year-old man. **B,** Intra-oral ulcer in the same patient as **A**. **C,** Lateral oblique radiograph showing a craterlike radiolucency with ragged ill-defined borders. **D,** Radiograph of the surgical specimen. **E,** Histopathologic appearance of the tumor showing features of a moderately well-differentiated SCC.

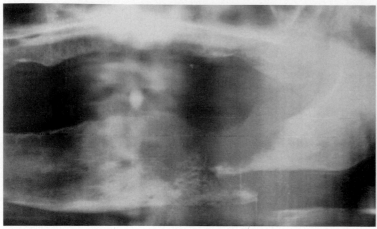
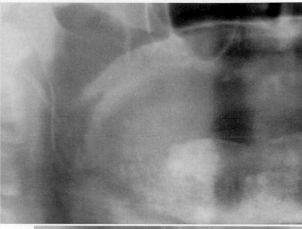
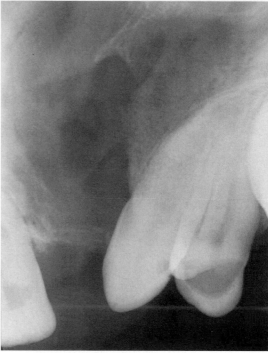

Fig. 21-4. **A** and **B,** Pathologic fractures of the mandible through areas of gross bone destruction caused by invasive SCCs. **C,** Ragged, ill-defined radiolucency between the maxillary canine and central incisor tooth. Although this appearance resembles malignancy, the missing bone represents an anterior cleft palate. (**A** and **B** courtesy W. Heaton, Chicago.)

If the advancing tumor has originated in the maxillary sinus, destroyed the sinus floor, and infiltrated the posterior maxillary ridge, its ragged and poorly defined borders are toward the ridge, away from the sinus. This is a useful feature for helping to differentiate between a tumor that has originated in the maxillary sinus and one that has developed on the ridge. If the maxillary sinus has been involved with a malignant tumor, the sinus walls are less well defined, and perhaps one or more are destroyed. The sinus itself shows increased density (clouding) where it is filled with tumor (see Fig. 21-5).

Enlarged regional lymph nodes are a frequent finding in oral SCC and may represent a benign lymphadenitis (caused by infection of the lesion by the oral flora) or metastatic spread. Inflamed nodes can usually be differentiated from nodes involved with metastatic tumor because the former tend to be enlarged, painful, firm, freely movable, and discrete, whereas the latter are enlarged, painless, very firm, immovable, and frequently matted to-gether. In advanced cases the lymph nodes are bound to adjacent structures by the infiltrating tumor and are not freely movable.

Central SCC is rare and frequently appears radiographically as a more or less rounded radiolucency completely surrounded by bone[8,9] (see Fig. 21-5). When its early appearance suggests that it originated in the wall of a cyst, the radiographic borders are evenly contoured and well defined. Later, when the malignancy has infiltrated the cyst wall and destroyed the bone, its borders become ragged and lose their sharp definition.[10,11]

The histologic picture of the central or peripheral type may be quite variable, ranging from a well-differentiated to a very anaplastic SCC (see Fig. 21-3).

Differential Diagnosis

The problems attending a differential diagnosis of SCC are discussed in the section on differential diagnosis at the end of the chapter.

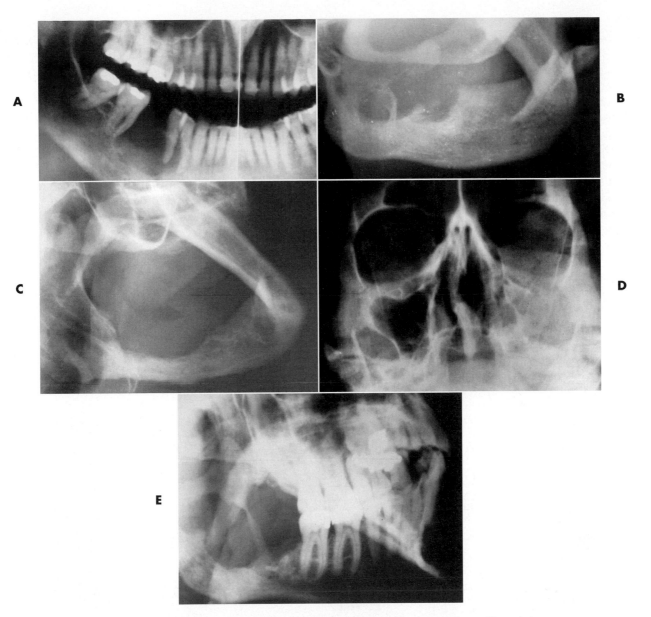

Fig. 21-5. SCC. **A** to **C,** Peripheral lesions in the mandible. **D,** Lesion in the maxillary sinus. Clouding of the left sinus with partial destruction of its walls is evident. **E,** Central lesion in the ramus. (**A** to **C** courtesy O.H. Stuteville, deceased; **E** courtesy R. Nolan, Williston, ND.)

Management

The management of patients with SCC is discussed in Chapter 35.

FIBROUS DYSPLASIA

Fibrous dysplasia (FD) is considered a hamartomatous fibroosseous lesion not of periodontal ligament origin.[12-14] The etiology is unknown, but it is a lesion of bone that produces lysis of bone with fibrous proliferation as a replacement (radiolucent) in its early stage. As it ages, immature bone is laid down in Chinese-character spicules (radiolucent-radiopaque [see Chapter 25]), which become larger and larger (radiopaque [see Chapter 28]). FD generally remodels into regular bone as the lesion regresses.

FD may involve a single bone (monostotic) or multiple bones (polyostotic). Some of the polyostotic cases are examples of McCune-Albright syndrome and are accompanied by skin pigmentation and endocrine disturbances.[12] The monostotic type is the most common and frequently involves the jaws and the skull.[12] Mandibular lesions are usually solitary, but maxillary lesions may involve neighboring bones, and this is referred to as *craniofacial FD.*

FD of the jaws is basically a disease of children, adolescents, and young adults that tends to stabilize and essentially stops growing as skeletal maturity is reached.[12] Malignant change in FD is rare, and most of the reported cases have been after radiation.[12]

Features

FD occurs equally in male and female patients and occurs in the maxilla slightly more often than the mandible. The molar, premolar, and canine areas; the ramus; and the symphysis are the most frequent sites in the mandible. In the maxilla the molar-premolar region is the most common, with the maxillary sinus being frequently involved. In the maxilla, FD may extend into the floor of the orbit, the zygomatic process, and backward toward the base of the skull, as well as through the maxillary sinus.

The lesion forms a painless expansion of the jawbone, which grows slowly over the years and then stops. The expansion is usually fusiform (low plateau) rather than nodular or dome shaped and is firm, smoothly contoured, and covered with normal mucosa. Teeth in the region remain firm and are not displaced.

Radiographically, early lesions of FD are usually an elongated rather than spherical radiolucency (Fig. 21-6). Margins are ragged and poorly defined, merging imperceptibly into normal bone.[14] These lesions are usually situated deep within the jawbone rather than superficially in the alveolus (see Fig. 21-6). The maturing changes that produce the ground-glass appearance may commence at the periphery of the lesion as shown in Fig. 21-6, *C*. This may be an early hint as to the lesion's correct identity. Gross displacement of the mandibular canal is frequently associated with FD of the mandible.[15]

Microscopically the immature trabeculae are of immature woven bone in fibroblastic stroma.[12] Many of these trabeculae are separate and have irregular shapes like Chinese characters and are not rimmed with osteoid tissue or osteoblasts (see Fig. 21-6, *D*).[12] More mature lesions develop lamellae that run parallel with each other.[12] Other features are discussed in detail in Chapter 25.

Differential Diagnosis

The differential diagnosis of FD is discussed in the section on differential diagnosis at the end of the chapter.

Management

In the usual course of FD of the jaws, a lesion occurs in a child or adolescent, grows slowly for a decade or so, stabilizes, and slowly returns to normal. Such cases require observation and perhaps orthodontic care. More exten-

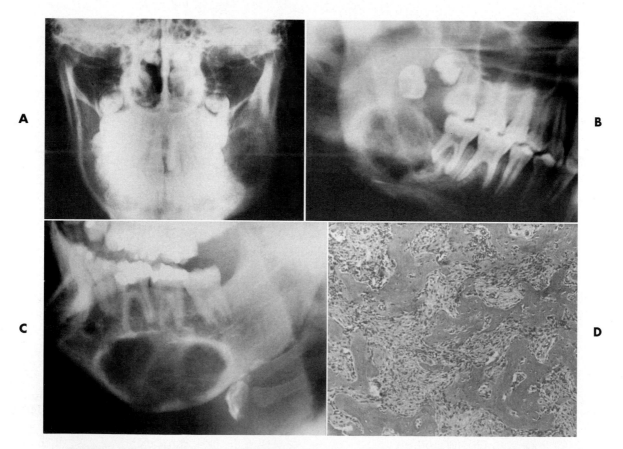

Fig. 21-6. Fibrous dysplasia. **A** and **B,** In a 16-year-old boy. The ill-defined margins of the radiolucency are evident. **C,** Advanced ossification at the periphery in this patient. The dense radiopaque appearance gives the illusion of well-defined borders. Periapical films of this peripheral region show a ground-glass pattern. **D,** Chinese-character spicules of woven osteoid tissue among the active fibrous stroma. Osteoblastic rimming is not a feature.

sive cases may require recontouring for cosmetic or functional improvement. Between 25% and 50% of patients may show some regrowth after recontouring, but this appears to be more common in younger patients.[12] It would seem to be advisable to delay surgery as long as possible unless there are other indications.[12]

METASTATIC TUMORS TO THE JAWS

Metastatic tumors to the jaws are second only to primary SCC as the most common group of malignant tumors in the jawbones. This group is discussed in detail in Chapter 20, where it is stated that the secondary jaw tumor may produce six different radiographic images. One possible image is a solitary radiolucency with ragged, poorly defined borders, which is the feature of metastatic tumors that explains their inclusion in this chapter.

Features

Although a secondary jaw tumor may occur at the periphery and expand into the oral cavity, it is usually situated deep in the bone. When it produces an expansion, the exophytic lesion is usually dome shaped and covered with normal-appearing mucosa. Later, because it increases in size and there is concomitant masticatory trauma, a mucositis commonly develops on its surface; if the trauma continues, the surface ulcerates and becomes necrotic (Fig. 21-7).

A radiolucent area that may vary greatly in size with ragged, poorly defined borders is one of the radiographic pictures produced by metastatic tumors in the jaws (Fig. 21-8). Pain and numbness are common complaints. If there are teeth in the affected section of bone, any combination of the loss of lamina dura, root resorp-

tion, and loosening and malposition of teeth may be found (see Fig. 21-8, *A*).

Findings from an extensive autopsy study of sectioned mandibles from patients with carcinoma have been reported.[16] Reporting on sites of metastatic tumors in the mandible, these authors indicate that 16% of total cases reveal metastatic involvement of this bone. They conclude that hematopoietic areas in the mandible appear to favor early deposition of tumor cells.[16]

Differential Dagnosis

A discussion of the differential diagnosis of metastatic tumors to the jaws is presented in the section on differential diagnosis at the end of the chapter.

Management

The management of metastatic tumors is discussed in Chapter 20.

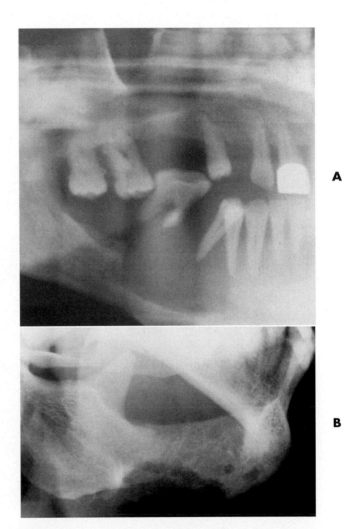

A

B

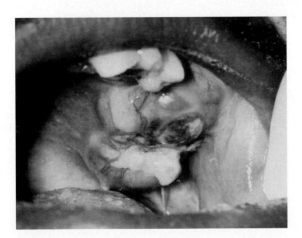

Fig. 21-7. Metastatic bronchogenic carcinoma to the maxillary molar and premolar region. Note the smoothly contoured, expanded alveolar process in this region. The surface ulceration recently occurred as a result of masticatory trauma. (Courtesy W. Heaton, Chicago.)

Fig. 21-8. Metastatic tumors. **A,** Metastatic bronchogenic carcinoma. **B,** Metastatic SCC from the lower lip. (**A** courtesy R. Latronica, East Amhurst, NY; **B** courtesy O.H. Stuteville, deceased.)

MALIGNANT MINOR SALIVARY GLAND TUMORS

Malignant minor salivary gland tumors (MMSGTs) are discussed in Chapter 10 as exophytic lesions and in Chapter 11 as mucosal ulcers. This chapter emphasizes the features produced by these tumors when they infiltrate and destroy jawbone. The more commonly occurring varieties are the pleomorphic and monomorphic adenocarcinoma, adenoid cystic carcinoma, mucoepidermoid tumor, and unclassified adenocarcinomas.

The incidence of MMSGT is much lower than that of SCC, and they may occur as peripheral or central lesions. Peripheral MMSGTs may occur anywhere in the soft tissue lining of the oral cavity but seldom in the gingiva or on the anterior hard palate because the minor salivary glands are not usually found in these sites.

The posterior hard palate, upper lip and anterior vestibule, retromolar regions, and base of the tongue are the peripheral sites most commonly affected. The glandular tissue is most proximal to bone on the hard palate and in the retromolar areas, so these are the main sites where MMSGTs invade the bone relatively early and produce poorly defined radiolucencies with ragged borders (Fig. 21-9).

The central variety occurs so seldom that it is not discussed here, other than to indicate that its features are similar to those produced by a central SCC or any radiolucent malignancy originating in the jawbones. An example that produced a multilocular radiolucency of the mandible is illustrated in Fig. 20-11.

Features

The benign minor salivary gland tumors and MMSGTs have been discussed in detail in Chapter 10. Early in development, these tumors are usually covered with smooth, normal-appearing mucosa. Later, the surface may demonstrate mucositis resulting from chronic trauma. If the trauma is severe or if a biopsy of the mass is performed, the surface ulcerates and may remain ulcerated; this occurrence frequently leads to the production of a necrotic surface.

When an MMSGT infiltrates bone, it produces a radiolucency identical to that produced by a peripheral SCC (i.e., a semicircular radiolucency with poorly defined, ragged borders advancing from the surface into the bone [see Fig. 21-9]). An undetected lesion on the posterolateral hard palate is apt to destroy the floor of the maxillary sinus and invade the air-filled cavity. Although the radiographic appearances of both tumors may be similar, the

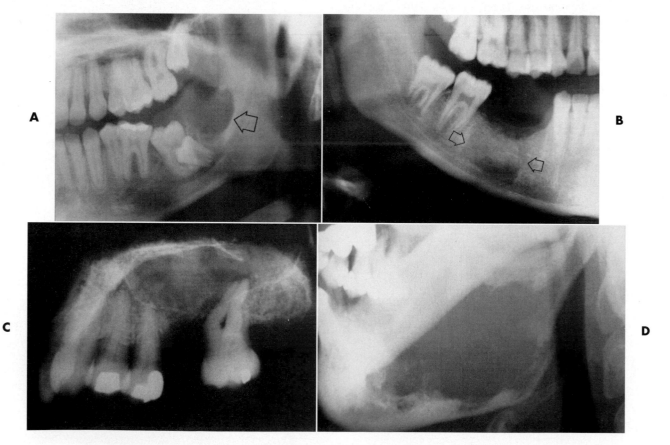

Fig. 21-9. Peripheral MMSGTs. **A,** Mucoepidermoid tumor in the retromolar region destroying the alveolar bone *(arrow).* **B,** Mucoepidermoid tumor *(arrows),* which originated in the floor of the mouth and infiltrated the lingual alveolar plate in the premolar and molar region. **C,** Radiograph of a surgical specimen of an adenocystic carcinoma. **D,** Adenocarcinoma of minor salivary gland origin. (**A** and **B** courtesy R. Kallal, Chicago; **C** courtesy O.H. Stuteville, deceased; **D** courtesy R. Goepp, Chicago.)

MMSGT seldom originates on the crest of the alveolar ridge, a fact that is useful in distinguishing this lesion from SCC. Magnetic resonance imaging and computed tomography are very helpful in giving additional detail on extent of bony invasion.[17]

Differential Diagnosis

The differential diagnosis of MMSGTs is discussed in the section on differential diagnosis at the end of the chapter.

Management

The management of MMSGTs is discussed with peripheral oral exophytic lesions in Chapter 10.

OSTEOGENIC SARCOMA—OSTEOLYTIC TYPE

Osteogenic sarcoma (OS) is second only to multiple myeloma as the most frequently encountered primary tumor of the jawbones. It is thought to arise from primitive undifferentiated cells and from malignant transformation of osteoblasts. OS occurs in approximately 1 per 100,000 persons, and about 6% to 7% of total cases occur in the maxillofacial region.[18] OS has three basic radiographic appearances: completely radiolucent, radiolucent with radiopaque areas, and predominantly radiopaque. The classic sunburst effect may be seen in the latter two types. The various radiographic appearances of osteosarcoma are listed in Table 21-1. Discussion in this chapter stresses the radiolucent variety.

Like other malignant tumors, OS is of unknown cause. However, bones that have been previously irradiated and bones affected with Paget's disease show an increased incidence. OS of the jaws differs in the following ways from that found in other bones:

1. The average age of onset is in the third to fourth decade, about a decade later that that observed in other bones.[18,19]
2. The jaw lesions have less tendency to metastasize.
3. The prognosis is better for jaw lesions.

OS metastasizes almost exclusively by hematogenous spread. Pulmonary metastasis, the most common, is frequently found at autopsy. Lymph node involvement is rare.

Juxtacortical OS is a rare variant that can be subdivided into parosteal and periosteal types.[20] The periosteal type is more malignant and radiolucent than the parosteal.[20]

Features

A patient with an OS may complain of intermittent local pain, swelling, paresthesia or anesthesia, tooth mobility, intraoral bleeding, asymmetry of the jaws, and in some cases a mass on the ridge or gingivae. The mandible is more frequently involved:[18,19,21] approximately 60%,[21] twice as often,[18] or about equal.[22] Overall, the most common sites are the body of the mandible and alveolar ridge of the maxilla.[22] The average age in reported series ranges from 34.2 to 36 years.[21,22] One study indicates a peak incidence of about 27 years of age.[18] Male patients show some predominance in some studies[18,22] but not in all.[21] The incidence of symptoms has been reported as pain, 40%;[18] paresthesia, 14%;[18,21] and dental symptoms, 25%.[18] There may be a history of recent tooth extraction with a nodular or polypoid, somewhat reddish, granuloma-like mass growing from the tooth socket.

As the tumor grows, eroding the cortical plates, the expansion is very firm because of the dense fibrous tumor tissue produced. Initially the swelling is smoothly contoured and covered with normal-appearing mucosa. Later, when the expansion becomes chronically traumatized, mucositis develops on the surface; still later the surface ulcerates, and a whitish-gray necrotic surface results. This surface can be removed with a tongue blade.

The bony lesion is radiolucent with poorly defined, ragged borders. Early in the course of the disease, it is usually located centrally in the jaws (Fig. 21-10), and changes are minimal and vague.[23] Sometimes, it is discovered as a radiolucency in the periapex or more toward the periphery of the ridge or cortical plates. It may originate adjacent to or seemingly in the periodontal ligament (pdl) space, and in such cases, it appears radiographically as a bandlike widening involving the complete length of the periodontal ligament space on one or both sides of the root[20,24] (Figs. 21-11 and 21-12, B). This bandlike widening is not pathognomonic for OS, however, and is seen with other types of malignancies in bone and in osteoblastoma,[25] in patients undergoing orthodontic therapy, and with unusual unilateral bone resorption in periodontal disease (Fig. 21-12, C and D). Cemental resorption may be present in some instances.[20,26] Involvement of the mandibular canal with widening of the canal evident on radiographic examination and by paresthesia occurs with some frequency.[26-28] The former finding is not pathognomonic for osteosarcoma because virtually any malignant tumor may cause pdl and canal widening. Specifically, SCC[29,30] and adenoid cystic carcinoma can produce this "broadening" by peripheral invasion.

On microscopic examination the radiolucent type of OS is basically fibroblastic, showing malignant cells, good vascularity, and a few areas of osteoid tissue. It may also form some cartilage. A tumor composed primarily of osteoid or cartilage may rapidly calcify in these areas and become evident as a mixed radiolucent-radiopaque area or as a predominantly radiopaque lesion. The latter two images are discussed in Chapter 25. It has been reported that chondroblastic osteosarcoma is the most frequent type in the jaws and is associated with the best survival rate.[22]

Differential Diagnosis

The differentiation of radiolucent lesions such as OS is discussed in the section on differential diagnosis at the end of the chapter.

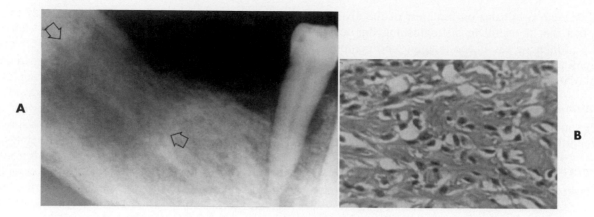

Fig. 21-10. **A,** OS (osteolytic variety) *(arrows).* **B,** Microscopy of the lesion showing scanty osteoid and malignant osteoblasts. (**A** courtesy R. Goepp, Chicago.)

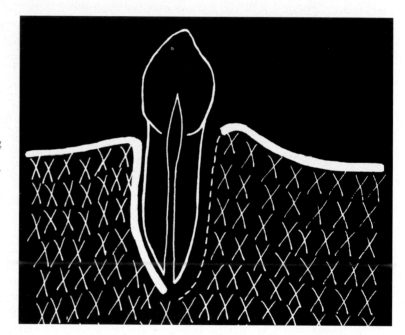

Fig. 21-11. Diagram of a periapical radiograph illustrating unilateral (asymmetric) bandlike widening along the right side of the root. Such a bandlike widening of the periodontal ligament, either unilateral or bilateral, suggests an intraosseous malignant tumor.

Management

Although a diagnosis of OS of the jaws is grave (approximately 25% of the patients survive 5 years), the prognosis is better than for OS of other bones of the skeleton,[18]). Lesions in the symphyseal region of the mandible have the best outlook, and those in the maxillary sinus have the poorest. Radical surgery (resection) by itself or in combination with chemotherapy offers the best chance of a cure.[21,22,31]

The osteolytic type is the least differentiated and carries the poorest prognosis.

CHONDROSARCOMA

Chondrosarcoma follows multiple myeloma and OS as the third most common primary malignant tumor of the jawbones. It is, however, an uncommon jaw tumor; OS is at least 3 times more common. Although the exact origin of the chondrosarcoma is obscure, it may be found developing in normal cartilage, chondromas, or osteochondromas. It may originate centrally or on the periphery of the bone.

Chondrosarcomas show two quite different radiographic images: a frank radiolucency (usually in an early stage) or a radiolucency containing various shapes and sizes of radiopaque shadows. These radiopaque shadows are the result of calcification or ossification in areas of cartilage formation and are a feature of relatively longstanding tumors; they are found in the older parts of the tumors. Chondrosarcoma may mimic the appearance of osteosarcoma on radiographs (see Table 21-1). Specifically, it may produce bandlike widening of the periodontal ligament.[32-34] The completely radiolucent type is accentuated in the context of this chapter.

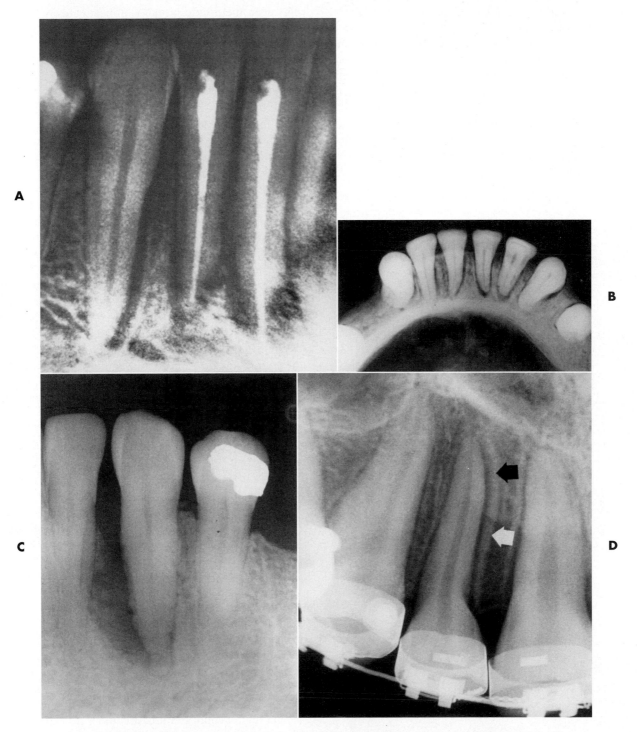

Fig. 21-12. Bandlike widening of the periodontal ligament. **A,** Chondrosarcoma of the anterior of the mandible in a young woman. **B,** Osteosarcoma of the anterior of the mandible. Symmetric and asymmetric bandlike widening of the periodontal ligament is evident in **A** and **B. C,** Asymmetric widening of the periodontal ligament on the mesial aspect of the canine tooth. This widening is caused by the presence of calculus. **D,** Asymmetric widening of the periodontal ligament on the mesial aspect of the upper lateral incisor tooth, which has been produced by recent orthodontic movement. (**A** courtesy O.H. Stuteville, deceased. **B** courtesy R. Goepp, Chicago.)

Features

The majority of chondrosarcomas of the jaws occur in patients between the ages of 20 and 60 years, with an average age of approximately 40 years.[35] The highest incidence occurs between the third and fifth decades[34] and peaks in the third decade.[33] More than 60% of chondrosarcomas are found in men, and the maxilla is involved more often than the mandible. Some of the maxillary tumors represent lesions that originated in the cartilages of the nasal cavity and invaded the maxillary bone. The premolar and molar region, symphysis, and coronoid and condyloid processes are the most frequent mandibular sites.[36]

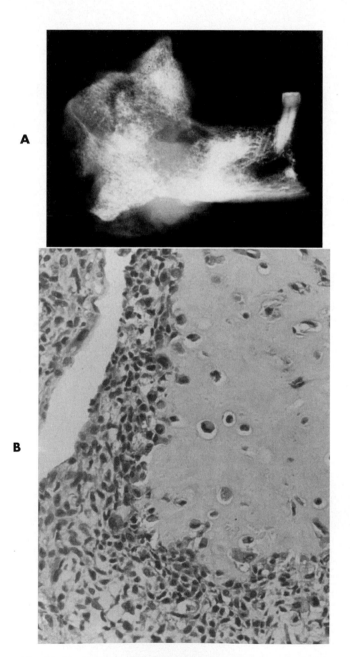

Fig. 21-13. Chondrosarcoma. **A,** Radiograph of a surgical specimen of a mandibular lesion. **B,** Photomicrograph of a chondrosarcoma. (**A** courtesy O.H. Stuteville, deceased.)

Unlike the OS, the chondrosarcoma metastasizes relatively rarely, especially in its early stages. As with OS, however, metastatic spread is almost entirely by vascular channels. Malignant cells may erode through the walls of a venule and extend along inside the venule without adhering to the vessel walls but still attached at their site of entry. When metastasis occurs, the lung is the organ most frequently involved.[33]

In the body, the common type of chondrosarcoma occurs more frequently than the mesenchymal type, but the mesenchymal type occurs more frequently in the jaws. The mesenchymal chondrosarcoma is a more malignant variety that grows faster and metastasizes earlier and more frequently; as a result, it has a much poorer prognosis.

Except for the mesenchymal variety, the chondrosarcoma behaves in a less aggressive fashion than the osteosarcoma. The patient frequently complains of a painful, slowly enlarging swelling in the affected region of the bone, often of several years' duration.

Until the chondrosarcoma causes expansion of the bone, pain may be the only clinical indication of the developing tumor. If it has eroded through the cortical plates, a tender or painful, smoothly contoured mass can be palpated over the bone. The mass is firm if the tumor or region contains substantial amounts of cartilage or fibrous tissue. If much myxomatous type of tissue is present near its periphery, however, the tumor feels soft. The mucosal covering appears normal in the early stage but later may ulcerate and develop a necrotic surface if it is chronically traumatized. Teeth in the affected region may demonstrate spreading, migration, increased mobility, and root resorption. A slowly increasing diastema may be the earliest clinical sign.[34] The most common symptoms in maxillary tumors are nasal problems.[35]

The earlier lesion in bone is usually radiolucent because the neoplastic cartilage has not yet become calcified (Figs. 21-12, *A,* and 21-13).

Radiographs show a central radiolucency bordered by a ragged, poorly defined perimeter of bone. Conversely, the peripheral type may show only one border in bone, and the rest of the tumor may be a vague, hazy mass peripheral to the uneven area of bony erosion. The peripheral lesion generally tends to be more circumscribed. A lesion involving the teeth may appear as a periapical radiolucency or as a symmetric or asymmetric broadening of the periodontal ligament space[33,34] (see Fig. 21-12, *A).*

On microscopic examination the lesion shows varying degrees of myxomatous type of tissue, atypical cartilage, endochondral bone, and nests of malignant chondrocytes (see Fig. 21-13, *B).* A low-grade chondrosarcoma is difficult to differentiate from an aggressive chondroma by microscopic study.

Differential Diagnosis

The discussion of the differential diagnosis of the chondrosarcoma is included in the section on differential diagnosis at the end of the chapter.

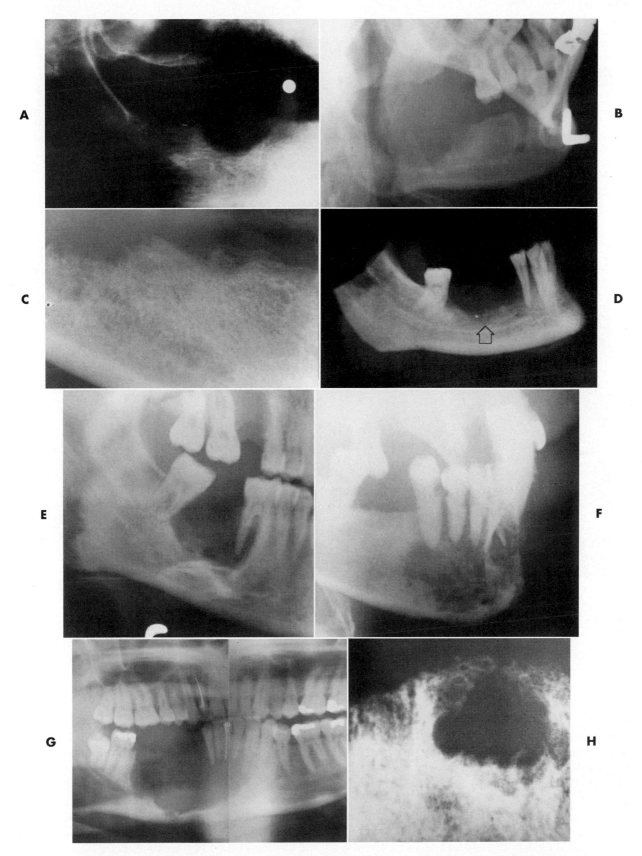

Fig. 21-14. Rare, ill-defined, ragged radiolucencies. **A,** Ameloblastoma. **B** and **C,** Lateral oblique and periapical radiographs of a reticulum cell sarcoma. **D,** Surgical specimen of a fibrosarcoma *(arrow)* of the mandible. **E,** Chronic localized type of Langerhans' cell disease (idiopathic histiocytoma) in the mandibular molar region. **F,** Central SCC. **G,** Ameloblastic carcinoma. **H,** Follicular ameloblastoma. (**A** courtesy D. Skuble, Hinsdale, Ill. **B** and **C** courtesy R. Goepp, Chicago. **D** courtesy R. Oglesby, East Stroudsburg, Pa. **E** courtesy N. Barakat, Beirut, Lebanon. **F** courtesy O.H. Stuteville, deceased. **G** courtesy R. Latronica, East Amhurst, NY. **H** courtesy R. Newman, Chicago.)

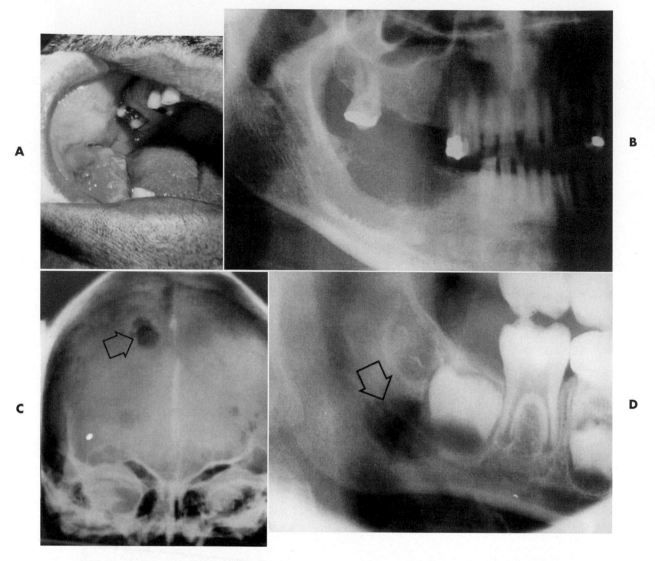

Fig. 21-15. **A** and **B,** Clinical and radiographic pictures of a solitary myeloma in a 55-year-old man. **C,** Radiograph of a solitary myeloma *(arrow)* in the frontal bone. **D,** Chronic localized type of Langerhans' cell disease (idiopathic histiocytoma) *(arrow)* in a 9-year-old child. (**A** and **B** courtesy N. Barakat, Beirut, Lebanon; **C** courtesy W. Heaton, Chicago; **D** courtesy R. Warpeha, Maywood, Ill.)

Management

Early resection is mandatory for a good cure rate. The chondrosarcoma is quite radioinsensitive, and radiation therapy is used only as a palliative procedure with large, inoperable tumors. Chemotherapy is also used as adjunctive therapy.

The prognosis for a jaw chondrosarcoma is not generally considered to be as good as for a chondrosarcoma of other bones.[33] At least 60% of cases have recurrences within 5 years of initial treatment, and some recur up to 10 to 20 years later.[33] Well-differentiated tumors involving the symphyseal region have the most favorable prognosis.[33]

RARITIES

A considerable number and variety of rare lesions of the jaws may appear as solitary radiolucencies with ragged, poorly defined borders. A partial list of such lesions may be found on the opening page of this chapter. These entities are considered rarities because they seldom occur or do not usually cause a solitary radiolucent lesion with poorly defined borders characteristic of this group (Figs. 21-14 to 21-16). Furthermore, benign lesions in rarefied jaws may appear to have ill-defined borders. For example, a giant cell lesion in a jaw that is rarefied by osteitis fibrosa cystica generalisata of hyperparathyroidism appears as an ill-defined lesion because of the overall radiolucent appearance of the bone (see Fig. 19-16).

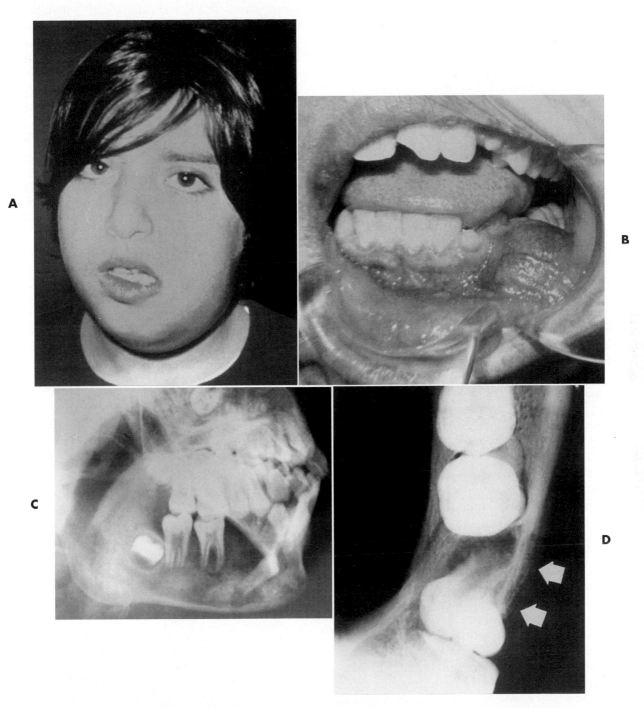

Fig. 21-16. Ewing's sarcoma in a 13-year-old girl. **A,** Full-face view showing asymmetry caused by a swelling in the left mandible. **B,** Intraoral view showing smoothly contoured bony expansion in the premolar and first molar region. **C,** Lateral oblique radiograph showing an ill-defined radiolucency and malposition of the premolar tooth. **D,** Occlusal view showing some central bone loss and also some destruction of the buccal plate *(arrows)*. Some bony spicules could be seen radiating from the bone at this location in the original radiograph. The posteroanterior view of the mandible (see Fig. 28-13, *A*) showed periosteal bone growth at the inferior border of the mandible with an onionskin appearance. (Courtesy N. Barakat, Beirut, Lebanon.)

DIFFERENTIAL DIAGNOSIS OF SOLITARY RADIOLUCENCIES WITH RAGGED, POORLY DEFINED BORDERS

The finding of a radiolucency with ill-defined, ragged borders must be regarded as an ominous sign. When such a picture is observed on good diagnostic films, additional radiographs of the suspected area from various angles should be obtained (1) to determine whether the radiolucency has ill-defined borders or whether it has produced the misleading impression because of the angle at which the original film was exposed and is actually an unusual variation in anatomic structure and (2) to ascertain the exact size, extent, and location of the lesion. The differential diagnosis of lesions included in this chapter is relatively difficult, since the clinical characteristics of most of the entities are so similar—an enlarging, tender or painful swelling of the jawbone accompanied by paresthesia or numbness. The radiographic appearances of these lesions are not unique during the radiolucent stage. Because of this similarity, the diagnostician must be alert to the more subtle features of each lesion: the relative frequency of occurrence, sexual predilection, age range of patients affected, incidence peaks, jaw regions usually involved, and accompanying systemic signs or symptoms.

An inflamed surface of an expanding jaw lesion or even the presence of purulent drainage from a sinus does not positively establish whether the pathosis is a chronic infection, since any of the tumors listed in this chapter may rarely be complicated by the superimposition of an osteomyelitis.[37,38]

Because the differential diagnosis of solitary, poorly defined, ragged radiolucencies in children are quite different from that of lesions having the same appearance in adults, this aspect is discussed separately for the two age-groups.

Solitary Lesion in an Adult

Peripherally located lesion A 59-year-old man complained of a tender swelling on the right side of the lower jaw in the molar area (Fig. 21-17). He also described a paresthesia of the lower lip on that side. He first noticed the swelling about 1 month before. He smoked and drank excessively and had poor oral hygiene. On examination the clinician found an ulcer on the mucosa over the edentulous mandibular alveolar ridge in the right molar region (see Fig. 21-17). The opposing posterior maxillary arch was also edentulous.

The ulcer had firm borders and was 2 cm in diameter. A firm, nontender expansion of soft tissue was present on the buccal and lingual surfaces of the ridge in the area of the ulcer. This soft tissue mass was tightly bound to the alveolar bone beneath. Several firm, nontender, enlarged, matted nodes were present in the right submandibular space. The hematologic examination revealed that although the patient was anemic, the total leukocyte count and differential count were within normal limits.

A broad, roughly semicircular, destructive lesion on the alveolar crest of the right mandibular molar region was apparent on a lateral oblique radiograph. The margin of this saucer-shaped erosion was ragged and poorly defined (see Fig. 21-17).

In evaluating this lesion the clinician can initially rule out FD because its early (radiolucent) stage would seldom if ever be seen at 59 years of age. Also, FD almost never causes pain or paresthesia, and enlarged lymph nodes are not a feature of the disease.

The more common metastatic tumors of childhood, neuroblastoma and retinoblastoma, may be assigned a low rank on the basis of the patient's age. Also, OS usually occurs in a younger age-group. Other metastatic tumors more common to the patient's age would be assigned a low priority because of the absence of symptoms suggestive of a distant primary tumor.

Chronic osteomyelitis and chronic osteitis are not prime suspects for consideration because there are no manifestations of infection, such as local pain, cervical lymphadenitis, or leukocytosis.

The patient's age would not exclude chondrosarcoma, but a chondrosarcoma that had reached this size would usually show some calcified foci within the radiolucency. Furthermore, chondrosarcomas seldom involve the regional lymph nodes and are more common in the maxilla.

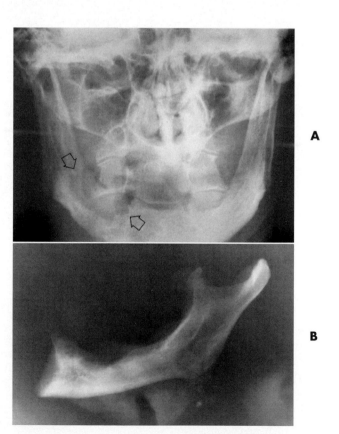

A

B

Fig. 21-17. Peripheral SCC. **A,** Bony destruction *(arrows).* **B,** Radiograph of the surgical specimen. (Courtesy E. Palacios, Maywood, Ill.)

SCC, MMSGT, and reticulum cell carcinoma (see Table 21-1) must be considered possible diagnoses on the basis of the patient's age and the fact that they may involve lymph nodes. On the basis of incidence, these entities would be ranked in the following order in the working diagnosis: (1) SCC, (2) MMSGT, and (3) reticulum cell sarcoma.

Peripheral SCC is the most likely diagnosis for this lesion, since minor salivary gland tissue is unlikely to be found on the crest of the alveolar ridge. Also, the radiographic appearance of the tumor suggests that it originated in the soft tissue and was invading the bone from the periphery, which would be atypical of the usual initial manifestation of a localized reticulum cell sarcoma (a rare lesion). Finally, the diagnosis of peripheral SCC is strongly supported by the fact that this oral lesion is frequently associated with poor oral hygiene, excessive smoking, and heavy alcohol consumption.

Centrally located lesion A 30-year-old man described appreciable pain of about 1 month's duration in the right body of his lower jaw. Shortly before this time, he had noticed a tingling in his lower lip on the right side. There was no history of trauma to the area.

During the examination, the clinician noticed a slight swelling on the buccal aspect of the alveolus between and beneath the first molar and second premolar. These two teeth were found to be abnormally mobile, but they were not sensitive to percussion, and they tested vital. The examination of the remainder of the oral cavity did not disclose additional significant abnormal conditions, and no cervical masses were found. A medical examination failed to disclose any systemic problems, and a skeletal radiographic survey revealed no other bony lesions. The results from all the appropriate laboratory tests were within normal ranges.

Periapical radiographs of the right mandible revealed a solitary radiolucency at the junction of the molar and premolar areas. It was approximately round with irregular, poorly defined borders. The first molar and second premolar were found to have advanced, uneven root resorption, although the crowns of both appeared to be free of caries and there were no restorations. The lower borders of the radiolucency appeared to be encroaching on the mandibular canal.

Chronic osteitis and osteomyelitis can be excluded as likely causes of this man's discomfort, since there were no local signs of infection and no apparent evidence of predisposing conditions, fractures, or teeth with probable pulpitis.

FD can be eliminated from further consideration on the basis of the patient's pain, lip paresthesia, tooth mobility, and root resorption, which point to the probability of a malignancy.

Peripheral SCC may be dismissed as an unlikely choice, since there is no mucosal involvement. The possibility that the lesion is a central SCC can be assigned a low rank, since this tumor is rare. Also, the peripheral and central SCCs are usually seen in an older age-group.

Because of the patient's age, Ewing's sarcoma, which occurs most commonly at a younger age; lymphosarcoma, which is seldom seen between the ages of 20 and 30 years; and metastatic lesions of childhood should be assigned a low ranking in the differential diagnosis.

Chondrosarcoma is more commonly seen in an older age-group, and it affects the maxilla more frequently than the lower jaw.

The patient is too young for adult metastatic disease to be strongly suspected, and there were no systemic symptoms to suggest a primary tumor elsewhere (although there could have been an occult primary lesion).

Central MMSGTs are rare and are usually found in older individuals.

Reticulum cell sarcoma of bone is a possibility, but it is also usually found in older people and occurs much less frequently than OS.

Finally, the location, signs and symptoms, age of the patient, and incidence prompt the clinician to assign a top ranking to OS (osteolytic type).

Solitary Lesion in a Child

A mother described the complaint of her 5-year-old daughter as a rapidly growing, painful swelling in the molar region of the right mandible. The mother reported that she had first noticed the swelling approximately 1 month before and that pain had initially been intermittent but soon became constant. The child had recently had a tingling sensation on the right side of the lower lip. A history of recent trauma could not be established. Vital signs, including temperature, were normal. Examination of the child's neck failed to reveal any abnormalities such as lymph node involvement or tender areas.

The intraoral swelling, which was clinically apparent to the examiner, was tender and firm on palpation, and the jaw was somewhat expanded both buccally and lingually. The smoothly contoured swelling was covered with normal-appearing mucosa, and no draining sinus was present. The two deciduous molars in the area of the swelling were mobile, and there was some bleeding from their gingival sulci.

A complete radiographic survey of the skeleton disclosed only a solitary radiolucent lesion in the right mandible. It was surrounded by bone measuring approximately 2 cm in diameter, and its ragged borders were poorly defined. An occlusal radiograph showed that, although there was minimal evidence of destruction of both lingual and buccal cortical plates, multiple layers of subperiosteal new bone were faintly evident. The first and second right deciduous molars were not carious and had not been restored, but their roots were almost entirely resorbed. The lamina dura surrounding the root and crypt of the developing first permanent molar was missing.

A detailed medical examination, including complete blood and urine tests, failed to provide any pathognomonic results.

Table 21-1 Solitary ill-defined radiolucencies

Lesion	Predominant gender	Usual age (years)	Predominant jaw	Predominant region	Additional features	Other radiographic appearances
Chronic osteitis	M > F	50-80 and 5-15			Usually associated with root of pulpless tooth Slow course	Cystlike radiolucency Radiopacity
Chronic osteomyelitis	$\frac{M}{F} = \frac{5}{1}$	30-80	Mandible:maxilla = 7:1	Premolar-molar Angle Symphysis	History of debilitating systemic disease and/or fracture Slow course	Radiolucency with radiopaque foci Radiopacity
Peripheral squamous cell carcinomas	$\frac{M}{F} = \frac{2\text{-}4}{1}$	40-80 (peak 65)	Mandible:maxilla = 3:1	Mandibular molar	Tobacco, alcohol Metastasizes—frequently early to regional lymph nodes Rapid growth	Radiolucency with radiopaque foci (sequestra)
Fibrous dysplasia (early stage)*	M ~ F	10-20 (peak 17)	Maxilla:mandible = 4:3	Rare in anterior maxilla and symphysis	No pain No paresthesia No root resorption Slow expansion	Mottled or smoky Ground glass
Metastatic tumors to jaws Adults	$\frac{F}{M} = \frac{3}{1}$	40-60	Mandible:maxilla = 7:1	Premolar-molar	Signs and symptoms from primary tumor Unpredictable course	Solitary cystlike radiolucency Multiple cystlike radiolucencies
Children	M ~ F	0-10	Mandible > maxilla	Premolar-molar	Signs and symptoms from primary tumor Usually rapid course	Generalized rarefaction Salt and pepper Radiopacity Radiolucency with smooth, well-defined borders

cystlik
marro
jaw (
wheth
condit
The
cal rac
radiol
same
bilater
If p
clinici
wheth
dioluc
the sai
viousl
a tootl
a reasc
separa
becula
quenco
wheth
is unu:
the ma
there :
pathol
Mu
separa
as patl
be exp
tractio
resenti
found
region
promir
parts l
upper

If tl
the soc
telltalc
the ex
only a
parent
the soc

MUL
(CON

From t
lomas
have a
these c

Entity	Sex	Age	Predilection	Location	Behavior / course	Radiographic features
Malignant minor salivary gland tumors	$\frac{F}{M} = \frac{2}{1}$	40-70	Mandible ~ maxilla	Posterior hard palate; Retromolar	Metastasizes to regional lymph nodes; Metastasizes to distant sites: lungs; Local extension by perineural space; Moderately slow but unpredictable course	
Osteogenic sarcomas	M > F	10-40 (peak 27)	Mandible:maxilla = 2:1	Mandibular body	Metastasizes by vascular route to lungs and other organs; Variable course	Radiolucency with radiopaque foci; Sunburst; Radiopacity
Chondrosarcomas	M > F	20-60 (avg. 30)	Maxilla > mandible		Metastasizes late by vascular route to lungs and other organs; Usually slow course	Broadening of periodontal ligament shadow; Widening of canals
Mesenchymal type	M > F	30-60 (peak 50s)			Metastasizes early by vascular route to lungs and other organs; Unpredictable course	Onionskin growth of periosteal bone; Codman's triangle; Cumulus cloud formation
Reticulum cell sarcomas	$\frac{M}{F} = \frac{2}{1}$	10-60 (avg. 37)	Rare in maxilla	Molar; Angle; Ramus	Metastasizes to bone or lymph nodes; Moderately slow course	Radiolucent and radiopaque
Ewing's sarcomas	$\frac{M}{F} = \frac{2}{1}$	5-24 (peak 14-18)	Rare in maxilla		Metastasizes to lymph nodes, lungs, and other bones; Rapid course	Onionskin growth of periosteal bone; Sunburst
Central squamous cell carcinomas	$\frac{M}{F} = \frac{2}{1}$	30-70 (peak 57)	Mandible:maxilla = 4.2:1	No predilection	Metastasizes to regional lymph nodes; Perhaps slow growth initially, then rapid growth	Cystlike radiolucency

*Pain, paresthesia, and root resorption are common features of all these lesions except fibrous dysplasia, although pain is not characteristically present in early lesions of peripheral squamous cell carcinoma and minor salivary gland tumors.
~, Approximately equal.

*In the co
cysts who

thalassemia. In fact, the maxillary enlargements resulting in prominent cheek bones and anterior displacement of the incisors produce a characteristic "rodent" facies, which when coupled with the sinus hypoplasia is pathognomonic of thalassemia.[43]

Although a range of changes may be apparent in the jaws of patients with thalassemia, not all the changes are evident in a particular patient. The cortices may be thinned and the tooth roots short and spike shaped (Fig. 23-4). In general, there is a blurring of the trabecula but with large, circular bone marrow spaces delineated by pronounced trabeculae. The lamina dura around the tooth roots and the opaque lamina around the crypts of developing teeth may be thin. There is a generalized rarefaction,[44] and occasionally a honeycomb pattern is seen throughout the jaws[45] (see Fig. 23-4).

Aspiration biopsy of the bone marrow reveals a specimen with very active, immature hematopoietic tissue.

Differential diagnosis The radiographic appearance of the thalassemias is distinct from that produced by osteoporosis, osteomalacia, and osteitis fibrosa generalisata but is similar to what might be seen in other hemolytic anemias. The mild changes that may be found in the minor form, however, do not differ greatly from the minor variations expected in normal marrow patterns (see Fig. 23-4). The history, clinical features, and blood studies are necessary to identify the general condition as thalassemia and to identify the specific form of it.

Management Treatment of thalassemia is limited to the administration of transfusions and other supportive therapy. The dental clinician must consult the patient's internist before initiating dental procedures because of the

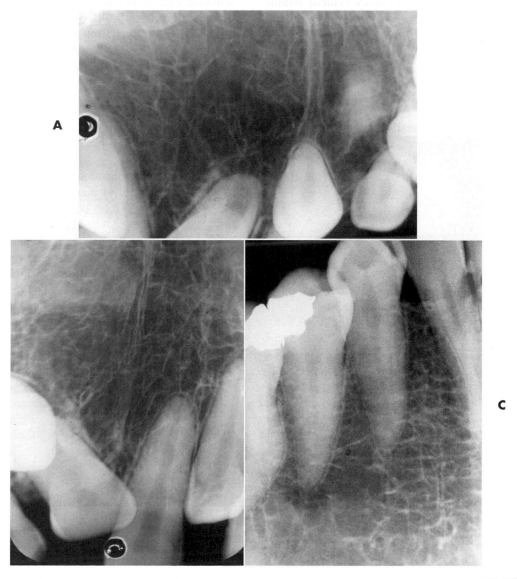

Fig. 23-4. Thalassemia. **A** and **B,** Honeycomb rarefaction in periapical radiographs. The lamina dura is present. **C,** Similar pattern in a healthy person. (**A** and **B** courtesy A.P. Angelopolous, Athens, Greece.)

potential problems of bleeding and hypoxia and the increased possibility of infection.

Sickle Cell Anemia

Sickle cell anemia is a hereditary disease affecting blacks almost exclusively. The disease apparent on clinical examination occurs in homozygotes; heterozygotes possess only the sickle cell trait, which does not (except in rare instances) produce any clinical manifestations. Approximately 10% of American blacks carry the sickle cell trait, whereas only 0.5% have the disease. The manifestations usually appear early in childhood.

The sickle cell defect lies in the inherited abnormal hemoglobin, which has diminished oxygen-carrying capacity and is less soluble in the reduced state than normal hemoglobin. Thus under conditions of low oxygen tension, the reduced abnormal hemoglobin crystallizes from solution within the red blood cells and causes the cells to take on abnormal shapes (especially crescents or sickles). The episode is termed a *sickle cell crisis;* during these phases, the sickled erythrocytes become physically trapped in small vessels, form thrombi, and cause the development of tiny infarctions. Thrombosis of vessels in the brain may cause severe neurologic deficiencies such as stroke, convulsions, coma, and drowsiness, as well as speech, visual, and hearing disturbances. Occlusion of smaller vessels results in headaches and cranial nerve neuropathies, including palsies, paresthesias, and neuralgias. The minor symptoms are usually transitory and disappear when the thrombus undergoes dissolution. Oral pain occurs in sickle cell patients and evidently is not related to common dental problems.[46] When these infarctions occur in bone, foci of dead bone develop and are then resorbed. Consequently the rarefaction related to the anemia-induced erythroblastic hyperplasia is intensified. Repeated infarctions are thought to produce sclerotic regions in the bone.

Features The patient with sickle cell disease may exhibit pallor, fatigue, weakness, dyspnea, retardation of growth, acute abdominal pain, and joint and muscle pains. An individual with sickle cell disease is quite susceptible to infection. Most patients with this disease die before reaching 40 years of age.

The sickle cell patient often has relatively long, gangling extremities, which are particularly striking when contrasted with the short, often rotund torso.[47]

Oral ulcers may be present, particularly on the gingivae; these oral ulcers represent infarcts that have become secondarily infected (see Fig. 11-14, *A*).

Splenomegaly is present in approximately 30% of adolescents with sickle cell anemia, but by adulthood the spleen has become fibrosed and small. The hemogram shows a mild to severe anemia, an increased reticulocyte count, and marked poikilocytosis. A special sickle cell preparation applied to a drop of blood on a glass slide demonstrates the sickling phenomenon (Fig. 23-5). Elec-

trophoretic analysis of hemoglobin is also used to establish the diagnosis.

Although one paper reports that 18 of 22 patients with sickle cell disease show generalized rarefaction of the skeleton,[48] most authors believe that bone changes are not found so frequently and are not so pronounced as those in thalassemia. The skull may show the hair-on-end appearance, which again is usually not so marked as in thalassemia. The following radiographic changes in the

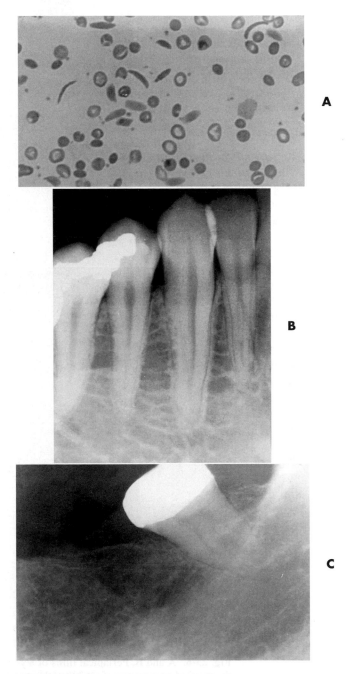

Fig. 23-5. Sickle cell anemia. **A,** Smear of peripheral blood showing sickle-shaped erythrocytes. **B,** Periapical radiograph showing the stepladder pattern. This pattern is also observed in healthy patients. **C,** Spherocytosis. Honeycomb radiolucency and the faint lamina dura are evident.

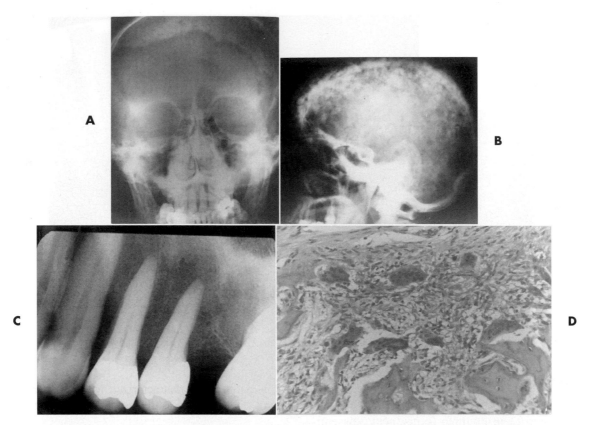

Fig. 23-9. Paget's disease, early stage. **A,** Osteoporosis circumscripta of the skull. **B,** Two stages of Paget's disease: intermediate stage in the skull and early osteolytic stage in the maxilla (which is almost completely radiolucent). **C,** Same patient as in **B.** Generalized rarefaction of the maxilla, loss of the lamina dura, and relative increase in the radiopacity of the teeth. (Photograph has been printed lighter than usual to bring out ground-glass pattern.) The mandible was unaffected. **D,** Photomicrograph of early Paget's disease showing the increased amount of fibrous tissue and the numerous osteoclasts resorbing thinned bony trabeculae. (**A** courtesy R. Moncada, Maywood, Ill.)

Management

The management of Paget's disease is discussed in Chapter 25.

MULTIPLE MYELOMA

Multiple myeloma is a disease characterized by the development of multiple malignant tumors of plasma cells. It originates in the bone marrow and represents the most common primary malignancy of bone. It is discussed in Chapter 22, where its radiographic appearance as multiple punched-out radiolucencies is emphasized.

Features

In advanced cases the gross destruction of the medullary portions of the bones, coupled with resorption of the cortices from within, is so extensive that a generalized rarefaction may be obvious (Fig. 23-10).

Differential Diagnosis

See the section on differential diagnosis at the end of the chapter.

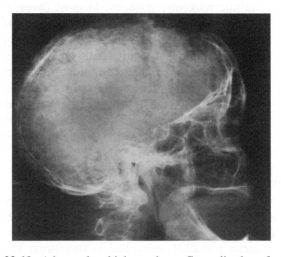

Fig. 23-10. Advanced multiple myeloma. Generalized rarefaction of the skull and jaws is evident. Most of the radiopaque appearance of the skull is produced by the brain. (Courtesy E. Palacios, Maywood, Ill.)

Management

The management of multiple myeloma is discussed in Chapter 22.

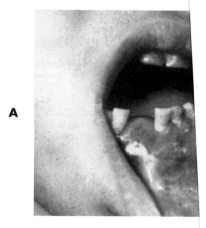

A

Fig. 23-13. Disseminated meta
ral view showing the tumorous
oblique radiographs showing the
tices and disruption of several d
Metastatic retinoblastoma of the

Table 23-1   Comparison of serum values

Disease	Calcium
Hyperparathyroidism	
Primary	Increase
Secondary	Normal
Tertiary	Increase
Osteoporosis	Normal
Osteomalacia	
Vitamin D deficiency	Decrease
Hypophosphatemia	Normal
Paget's disease	Normal
Multiple myeloma	Normal t

contrast, those of leukemia characteristically or
the deeper, medullary portion.

Several diseases that occur primarily in youn
are thalassemia, sickle cell anemia, acute leuke
acute disseminated Langerhans' cell disease. Olde
(over 40 years) are affected primarily by hype
roidism (especially secondary or tertiary), osteopo
teomalacia, Paget's disease, and multiple myeloma

Laboratory values may be particularly useful i
entiating among the preceding diseases, but the
tions of these parameters must be kept in mind. T
chemical indices and morphologic characteristic

RARITIES

As shown in the list of rarities at the beginning of this chapter, a varied group of diseases may produce generalized rarefactions of the skeleton, including the jaws (Figs. 23-11 to 23-13). Either these diseases occur rarely, or they seldom produce rarefactions of the bone or jaws. Nevertheless, the clinician must know of them when developing a differential diagnosis for a particular case. Usually the other symptoms coincidental with the rarefaction direct the clinician to include the appropriate diseases in the working diagnosis.

DIFFERENTIAL DIAGNOSIS OF GENERALIZED RAREFACTIONS OF THE JAWBONE

Distinguishing the radiographic appearance of normal jawbone from changes produced by disease is frequently difficult because of the wide range of naturally occurring anatomic variations in healthy bone. The jawbones of frail but healthy persons with delicate structures may appear more radiolucent than usual. Some persons may normally have relatively large marrow spaces, whereas others normally have faint laminae durae. As a rule, if the patient is

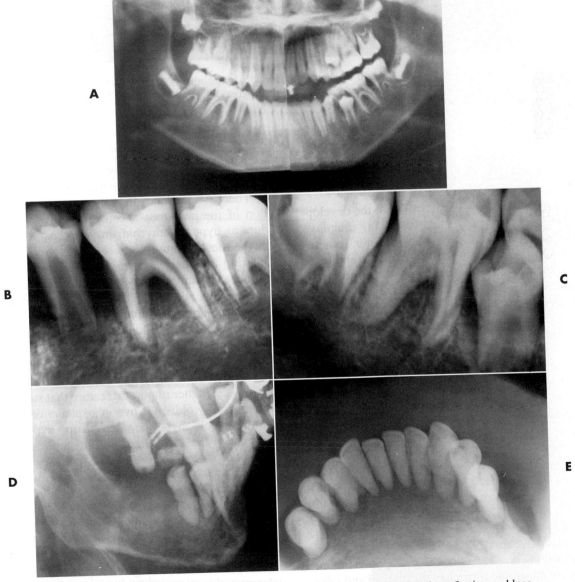

A   **B**   **C**   **D**   **E**

Fig. 23-11. Rarities. **A** to **C**, Lymphosarcoma. Radiographs show generalized rarefaction and loss of the lamina dura around the roots (**A**) as well as the blurred appearance of bone and loss of lamina dura (**B** and **C**). **D** and **E**, Diffuse squamous cell carcinoma of the anterior mandible showing loss of the lamina dura and generalized rarefaction.

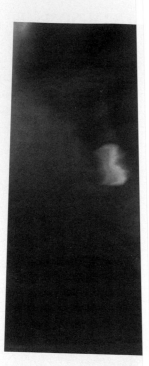

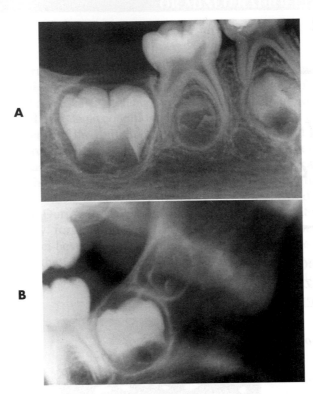

Fig. 24-1. Calcifying crowns of developing teeth. **A,** Mandibular right second premolar. **B,** Mandibular left third molar.

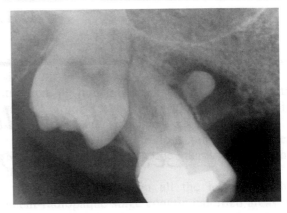

Fig. 24-2. Root tip with accompanying rarefying osteitis.

Fig. 23-12. Panorex radiogra[ph] almost complete loss of the bo[ne] Detroit.)

well and changes are not evident on serial ra[d] appearance of the bone is most likely withi[n] normal variation.

The ensuing discussion, which pertains t[o] ment of a differential diagnosis and a work[up] for the disorders included in the present cha[pter] some initial qualification, since it is unique [in] other discussions of differential diagnosis in [that] the pathoses discussed in this chapter are s[ystemic dis]eases, and needless to say, the differential [diagnosis of] bone diseases requires a detailed history [and] physical examination. To describe all the m[inute and] subtle differences that characterize these enti[ties is an en]deavor beyond the scope of this text.

An effort has been made, however, to prese[nt enough] detail that the dental practitioner can appreci[ate the rela]tionships between the oral and systemic ma[nifestations] and thereby be prepared for a consultation wit[h a physi]cian; that is, the dental practitioner can, first, re[cognize the] need for the consultation and, second, be prep[ared to pro]vide the most appropriate dental therapy when [indicated.]

In addition to causing rarefactions of the sk[eleton, the] conditions listed here (except two or three of t[hem) usually] produce other systemic changes. These feature[s are identi]fied by the general clinical examination and [laboratory] tests, supplementing the radiographic finding[s. Even] though there are no simple formulae, the clinica[l and labo]ratory examinations help the clinician establish [the rank]ings of the probable entities in the differential d[iagnosis.]

Before calcification, permanent tooth buds may appear in the periapical regions of deciduous teeth and in a few months undergo sufficient mineralization to appear as periapical radiolucencies with radiopaque foci. The clinician should therefore be familiar with the normal positions, chronologies, and radiographic appearances of the tooth buds with calcifying crowns. If there is a question, the clinician can compare the appearances of developing contralateral teeth to confirm identity of these calcifying crowns.

The radiographic appearance in certain cases may not be definite enough to allow the clinician to make a firm diagnosis of calcifying crown (e.g., when the developing tooth's formation or calcification is delayed, when the tooth is not in its normal position, when the tooth is supernumerary and not immediately identifiable). Subsequent periodic radiographs reveal the nature of the suspect region as the form of the calcifying crown becomes more typical.

TOOTH ROOT WITH RAREFYING OSTEITIS

Retained roots and root tips are the abnormal radiopacities most commonly found in edentulous regions of the jaws. Retained roots may be present in the jaws of one of every four edentulous persons; 80% of these retained roots are in the posterior region of the jaws, and 6% of all retained root tips are associated with radiolucent areas. (The latter statistic is a corollary to the observation that

the root canal of a retained root is frequently continuous with the oral cavity at its coronal end.) Thus the root canal may become the channel for infection, with a resulting rarefying osteitis in the periapex and the production of a radiolucent-radiopaque jaw lesion. Such root tips are surrounded by granulation tissue; they may be totally asymptomatic, or the patient may complain of intermittent slight pain or swelling. When the patient's resistance becomes depressed, an acute infection may ensue and produce a fluctuant, painful, smooth-surfaced mass (abscess). On microscopic examination a cross section of the tooth root (with perhaps a purulent root canal) is surrounded by chronic granulation.

The retained root is relatively easy to identify when the shape of the root has persisted with the linear radiolucent shadow of the root canal, a portion of the periodontal membrane space, and the surrounding lamina dura. In other instances, when the root fragment has been resorbed to some extent, the root canal is not discernible, the lamina dura is no longer present, and chronic inflammation has produced a rarefaction of the surrounding bone (Fig. 24-2), the clinician's diagnostic problem is more difficult.

Differential Diagnosis

Root tips that are atypical in appearance (partially resorbed, with the root canal and lamina dura obscured) and surrounded by rarefying osteitis may be confused with intermediate-stage cementoosseous dysplasia or odontoma, chronic osteomyelitis, cementoossifying fibroma, osteogenic sarcoma, chondrosarcoma, or metastatic osteoblastic carcinoma. Recent preextraction radiographs usually help identify the lesion as a root tip.

The metastatic osteoblastic carcinoma, chondrosarcoma, and osteogenic sarcoma may share two characteristics with a retained root tip whose identity is obscured by rarefying osteitis: local discomfort and a radiolucency with usually ill-defined, ragged margins. The malignant tumors all show moderate to rapid growth, as evidenced by an enlargement of the region that may become appar-

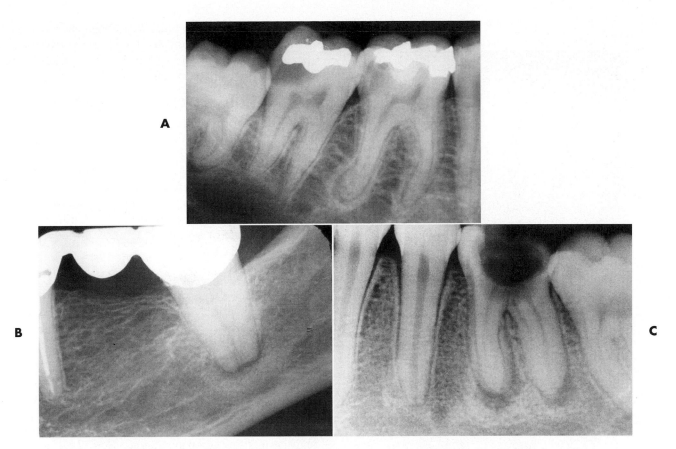

Fig. 24-3. Combined periapical rarefying and condensing osteitis. The teeth in the three cases were nonvital. The rarefying osteitis contacts the root end, and the condensing osteitis (radiopaque halo) is located around the periphery of the rarefied area.

ent on clinical examination within a few weeks. An acute abscess originating from an infected root tip, however, usually enlarges rapidly within a few days and becomes quite painful, inflamed, and perhaps fluctuant. If the infection is chronic, a draining sinus may develop. A medical history indicating that the patient has a primary malignancy elsewhere or has symptoms that suggest such a tumor prompts the examiner to suspect a metastatic osteoblastic tumor.

If the patient has no predisposing systemic disease and no history of trauma to the area and if the lesion is in the maxilla, osteomyelitis may be assigned a low rank in the differential diagnosis. An absence of pain, swelling, or drainage further deemphasizes osteomyelitis.

If the patient is over 20 years of age, the radiolucent-radiopaque lesion is unlikely to be an odontoma that has yet to develop beyond the intermediate stage.

The radiopacities in fibroosseous lesions of periodontal ligament origin (PDLO) (such as a periapical cementoosseous dysplasia [PCOD]) are frequently multiple and have a more uneven density. Also, if the lesion is single, asymptomatic, and situated in the maxilla or molar region of a white man, it is unlikely to be a PCOD.

On the basis of incidence alone, the working diagnosis for a relatively small, well-defined, smoothly outlined,

homogeneously dense radiopaque image surrounded by an ill-defined, ragged radiolucency in a tooth-bearing area of the jaws would be a root tip surrounded by rarefying osteitis.

Management

Retained root tips that are infected generally should be removed, the surrounding soft tissue enucleated, the bone defect curetted, and the tissue microscopically examined.

RAREFYING AND CONDENSING OSTEITIS

Frequently, rarefying and condensing osteitis occurs at the apex of a nonvital tooth or a retained root (Fig. 24-3). Chronic infection acts as an irritating factor (causing resorption of bone) and as a stimulating factor (producing dense bone, perhaps as a defense mechanism to contain the local problem.

Bone resorption occurs about the apex, where irritating products of chronic infection are most concentrated. On the other hand, bone apposition occurs at the periphery of the rarefying lesion.

When the chronic infection has run a steady course, a reasonably well-defined, somewhat homogeneous radiopacity is seen more or less circumscribing the radiolucency

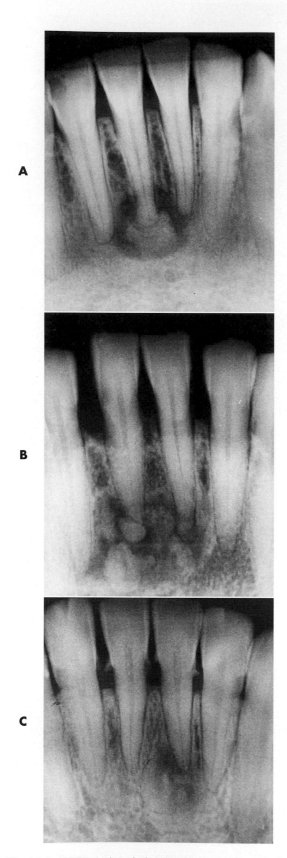

Fig. 24-4. PCOD lesions in intermediate stage in periapices of teeth with vital pulps.

around the root end (see Fig. 27-2). When the course of the chronic infection is punctuated by acute exacerbations, the radiographic picture is less orderly and the sclerosis more diffuse and less homogeneous.

Features, Differential Diagnosis, and Management

The features, differential diagnosis, and management of rarefying and condensing osteitis are similar to those for a root tip with rarefying osteitis. An incidence of approximately 9.5% has been reported in a randomly selected population.[3] The differential diagnosis is further discussed in this chapter in the sections on differential diagnosis of benign fibroosseous lesions of PDLO and the intermediate stage of odontoma.

PCOD—INTERMEDIATE STAGE

PCOD (periapical cementoosseous dysplasia) is thought to be a reactive phenomenon that arises from elements within the periodontal ligament.[4-11]

PCOD is discussed in detail in Chapter 16 as a periapical radiolucency, in Chapter 19 as a cystlike radiolucency, and in Chapter 27 as a periapical radiopacity. In this chapter the emphasis is on its intermediate radiolucent-radiopaque stage, which embraces a spectrum of radiographic appearances between the totally radiolucent and the mature radiopaque stage (Figs. 24-4 and 24-5). Some authors subdivide these lesions into two groups: those that occur in the mandibular incisor region (PCOD) and those that occur in the premolar molar region (focal cementoosseous dysplasia [FCOD]) (see Fig. 24-5).[10]

Features

The features of PCOD are described in Chapter 16. In addition, an incidence of approximately 0.5% has been reported in 889 randomly chosen patients at The Hebrew University–Hadassa Faculty of Dental Medicine.[3] It has also been reported that 5.9% of black women have at least one PCOD.[8]

The initial PCOD lesion is osteolytic; as it matures, particles or spicules of calcified material develop in the cystlike radiolucency (see Figs. 24-4 and 24-5). When these foci of calcification become radiographically apparent, the lesion is in its intermediate stage of maturation. The size, shape, number, and discreteness of the radiopacities vary greatly as the calcified components become larger and coalesce and the lesion becomes more radiopaque.

Regardless of its stage of development, the PCOD usually has well-defined, smoothly contoured radiolucent borders (see Figs. 24-4 and 24-5). Sometimes, sclerosis is induced in the bone at the periphery of the radiolucent border and appears on the radiograph as a hyperostotic collar.

The microscopic appearance reflects what is seen on the radiograph. At the intermediate stage a PCOD is made up of a fibroblastic type of matrix that is moderately vascular and contains a varied number of calcified zones of cementum or bone, or cementum and bone in varying combinations (see Fig. 24-5).

Differential Diagnosis

Entities that should be included in the differential diagnosis of the intermediate stage of PCOD are rarefying osteitis in combination with condensing osteitis, chronic osteomyelitis, fibrous dysplasia, calcifying crowns, cementoossifying fibroma, postsurgical calcifying bone defect, odontoma (intermediate stage), juxtaposed pericoronal mixed lesions, osteogenic sarcoma, chondrosarcoma, and metastatic osteoblastic carcinoma.

The PCODs are slow growing, which distinguishes them from the more rapidly growing malignant metastatic osteoblastic carcinoma, chondrosarcoma, and osteogenic sarcoma. Like the PCOD, these malignancies may appear as mixed radiolucent-radiopaque lesions, but unlike the smooth, well-defined fibroosseous lesions, they are usually irregular and ill defined. Furthermore, these malignancies (with the chondroma) frequently cause root resorption, whereas PCODs characteristically do not.

The mass or masses of calcified material within an intermediate-stage odontoma, especially of the compound variety, frequently show a somewhat orderly relationship of the radiodense enamel to the dentin and pulp spaces. The complex odontoma, on the other hand, is more difficult to recognize because the hard dental tissues may be so disorganized that they appear as irregular masses of calcified material. Even in these lesions, however, the more radiopaque enamel component may be discernible and often provides a clue to the identity of the lesion. In addition, the odontoma is usually located above the crown of an unerupted tooth, sometimes between teeth but seldom in the periapex.

The scattered calcifying foci in a healing postsurgical bone defect may be identified by a history of a recent enucleation.

Calcifying crowns, which are present in the jaws of patients under 20 years of age, are easily identified by their anticipated location in the jaw, the radiographically distinguishable tissues of the tooth, and usually the presence of a similar picture in the contralateral jaw.

These considerations narrow the working diagnosis to PCOD, cementoossifying fibroma, rarefying osteitis combined with condensing osteitis, chronic osteomyelitis, and fibrous dysplasia.

The current, generally accepted concept of fibrous dysplasia of the jaws supposes several obvious differences between this entity and the fibroosseous lesions originating from the periodontal ligament (PCOD and cementifying and ossifying fibroma):

1. Fibrous dysplasia is slightly more common in the maxilla, whereas 90% of fibroosseous lesions of PDLO are found in the mandible.
2. Fibrous dysplasia has a definite tendency to develop during the first and second decades of life, whereas PCOD is seldom observed in patients under 30 years of age.

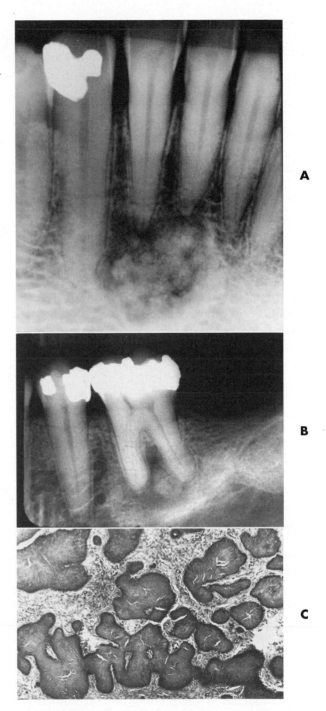

Fig. 24-5. Intermediate-stage fibroosseous lesions of PDLO. **A,** PCOD. **B,** FCOD at the periapex of the first molar. **C,** Microscopic study showing the small, separate masses of a cellular cementum characteristic of these lesions. (**A** courtesy M. Smulson, Maywood, Ill.)

3. Fibrous dysplasia affects men and women equally, whereas PCOD has a high predilection for women.
4. Jaw expansion caused by lesions of fibrous dysplasia is usually of the elongated fusiform type, whereas jaw expansion caused by fibroosseous lesions of PDLO is less common and is usually more nodular or dome shaped.

5. The radiographic borders of the lesions of fibrous dysplasia are characteristically poorly defined (i.e., they merge imperceptibly with normal bone), whereas the radiographic borders of fibroosseous lesions of PDLO are well defined.[7,9]

Application of these differences should enable the clinician to distinguish between most of the lesions of fibrous dysplasia and PDLO that are encountered.

Fibrous dysplasia containing only mottled areas of calcification is more difficult to differentiate. However, this mottled appearance represents an immature stage seldom seen in persons over 20 years of age; this consideration contributes to the differentiation.

If the patient is a young girl with a known case of Albright's syndrome and if she has jaw lesions, the clinician would have to rank fibrous dysplasia as a likely diagnosis.

If the lesions are periapical and the tooth is vital, the possibility is minimized that a pathosis has resulted from an infection of a root canal, such as might produce the combination of rarefying and condensing osteitis and chronic osteomyelitis. The absence of pain, drainage, inflammation, and tenderness on palpation, as well as the absence of regional lymphadenitis, further prompts the examiner to assign a lower ranking to these entities, which are a direct result of infection. In addition, it is helpful to consider that in cases of combined periapical rarefying and condensing osteitis, the radiolucent zone always lies next to the root end, whereas the radiopaque zone (condensing) forms a halo outside the radiolucency.

It may be difficult to differentiate between a PCOD and a cementoossifying fibroma because both lesions occur at the apices of vital teeth, are basically round with well-defined borders, and mature through the three stages. It is necessary to differentiate between the two lesions because the cementoossifying fibroma has very significant growth potential and requires excision, whereas the PCOD seldom requires removal.

The following characteristics help the clinician differentiate the two lesions. The PCOD (1) is a common lesion, (2) has a predilection for the lower incisor teeth, (3) has a marked predilection for female patients, (4) almost invariably occurs in patients over 30 years of age, (5) seldom attains a diameter of more than 1 cm, (6) seldom produces clinically discernible expansion, and (7) often occurs as multiple lesions. In contrast, the cementoossifying fibroma (1) is an uncommon lesion, (2) has a predilection for the premolar and molar area of the mandible,[9] (3) has less of a female predilection, (4) occurs in patients under 30 years of age (average age is 26.4 years), (5) frequently attains a diameter of 2 to 4 cm (Fig. 24-6), (6) frequently produces a clinically discernible expansion, and (7) occurs as a single lesion.

Occasionally, unerupted malposed teeth with mixed radiolucent-radiopaque lesions are positioned in such a fashion that the mixed image contacts the image of the periapex of neighboring teeth (see Fig. 24-11). The diagnostician then faces the difficulty of deciding whether the lesion was primarily a periapical or a pericoronal lesion. The correct decision in such a case often greatly facilitates the differential diagnosis process. Additional radiographic views frequently separate the lesion from the periapex or from the crown of the unerupted tooth.

CEMENTOOSSIFYING FIBROMA

Cementoossifying fibromas are thought to be uncommon neoplastic processes that originate from elements in the periodontal ligament.[4-9] These authors explain that in response to a variety of stimuli, cells of the periodontal ligament are capable of producing lesions composed of cementum, lamellar bone, fibrous tissue, or any combination of these tissues.

Features

The cementifying and ossifying fibromas usually occur as periapical lesions that are basically round and well marginated (see Fig. 24-6). Some 70% to 80% occur in the mandible, primarily in the premolar and molar region.[9,12] Although the reported range is 7 to 57 years,[4] they are most commonly found in adults in their 20s and 30s.[9] There is a definite female predilection.[9,12] The cementoossifying fibromas usually occur as solitary entities; go unnoticed when small; and frequently reach a size of 2 to 4 cm in diameter, expanding the jaws as they grow.

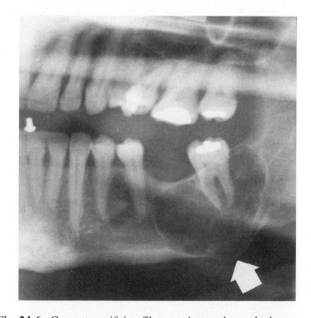

Fig. 24-6. Cementoossifying fibroma. Arrow shows the large, well-marginated radiolucent lesion with radiopaque foci involving the roots of the mandibular second molar tooth. (Courtesy W. Schoenheider, Oak Lawn, Ill.)

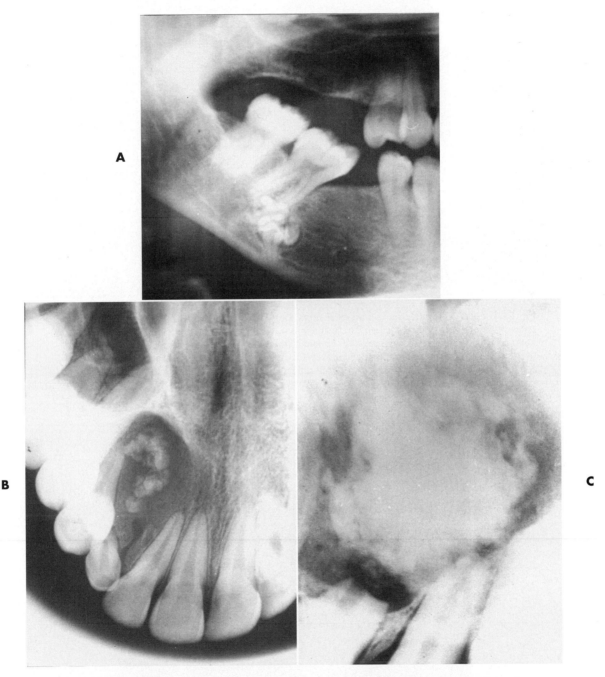

Fig. 24-7. Rare periapical mixed lesions. **A,** Compound odontoma at the apices of a second molar tooth, a most unusual location. **B** and **C,** Calcifying odontogenic cysts. In the canine region of a 14-year-old girl (**B**) and in the maxillary incisor region (**C**). The unusually radiopaque lesion has caused root resorption. (**B** from Seeliger JE, Regneke JP: The calcifying odontogenic cyst: report of case, *J Oral Surg* 36:469-472, 1978; **C** courtesy K. Kennedy, Chicago.)   *Continued.*

D

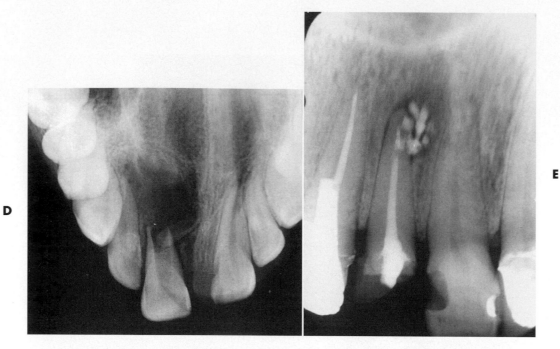

E

Fig. 24-7, cont'd. Rare periapical mixed lesions. **D,** A mixed radiolucent-radiopaque lesion at the apex of the nonvital central incisor. The lesion was basically a pulpoperiapical lesion, and the rectangular radiopaque image was the mesial segment of the crown of the other central incisor, which had been broken off in a traumatic incident and driven up into the tissue. **E,** Several radiopaque foci (root canal–filling material) within a periapical radiolucency. (**E** courtesy M. Smulsen, Maywood, Ill.)

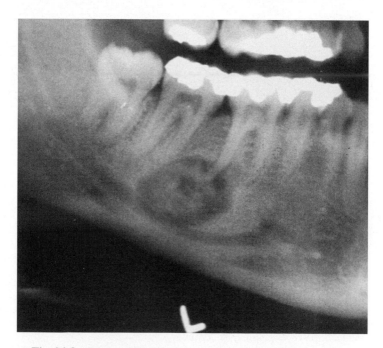

Fig. 24-8. Cementoblastoma in the intermediate stage at the apex of the distal root of the vital first molar tooth. (Courtesy N. Barakat, Beirut, Lebanon.)

Differential Diagnosis

The differential diagnosis of cementoossifying fibromas is discussed with the differential diagnosis of PCODs.

Management

Cementoossifying fibromas are well demarcated from surrounding bone[9] and therefore are amenable to enucleation. Large lesions may present continuity problems. Recurrence has been reported at about 6%.[13]

RARE PERIAPICAL MIXED LESIONS

There is a vast array of rare lesions and lesions that are common but rarely appear to be primarily associated with the periapex. For instance, a mixed periapical lesion seen at the root end of a tooth in a periapical film could represent a generalized condition such as FCOD or Paget's disease. Figs. 24-7 and 24-8 illustrate some of the rare mixed periapical lesions. Features of mixed radiolucent-radiopaque periapical lesions are shown in Table 24-1.

PERICORONAL MIXED LESIONS

Chapter 17 discusses the more common pericoronal radiolucencies. In the present context of pericoronal mixed lesions, less common entities are considered. Recent publications have dealt with pathology associated with impacted third molars as well. The incidence of pericoronal pathology ranged from 0.81% to 4.6%.[14-16]

ODONTOMA—INTERMEDIATE STAGE

The odontoma is a benign tumor containing all the various component tissues of teeth. It is the most common odontogenic tumor, representing 67% of all odontogenic tumors.[17,18] The odontoma seems to result from a budding of extra odontogenic epithelial cells from the dental lamina. This cluster of cells forms a large mass of tooth tissue that may be deposited in an abnormal arrangement but consists of normal enamel, dentin, cementum, and pulp.

The more common compound odontoma[17,18] comprises odontogenic tissues laid down in a normal relationship, and the resulting structure bears considerable morphologic resemblance to teeth. When the tooth components are less well organized and toothlike structures are not formed, the lesion is termed a *complex odontoma.* Some tumors are a combination of both types (i.e., they contain not only multiple toothlike structures, but also calcified masses of dental tissue in haphazard arrangement). Such lesions are called *compound-complex odontomas.* Another type, the ameloblastic odontoma, is an uncommon tumor and represents what the name implies.

The odontoma passes through the same stages as a developing tooth. First, there is a resorption of bone, so the lesion is radiolucent. An intermediate stage then follows; because of the partial calcification of the odontogenic tissues, this stage is characterized by a radiolucent-radiopaque image. This process continues to the most radiopaque stage, in which the calcification of the dental tissues is completed.

Table 24-1   Mixed radiolucent-radiopaque periapical lesions

Entity	Predominant gender	Predominant age	Predominant jaw	Predominant region	Distinguishing features
Calcifying crowns	M = F	Under 20	—	Tooth-bearing areas	Compare with appearance in contralateral and opposing arches
Tooth root with rarefying osteitis	M = F	10-60	—	80% posterior	Position of tooth root on preextraction radiograph
Rarefying and condensing osteitis	M = F	20-60	Mandible	Premolar-molar	—
Calcifying postsurgical bone defect	M	—	Mandible	—	History of surgery
PCOD	F—80%	Over 30	Mandible 90%	Tooth-bearing areas (especially anterior mandible)	Vital teeth; circular; size < 1 cm; well-defined margins with radiolucent rim; often multiple
Cementoossifying fibromas	F	20s, 30s	Mandible 70%-80%	Premolar-molar	Circular; 2-5 cm; well marginated; solitary

olucency with many radiopaque foci that vary greatly in size, shape, and prominence (see Figs. 24-9 and 24-10).

The microscopic appearance of the compound odontoma corresponds to the histologic structure of normal teeth, whereas the intermediate stage of a complex odontoma reveals deposits of dentin, enamel, enamel matrix, cementum, and pulp tissue arranged in a completely haphazard relationship.

Differential Diagnosis

The compound odontoma seldom presents a problem in differential diagnosis, even in the intermediate stage, because of its characteristic radiographic appearance. Despite this statement, on microscopic examination a particular tumor may show areas of ameloblastic proliferation and thus prove to be an ameloblastic odontoma. It is impossible to distinguish these two lesions by clinical or radiographic examination or on the basis of the history.

On the contrary, the complex odontoma in its intermediate stage may mimic several other lesions: fibroosseous lesions of PDLO, calcifying odontogenic cyst (COC), adenomatoid odontogenic tumor (AOT) (intermediate stage), calcifying epithelial odontogenic tumor (CEOT), postsurgical calcifying bone defect, fibrous dysplasia, rarefying osteitis with condensing osteitis, and chronic osteomyelitis.

Chronic osteomyelitis and rarefying osteitis with condensing osteitis may be initially ruled out because of the absence of pain, tenderness, inflammation, drainage, regional lymphadenopathy, or obvious etiology. The radiographic margins of these entities are usually poorly defined and roughly contoured, whereas the radiolucent borders of the complex odontoma are as well contoured and defined as the margins of a crypt about a developing tooth. Periodic radiographs of untreated infectious lesions frequently show the lesions to be increasing in size, whereas the complex odontoma does not increase in size after calcification of the odontogenic tissues has commenced.

Even when fibrous dysplasia appears mottled or has a smoky pattern on the radiograph, it has poorly defined borders, so it can be deemphasized as a possible diagnosis.

These comparisons narrow the clinician's working diagnosis to include fibroosseous lesions of PDLO, COC, AOT, CEOT, and postsurgical calcifying bony defect. All these entities produce well-defined radiolucencies containing radiopaque foci that may be located pericoronally.

The postsurgical calcifying defect is easily eliminated from consideration if there is no recent surgical procedure in the patient's history.

The CEOT (Pindborg tumor) is the rarest of these conditions. Unlike the odontoma, which develops in the first and second decades of life, the CEOT occurs at an average patient age of 40.41 years.[21] As with the complex odontoma, the molar region of the mandible is the preferred site, and a large percentage are associated with unerupted teeth. In view of this information, a radiolucency with radiopaque foci associated with the crown of an unerupted mandibular molar tooth in a child or adolescent is much more likely to be an intermediate-stage odontoma than a CEOT. After a considerable amount of mineralization has taken place in the odontoma, the differentiation is easier to establish because the CEOT does not often produce large, dense masses of calcified tissue.

In its intermediate stage of development, the AOT is radiographically indistinguishable from the fibroosseous lesions of PDLO, COC, and the complex odontoma; like the odontoma, it occurs most often in the first two decades of life. Unlike the complex odontoma, which is relatively common and is most often found in the molar region of the mandible, the AOT is relatively uncommon and usually is found in the anterior maxilla.

The COC, is an uncommon lesion. Some 75% occur anterior to the first molars; 47% occur in patients under 31 years of age. Like the complex odontoma, it has a predilection for the mandible. The aspiration test is often helpful in differentiating the COC from the odontoma. Whereas aspiration of a COC may yield a thick, granular, yellow fluid (keratin), aspiration of an odontoma is nonproductive.

In the intermediate stage of development, a fibroosseous lesion of PDLO shares several characteristics with a complex odontoma: both usually develop in the mandible, both are asymptomatic (except in unusual instances when they attain a large size), and both may have a similar radiographic appearance at this stage of development. However, the fibroosseous lesion of PDLO is usually situated in a more inferior position in the mandible and frequently appears as a periapical lesion, whereas the complex odontoma is usually situated in a more superior position between the crown of a tooth and the crest of the ridge. PCOD is seen more in women over 30 years of age, and the intermediate-stage complex odontoma is seen in patients under 30 years of age; these characteristics further contribute to the differential diagnosis. A rare condition just reported, calcifying hyperplastic dental follicles, needs to be considered also as a possibility.[1]

Management

Because of its capsule of peripheral fibrous connective tissue, which is really the follicle or periodontal ligament of the abnormal dental structure, the odontoma is easily enucleated. Such treatment is curative. Nevertheless, suitable periodic postoperative examination is necessary to ensure that complete healing has taken place. Microscopic examination is especially necessary to ensure the diagnosis.

ADENOMATOID ODONTOGENIC TUMOR

The AOT is an uncommon tumor that may undergo different stages of development. It represents approximately 3% of odontogenic tumors.[17,18] It may occur as a well-circumscribed radiolucency, or it may contain radiopaque foci. The lesion is discussed in detail in Chapter 16, where its pericoronal radiolucent appearance is stressed. The mixed radiolucent-radiopaque stage is emphasized in this chapter. The AOT may also occur in locations other than the pericoronal region. These represent 25% of the total number.[22]

Features

The AOT is a slow-growing lesion that occurs most often in patients between 10 and 30 years of age. Approximately 95% occur in the anterior regions of the jaws (64% in the maxilla), and 72% are associated with an impacted tooth (most often a canine[22]). Approximately 65% of the lesions occur in women and girls.[22] Delayed eruption of a permanent tooth or a regional swelling of the jaws may be the first symptom. Pain or other neurologic signs are not characteristic.

On radiographs the AOT is a pericoronal cystlike radiolucency that mimics the radiographic appearance of a dentigerous cyst. In the maturing stage (which represents 65% of the lesions[23]), sharply defined radiopaque foci are seen within the radiolucency (Fig. 24-11).

On microscopic examination, small deposits of calcified material are present and scattered over a background of odontogenic cells that form cords and swirls of ductlike structures and pseudoacini (see Fig. 24-11).

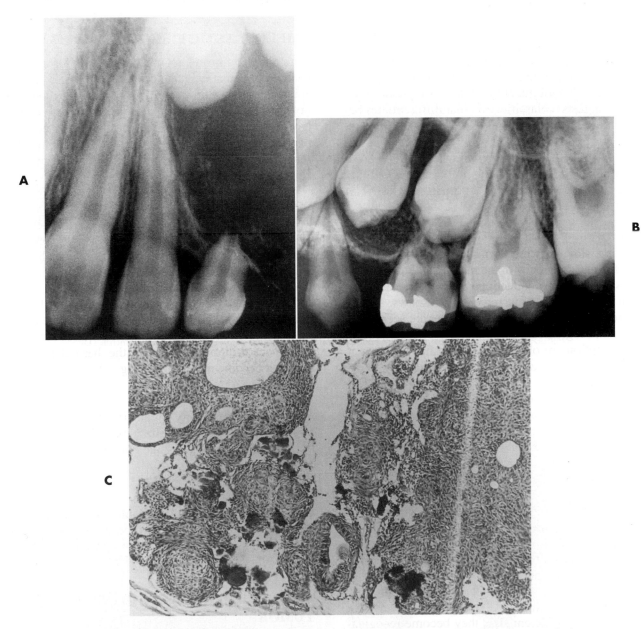

Fig. 24-11. AOTs in the intermediate stage seen as pericoronal radiolucencies with radiopaque foci. **A,** Case in the maxillary canine region. **B,** Different case in the upper premolar region. **C,** Photomicrograph. Dark foci of calcified material are evident. (**A** courtesy K. Giedt, Aberdeen, SD; **B** from Abrams AM, Melrose JR, Howell FV: Adenoameloblastoma: a clinical pathological study of 10 new cases, *Cancer* 22:175-185, 1968.)

coronal radiolucency, (2) a pericoronal radiolucency with radiopaque foci (Fig. 24-14), (3) a mixed radiolucent-radiopaque lesion not associated with an unerupted tooth, (4) a "driven snow" appearance, and (5) a dense radiopacity (occasionally). The most common are of a pericoronal radiolucency and of diffuse radiopacities within radiolucent areas.[21]

Features

From a review of 113 cases, the following statistics have been reported.[21] All but five of the lesions are intraosseous. The intrabony lesions occur in patients from 9 to 92 years of age, and the mean age at initial diagnosis is 40.41 years. Male and female patients are equally affected. Some 68% of the tumors occur in the mandible, with a marked predilection for the molar region (see Fig. 24-14). The molar region of the maxilla and the premolar region of the mandible are the next most common sites. A total of 52% of cases are undoubtedly associated with an unerupted tooth. The CEOT commonly occurs as a painless, slowly increasing expansion of the jaws. Small lesions are usually entirely asymptomatic.[21]

Microscopic study shows abundant sheets of polyhedral epithelial cells, which usually have prominent intracellular bridges. A variable amount of pleomorphism is present, and there are rare mitotic figures (see Fig. 24-14, *C*). Circular areas within these epithelial cells are filled with a

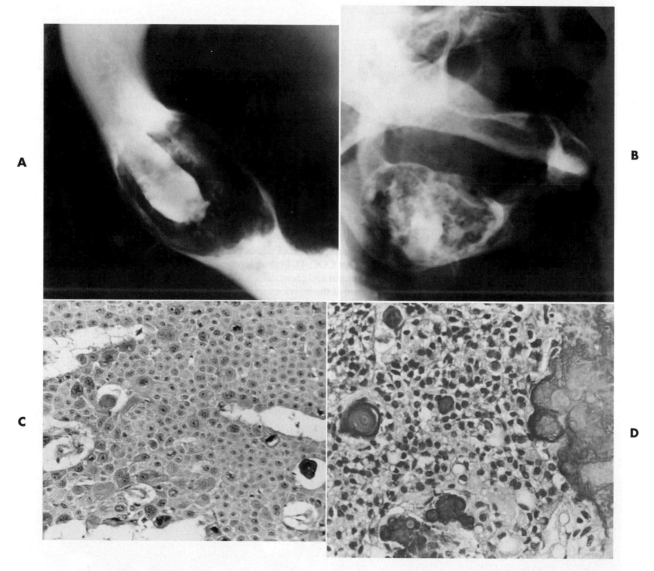

Fig. 24-14. Pericoronal CEOT. **A,** An embedded premolar tooth and small radiopaque foci are seen within the radiolucency in this occlusal view of the mandible of a 57-year-old man. **B,** Lateral oblique radiograph of a 77-year-old woman showing a mixed radiolucent-radiopaque image in association with an embedded molar tooth. **C** and **D,** Photomicrographs of CEOT. The pleomorphism of epithelial cells is evident in **C.** In **D,** clear epithelial cells and calcified material can be seen. (**A** and **B** from Franklin CD, Hindle MO: The calcifying epithelial odontogenic tumor, *Br J Oral Surg* 13:230-238, 1976; **D** courtesy S.O. Raibley, Maywood, Ill.)

homogeneous eosinophilic material. This eosinophilic material becomes calcified and follows a pattern of concentric deposition known as Liesegang's rings.

Differential Diagnosis

The differential diagnosis of the pericoronal radiolucent-radiopaque image of CEOT is included in the discussion of the differential diagnosis of the odontoma.

Management

Surgical resection that includes a satisfactory border of apparently normal tissue is the recommended treatment for the CEOT. The recurrence rate is considerably lower than that of the ameloblastoma; however, careful patient follow-up is mandatory.

RARITIES

Virtually any mixed radiolucent-radiopaque lesion that occurs in the jaw may contact the crown of an unerupted tooth and thus appear as a mixed pericoronal lesion. Because of the many unerupted teeth in the jaws of patients under 15 years of age, a greater incidence of such a "coincidental" appearance can be expected during these early years. Figs. 24-15 and 24-16 illustrate two examples of these rare conditions.

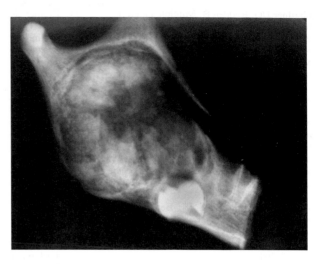

Fig. 24-15. Cementoossifying fibroma. Radiograph of a surgical specimen hows the well-defined borders of the fibroma and the displaced third molar.

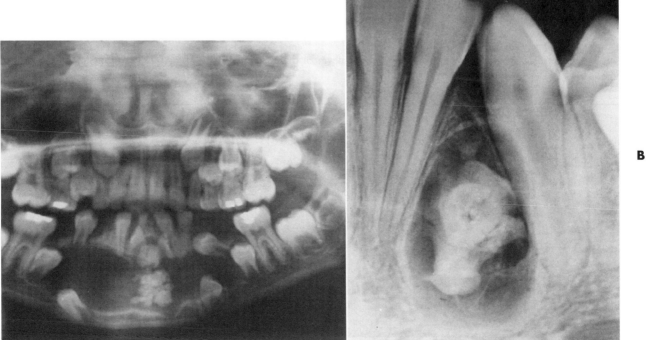

Fig. 24-16. Cystic odontomas. **A,** Orthopantomograph showing an odontoma within a large dentigerous cyst. **B,** Cystic odontoma in an intraradicular location between the lateral incisor and canine tooth. (**A** courtesy M. Kaminski, deceased, and S. Atsaves, Chicago; **B** courtesy W. Kinsler, Chicago.)

they require no further description. Extruded endodontic sealer has been observed in 5.1% of adolescent and adult patients.[14]

HYPERCEMENTOSIS

Hypercementosis (cemental hyperplasia) has been defined by Stafne[21] as "excessive formation of cementum on the surface of the root of the tooth." The early stages are only microscopically detectable, but as additional layers of cementum are added, the accumulation becomes apparent on the radiograph (Fig. 27-8).

The etiology of hypercementosis is not well understood, but repeated observations seem to indicate that this lesion is sometimes associated with the development of periapical inflammatory conditions, PCOD, and systemic disease (such as Paget's disease, acromegaly, and giantism).

Features

Hypercementosis is completely asymptomatic and is usually discovered on routine radiographic surveys. It has been reported to occur in 7.6% of patients.[14] The premolars are more often affected than the remaining teeth (6:1), and the first molars are next in order of involvement. Hypercementosis may be confined to just a small region on the root, producing a nodule on the surface, or the whole root may be involved. In multirooted teeth, one or two or all roots may show hypercementosis. Often, teeth are bilaterally involved, and a generalized form with hyperplasia of cementum on all root surfaces has been reported. The teeth affected are usually vital and are not sensitive to percussion.

On radiographs the altered shape of the root is apparent if there has been a reasonable amount of cemental hyperplasia. An isolated nodule or the characteristic club-shaped root may be seen. In either case the root is surrounded by a normal periodontal ligament space and lamina dura. The different densities of the excess cementum and root dentin are such that the original outline of the dentin root is discernible on the radiograph (see Fig. 27-8). Hypercementosis on anterior teeth may appear as a spherical mass of cementum attached to the root end.

On histologic study the cementum may be acellular (primary) or cellular (secondary). It is usually deposited in layers but may be arranged in an irregular fashion with fibrovascular inclusions.

Differential Diagnosis

Hypercementosis may be differentiated from the false radiopaque images that are projected over the apex by two features of the projected images:

1. The projected radiopacities are not delineated by a periodontal ligament space and lamina dura like hypercementosis is.
2. The projected images may be shifted in relation to the apex by altering the angle at which additional radiographs are exposed.

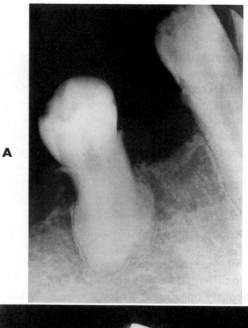

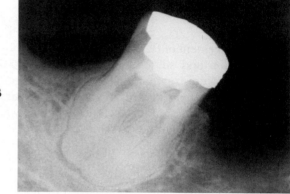

Fig. 27-8. Hypercementosis. **A,** On a mandibular premolar. **B,** On a mandibular molar.

The true periapical radiopacities are more difficult to differentiate from hypercementosis. They include PCOD, condensing osteitis, periapical idiopathic osteosclerosis, and developmental anomalies such as fused roots, dilacerations, and similar images caused by multirooted teeth.

The club-shaped images cast by multirooted teeth and the shadows of dilacerated roots can be identified by making successive radiographs exposed from different angles.

Sometimes the fused roots of multirooted teeth have a bulbous shape, but these fused roots can be recognized by the apparently expanded region of the root that does not have the relatively lower radiodensity of hyperplastic cementum.

Periapical idiopathic osteosclerosis, condensing osteitis, and PCOD lie outside the shadow of the periodontal ligament and lamina dura, whereas hypercementosis forms an integral part of the root surface and is therefore enclosed by a normal periodontal ligament space and lamina dura. Nevertheless, there may be difficulty in distinguishing these entities when the periodontal ligament space and lamina dura are indistinct. Differentiation may

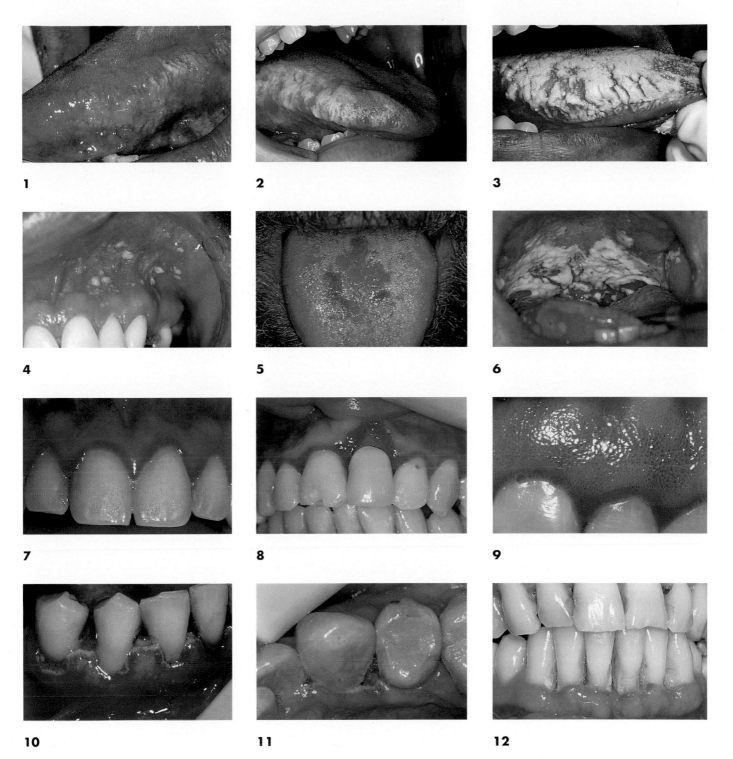

Plate E. **1,** Hairy leukoplakia in a patient who tested positive for the human immunodeficiency virus. **2,** Hairy leukoplakia in a patient who tested positive for the human immunodeficiency virus. **3,** Hairy leukoplakia in a patient who tested positive for the human immunodeficiency virus. **4,** Candidiasis in a patient who tested positive for the human immunodeficiency virus. **5,** Candidiasis in a patient who tested positive for the human immunodeficiency virus. **6,** Candidiasis in a patient who tested positive for the human immunodeficiency virus. **7,** Marginal gingivitis in a patient who tested negative for the human immunodeficiency virus. **8,** HIV-associated gingivitis and periodontitis. **9,** HIV-associated gingivitis. **10,** HIV-associated acute necrotizing gingivitis. **11,** HIV-associated acute necrotizing gingivitis and periodontitis. **12,** HIV-associated periodontitis. (**1** courtesy J. Guggenheimer, Pittsburgh; **2** courtesy S. Silverman, San Francisco; **3** courtesy E. Cataldo, Boston; **4** to **6,** and **11** courtesy M. Glick, Philadelphia; **8** and **9** from Glick M: *Dental management of patients with HIV,* Carol Stream, Ill, 1994, Quintessence; **10** and **12** courtesy J. Epstein, Vancouver, British Columbia, Canada.)

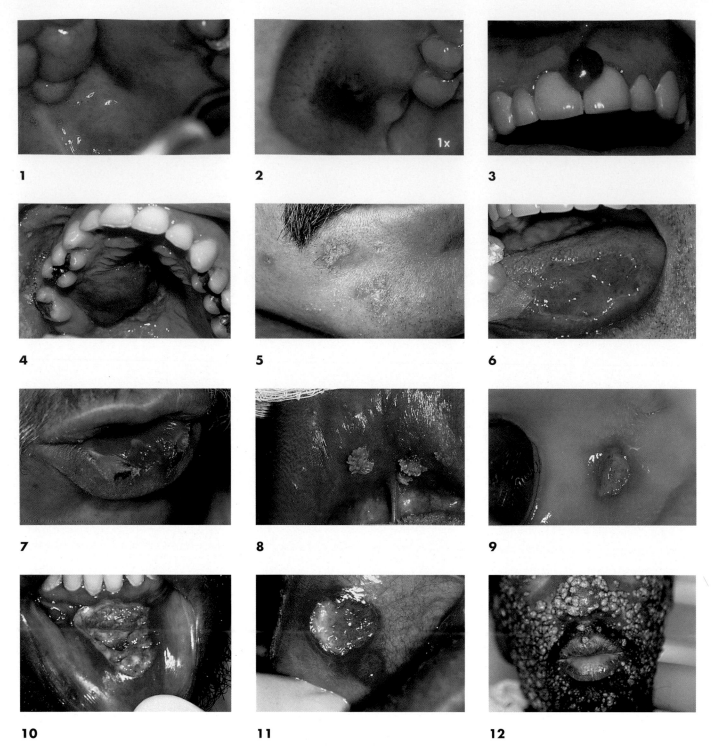

Plate F. 1, Kaposi's sarcoma in a patient who tested positive for the human immunodeficiency virus. **2,** Kaposi's sarcoma in a patient who tested positive for the human immunodeficiency virus. **3,** Kaposi's sarcoma in a patient who tested positive for the human immunodeficiency virus. **4,** Kaposi's sarcoma in a patient who tested positive for the human immunodeficiency virus. **5,** Herpes simplex virus in a patient who tested positive for the human immunodeficiency virus. **6,** Herpes simplex virus in a patient who tested positive for the human immunodeficiency virus. **7,** Herpes simplex virus in a patient who tested positive for the human immunodeficiency virus. **8,** Multiple condyloma acuminata in a possible HIV case. **9,** Minor aphthous ulcer in a patient who tested positive for the human immunodeficiency virus. **10,** Major aphthous ulcer in a patient who tested positive for the human immunodeficiency virus. **11,** Cytomegalovirus lesions in a patient who tested positive for the human immunodeficiency virus. **12,** Molluscum contagiosum in a patient who tested positive for the human immunodeficiency virus. (**1** courtesy J D'Ambrosio, Hartford, Conn; **2** courtesy S. Fischman, Buffalo, NY; **3** and **8** courtesy J. Guggenheimer, Pittsburgh; **4** to **6** courtesy J. Epstein, Vancouver, British Columbia, Canada; **7, 10,** and **11** courtesy M. Glick, Philadelphia; **9** from Glick M: *Dental management of patients with HIV,* Carol Stream, Ill, 1994, Quintessence; **12** courtesy R. Holloway, Maywood, Ill.)

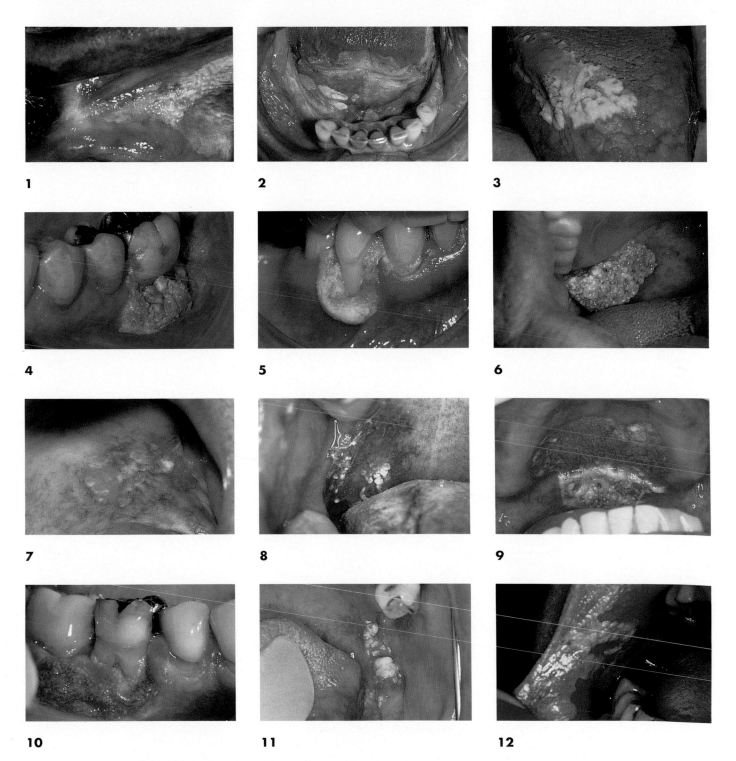

Plate G. **1,** Homogenous leukoplakia. **2,** Proliferative verrucous leukoplakia. **3,** Verrucous leukoplakia. **4,** Verrucous carcinoma. **5,** Verrucous carcinoma. **6,** Verrucous carcinoma. **7,** Speckled leukoplakia and squamous cell carcinoma. **8,** Speckled erythroplakia and squamous cell carcinoma. **9,** Speckled leukoplakia, proliferative verrucous leukoplakia, and squamous cell carcinoma. **10,** Squamous cell carcinoma. **11,** Squamous cell carcinoma. **12,** Erythroleukoplakia and carcinoma in situ. (**4** and **9** courtesy S. Silverman, San Francisco; **5** and **10** courtesy R. Priddy, Vancouver, British Columbia, Canada, and teaching collection, Faculty of Dentistry, Dalhousie University, Halifax, Nova Scotia, Canada; **6** from Claydon PJ, Jordon JE: Verrucous carcinoma of Ackerman, a distinctive clinicopathologic entity: report of two cases, *J Oral Surg* 36:564-567, 1978; **7** courtesy M. Lehnert, Minneapolis; **8** courtesy G. Blozis, Columbus, Ohio; **12** courtesy O.H. Stuteville, deceased.)

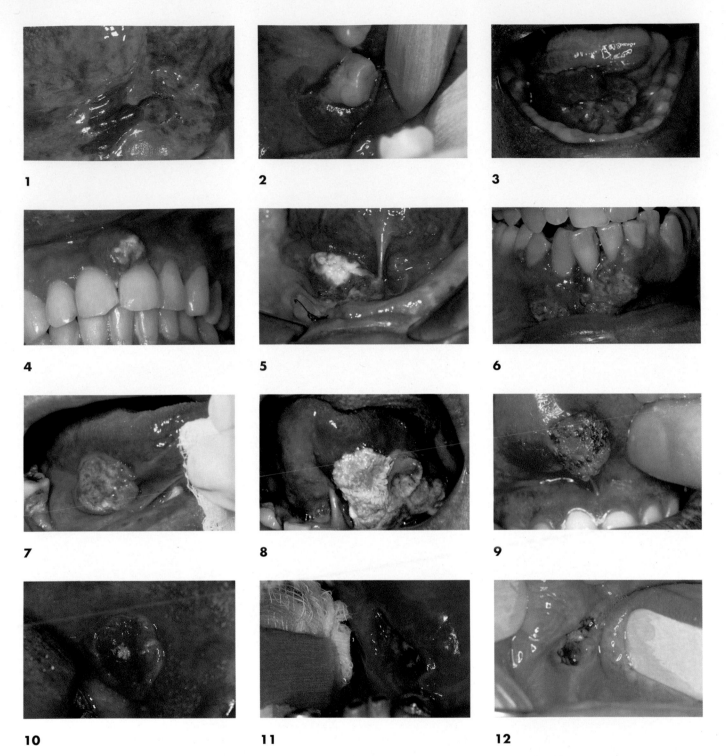

Plate H. 1, Erythroplakia (squamous cell carcinoma). **2,** Erythroplakia (squamous cell carcinoma). **3,** Squamous cell carcinoma. **4,** Squamous cell carcinoma. **5,** Squamous cell carcinoma. **6** Squamous cell carcinoma. **7,** Squamous cell carcinoma. **8,** Squamous cell carcinoma. **9,** Squamous cell carcinoma. **10,** Squamous cell carcinoma. **11,** Squamous cell carcinoma. **12,** Squamous cell carcinoma. (**2** from Lovas JGL: Oral precancer patterns, complexities and clinical guidelines, *J Can Dent Assoc* 55:209-214, 1989; **4** and **6** courtesy S. Silverman, San Francisco; **5** courtesy P. Akers, Chicago; **7** courtesy V. Saunders, Richmond, Va; **8** courtesy W. Schoenheider, Chicago; **9** courtesy R. Nolan, Williston, ND.)

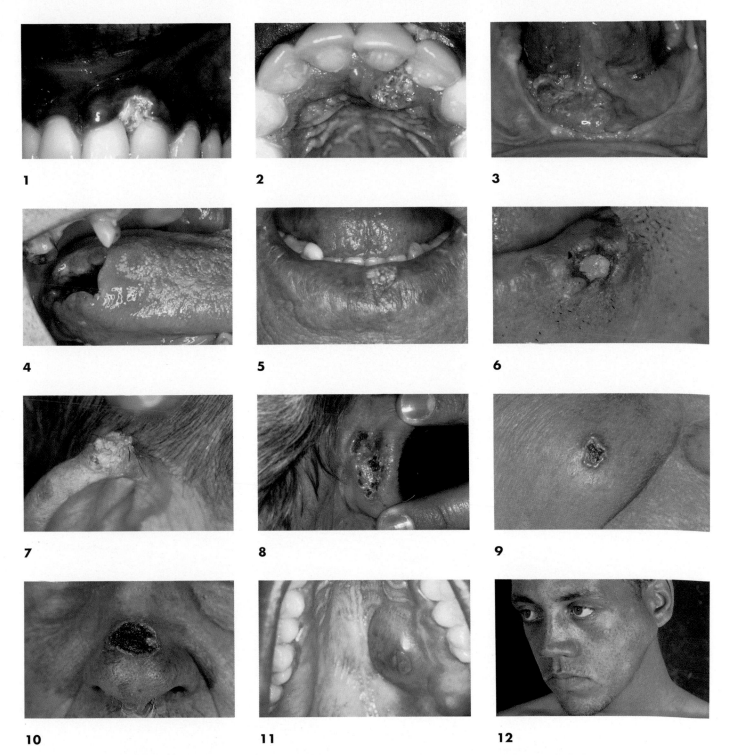

Plate I. **1,** Squamous cell carcinoma. **2,** Same lesion as **1. 3,** Squamous cell carcinoma. **4,** Squamous cell carcinoma. **5,** Squamous cell carcinoma. **6,** Squamous cell carcinoma. **7,** Squamous cell carcinoma. **8,** Basal cell carcinoma. **9,** Basal cell carcinoma. **10,** Basal cell carcinoma. **11,** Adenoid cystic carcinoma. **12,** Malignant mixed tumor of the parotid gland. (**5** courtesy S. Silverman, San Francisco; **11** courtesy D. Smith, North Conway, NH.)

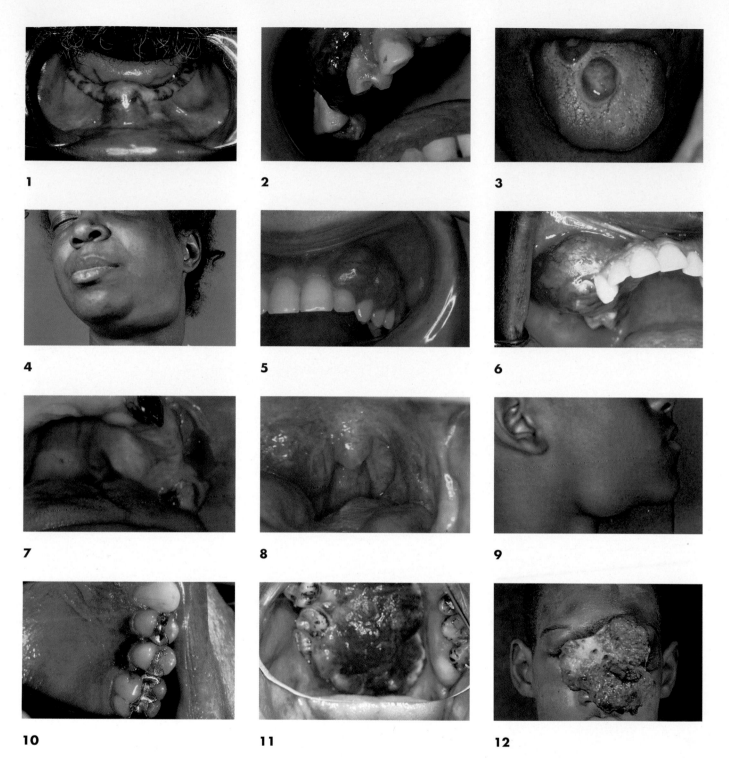

Plate J. 1, Metastatic carcinoma of the prostate. **2,** Metastatic adenocarcinoma of the lung. **3,** Metastatic carcinoma of the esophagus. **4,** Metastatic cancer of the oral cavity to cervical lymph nodes. **5,** Osteogenic sarcoma. **6,** Chondrosarcoma. **7,** Carcinoma of the maxillary sinus. **8,** Lymphoma. **9,** Lymphoma. **10,** Superficial melanoma. **11,** Melanoma. **12,** Transitional cell carcinoma of the nasal cavity. (**1** courtesy R. Kallal, Chicago; **2** from Ellis G, Jensen J, Reingold IM, et al: Malignant neoplasms metastic to gingivae, *Oral Surg* 44:238-245, 1977; **3** courtesy E. Robinson, Toledo, Ohio; **5** courtesy V. Barresi, De Kalb, Ill; **9** courtesy J. Laviere, Chicago; **10** from Robertson GR, et al: *J Oral Surg* 37:349-352, 1979.)

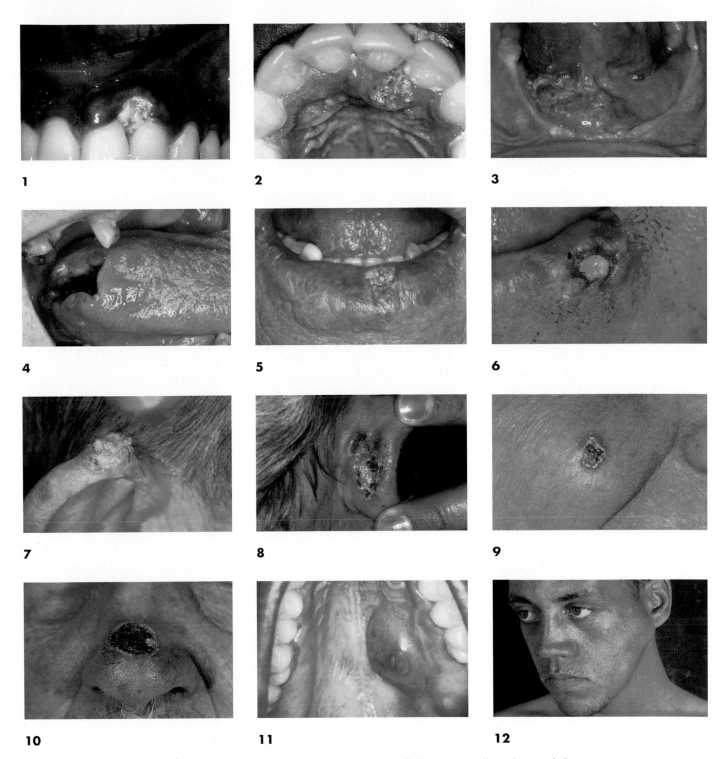

Plate I. 1, Squamous cell carcinoma. **2,** Same lesion as **1. 3,** Squamous cell carcinoma. **4,** Squamous cell carcinoma. **5,** Squamous cell carcinoma. **6,** Squamous cell carcinoma. **7,** Squamous cell carcinoma. **8,** Basal cell carcinoma. **9,** Basal cell carcinoma. **10,** Basal cell carcinoma. **11,** Adenoid cystic carcinoma. **12,** Malignant mixed tumor of the parotid gland. (**5** courtesy S. Silverman, San Francisco; **11** courtesy D. Smith, North Conway, NH.)

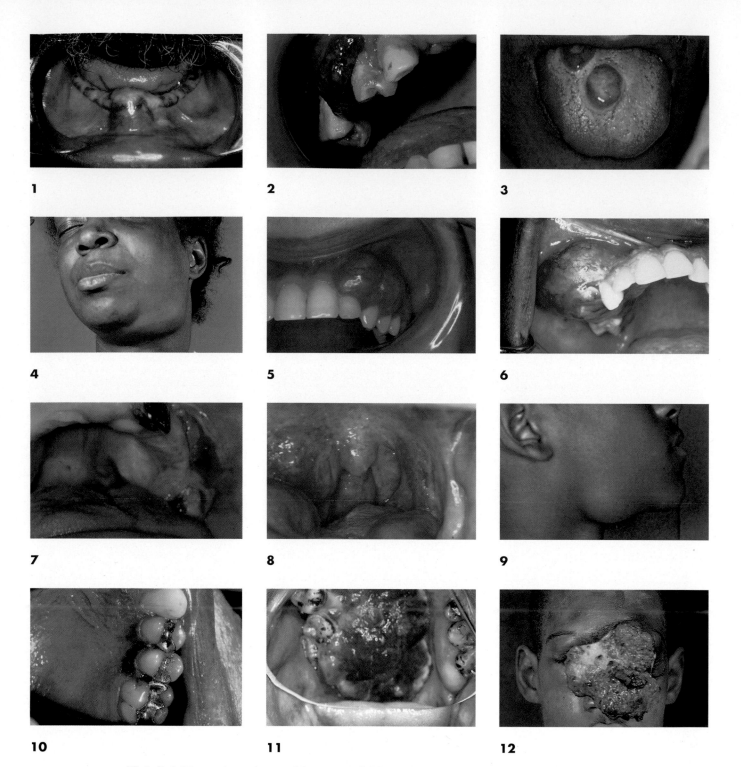

Plate J. **1,** Metastatic carcinoma of the prostate. **2,** Metastatic adenocarcinoma of the lung. **3,** Metastatic carcinoma of the esophagus. **4,** Metastatic cancer of the oral cavity to cervical lymph nodes. **5,** Osteogenic sarcoma. **6,** Chondrosarcoma. **7,** Carcinoma of the maxillary sinus. **8,** Lymphoma. **9,** Lymphoma. **10,** Superficial melanoma. **11,** Melanoma. **12,** Transitional cell carcinoma of the nasal cavity. (**1** courtesy R. Kallal, Chicago; **2** from Ellis G, Jensen J, Reingold IM, et al: Malignant neoplasms metastatic to gingivae, *Oral Surg* 44:238-245, 1977; **3** courtesy E. Robinson, Toledo, Ohio; **5** courtesy V. Barresi, De Kalb, Ill; **9** courtesy J. Laviere, Chicago; **10** from Robertson GR, et al: *J Oral Surg* 37:349-352, 1979.)

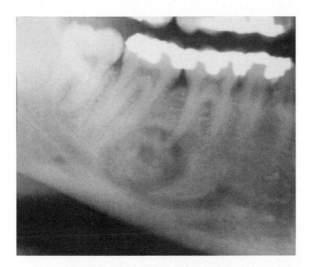

Fig. 27-9. Cementoblastoma at the apices of the distal root of the first molar tooth, which has a vital pulp. The symmetric, round radiopacity and the radiolucent rim are evident. (Courtesy N. Barakat, Beirut, Lebanon.)

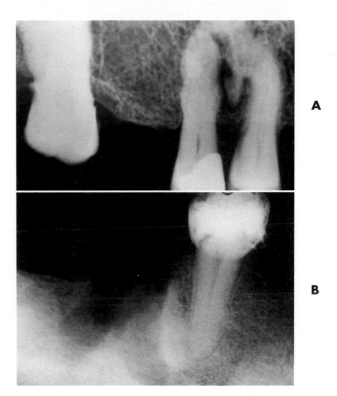

Fig. 27-10. Paget's disease. (**A** courtesy R. Goepp, Chicago.)

also be a problem when the clinician is confronted by the spherical type of hypercementosis occasionally seen on the anterior teeth. In hypercementosis, continuity with the root surface is discernible if the radiograph is carefully examined.

Management

Hypercementosis does not require special treatment, although the obvious surgical problem is encountered during removal of the involved tooth. When many teeth show hypercementosis, the patient should be examined for diseases such as Paget's disease, acromegaly, and giantism.

RARITIES

A number of entities may cause true periapical radiopacities (Figs. 27-9 and 27-10), but since they are rare or are only rarely homogeneously radiopaque, they are merely listed on the first page of the chapter.

The complex odontoma is included in this list of rarities because it usually occurs supracoronally or between the roots of adjacent teeth, so it only rarely produces a periapical radiopacity. It is listed with true periapical radiopacities because its image cannot usually be shifted from the apex, since its buccolingual dimension is relatively large.

The reader is directed to the references at the end of the chapter for sources of further information concerning these disorders.

FALSE PERIAPICAL RADIOPACITIES

False (projected) periapical radiopacities, which are produced by a large number of entities, may be categorized into (1) radiodense bodies within the bone, situated either bucally or lingually to the apex, and (2) hard or soft tissue situated on the periphery of the bone or in the adjacent

soft tissue. A normal or pathologic soft tissue mass projected over bone may impart a considerably denser quality to the shadow of the bone.

False periapical radiopacities have a characteristic that is diagnostically useful: Their relationship to the apex is such that the radiopaque images can be shifted from the apex by altering the angle of projection.[9-11] Additional views (such as occlusal, lateral oblique, posteroanterior, Waters', and panographic) may be necessary to establish the true location of the entities that produce these radiopacities.

ANATOMIC STRUCTURES

Soft tissue or bony anatomic structures may be projected as radiopaque shadows over tooth apices. Examples of such configurations include the anterior nasal spine, ala of the nose, malar process of the maxilla, external oblique ridge, mylohyoid ridge, mental protuberance, and hyoid bone (Fig. 27-11).

Identification of these structures depends on an awareness of the regional anatomy, a general understanding of the geometry required to radiographically visualize the area, and usually at least two different radiographic projections of the area.

IMPACTED TEETH, SUPERNUMERARY TEETH, AND COMPOUND ODONTOMAS

Since it is unusual for impacted or supernumerary teeth or those in a compound odontoma to be situated directly

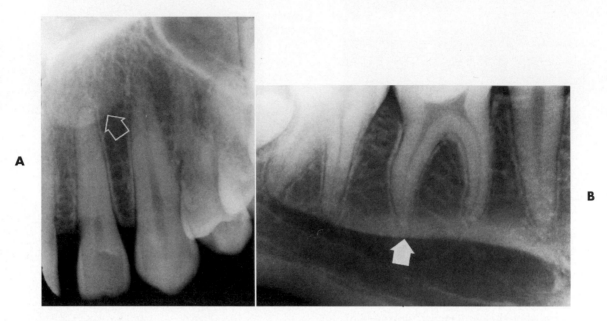

Fig. 27-11. Projected anatomic periapical radiopacities. **A,** Ala of the nose *(arrow).* **B,** Mylohyoid ridge *(arrow).*

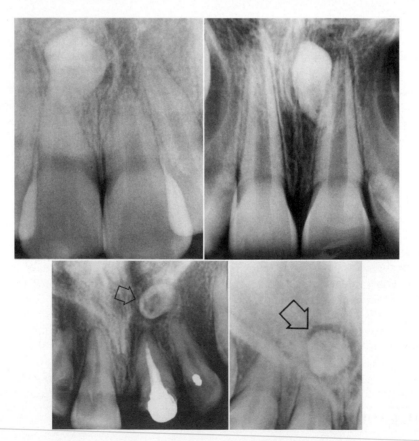

Fig. 27-12. Impacted supernumerary teeth as projected periapical radiopacities.

at the apex of an erupted tooth, these entities are classified as false periapical radiopacities.

The periapical radiopaque images produced by an impacted or supernumerary tooth or an odontoma are readily identified by their density and shape (Fig. 27-12). In most cases the images can be shifted from the apex by the Clark tube-shift technique.

TORI, EXOSTOSES, AND PERIPHERAL OSTEOMAS

Tori, exostoses, and less frequently, osteomas are situated at the periphery of the jaws and may vary greatly in size, shape, and location. They are all discussed in detail in Chapter 10 as examples of exophytic lesions. Because they originate deep to the surface epithelium and are slow growing, they have a smoothly contoured surface.

On radiographic examination, tori, exostoses, and periosteal osteomas may appear as single or multiple, smoothly

contoured, somewhat rounded, dense radiopaque masses (Fig. 27-13). Since they are peripheral, if their shadows happen to fall in an apical area on the radiograph, shifting the tube on a subsequent exposure (Clark tube-shift technique) readily demonstrates that these images are false periapical radiolucencies. In addition, these radiopaque images are not circumscribed by a periodontal ligament space and lamina dura. Such information from the radiographs, corroborated by clinically apparent intraoral bony protuberances, render the diagnosis obvious.

RETAINED ROOT TIPS

Retained root tips, especially in the molar regions, may be situated so that their radiopaque shadows are projected over the apex of an adjacent tooth (Fig. 27-14). When this happens, the root tip's position relative to the apex in question can be demonstrated on subsequent films by the Clark tube-shift technique. If the shapes of the root, its root canal, the surrounding periodontal ligament, and the lamina dura remain, unaltered, the identification is relatively easy; if these features are obliterated, however, the nature of the radiopacity may not be as obvious. Furthermore, a condensing osteitis may develop around the root tip and obscure it on the radiograph. Retained roots have been reported to occur in 6.1% of patients.[14]

FOREIGN BODIES

A variety of foreign materials within the jawbone or in the surrounding soft tissue may be projected over apices and cause periapical radiopacities on the radiograph (Fig. 27-15). A list of such objects includes metal fragments, buttons, zippers, hooks, other metal dress accessories, jewelry, and various dental materials and fragments of instruments. Usually the images cast by such items are distinctive and readily identifiable.[22-24] If there is a history of trauma to the region, the clinician may anticipate

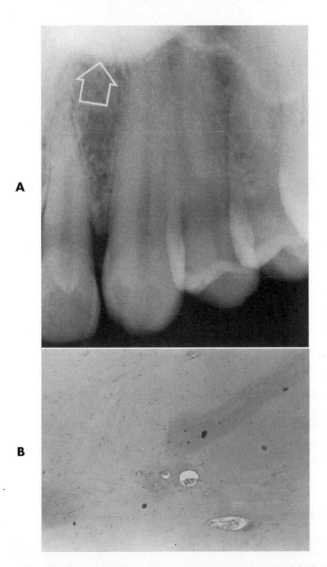

A

B

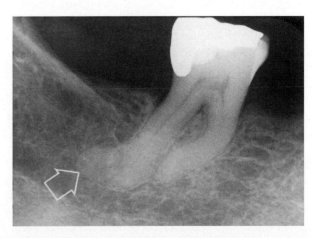

Fig. 27-13. A, Maxillary torus *(arrow)* as a projected periapical radiopacity. **B,** Microscopy of the torus.

Fig. 27-14. Retained root tip of the mesial root of the third molar *(arrow)* projected onto the periapex of the second molar.

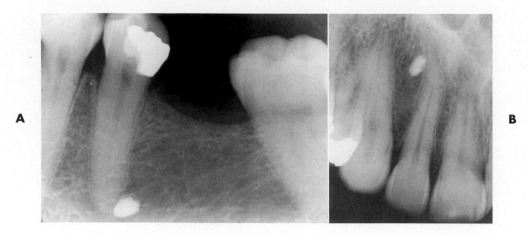

Fig. 27-15. Metal fragments projected as periapical radiopacities. **A,** This foreign body proved to be in the buccal cortical plate. **B,** This foreign body proved to be in the upper lip.

finding a foreign body embedded in the tissue and even look for its appearance on the radiograph. Price[25] discusses the problem presented when dental materials become foreign bodies in the tissue, because not all of these materials are radiopaque.

MUCOSAL CYST OF THE MAXILLARY SINUS

The mucosal cyst of the maxillary sinus occurs in approximately 2% of the population. This entity represents a retention cyst in the lining mucosa of the maxillary sinus.

Features

The incidence of a mucosal cyst of the maxillary sinus, which affects men and women equally and may be bilateral, peaks during the third decade of life. Although most of these cysts are symptomless, a significant number produce accompanying symptoms of a sinusitis.

On radiographs the cyst usually appears as a relatively dense, dome-shaped mass with its base on the floor of the maxillary sinus; the apices of the maxillary first and second molars may appear to be within the opaque image of the cyst (Fig. 27-16).

The location and appearance of the dome-shaped radiopaque structure of the mucosal cyst of a maxillary sinus are almost diagnostic. Although the cyst may remain constant in size for a long time, it also may spontaneously empty slowly or rapidly; thus periodic radiographic examinations frequently reveal a radiopacity of varying dimensions.

Differential Diagnosis

When a mucosal cyst of the maxillary sinus appears as a periapical radiopacity, it must be differentiated from the true radiopacities: a condensing or sclerosing osteitis, a periapical idiopathic osteosclerosis, and a PCOD. Additional radiographic views (such as panographic, Waters', and posteroanterior) usually identify it as a mass situated in the maxillary sinus.

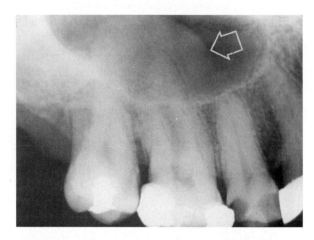

Fig. 27-16. Tentative diagnosis of a benign mucosal cyst *(arrow)* of the maxillary sinus projected as a radiopacity over the molar roots.

The smooth dome shape of the mucosal cyst of the maxillary sinus often differentiates it from a malignant tumor of the sinus.

Occasionally, fibrous dysplasia originating on the floor of the maxillary sinus mimics a maxillary sinus retention phenomenon, but the ground-glass appearance of the former entity helps distinguish this lesion from the mucosal cyst.

Management

When the clinician discovers what appears to be a mucous retention cyst in the maxillary sinus and it is asymptomatic, periodic radiographs are in order.

ECTOPIC CALCIFICATIONS

Ectopic calcifications* in the soft tissues surrounding the jaw may be mistaken on radiographs for calcified odonto-

_____

*Pathologic deposits of calcium salts in tissues that are normally uncalcified.

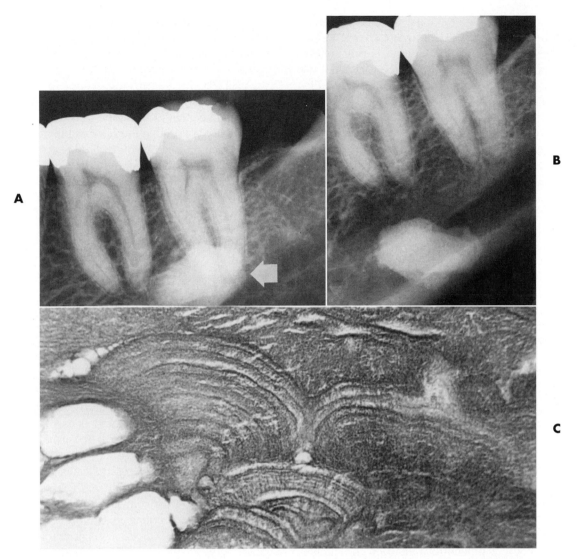

Fig. 27-17. Sialolith. **A,** Sialolith in the submandibular salivary gland projected over the apex of the mandibular second molar *(arrow).* **B,** Shift in the image of the stone caused by an altered vertical angle of exposure. **C,** Photomicrograph.

genic structures. Such deposits of abnormal calcific salts may be readily distinguished from calcified odontogenic structures and lesions by considering that the latter radiopacities are usually surrounded by a periodontal ligament type of space and a lamina dura, whereas the former do not have such characteristic borders. Also, the location of these ectopic calcifications can be shown to be some distance from the teeth by Clark's tube-shift technique. Katz, Langlais, Underhill, and Kimura[11] describe the tube-shift technique in extraoral radiography.

Sialoliths (Salivary Gland Calculi)

Sialoliths are calcareous (radiopaque) deposits in the ducts of the major or minor salivary glands or within the glands themselves. They are thought to form from a slowly calcifying nidus of tissue or bacterial debris (organic matrix).

In their early stages the sialoliths may be too small or insufficiently mineralized to be visible on radiographs. If they are not expelled from the duct, however, they eventually become large enough to be visible as radiopacities (Fig. 27-17).

Major Salivary Gland Sialoliths

Sialolithiasis, a common finding, occurs mainly in the submandibular gland (80% to 90%) and to a lesser degree in the parotid gland (5% to 20%).[26] Predilection for the submandibular gland and duct may result from gravity and the fact that the oral terminus is superior to the gland. The sublingual gland is involved in less than 1% of cases.[26]

When sialoliths reach a critical size or position, they effect a partial or complete obstruction of the duct. This results in a sialadenitis, which is manifested as a painful swelling of the gland that is most pronounced just before, during, and immediately after meals. The enlargement usually is minimal when the patient awakes in the morning. Often, several episodes of sialadenitis occur before the patient seeks professional help. Since the major or collecting ducts are usually completely occluded, milking the gland and duct is nonproductive.

Sialoliths vary greatly in size, shape, density, contour, and position, and they may be solitary or multiple (see Fig. 27-18). They are frequently seen within the substance of the submandibular gland and may be one solid mass or many smaller masses.

Although sialoliths in the submandibular gland and duct may be seen on periapical films, they are best visualized on occlusal, lateral oblique, and panoramic radiographs. When present in the parotid duct, on periapical films, they may be superimposed over the maxillary molars or the posterior maxillary alveoli. Sialoliths located in the anterior two-thirds of the Wharton's duct may be palpated intraorally.[27] Haug, Bradrick, and Indresano[28] describe the successful use of xeroradiography in the identification of nonradiopaque sialoliths by distinguishing only slightly different densities.

On histologic examination a sialolith resembles a calculus, showing concentric rings of alternating light and dark bands (Fig. 27-17, *C*).

Differential diagnosis The first step in the diagnostic procedure is to obtain another radiographic view of the stone taken at a different angle from the first. This step verifies that the radiopacity in question is actually a false (projected) periapical radiopacity.

Once the radiopacity is established to be a projected radiopacity, the sialolith must be distinguished from several entities—a calcified lymph node, an avulsed or embedded tooth, a foreign body, a phlebolith (calcified thrombus), calcification in the facial artery, myositis ossificans, and an anatomic structure (such as the hyoid bone).

The radiopaque image of the hyoid bone is frequently projected over the region of the submandibular gland and duct and mandible on lateral oblique radiographs but appears bilaterally on panoramic films. Consequently, if the mass is single on the lateral oblique and the panographic radiograph, it is unlikely to be the hyoid bone. The shape of the hyoid bone (V) is actually so diagnostic that clinicians do not mistake this structure for pathosis.

Myositis ossificans is a rare disturbance characterized by the formation of bone in the interstitial tissue of muscle. It has also been observed in the superficial tissues away from muscle, even in the skin. When muscles of the face are involved, the masseter muscle is most frequently affected. This results in a restriction of mandibular movements, which should alert the clinician to the possibility of myositis ossificans.

Calcification in the walls of the facial artery may also be projected over the apex of teeth and produce a suspect area. If a significant length of the artery is involved, the resultant serpentine, calcified image is diagnostic, but if there are calcific deposits in just a short section of the vessel, the resultant image may be mistaken for a sialolith, especially if the section of facial artery that courses through the submandibular space is involved.

A phlebolith sometimes occurs in the floor of the mouth and may be seen on an occlusal radiograph; it usually accompanies a clinically discernible varicosity. If a radiopacity is found in the floor of the mouth and there is no sialadenitis, the clinician should favor phlebolith as a diagnosis. The final differentiation between these two entities may have to await surgery.

A foreign body is usually readily diagnosed by its characteristic shape and by the history of a traumatic incident to the region.

Similarly an avulsed tooth lying in the soft tissues should be recognized by its shape and relative density, and the clinician should be able to obtain a history of a traumatic incident.

A calcified submandibular lymph node may be difficult to distinguish from a sialolith occurring within the submandibular gland, since some of the lymph nodes in the submandibular space rest on the surface of the submandibular gland (some are even inside the capsule of the gland). Also a calcified lymph node and a sialolith would be projected into the same general region on the radiograph. The relative incidences of the two entities favor the diagnosis of sialolith; furthermore, a painful swelling accompanying a calcified mass in the submandibular space strongly indicates a sialolith, since a calcified node represents an old, burned-out, asymptomatic lesion. On the contrary, if the calcified mass has a smooth, rounded contour, it is more apt to be a calcified lymph node than a sialolith. A sialogram may help distinguish between these entities. When painful swelling is not present, the examiner may be able to determine by careful bimanual palpation whether the firm mass is within the submaxillary salivary gland.

Management When a stone is discovered in the duct or the gland proper, it should always be removed. If the sialolith is impacted in the duct and the case is complicated by secondary infection, the infection should be eliminated before the stone is surgically removed. If the stone is in Wharton's duct, it may be approached and removed intraorally.

When the sialolith is small and located within the gland, it can ordinarily be removed by simple incision. If it is large, however, the gland must be excised; when a sialolith is in the gland, surgery may have to be performed even though there is a concurrent sialadenitis.

Minor Salivary Gland Sialoliths

Sialoliths in minor salivary glands are more common than previously believed.[29-31] They are usually solitary, small, painless submucosal nodules that are fully movable in the tissue.[30] They occur most often on the buccal mucosa and upper lip of people in the fifth to seventh decade and rarely occur on the palate or lower lip.[30] They vary greatly in size, shape, and morphologic appearance.[29] On rare occasions, multiple sialoliths may be seen.[31]

Differential diagnosis Small mucous cysts, lymph nodes, and salivary gland tumors[29] need to be considered in the differential diagnosis of sialoliths of minor salivary glands. Radiographs show the small radiopacity if sufficient mineral content is present (see Fig. 28-25). Xeroradiography is helpful in showing nonradiopaque sialoliths.[28]

Management The lesion should be excised in its entirety and studied microscopically.

Rhinoliths and Antroliths

Rhinoliths and antroliths are calcified masses occurring in the nasal cavity and maxillary sinus, respectively. Their development is similar to that of a sialolith: commencing with the calcification of a nidus of tissue debris or concentrated mucus, which continues to grow because of the precipitation of calcium salts in concentric layers. Beads and buttons have been identified as the nidus in two interesting cases.[32,33]

Rhinoliths and anthroliths are included in this chapter because their images may be cast over the apices of adjacent maxillary teeth on periapical radiographs.

Features Usually, no symptoms accompany the smaller rhinoliths or antroliths, but the larger stones may be associated with a sinusitis or nasal obstruction.

These calcifications are usually found on routine radiographs of the region and are of various shapes, from round to oval to irregular, with outlines that may be smooth or ragged (Fig. 27-18). They may appear as a dense, homogeneous radiopacity or may show concentric rings of radiopaque and radiolucent material. In some instances, small radiolucent areas are distributed haphazardly throughout the radiopaque mass.

Rhinoliths and antroliths may contain so little mineral that their image is quite faint. On microscopic examination, they resemble sialoliths and calculi.

Differential diagnosis When solitary radiopacities are seen in the superior aspect of a maxillary periapical film, antroliths and rhinoliths must be considered possible diagnoses. It is then particularly important to obtain additional maxillary views (such as panoramic, occlusal, Waters', and posteroanterior), as well as several additional periapical views, to facilitate the differential diagnosis, since these projections show the complete lesion or structure and demonstrate whether the mass is in the sinus, nasal cavity, or adjacent maxillary alveolar bone.

Different projections further enable the clinician to determine the relative location of the object by its apparent shift in position according to the varying angles of exposure.

Knowledge of the anatomy of the area and the information obtained from a complete radiographic examination enable the clinician to identify and differentiate the following entities, which can be confused with antroliths and sialoliths: a cone cut, eyeglasses, a complex odontoma, a mature cementoma, a periapical condensing osteitis, a buccal exostosis, a palatine torus, an impacted tooth, the ala of the nose, and the malar process of the maxilla.

A cone cut in the superior aspect of a periapical film appears as a homogeneous radiopacity containing no detail. However, its contour is convex like that of the rhinolith.

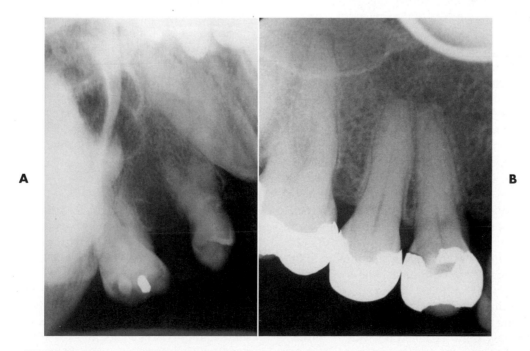

Fig. 27-18. A, Large antrolith projected over the roots of a molar. **B,** Lens of the patient's eyeglasses projected as a radiopacity.

Such cone cuts are not likely to be present or similarly positioned on additional films.

Eyeglasses occasionally show on radiographs as a solid, homogeneous radiopacity rather than a radiopaque rim (see Fig. 27-18). Although antroliths are not likely to occur bilaterally and with such symmetry, additional radiographs should be taken after the removal of the eyeglasses to determine the identity of the opacities.

The radiopaque images of a complex odontoma and a mature cementoma may mimic those produced by an antrolith, but the former images have characteristically radiolucent borders. When these odontogenic tumors become large enough to cause a bulge in the floor of the antrum, differentiation from an antrolith may be difficult; fortunately, the complex odontoma and the mature cementoma rarely reach such a size in this location.

Periapical condensing osteitis at the apices of a maxillary premolar may simulate an antrolith on periapical films. However, the adjacent teeth test nonvital in the case of periapical condensing osteitis, and additional films show that the mass is not encroaching on the antrum. These considerations help identify the radiopacity as a periapical condensing osteitis.

The dense, rounded radiopacity produced by a buccal exostosis or a palatine torus is frequently seen in the superior aspect of a maxillary periapical radiograph and may closely resemble the image produced by an antrolith or a sialolith. Clinical detection of the torus or the exostosis provides the correct diagnosis.

An impacted tooth may be confused with an antrolith or a rhinolith, especially when it is projected high on the film or when it is positioned in the jaw so that its image is not characteristic of a tooth. Good, properly positioned films, show the typically clear outlines of the impacted tooth.

The ala of the nose may be projected over the periapices of the upper incisors or canines and appear as a partially mineralized rhinolith (see Fig. 27-11, *A*). Again, additional films and a familiarity with the regional anatomy suggest the correct diagnosis.

The inferior portion of the malar process of the maxilla or the zygomatic bone on some periapical films appears identical to an antrolith (see Fig. 28-21). Additional projections enable the clinician to correctly identify this structure.

When a mature cementoma or a complex odontoma produces a bulge in the floor of the maxillary sinus, differentiating it from an antrolith or some other pathosis of the maxillary sinus (such as a mucosal retention cyst, fibrous dysplasia, a tumor, and root tips) is more difficult.

Root tips in the maxillary sinus may be difficult to differentiate from a small antrolith unless the root canal is evident.

Except for the rare osteoma, a tumor of the maxillary sinus usually is less radiopaque than an antrolith.

Although possibly quite opaque on a Waters' projection, fibrous dysplasia usually has a ground-glass appearance on periapical films.

The dome-shaped appearance of a mucosal retention cyst usually distinguishes this phenomenon from the more spherical-appearing antroliths. Also, its less dense opacity usually permits normal landmarks to be seen through its image.

Management Patients with antroliths and rhinoliths should be referred to an otolaryngologist for evaluation and management.

Calcified Lymph Nodes

Calcified lymph nodes occur in the cervical and submaxillary regions (Fig. 27-19). The majority are calcified tuberculous nodes. On certain radiographic views, their images are projected over the mandibular bone and occasionally over the apex of a mandibular tooth.

Features Calcified lymph nodes are asymptomatic and are usually found on a routine radiographic survey. The patient may have a history of successful treatment for tuberculosis. Any of the cervical and submandibular nodes may be involved. In some cases, just an isolated node has been calcified; in others, several nodes or perhaps a whole chain of nodes has become calcified. If the nodes are superficial, they may be palpated as bony hard, round or linear masses with variable mobility.

On radiographs a single round, oval, or linear calcified radiopaque mass may be seen (see Fig. 27-19). Frequently the outlines are well contoured and well defined, depending on whether the original inflammatory process was contained within the capsule of the lymph node.

Differential diagnosis The differential diagnosis between calcified lymph nodes and a sialolith in the submandibular salivary gland is discussed in the section on the differential diagnosis of the sialolith. In addition a tubercular calcified node needs to be differentiated from that of histoplasmosis, bacillus Calmette-Guérin vaccination, coccidioidomycosis, filariasis, lymphoma, metastatic calcifying tumor, and idiopathic calcification.[34] Superimposed myositis ossificans needs to be considered as well.[35]

Management Calcified lymph nodes do not require treatment, although they may be indicators of diseases in the latent stage.

Phleboliths

Phleboliths (angioliths) are calcified thrombi occurring in venules, veins, or sinusoidal vessels of hemangiomas. They are always coincidental with vascular stasis.[26] They may occur singly or as multiple calcifications, are usually small radiopacities, may be round or oval, and may show concentric light and dark rings (see Fig. 28-22). When they are projected over the mandibular bone or the periapices of mandibular teeth, they may easily be confused with sialoliths. They should also be differentiated from tonsilloliths, calcified acne, cysticerosis, myositis ossificans, and arterial calcifications.[36]

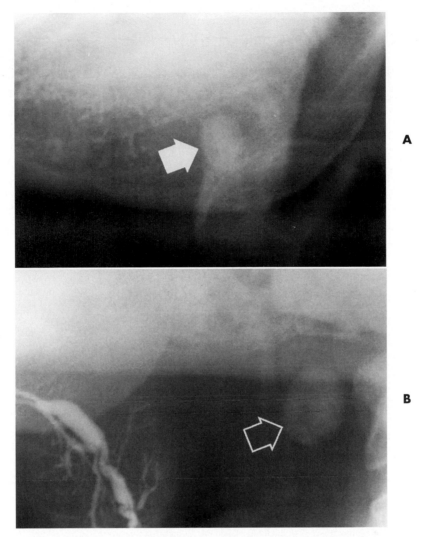

Fig. 27-19. Solitary calcified cervical lymph node *(arrow).* **A,** Projected over the mandible as a radiopacity. **B,** Another view of the same node showing the image shifted away from the mandible. A sialogram of the submandibular salivary gland proved that the calcified lesion was not a sialolith. (Courtesy R. Goepp, Chicago.)

Arterial Calcifications

Calcification frequently accompanies arteriosclerosis, and the facial artery is sometimes affected. When a considerable length of this artery is involved, the serpentine outline and the position of the faint radiopacity are pathognomic. When just a small segment of the artery is involved, however, and the radiopaque image of this segment is cast over the body of the mandible near the inferior border, the artery may simulate a sialolith within the submaxillary gland or duct or a small, calcified lymph node.

RARITIES

Rarities of soft tissue calcifications that occur as single or multiple entities are listed on the first page of this chapter.

REFERENCES

1. McDonald M, Pogrel MA: Calcification of the cricoid cartilage mistaken for a foreign body: report of a case, *J Oral Maxillofac Surg* 50:62-63, 1992.
2. De Leon ER, Aguirre A: Oral cysticerosis, *Oral Surg* 79:572-577, 1995.
3. Mc Donnell D: Dense bone island: a review of 107 patients, *Oral Surg* 76:124-128, 1993.
4. Eversole LR, Stone CE, Straub D: Focal sclerosing osteomyelitis/focal periapical osteopetrosis: radiographic patterns, *Oral Surg* 58:456-460, 1984.
5. Douglass GD, Towbridge HO: Chronic focal sclerosing osteomyelitis associated with a cracked tooth: report of a case, *Oral Surg* 76:351-355, 1993.
6. Farman AG, Joubert JJ, Nortje CJ: Focal osteosclerosis and apical periodontal pathosis in "European" and Cape coloured dental outpatients, *Int J Oral Surg* 7:549-557, 1978.
7. MacDonald-Janowski DS: The detection of abnormalities in the jaws: a radiological survey, *Br Dent J* 170:215-218, 1991.
8. Eliasson S, Halvarsson C, Ljungheimer G: Periapical condensing osteitis and endodontic treatment, *Oral Surg* 57:195-199, 1984.
9. Clark CA: A method of ascertaining the relative position of unerupted teeth by means of film radiographs, *Proc R Soc Med* 3:87-90, 1910.
10. Ludlow JB, Nesbit SP: Teaching radiographic localization in dental schools in the United States and Canada, *Oral Surg* 79:393-397, 1995.
11. Katz JO, Langlais RP, Underhill TE, Kimura K: Localization of paraoral soft tissue calcifications: the known object rule, *Oral Surg* 67:459-463, 1989.
12. Jordan RE, Suzuki M, Skinner DH: Indirect pulp-capping of carious teeth with periapical lesions, *J Am Dent Assoc* 97:37-43, 1978.
13. Marmary Y, Kutiner G: A radiographic survey of periapical jawbone lesions, *Oral Surg* 61:405-408, 1986.
14. White SC, Atchison KA, Hewlett ER, Flack VF: Efficacy of FDA guidelines for prescribing radiographs to detect dental and intraosseous conditions, *Oral Surg* 80:108-114, 1995.
15. Geist JR, Katz JO: The frequency and distribution of idiopathic osteosclerosis, *Oral Surg* 69:388-393, 1990.
16. Kaffe I, Rosen P, Horowitz I: The significance of idiopathic osteosclerosis found in panoramic radiographs of sporadic colorectal neoplasia patients and their relatives, *Oral Surg* 74:366-370, 1992.
17. Waldron CA: Fibro-osseous lesions of the jaws, *J Oral Maxillofac Surg* 51:828-835, 1993.
18. Summerlin D-J, Tomich CE: Focal cemento-osseous dysplasia: a clinicopathologic study of 221 cases, *Oral Surg* 78:611-620, 1994.
19. Neville BW, Albenesius RJ: The prevalence of benign fibro-osseous lesions of periodontal ligament origin in black women: a radiographic survey, *Oral Surg* 62:340-344, 1986.
20. Alantar A, Tarragano, H, Lefèvre B: Extrusion of endodontic filling material into the insertions of the myohyloid muscle: a case report, *Oral Surg* 78:646-649, 1994.
21. Stafne EC: *Oral roentgenographic diagnosis,* ed 3, Philadelphia, 1969, WB Saunders.
22. Oikarinen KS, Nieminen TM, Mäkäräinen H, Pyhtinen J: Visibility of foreign bodies in soft tissue in plain radiographs, computed tomography, magnetic resonance imaging, and ultrasound, *Int J Oral Maxillofac Surg* 22:119-124, 1993.
23. Steele J, Khan Z, Steiner M, et al: Stent-aided imaging for osseointegrated implants, *Oral Surg* 70:243, 1990.
24. Scully C, Chen M: Tongue piercing (oral body art), *Br J Oral Maxillofac Surg* 32:37-38, 1994.
25. Price C: A method of determining the radiopacity of dental materials and foreign bodies, *Oral Surg* 62:710-718, 1986.
26. Raymond AK, Batsakis JG: Pathology consultation: angiolithiasis and sialolithiasis in the head and neck, *Ann Otol Rhinol Laryngol* 101:455-457, 1992.
27. Lustmann J, Regev E, Melamed Y: Sialolithiasis: a survey on 245 patients and a review of the literature, *Int J Oral Maxillofac Surg* 19:135-138, 1990.
28. Haug RH, Bradrick JP, Indresano AT: Xeroradiography in the diagnosis of nonradiopaque sialoliths, *Oral Surg* 67:146-148, 1989.
29. Yamane GM, Scharlock SE, Jain R, et al: Intraoral salivary gland sialolithiasis, *J Oral Med* 39:85-90, 1984.
30. Ho V, Currie WJR, Walker A: Sialolithiasis of minor salivary glands, *Br J Oral Surg* 30:273-275, 1992.
31. Anneroth G, Hansen LS: Minor salivary gland calculi: a clinical and histopathological study of forty-nine cases, *Int J Oral Surg* 12:80-89, 1983.
32. Appleton SA, Kimbrough RE, Engstrom HIM: Rhinolithiasis: a review, *Oral Surg* 65:693-698, 1988.
33. Damm DD, Ziegler RC: Roentgeno-oddities: factitious rhinolith, *Oral Surg* 59:662, 1985.
34. Hirschfeld JJ: Roentgeno-oddities: calcifications in lymph nodes, *Oral Surg* 61:412, 1986.
35. Woolgar JA, Beirne JC, Triantafylou A: Myositis ossificans traumatica of sternocleidomastoid muscle presenting as cervical lymph-node metastasis, *Int J Oral Maxillofac Surg* 24:170-173, 1995.
36. Zachariades N, Rallis G, Papademetriou J, et al: Phleboliths: a report of three unusual cases, *Br J Oral Maxillofac Surg* 29:117-119, 1991.

CHAPTER 28

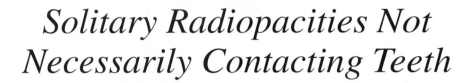

Solitary Radiopacities Not Necessarily Contacting Teeth

NORMAN K. WOOD

PAUL W. GOAZ

A list of radiopacities that may not be in contact with the roots of teeth follows:

TRUE INTRABONY RADIOPACITIES
TORI, EXOSTOSES, AND PERIPHERAL
  OSTEOMAS
UNERUPTED, IMPACTED, AND
  SUPERNUMERARY TEETH
RETAINED ROOTS
IDIOPATHIC OSTEOSCLEROSIS
CONDENSING OR SCLEROSING OSTEITIS
MATURE FOCAL CEMENTOOSSEOUS
  DYSPLASIA
FIBROUS DYSPLASIA
FOCAL SCLEROSING OSTEOMYELITIS
DIFFUSE SCLEROSING OSTEOMYELITIS
PROLIFERATIVE PERIOSTITIS (GARRÉ'S
  OSTEOMYELITIS)
MATURE COMPLEX ODONTOMA
OSSIFYING SUBPERIOSTEAL HEMATOMA

RARITIES
  Cementifying and ossifying fibroma
  Chondromas and chondrosarcomas—
    radiopaque variety
  Mature osteoblastoma
  Metastatic osteoblastic carcinomas—
    radiopaque variety
  Osteoblastoma
  Osteochondroma
  Osteogenic sarcoma—radiopaque variety
PROJECTED RADIOPACITIES
ANATOMIC STRUCTURES[1]
FOREIGN BODIES
PATHOLOGIC SOFT TISSUE MASSES
ECTOPIC CALCIFICATIONS
  Sialoliths of major and minor salivary glands
  Rhinoliths and antroliths

  Calcified lymph nodes
  Tonsilloliths
  Phleboliths
  Arterial calcifications
RARITIES
  Calcified acne lesion
  Calcified hematoma (soft tissue)
  Calcinosis cutis
  Cysticercosis[2]
  Hamartoma
  Myositis ossificans
  Peripheral fibroma with calcification
  Pilomatricoma (calcifying epithelioma of
    Malherbe)
  Tumoral calcinosis

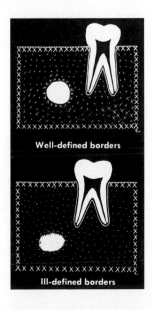

Well-defined borders

Ill-defined borders

Many of the radiopacities included in this chapter are discussed in Chapter 27. It seems expedient, however, to repeat the listing of these entities and reconsider some of them, since they may also occur as solitary radiopacities not contacting the roots of teeth. Such an arrangement is appropriate, since there is a difference in the incidence of these entities, which correlates with their contacting the roots of teeth.

Certainly, this consideration affects the development of a valid differential diagnosis. Condensing or sclerosing osteitis is a good case in point: As a periapical radiopacity, the lesion occurs quite commonly, but its occurrence as a solitary radiopacity not contacting the roots of teeth is uncommon. Thus the two entities are discussed in both chapters.

In this chapter, solitary radiolucencies not contacting the roots of teeth are discussed as true intrabony radiopacities and projected radiopacities.

TRUE INTRABONY RADIOPACITIES

TORI, EXOSTOSES, AND PERIPHERAL OSTEOMAS

Tori, exostoses, and peripheral osteomas are discussed in Chapter 10 as exophytic lesions and in Chapter 27 as projected (false) periapical radiopacities.

Features

The well-defined radiopaque shadows of these bony protuberances are projected over the images of tooth roots on radiographic films and not on others (Fig. 28-1). Usually a torus on the mandible, an exostosis, and sometimes an osteoma (in either jaw) cast radiopaque shadows over the images of tooth roots if the jaw segments in which they occur are bearing teeth.

Differential Diagnosis

Correlating the clinical finding of a smooth, nodular, hard protuberance with the radiographic finding of a smoothly contoured radiopacity establishes the correct diagnosis and eliminates the need for additional radiographs or an extensive differential diagnosis (see Fig. 28-1). Nevertheless, as shown in Fig. 28-2, a case of a mature cemento-ossifying fibroma can mimic an exostosis. However, in this case, periapical films show a thin radiolucent rim surrounding the mature fibroosseous lesion. In addition, an early osteogenic sarcoma or a small chondrosarcoma can mimic a torus or exostosis.

Management

Tori, exostoses, and peripheral osteomas may not have to be treated, but they may be removed surgically for phonetic, psychologic, or prosthetic reasons or if they are being chronically irritated.

UNERUPTED, IMPACTED, AND SUPERNUMERARY TEETH

Unerupted permanent molars and impacted and supernumerary teeth are the next most common solitary radiopacities after tori, exostoses, and osteomas, whose images may not overlap the roots of other teeth. These are common findings, since one study from the United Kingdom has shown that 25% of adults have at least one unerupted tooth.[3] The lower third molars were the most common, followed closely by the upper third molars, with canines, premolars, and supernumeraries a distant third.[3] In contradistinction, a study of patients applying to a dental school clinic in Australia found only

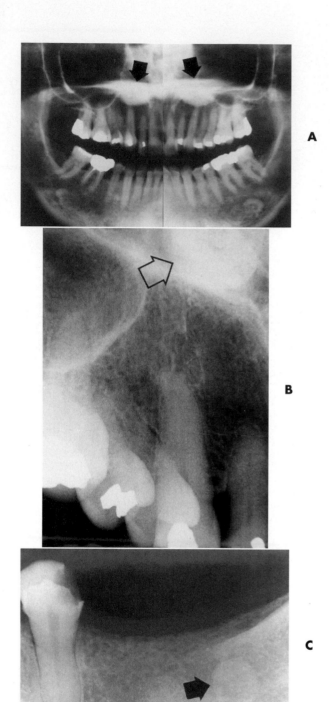

Fig. 28-1. A, Palatine torus *(arrows)* appears as bilateral radiopacities in this panograph. **B,** Palatine torus *(arrow)* projected superior to the apex of the canine. **C,** Small lingual mandibular torus *(arrow)* appearing as a rounded radiopacity.

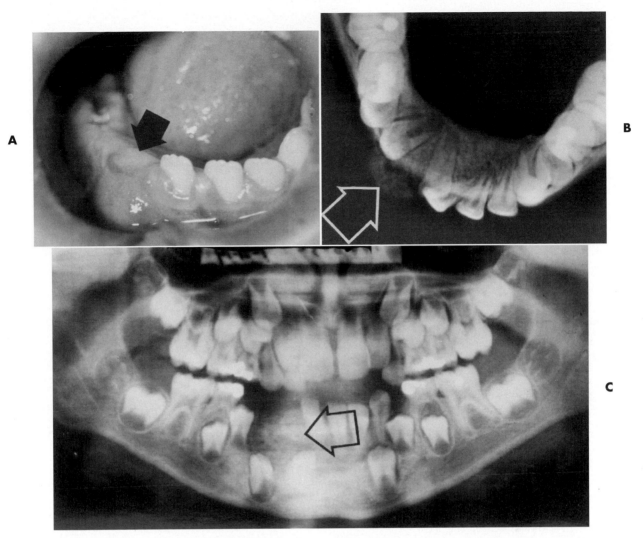

Fig. 28-2. Cementoossifying fibroma in an 8-year-old boy that resembled an exostosis on clinical examination (**A**) and in the occlusal radiograph (**B**). **C,** Orthopantomograph showing that the radiopaque lesion has blocked the eruption of the lower right permanent incisor and canine tooth. (Courtesy N. Choukas, Barrington, Ill.)

unerupted teeth in 2% of cases.[4] In Athens, Greece, unerupted teeth (mostly maxillary canines) were found on 9% of edentulous dental school patients.[5] If good radiographs are obtained, the recognizable outline of a tooth and the radiolucent shadows of the pulp canal, periodontal ligament, and follicular space establish the identity of these entities (Fig. 28-3). Bizarre shapes of malformed teeth coupled with technically poor films may complicate the identification of the entities.

RETAINED ROOTS

Retained roots are a common finding in edentulous regions of the jaws, and the images of retained roots usually do not contact those of other roots. Surveys of edentulous patients disclose that approximately 25% to 50% of these

patients have retained roots.[5-7] Some 80% of the roots are located in the posterior regions of the alveolar processes.[6] Most are found in the maxilla.[5,7] Approximately 6% of the retained roots have an accompanying radiolucency. This last group is classified under mixed radiolucent-radiopaque lesions, which is discussed in Chapter 24.

Features

The majority of retained roots are quiescent and asymptomatic, and they are found on routine radiographs. If they are unaltered, their identification is relatively easy (Fig. 28-4), but if chronic infection has caused the root canals to be obliterated or has resulted in some peripheral resorption or enveloping condensing osteitis, their recognition may be difficult. A careful study of the radiograph, however, usually discloses the homogeneous quality of

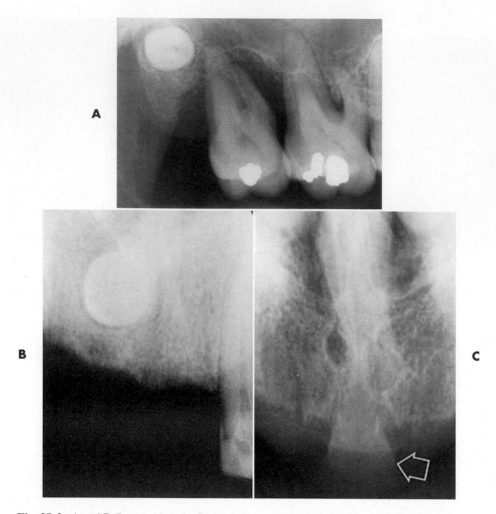

Fig. 28-3. A and **B,** Impacted teeth. **C,** Cartilage of the nasal septum *(arrow)* that resembles the crown of a developing incisor.

the root tip's shadow, which is in contrast to the somewhat obscure trabecular character of the sclerotic bone. Thus differentiation is possible.

On occasion, retained roots become infected, or longstanding chronic infection is exacerbated. In this case, local swelling, pain, regional lymphadenitis, space infections, and even osteomyelitis ensue.

Differential Diagnosis

The differential diagnosis for retained roots is discussed later in the section on the differential diagnosis of condensing osteitis.

Management

The management of a retained root tip depends on the circumstances of the individual case. If the root tip is small, asymptomatic, and situated relatively deep so that its removal would require excising an unacceptable amount of bone or if it is so close to an important structure that the structure could be significantly damaged during the root's removal, it should not be excised unless a serious pathologic condition appears to be associated with it. The patient

should simply be apprised of its presence, and its status should be periodically evaluated by serial radiographs. Roots that are near the surface and beneath the site of a proposed artificial denture or bridge, roots associated with a pathologic lesion, or roots causing pain should be removed.

IDIOPATHIC OSTEOSCLEROSIS

Idiopathic osteosclerosis is discussed in Chapter 27 as a periapical radiopacity. The objective of its inclusion in this chapter is to emphasize and illustrate that this entity is not always found in association with the roots of teeth.

Features

Idiopathic osteosclerotic lesions may occur in the alveolus, between the roots of teeth, just below the crest of the ridge, or in the body of the mandible (Fig. 28-5).

Usually the cause is obscure. When the lesion is present in the alveolus between the first and second premolars or between the second premolar and the first molar, its occurrence is generally described as a sequela of retained deciduous molar roots. These retained roots are resorbed

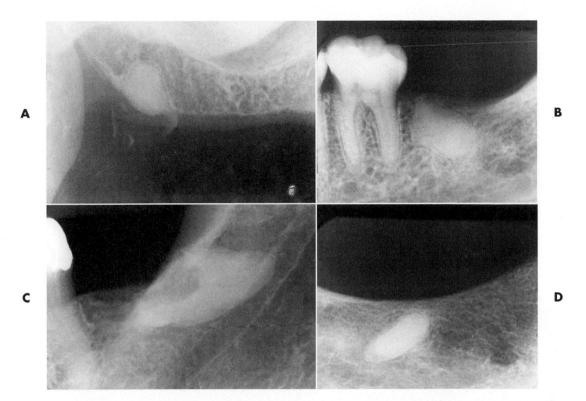

Fig. 28-4. Retained roots. The periodontal ligament space and lamina dura cannot be clearly detected around some of the root fragments. The root canal shadows are not apparent.

and replaced by sclerotic bone, or fragments of the roots are surrounded and obliterated by the condensed bone.

Because the radiopaque areas of periapical condensing osteitis frequently do not resolve after extraction of a tooth, many such residual areas may be diagnosed as idiopathic osteosclerosis if the clinician is unaware that teeth with infected or nonvital pulps have been removed from the area. This possibility should be considered when a suspect area is encountered. Postextraction wounds and other surgical defects may result in idiopathic osteosclerosis (see Fig. 28-5).

The sclerotic lesion is usually solitary but may be multiple or even bilateral; however, its bilateral occurrence is only incidental and should not be considered a significant diagnostic feature.

On microscopic examination, thickened trabeculae with few lacunae and greatly reduced marrow and fibrovascular spaces are seen.

Differential Diagnosis

The differential diagnosis of idiopathic osteosclerosis is discussed later in the section on the differential diagnosis of condensing osteitis.

Management

The identification of idiopathic osteosclerosis is all that is necessary. However, the clinician should observe the course of the lesion by taking serial radiographs.

CONDENSING OR SCLEROSING OSTEITIS

Condensing or sclerosing osteitis is an osteosclerosis that can be explained as a sequela of an inflammatory process.

It occurs much less frequently as a periapical radiopacity in edentulous regions, of course. In edentulous regions, it is usually a residual lesion or is limited to reactions around retained roots or root tips. Its appearance as a periapical radiopacity is described in detail in Chapter 27.

Features

On radiographs, condensing or sclerosing osteitis resembles the radiopacity of idiopathic osteosclerosis except that root tips are usually identifiable within the radiopaque lesion, or there may be a history or some presumptive evidence that an infected tooth was previously removed from the area. The borders may be ragged or smoothly contoured, and vague or well defined (Fig. 28-6).

The microscopic appearance is identical to that of idiopathic osteosclerosis except that if the lesion is still active, an extensive examination of the specimen discloses restricted areas of chronic inflammation. If the source of infection was removed some time before the specimen was taken, the inflammatory reaction may have completely subsided, with only the dense mass of trabeculae remaining.

Differential Diagnosis

Many of the entities discussed in this chapter must be included in the differential diagnosis. The lesions that may

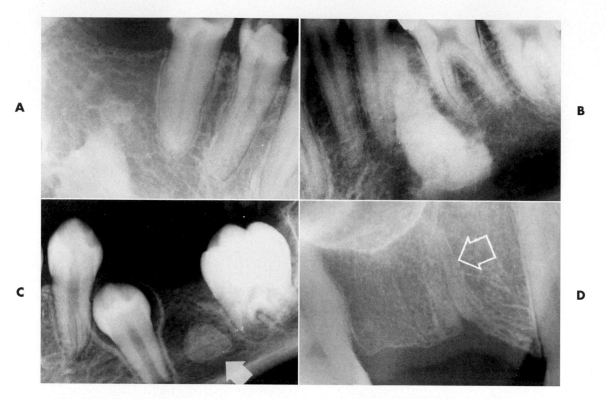

Fig. 28-5. **A** to **C,** Idiopathic osteosclerosis. The second premolar pulp in **B** was vital. **C,** Idiopathic osteosclerosis *(arrow).* **D,** Socket sclerosis *(arrow).* The central linear radiolucent shadow resembles a root canal.

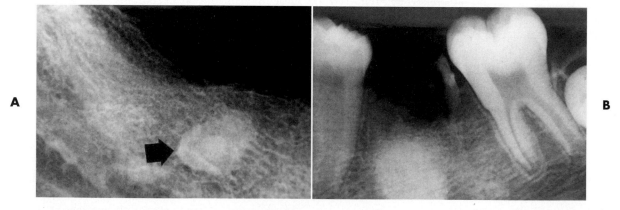

Fig. 28-6. Condensing osteitis. **A,** Surrounding a small, round root tip *(arrow).* **B,** Surrounding the mesial root of a grossly decayed molar.

be confused with condensing or sclerosing osteitis are a variety of the projected radiopacities that are not attached to or within the alveoli or jawbone under scrutiny. They include the following: focal cementoosseous dysplasia (FCOD), retained roots, unerupted tooth, mature complex odontoma, osteoblastic malignant tumor, focal sclerosing osteomyelitis, tori, exostoses, peripheral osteomas, and idiopathic osteosclerosis.

As discussed in Chapter 27, the projected radiopacities can be readily identified by obtaining additional radiographs of the area using Clark's tube-shift technique.

The opacities produced by hard odontogenic tissue, including the mature FCOD, retained roots, unerupted tooth, and mature complex odontoma, may be recognized by their distinctive shapes and densities and their radiolucent borders. A partially resorbed root tip or root fragment is usually relatively small and, if not surrounded by condensing osteitis, in most cases retains enough of its shape to be recognizable. It should be found only in tooth-bearing areas of the jaws.

Although an osteoblastic malignancy producing a completely radiopaque lesion in this area is very rare, in the event of such an occurrence, the examining clinician must consider osteogenic sarcoma, metastatic prostatic carcinoma, or metastatic mammary carcinoma. A case of lymphoma of the mandible that closely resembled condensing osteitis has been reported.[8] In addition to the symptoms of the primary tumor or the history of its treatment, the tumor is usually accompanied by pain, swelling, and frequently paresthesia. Paresthesia, if present, strongly suggests that the lesion is malignant.

Focal sclerosing osteomyelitis is a moderate proliferative reaction of the bone to a mild type of infection. The patient usually has a history of a prolonged, tender swelling with, in some cases, intermittent drainage through a sinus from the body of the mandible. Osteomyelitis seldom becomes established in healthy persons who do not have a history of jaw fracture. Condensing osteitis, by comparison, is common and usually asymptomatic.

The opacities produced by tori, exostoses, and peripheral osteomas can be identified promptly if the characteristic painless, smooth nodular swelling on the jaws is detected during the clinical examination.

Differentiating between condensing or sclerosing osteitis and idiopathic osteosclerosis is often difficult, if not impossible, when the suspect lesion is in an edentulous region and cannot be related to a specific tooth. Of course, if a root tip can be observed within the region of sclerotic bone, the diagnosis is condensing osteitis. Thus if the sclerotic area does not contain root tips and the lesion has not formed at the apex of a tooth with an infected or nonvital pulp, the diagnosis of idiopathic osteosclerosis is appropriate.

Management

The treatment of condensing or sclerosing osteitis surrounding a root tip must be tailored to the individual situation. As with root tips, lesions that are in the superficial alveolar crest should be removed to prepare for a prosthesis and to prevent the occurrence of active infection. Deeper lesions that are asymptomatic are usually not disturbed but are observed with serial radiographs. Lesions complicated by acute or chronic infection should be enucleated, and the patient should receive appropriate presurgical and postsurgical antibiotic therapy.

MATURE FCOD

The periapical cementoosseous dysplasia (PCOD) or FCOD that develops from cells of the periodontal ligament is discussed in Chapter 16 as a periapical radiolucency, in Chapter 24 as a mixed radiolucent-radiopaque lesion, and in Chapter 27 as a periapical radiopacity. In this chapter, its occurrence as a solitary radiopaque mass away from periapices or in edentulous regions of the jaws is discussed as FCOD.[9,10]

Features

When these mature fibroosseous lesions occur without apparent relation to teeth, they have the following features:

1. They are ordinarily found at the apices of vital teeth but also occur with significant frequency in edentulous regions. Many of these latter lesions may be residual (i.e., they were left in place when the involved tooth was removed).
2. They may be solitary or multiple, and their radiographic appearance is similar to that of the periapical variety. The mature lesions are uniformly radiopaque and often have a radiolucent border. Most of the lesions are round to oval but occasionally have irregular shapes (Fig. 28-7).
3. Bone peripheral to the radiolucent rim may show a sclerotic or ground-glass appearance.
4. On histologic study, they consist almost entirely of varying proportions of dense cementum and bone with few lacunae or vascular spaces and fibrous tissue.

Differential Diagnosis

The differential diagnosis of an FCOD is discussed earlier, in the section on the differential diagnosis of condensing osteitis.

Management

The proper management of an FCOD entails only its recognition and periodic observation by serial radiographs. It is important to identify the FCOD so that surgical removal is not mistakenly undertaken.

Lesions situated in the crest of the ridge, however, are usually removed if a denture is to be placed over the area (see Fig. 28-7, *D*). Lesions that continue to enlarge should be enucleated. This procedure enables the clinician to establish the correct diagnosis by microscopic examination of the tissue removed.

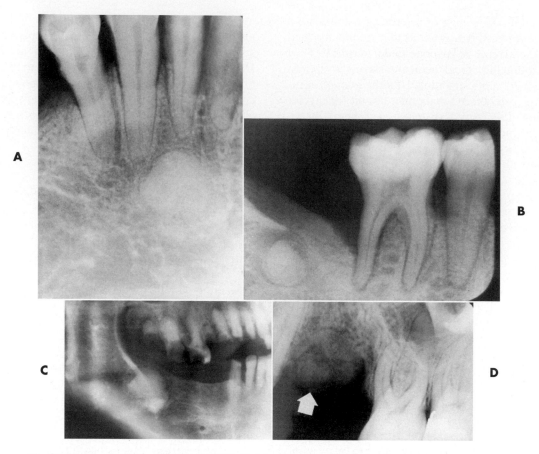

Fig. 28-7. **A** to **C,** Mature PCOD or FCOD. **D,** Mature cementoossifying fibroma *(arrow).* (Courtesy N. Barakat, Beirut, Lebanon.)

FIBROUS DYSPLASIA

Fibrous dysplasia appears to be a lesion that matures from radiolucent to radiopaque stages and then returns to normal architecture in patients in their 30s. It is discussed with ill-defined radiolucencies in Chapter 21 and in Chapter 25 as a mixed radiolucent-radiopaque lesion. In this chapter, its more radiopaque, classic, ground-glass appearance is emphasized.

Features

Fibrous dysplasia is basically a bony lesion of children, adolescents, and young adults that may involve the jawbones. The majority of the enlargements measure between 2 and 8 cm in length.

The radiographic image cast by these lesions is generally uniform and of the classic ground-glass* type (Fig. 28-8). In an earlier stage, there may be a mixed pattern with irregular radiodense foci distributed throughout a lesion of ground-glass appearance or through a radiolucent area. As the lesion matures, the foci become more radiopaque. The margins of the lesion are vague on the radiograph because there is a gradual transition between the pathosis and the surrounding normal bone. Mature lesions on extraoral radiographs often appear completely radiopaque, but usually on periapical films the region shows the ground-glass feature.

On histologic study, spicules of woven bone that appear in Chinese letter–like (retiform) patterns are scattered throughout a fibrous tissue stroma. Osteoblastic rimming of the bony spicules is usually missing. More mature lesions show a larger proportion of bone to fibrous tissue and frequently contain some lamellar type of bone with osteoblastic rimming.[10] Diagnosis must be based on considerations of history, clinical, radiographic, and gross appearance in conjunction with histopathologic findings.

Differential Diagnosis

A solitary, painless fusiform enlargement is almost certainly fibrous dysplasia when it is firm, smooth, and covered with normal mucosa; has a radiopaque, ground-glass appearance; and occurs in the jawbone of a relatively young person.

Other diseases such as Paget's disease in the radiolucent stage and hyperparathyroidism may produce a ground-glass appearance of the bone, but the overall effect is one of rarefaction, not of radiopacity. Also, the radiographic pattern in these two diseases is generalized, not localized and solitary as in fibrous dysplasia. Occa-

---

*The terms *orange peel, stippled,* and *salt-and-pepper* are used synonymously with *ground-glass* to describe the image produced by many closely arranged, small trabeculae.

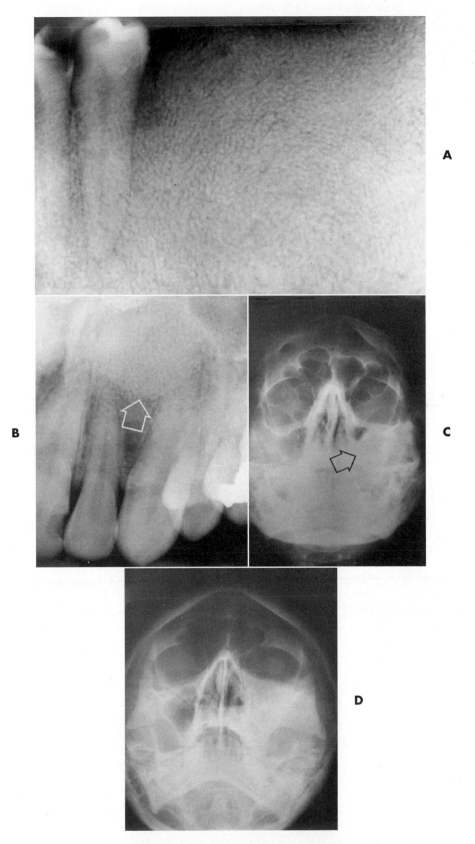

Fig. 28-8. Fibrous dysplasia. **A** and **B,** The opaque ground-glass appearance in two patients. **C** and **D,** Waters' views of two other patients with fibrous dysplasia of the left maxillary sinus. A ground-glass appearance was seen on periapical films. The arrows in **B** and **C** show the lesions. (**D** courtesy E. Palacios, Maywood, Ill.)

sionally, radiopaque ground-glass patterns may be seen in Paget's disease and hyperparathyroidism (Fig. 28-9).

Diffuse sclerosing osteomyelitis (DSO) can also mimic fibrous dysplasia radiographically, but usually the ground-glass pattern is not present. In addition, periodic episodes of pain and swelling are seen with DSO but not with fibrous dysplasia.

Although several bones may be involved with fibrous dysplasia in Albright's syndrome, which occurs in young girls, this syndrome is readily identified by its accompanying features of precocious puberty and café–au-lait spots.

Occasionally, mature cementoossifying fibromas may assume a radiopaque ground-glass appearance, as may calcifying postsurgical bone defects (see Fig. 28-9).

Management

Fibrous dysplasia should be managed by close clinical and radiographic observation, since the lesions may undergo surges of growth during hormonal changes. Recontouring of the bone to correct a deformity is occasionally necessary for esthetic or prosthetic reasons, but block resection is seldom if ever indicated. Radiation therapy is not recommended because of the possibility of radiation-induced sarcomas.

FOCAL SCLEROSING OSTEOMYELITIS

Osteomyelitis is discussed in Chapter 16 as a periapical radiolucency, in Chapter 21 as a ragged radiolucency, and in Chapter 24 as a mixed radiolucent-radiopaque lesion. The focal sclerosing variety of osteomyelitis, which represents a reaction to a low-grade infection, is included in this chapter because it sometimes occurs as a totally radiopaque lesion.

Features

The borders of the radiopaque lesions may be ragged or smooth and well defined or vague (Fig. 28-10).

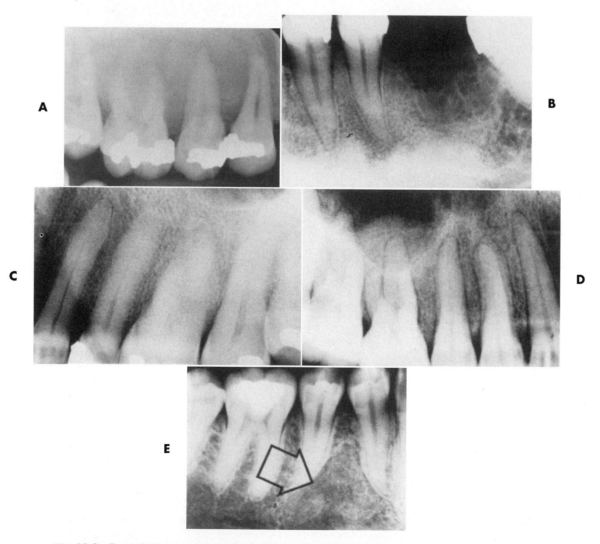

Fig. 28-9. Ground-glass lesions. **A** and **B,** Fibrous dysplasia. **C,** Paget's disease. **D,** Secondary hyperparathyroidism. **E,** Resolving traumatic bone cyst *(arrow).* Note that **C** and **D** have been printed lighter to bring out detail. (**D** courtesy P. O'Flaherty, Chicago.)

Identification of a focal sclerosing osteomyelitis in the bone usually depends on detecting symptoms of chronic infection such as tenderness, pain, or local swelling. A regional lymphadenitis is a frequent complaint, and a draining sinus may accompany some cases.

On microscopic examination, dense, sclerotic, nonvital bone is seen. Acute inflammation is present in some areas, and occasionally, focal collections of pus are found (see Fig. 28-10).

Differential Diagnosis

The lesions included in the differential diagnosis for a solitary intrabony area of sclerosis are an osteoblastic or sclerosing malignancy, condensing osteitis, fibrous dysplasia, and FCOD.

A totally radiopaque osteoblastic or sclerosing malignancy is rare—possibly an osteogenic sarcoma or a metastatic osteoblastic prostatic, bronchogenic, or mammary carcinoma. If one occurs, however, rapid growth, frequent pain without symptoms of infection, and paresthesia (frequently produced by malignant lesions of bone) help distinguish it from the more common focal sclerosing osteomyelitis. Nevertheless, a malignant tumor with superimposed osteomyelitis may be difficult to identify because of the overlapping signs and symptoms. Lesions occurring after radiation may also present a problem in differentiating between sclerosing osteoradionecrosis and a recurrent tumor.

Condensing osteitis can usually be eliminated from the differential diagnosis by the presence of the more subjective symptoms of chronic infection that frequently accompany chronic osteomyelitis and that are not features of condensing osteitis.

FCOD can usually be identified by its radiolucent rim, a greater uniformity (radiographic), and its lack of symptoms. However, both occur predominantly in the mandible.

Management

The first step in managing sclerosing osteomyelitis is to control the contributing systemic disease, if one is present. A protracted course of antibiotics, judiciously selected and administered, is indicated; however, some cases require incision and drainage and possibly enucleation or saucerization and recontouring if the antibiotic therapy fails to eliminate the bone infection. The use of hyperbaric oxygen may be beneficial.

DIFFUSE SCLEROSING OSTEOMYELITIS

DSO is an entirely different entity from focal sclerosing osteomyelitis, which usually has an obvious cause. DSO is an uncommon disease that affects a broad area of the body of the mandible, most frequently the molar, angle, and lower ramus region. An etiology has not been firmly established. One theory favors chronic infection by bacteria of low virulence, perhaps from the skin, oral cavity, or blood.[11-13] Bacterial types such as *Propionibacterium acnes,*[12] *Actinomyces* species,[13] and *Eikenella corrodens*[13] have been cultured from cases in support of an infectious etiology. Kahn, Hayem, Hayem, and Grossin[14] suggested that DSO may be related to the synovitis, acne, pustulosis, hyperostosis, and osteitis (SAPHO) syndrome, in which pustular skin lesions are associated with similar bony lesions. Another theory suggests that DSO is an expression of chronic recurrent multifocal osteomyelitis.[15] Genetics may play a role as well.[16] Another theory links DSO to chronic tendoperiostitis.[17,18] Hyperactive immune response has been postulated as well.[19]

Features

DSO characteristically follows a protracted course of recurrent pain, swelling of the inferior aspect of the cheek, and trismus.[20] There is a wide age span; the average age is approximately 40 years.[20] One series reports that both genders are equally affected,[20] whereas another indicates a 73% predilection for female patients.[13] The disease has cyclic episodes over the months and years.[21] During exacerbations, subfebrile temperatures and elevated sedimentation rates are found.[20] The cervical lymph nodes are variably affected, and those affected are usually the

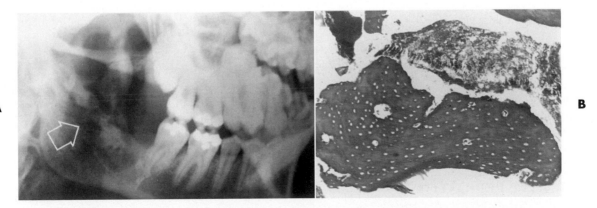

Fig. 28-10. Focal sclerosing osteomyelitis after a jaw fracture. Some of the radiopaque areas are sequestra. **A,** Radiopaque lesion *(arrow)* in the ramus. **B,** Photomicrograph. (**A** courtesy O.H. Stuteville, deceased.)

submandibular group.[18] Yield from bone cultures varies significantly in reported studies.[12-20]

Radiographically the process is characteristically limited to half the mandible. Large sections of the bone are involved, most commonly the molar, angle, and lower ramus region (Fig. 28-11). Changes occur slowly over several years. Osteolytic areas may predominate at first, when symptoms are at their worst. As episodes become less frequent and less severe, dense diffuse bony sclerosis predominates, and the radiolucent component diminishes (see Fig. 28-11). Endosteal sclerosis may be so dense that the cortex loses definition. Subperiosteal bone and external cortical erosion are observed in some cases.[17] Scintigraphy is very positive in the bony segment involved with DSO.

Histologically the overall bony changes are reactive. There is formation of subperiosteal bone, with dense remodeling of cortical and subcortical bones resulting in an increased bony volume.[20] Foci of granulocytes, lymphocytes, or both may be seen, especially in the larger cortical resorptive defects.[20] Necrotic foci have also been reported.[13]

Differential Diagnosis

The following conditions that produce a large, diffuse radiopaque involvement of a large section of the mandible must be included in the differential diagnosis: florid cementoosseous dysplasia,[21] Paget's disease, osteopetrosis fibrous dysplasia, dysosteosclerosis.[22] Characteristically, all of these conditions except florid cementoosseous dysplasia and fibrous dysplasia affect multiple bones in the same patient. (Fibrous dysplasia can affect two or more bones in Albright's syndrome.) Atypical cases that may affect only a segment of the mandible are seen occasionally. See Chapter 30 for information on these entities.

Fibrous dysplasia in its mature dense radiopaque stage could be mistaken for DSO, but fibrous dysplasia is painless and seldom causes trismus. Usually the ground-glass pattern can be identified on radiographs.

Florid cementoosseous dysplasia characteristically has large, usually separate somewhat circular radiopacities that are marginated by a radiolucent border. This condition is painless unless infected with the production of a secondary osteomyelitis.[21]

Management

DSO usually follows a protracted course and responds variably to treatment. Decortication of the buccal aspect of the mandible with use of gentamicin-impregnated beads in the surgical bed, followed by long-term antibiotic coverage, has been used.[11] Antibiotic coverage alone and muscle relaxation techniques have also been used.[17,18]

PROLIFERATIVE PERIOSTITIS

Proliferative periostitis (periostitis ossificans, Garré's osteomyelitis), a particular type of osteomyelitis, is so distinctive that it has been considered a separate entity. For many years, this entity has been referred to as Garré's osteomyelitis. (It is interesting that a 1988 review of the original paper by Garré found not only that Garré's name has been consistently misspelled in the literature but also that Garré did not describe this type of osteomyelitis at all.[23]) This condition is characterized by the formation of new bone on the periphery of the cortex over an infected area of spongiosa. The formation of new bone is a response of the inner surface of the periosteum to stimulation by a low-grade infection that has spread through the bone and penetrated the cortex.

Strains of staphylococci and streptococci are the microorganisms most commonly cultured. Periapical odontogenic infection is a frequent cause of proliferative periostitis of the jaws, although an occasional case can be traced to a pericoronitis.

We infer, from the paucity of reports in the dental literature that recount the occurrence of this disease and from our own experience, that proliferative periostitis of the jaws is a relatively uncommon dental complication. For this lesion to develop, the following peculiar combination of circumstances must coexist:

1. The periosteum must possess a high potential for osteoblastic activity (this requirement is satisfied in young patients).
2. A chronic infection must be present.
3. A fine balance must be maintained between the resistance of the host and the number and virulence of present organisms so that the infection can continue at a low, chronic stage: invasive enough to stimulate new periosteal bone formation but not severe enough to induce bone resorption.

Proliferative periostitis is included in this chapter because it may produce a solitary radiopacity that does not contact the roots of teeth.

Features

Proliferative periostitis is seen almost exclusively in children and rarely occurs in patients over 30 years of age. Reports indicate that the mean age varies from 12 to 13.3 years,[24,25] and that there is a male predominance of 1.4 to 1.[24] An infected mandibular first permanent molar is the most common etiologic factor.[24,25]

The patient may complain of the pain of odontogenic infection before the intermittent, usually nontender swelling develops at the inferior border or other peripheries of the mandible. The most frequent site is the inferior border of the mandible below the first molar (Fig. 28-12). The maxilla is seldom affected. Facial asymmetry is present, the swelling is bony hard and usually nontender, and the overlying skin or mucosa appears normal.[25] Although the condition is characteristically solitary, a case that occurred simultaneously in all four quadrants has been reported.[26]

If the chronic infection becomes established just beneath the periosteum and is not treated, the swelling per-

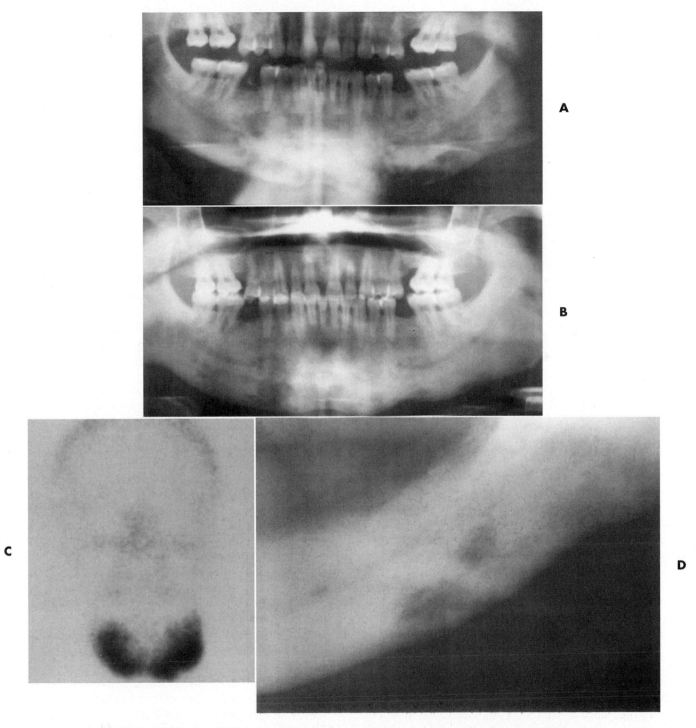

Fig. 28-11. DSO. **A** to **C,** The same bilateral case. **A,** Mixed radiolucent-radiopaque appearance. **B,** More mature radiopaque appearance in panoramic film taken some years later. **C,** Technetium-99m film showing bony activity on both sides of the mandible but with a wider distribution of labeling of the left. **D,** Unilateral mandible of DSO. (**A** to **C** courtesy D. Stoneman, Toronto; **D** courtesy C. Baker, Edmonton, Alberta, Canada.)

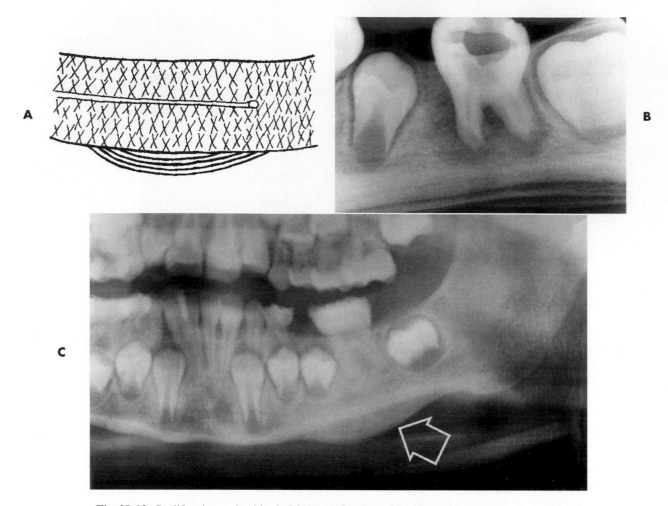

Fig. 28-12. Proliferative periostitis. **A,** Diagram of periosteal new bone formation in a layered or "onionskin" appearance. The integrity of the original cortex is usually maintained. **B** and **C,** Two cases of proliferative periostitis in the first molar region of the mandible. **B,** The definite layering effect and the rarefying osteitis are evident at the apex of the pulpless molar. **C,** The layering effect is not as noticeable in this more radiopaque periostitis *(arrow),* which was caused by a chronically infected second deciduous molar tooth that had been extracted recently. (**B** courtesy N. Barakat, Beirut, Lebanon; **C** courtesy J. Baird, Evanston, Ill.)

sists and soon becomes hard as new bone is laid down. After the infection has been eliminated, the hard elevation usually disappears slowly as the bone is recontoured by the functional forces.

The swelling is characteristically convex, varying in length and depth of bone deposits. It may range from 2 cm to involvement of the whole length of the mandibular body on the affected side. The covering skin or overlying mucosa may appear normal or be moderately inflamed. Occasionally, fever and leukocytosis are present.

On radiographs a smoothly contoured, moderately convex bony shadow can be seen extending from the preserved cortex of the jaw (see Fig. 28-12). The space between this new, thin shell of bone and the cortex may be quite radiolucent without images of trabeculae. Later an alternating light and dark, laminated appearance may be seen, and when the whole lesion mineralizes, the lesion may be completely ra-

diopaque (see Fig. 28-12). From 1 to 12 separate laminations have been found by investigators.[24]

In most cases the adjacent jawbone appears normal on the radiograph, but sometimes, there may be accompanying radiolucent or osteosclerotic osteomyelitis changes, and small sequestra can often be seen.[24]

Histologic examination shows dense new bone with minimal vascular spaces. The periosteum is thickened and shows an overactive osteoblastic layer. Scattered regions of chronic inflammation may be present.

Differential Diagnosis

Lesions included in the differential diagnosis for a condition that resembles proliferative periostitis are Ewing's sarcoma, fibrous dysplasia, osteogenic sarcoma, infantile cortical hyperostosis, callus, ossifying hematoma, tori, exostoses, and peripheral osteomas.

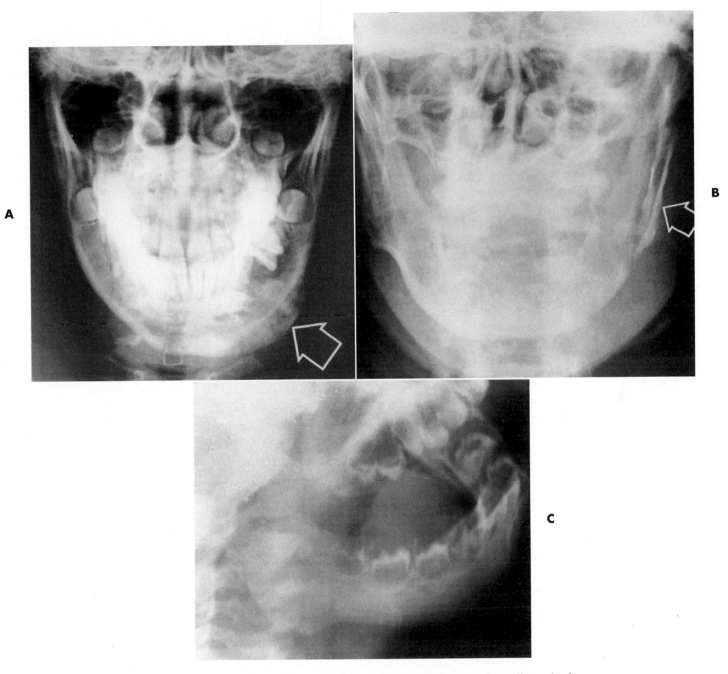

Fig. 28-13. Other lesions that produce cortical duplication. **A,** Posteroanterior radiograph of Ewing's sarcoma in the left mandible of a young girl. The cortical redundancy and layering effect *(arrow)* can be seen at the inferior border of the mandible. (Fig. 21-16 shows the extent of bone destruction of this lesion in a lateral view.) **B,** Posteroanterior radiograph showing a cortical redundancy in the left ramus *(arrow)*. This appearance was produced in a 56-year-old man by a large segment of bone being fractured and displaced to the buccal area during a traumatic episode. A chronic osteomyelitis had become established here at the time this radiograph was taken, so the segment represents a large sequestrum. **C,** Redundancy of the inferior border of the mandible in a case of cortical infantile hyperostosis. (**A** courtesy N. Barakat, Beirut, Lebanon; **C** courtesy R. Moncada, Maywood, Ill.)

Ewing's sarcoma may produce a radiolucent lesion with a convex peripheral radiopaque lesion with laminations (Fig. 28-13) somewhat similar to that of proliferative periostitis. However, the periosteal reaction is usually not laminated but more like the sun-ray appearance of osteogenic sarcoma.[27] The predilection for children and the symptoms of tender swellings are shared by Ewing's sarcoma and proliferative periostitis. Further, in both diseases the adjacent bone may show osteolytic changes, although a moth-eaten type of destruction is more typical of Ewing's sarcoma.[28] Ewing's sarcoma also shows rapid, unrestricted growth and often produces a paresthesia of the lip.

Fibrous dysplasia may appear to be located on the periphery, but a careful inspection of the radiograph usually reveals that the complete thickness of bone, which has the ground-glass appearance, is altered.

Osteogenic sarcoma may cause a peripheral radiopacity, and it occurs predominantly in generally the same age-group as proliferative periostitis. The radiographic image of this tumor, however, usually appears more irregular, and the sunburst effect (if present) is so characteristic that the two entities are not likely to be confused.

Although infantile cortical hyperostosis occurs in the same age-group of children, it differs from proliferative periostitis in that it is a generalized expansion of the cortices of several bones (see Fig. 28-13), usually including the mandible, whereas proliferative periostitis is a single local expansion.

A callus developing around a healing fracture may also appear as a peripheral radiopacity, but it is usually not radiodense. A history of trauma and radiographic evidence of the fracture line help identify the callus.

A hematoma may develop subperiosteally after trauma to a bone. This collection of extravasated blood occasionally ossifies, resulting in a peripheral radiopaque enlargement of the bone. The hematoma may then be confused with proliferative periostitis, but its radiopacity is not as uniform; rather, a more mottled appearance, coupled with a history of trauma to the suspect area, should identify the ossifying hematoma.

Since tori, exostoses, and peripheral osteomas also occur at peripheral borders of the mandibular body, they might be confused with proliferative periostitis. These entities are distinguishable from proliferative periostitis since they do not show a predilection for patients under 20 years of age, are more nodular (even polypoid in some cases), and require months and years to increase appreciably in size.

Eversole, Leider, Corwin, and Karian[28] have reviewed six cases of proliferative periostitis and have outlined criteria for its differentiation from the other neoperiostoses. These criteria include (1) facial asymmetry resulting from localized osseous enlargement, (2) histologic findings showing a benign periosteal fibroosseous lesion, and (3) complete or partial resorption (remodeling) of excess bone after eliminating the course.

Management

In most cases, proliferative periostitis can be successfully treated by simply removing the source of infection (usually an infected tooth) and administering an appropriate antibiotic. The periosteal lesion then gradually regresses until the original bone contour has been reestablished. Endodontic treatment may circumvent the need for extraction.[29]

Sometimes the projecting mass is extensive, and surgical contouring for esthetics may be in order. This procedure in turn provides a specimen for microscopic study and a final diagnosis can be established more quickly.

MATURE COMPLEX ODONTOMA

The complex odontoma is a developmental anomaly of tooth tissue that, like teeth, is completely radiolucent in the initial stage, passes into a mixed radiolucent-radiopaque stage, and may mature as a completely radiopaque lesion surrounded by a radiolucent halo of varying width. The tumor is made up of the three calcified dental tissues, but these are laid down in a disorganized, irregular mass without normal morphologic relationships of one tissue to another.

Odontomas are discussed in detail in Chapter 24, which describes them as radiolucent images containing radiopaque foci.

Features

The mature complex odontoma is seldom seen in patients under 6 years of age. When it occurs, it most commonly affects the first and second permanent mandibular molars, often forming in the alveoli just superior to the crowns of these teeth and effectively preventing their eruption (Fig. 28-14). Pain or paresthesia is not characteristic of these tumors, which may vary in diameter from 1 to approximately 6 cm and may produce a bulge on the mandible.

On radiographic examination the mature lesion of considerable buccolingual width appears as a homogeneously dense radiopacity; the earlier lesion of less width may show irregular radiodense patterns throughout and may even cast a cotton-wool image on the radiograph. Although the outline of the calcified mass within the odontoma may be quite irregular, the radiolucent rim surrounding the lesion has a well-defined and smooth outer periphery.

On histologic study the lesion is composed of varying proportions of enamel, dentin, cementum, and pulp tissue in a disorganized arrangement.

Differential Diagnosis

Because mature fibroosseous lesions of periodontal ligament origin (e.g., PCOD or FCOD) may be solitary and are dense radiopacities with radiolucent rims, they are the entities most frequently confused with the mature complex odontoma. Usually, PCOD or FCOD forms in persons over 30 years of age, whereas an odontoma develops in much younger patients (although both lesions may persist and be found in late adulthood). PCOD or FCOD usually is situated deep in the alveolar bone, whereas the complex odontoma often extends high into the alveolus, toward the crest of the ridge.

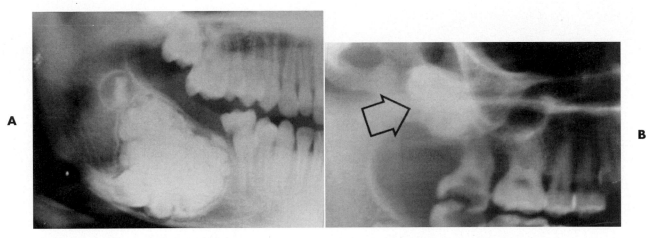

Fig. 28-14. Complex odontoma. **A,** Causing impaction of a mandibular molar. **B,** In the maxillary third molar region *(arrow).* (**A** courtesy V. Barresi, DeKalb, Ill, and D. Bonomo, Flossmoor, Ill; **B** courtesy B. Saunders, Los Angeles.)

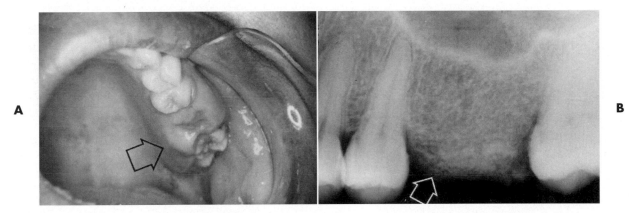

Fig. 28-15. Calcified subperiosteal hematoma *(arrow)* after tooth extraction with primary closure of the mucosa. **A,** Clinical appearance. **B,** Periapical radiograph of the hematoma *(arrow).*

Management

Surgical enucleation of the odontoma is the treatment of choice, and the excised material should be microscopically examined.

OSSIFYING SUBPERIOSTEAL HEMATOMA

Occasionally a subperiosteal hematoma sustained as the result of trauma ossifies instead of resolves. Early in the course of its ossification, it appears as a mixed radiolucent-radiopaque lesion, but as ossification is completed, it becomes a dense, radiopaque, smoothly contoured convex expansion on the periphery of the bone (Fig. 28-15). The swelling is nontender. This may be the same lesion reported as subpontic osseous dysplasia.[30]

Differential Diagnosis

The differential diagnosis of the ossifying subperiosteal hematoma is discussed in the section on the differential diagnosis of proliferative periostitis.

Management

Functional forces reshape the deformed bone and reestablish normal contour if the lesion is subjected to the vectors of these forces. If the bone enlargement persists for a few months, recontouring may be necessary for improved function and esthetics and in preparation for the construction of a prosthetic appliance.

RARITIES

The rare solitary completely radiopaque lesions are listed on the first page of this chapter.

PROJECTED RADIOPACITIES

Radiopaque shadows that may be projected over the roots of teeth are discussed in detail in Chapter 27. The radiopacities that may be projected over the jawbone but not necessarily over a periapex are essentially the same. Consequently, illustrations of these entities are included in this chapter without further discussion (Figs. 28-16 to 28-26).

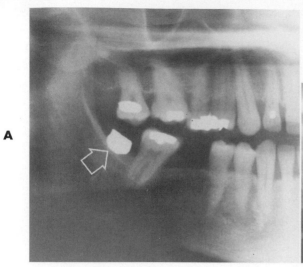

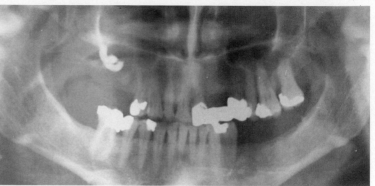

Fig. 28-16. Foreign bodies. **A,** Bullet in the cheek *(arrow)*. **B,** Endodontic filling material in the right maxillary sinus. (**B** courtesy N. Barakat, Beirut, Lebanon.)

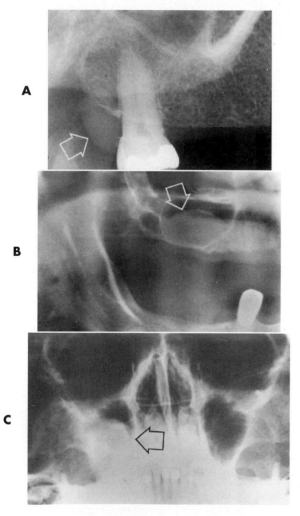

Fig. 28-17. Soft tissue shadows. **A,** Fibrous tuberosity *(arrow)* superimposed over the coronoid process. **B** and **C,** Retention cysts of the maxillary sinus *(arrows).* (**C** courtesy E. Palacios, Maywood, Ill.)

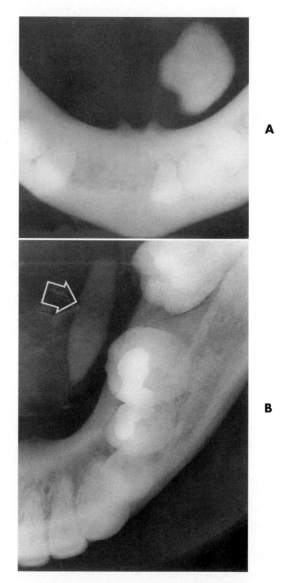

Fig. 28-18. Sialoliths in Wharton's ducts. (Courtesy R. Latronica, East Amherst, NY.)

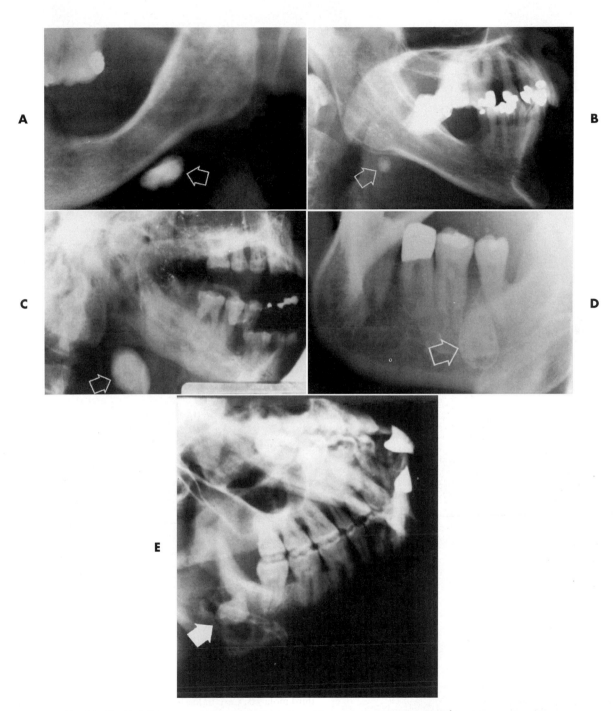

Fig. 28-19. Sialoliths *(arrows)*. **A-D,** In the submaxillary glands. **E,** Resembling an impacted tooth. (**B** and **C** courtesy O.H. Stuteville, deceased; **D** courtesy R. Goepp, Chicago; **E** courtesy D. Bonomo, Flossmoor, Ill.)

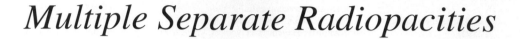

CHAPTER 29

Multiple Separate Radiopacities

NORMAN K. WOOD

PAUL W. GOAZ

Most of the lesions that appear as multiple but separate radiopacities occur more frequently as solitary radiopacities. They include the following:

TORI AND EXOSTOSES
MULTIPLE RETAINED ROOTS
MULTIPLE SOCKET SCLEROSIS
MULTIPLE PERIAPICAL OR FOCAL
   CEMENTOOSSEOUS DYSPLASIA
MULTIPLE PERIAPICAL CONDENSING
   OSTEITIS
MULTIPLE EMBEDDED OR IMPACTED
   TEETH
CLEIDOCRANIAL DYSPLASIA
MULTIPLE HYPERCEMENTOSES

RARITIES
   Calcinosis cutis
   Chronic recurrent multifocal osteomyelitis[1]
   Cretinism (unerupted teeth)
   Cysticercosis[2]
   Familial adenomatosis coli (Gardner's
      syndrome)[3,4]
   Idiopathic hypoparathyroidism
   Klippel-Feil syndrome
   Maffucci's syndrome
   Multiple calcified acne lesions

Multiple calcified nodes
Multiple chondromas (Ollier's disease)
Multiple odontomas
Multiple osteochondromas
Multiple osteomas of skin
Multiple phleboliths
Multiple sialoliths
Myositis ossificans
Oral contraceptive sclerosis
Paget's disease—intermediate stage
Sickle cell sclerosis
Tumoral calcinosis

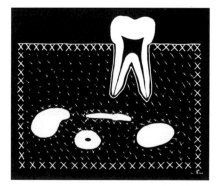

The majority of the entities included here are discussed in Chapter 27 as periapical radiopacities or in Chapter 28 as solitary radiopacities not contacting the roots of teeth. As described in those two chapters, radiopaque lesions that appear to be within the jaw may actually be in or on the periphery (cortex) of the jawbone or in the adjacent soft tissues. The radiopaque shadows may also represent ghosting or images of multiple artifacts on the film, so it is important to rule out those possibilities.[5]

TORI AND EXOSTOSES

Tori and exostoses are described as exophytic lesions in Chapter 10 and as single radiopacities in Chapters 27 and 28. In the context of this chapter, therefore, it remains only to note that tori (especially the lingual mandibular type) frequently develop as multiple nodules that may be contiguous or separate. Exostoses may also be multiple, especially those occurring on the buccal surfaces of the jaws. In either case, they appear as relatively dense, smoothly contoured multiple radiopacities on radiographs of the jaws (Fig. 29-1).

Differential Diagnosis

Multiple tori or exostoses must be differentiated from any of the other similar-appearing entities included in this

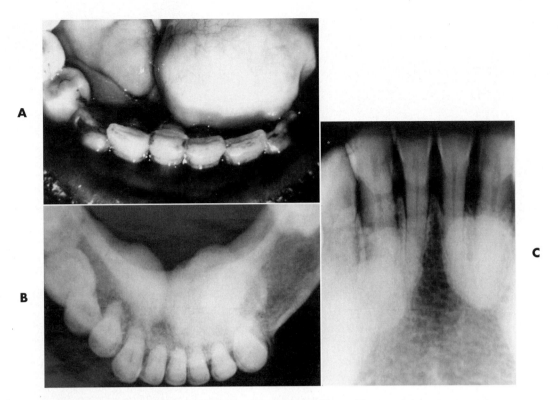

Fig. 29-1. Multiple large tori. **A** and **B,** Clinical and radiographic appearances in one patient. **C,** Periapical radiograph of another patient. (**A** and **B** courtesy P. Akers, Chicago.)

chapter. If multiple smoothly contoured radiopacities are present on periapical radiographs and the typical peripheral nodules are palpable on the buccal or lingual alveolar surfaces, the diagnosis is clear-cut.

Rare diseases such as adenomatosis coli, Maffucci's syndrome, Ollier's disease, and multiple osteochondromas should sometimes be considered, but a detailed discussion of these entities is beyond the scope of this text.

Management

Multiple tori and exostoses require surgical excision (1) for psychologic reasons, (2) if they are continually being traumatized, (3) if they are interfering with speech or mastication, or (4) if they will interfere with the fabrication of a prosthetic appliance.

MULTIPLE RETAINED ROOTS

Solitary retained roots are extensively discussed in Chapter 28. Retained roots are usually asymptomatic (Fig. 29-2) but may cause pain if they become infected.

Differential Diagnosis

The radiographic appearance of multiple retained roots is diagnostic. If the root fragments have been fractured at the level of the alveolar crest and the radiolucent images of the periodontal ligaments are indistinct, multiple retained roots may be difficult to distinguish from multiple sclerosed sockets (Fig. 29-3). The study of radiographs taken shortly after the extractions were performed enables the clinician to distinguish between retained roots and sclerosed sockets.

Retained root tips may not be readily recognized when the root tips are chronically infected and condensing osteitis has developed around them. Where there are multiple retained roots, however, all the roots are unikely to be involved with sclerosed bone; one or two fragments retain their typical appearance, and these suggest the correct diagnosis. A detailed discussion of the differentiation of retained root fragments may be found in the discussion of the differential diagnosis of condensing osteitis in Chapter 28.

Management

Since it is not safe to assume on the basis of radiographic evidence alone that retained roots are free of infection, removal of retained roots should be considered. If the root tips are small, asymptomatic, and apparently free of pathosis and if a relatively large amount of alveolar bone may have to be removed, it is best to leave them undisturbed. Periodic radiographic surveillance is required.

MULTIPLE SOCKET SCLEROSIS

Tooth socket sclerosis is a special form of osteosclerosis that occasionally develops in a socket after tooth removal.

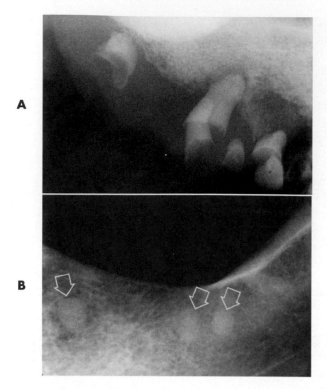

Fig. 29-2. Multiple root fragments. **A,** Readily identified. **B,** Not so readily identified *(arrows).*

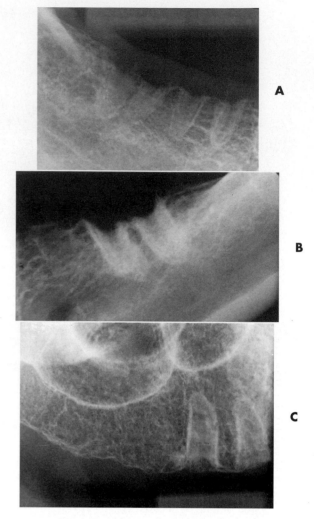

Fig. 29-3. Multiple socket sclerosis. (**A** courtesy R. Goepp, Chicago.)

Examples of the sclerosis of solitary sockets are described in Chapter 28. Since multiple sclerotic lesions may also occur when a number of tooth sockets are healing after multiple extraction, this entity is included in this chapter as well (see Fig. 29-3).

Although the specific cause is unknown, socket sclerosis is believed to be the result of a sudden disturbance of the osteogenic-osteolytic balance in bone metabolism. An increased incidence of socket sclerosis has been reported among patients with problems of gastrointestinal malabsorption or kidney disease.[6] Some 2.7% of patients had one or more sclerosed tooth sockets, an incidence much higher than that found in the general population.

Features

Since the development of sclerosed bone in healing sockets is not accompanied by local symptoms, the radiopaque lesion is discovered on routine radiographs. Sclerosis of tooth sockets is found more often in older adults and seldom, if ever, in persons under 16 years of age. Sequential radiographs made when the sclerosis is active reveal the successive stages of development.

When a socket is healing normally, the lamina dura usually disappears within 4 months, and the socket is completely obliterated by 8 months. When socket sclerosis is developing, however, the lamina dura fails to resorb. The deposition of sclerotic bone begins in the depth of the socket and continues along the socket walls.

As the lateral walls of sclerotic bone approximate each other, the thin, vertical radiolucent shadow of the void between them resembles the image of a pulp canal on periapical radiographs (see Fig. 29-3). At this stage the sclerosed socket can be easily mistaken for a retained, ankylosed root.

On histologic study, socket sclerosis is identical to the osteosclerosis that occurs in other locations. Dense, broad trabeculae of bone with few lacunae and few vascular marrow spaces are characteristic of the microscopic appearance.

Differential Diagnosis

Socket sclerosis may be mistaken for retained roots because both have identical shapes. Differentiating between the two is especially difficult when the socket has not yet completely calcified and a thin, central core resembles a root canal. Since osteosclerosis of a tooth socket usually involves the length of the socket, the radiopaque images of roots fractured well below the alveolar crest are not

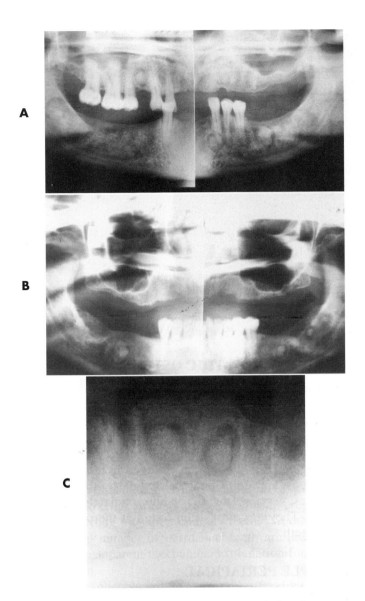

Fig. 29-4. **A** and **B,** Multiple PCOD or FCOD lesions in two patients. **C,** Two mature FCOD lesions in the mandibular incisor region of another patient. Mature PCOD or FCOD have radiolucent rims, but surrounding bone beyond the rims may show a sclerotic margin.

confused with this dense remodeling of the socket. If the periodontal ligament space is not apparent, the radiopacity should be identified as socket sclerosis. The uncommon ankylosed roots are exceptions. If radiographs of the area are available and were made shortly after the extractions were performed, the identity of the opaque material in the sockets should not be in doubt; the retained root tips are apparent from the time of the extractions, whereas the osteosclerotic healing of the sockets requires months to become obvious.

Management

Once the diagnosis of socket sclerosis has been established (biopsy may be necessary in some cases), consul-

tation with the patient's physician is recommended, since there is reason to suspect that the patient may have a gastrointestinal malabsorption problem or a kidney malady.[6] The sclerosed tooth socket does not require definitive treatment.

MULTIPLE MATURE PERIAPICAL OR FOCAL CEMENTOOSSEOUS DYSPLASIA

Variations in the appearance and nature of periapical cementoosseous dysplasia (PCOD) or focal cementoosseous dysplasia (FCOD) are discussed in Chapters 16, 21, 24, 25, and 27. In this chapter, multiple PCODs or FCODs that occurr in the jaws are emphasized (Fig. 29-4).

Although multiple PCODs or FCODs are most frequently found in the periapices of mandibular incisors, they may occur in the periapices of any of the mandibular teeth, as well as in nonperiapical locations and (less frequently) in the maxilla. Multiple PCODs or FCODs in Japanese women occur predominantly in the premolar and molar region of the mandible.[7] The features of multiple PCOD or FCOD are similar to those of the solitary PCOD or FCOD (see Chapters 27 and 28).

Differential Diagnosis

Multiple mature PCODs or FCODs should be differentiated from the intermediate stage of Paget's disease, florid cementoosseous dysplasia, complex odontoma, idiopathic osteoscleroses, toris, exostoses, osteomas, and multiple retained root fragments, as well as some of the rare lesions listed at the beginning of this chapter.

In some cases of intermediate-stage Paget's disease, separate round radiopaque areas are scattered throughout the jaws. The margins of these radiopaque osteoblastic areas are not as well defined as those of mature PCOD or FCOD, however. They also do not have uniform radiolucent rims. Further radiographic examination of the patient reveals the deformation of the skull and other bones, and these findings help the clinician recognize Paget's disease.

The features of florid cementoosseous dysplasia are quite different from those of mature PCOD or FCOD. The former condition is less common, and the radiopaque lesions are relatively large and multiple; the lesions merge and occupy much of the body of the mandible and maxilla. They appear as large radiopaque masses, usually with radiolucent borders, and have the cotton-wool appearance often seen in the late stages of Paget's disease.

The complex odontoma may resemble a mature PCOD or FCOD in that it often appears as a dense radiopacity surrounded by a radiolucent border; however, it is usually larger and occurs almost invariably as a solitary lesion. Furthermore, most complex odontomas do not have a homogeneous opacity like the mature cementomas

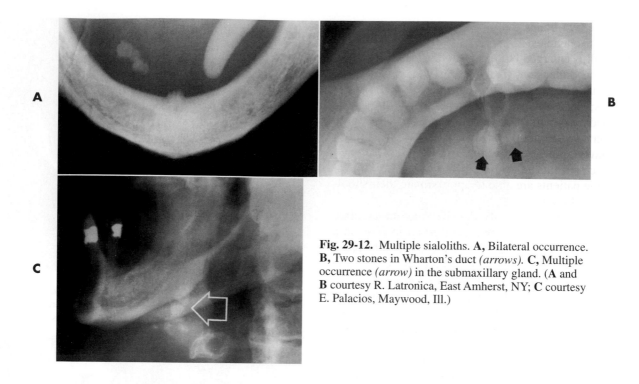

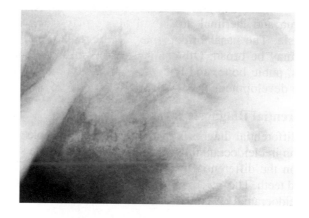

Fig. 29-12. Multiple sialoliths. **A,** Bilateral occurrence. **B,** Two stones in Wharton's duct *(arrows).* **C,** Multiple occurrence *(arrow)* in the submaxillary gland. (**A** and **B** courtesy R. Latronica, East Amherst, NY; **C** courtesy E. Palacios, Maywood, Ill.)

Fig. 29-13. Multiple radiopaque appearance of Paget's disease in the maxillary premolar region.

REFERENCES

1. Suei Y, Tanimoto K, Taguchi A, et al: Chronic recurrent multifocal osteomyelitis involving the mandible, *Oral Surg* 78:156-162, 1994.
2. De Leon ER, Aguirre A: Oral cysticercosis, *Oral Surg* 79:572-577, 1995.
3. Yuasa K, Yonetsu K, Kanda S, et al: Computed tomography of the jaws in familial adenomatosis coli, *Oral Surg* 76:251-255, 1993.
4. Takeuchi T, Takenoshita Y, Kubo K, Iida M: Natural course of jaw lesions in patients with familial adenomatosis coli (Gardner's syndrome), *Int J Oral Maxillofac Surg* 22:226-230, 1993.

5. Kaugers GE, Collett WK: Panoramic ghosts, *Oral Surg* 63:103-108, 1987.
6. Burrell KH, Goepp RA: Abnormal bone repair in jaws, socket sclerosis: a sign of systemic disease, *J Am Dent Assoc* 87:1206-1215, 1973.
7. Tanaka H, Yoshimoto A, Toyama Y, et al: Periapical cemental dysplasia with multiple lesions, *J Oral Maxillofac Surg* 16:757-763, 1987.
8. Leider AS, Garbarino VE: Generalized hypercementosis, *Oral Surg* 63:375-380, 1987.

9. Kantor ML, Bailey CS, Burkes DJ: Duplication of the premolar dentition, *Oral Surg* 66:62-64, 1988.
10. Loevy HT, Aduss H, Rosenthal IM: Tooth eruption and craniofacial development in congenital hypothyroidism: report of case, *J Am Dent Assoc* 115:429-431, 1987.

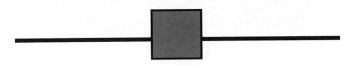

CHAPTER 30

Generalized Radiopacities

THOMAS E. EMMERING
NORMAN K. WOOD

A multitude of diseases are capable of causing osseous changes in the jaws and skull. Discussion in this chapter is limited primarily to those that at one stage or another appear as generalized radiopacities of the jawbones. In addition, the degree of jaw radiodenseness of normal people is interesting; this ranges from light in frail, nonvigorous individuals to dense in strong, vigorous individuals.

FLORID CEMENTOOSSEOUS DYSPLASIA
PAGET'S DISEASE—MATURE STAGE
OSTEOPETROSIS
RARITIES
  Albright's syndrome
  Caffey's disease (infantile cortical
    hyperostosis)
  Camurati-Engelmann disease

Craniometaphyseal dysplasia
Craniodiaphyseal dysplasia
Diffuse sclerosing osteomyelitis, atypical
Dysosteosclerosis[1]
Familial gigantiform cementomas[2]
Fluorosis
Familial adenomatosis coli (Gardner's
  syndrome)

Hyperostosis deformans juvenilis
Melorheostosis
Metastatic carcinoma of prostate
Multiple large exostoses and tori
Osteogenesis imperfecta
Osteopathia striata
Pyknodysostosis
van Buchem's syndrome

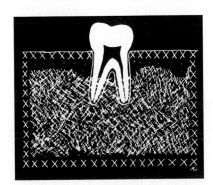

Diseases of bone that can produce generalized radiopacities are not frequently encountered in the general population. Florid cementoosseous dysplasia (FLCOD), Paget's disease, and osteopetrosis are the most common of these and are listed in order of diminishing frequency. They are discussed, whereas the rarer disorders are only listed.

FLORID CEMENTOOSSEOUS DYSPLASIA

FLCOD is the most common cause of pathologic generalized radiopacity of the jaws (Figs. 30-1 and 30-2). This benign condition usually involves multiple quandrants of the tooth-bearing regions of the jaws. FLCOD belongs to the spectrum of benign reactive fibrocementoosseous lesions of periodontal ligament origin[3,4] and probably represents the most extensive manifestation of these reactive processes.[5]

Features

In the United States, FLCOD is seen almost exclusively in middle-aged to elderly black women.[4-6] FLCOD also develops in Chinese[7] and Japanese[8] women in the same age group, and at least one case has been reported occurring in an Indian.[7] The lesions are basically restricted to the tooth-bearing regions of the jawbones[4-7] and are often bilaterally and symmetrically positioned. The radiopaque cloud-like masses vary greatly in size and shape and may be so dense and disseminated that they appear as generalized

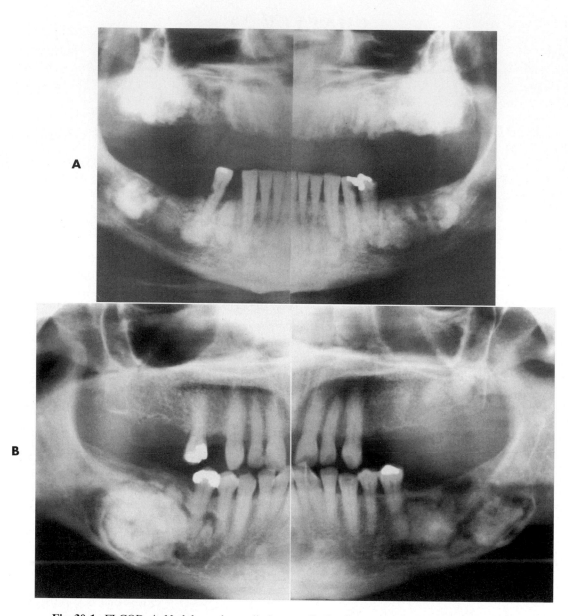

Fig. 30-1. FLCOD. **A,** Nodular, rather well-circumscribed radiopaque masses are distributed throughout the maxilla and mandible. This panograph is of a 45-year-old black woman. **B,** Panograph of nodular masses in another black woman, 42 years of age, shows greater involvement of the mandible than of the maxilla. (**B** courtesy R. Kallal, Chicago.)

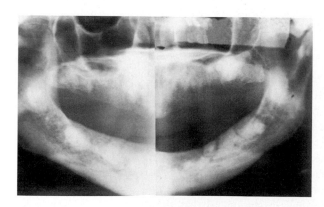

Fig. 30-2. FLCOD in a middle-aged black woman who was asymptomatic. The particular pattern prevalent in this case is more diffuse, less nodular, and less well defined than usual.

radiopacities. Some are somewhat spherical, whereas others are lobular, suggesting coalescence. Hypercementosis may be a feature.[7]

Often, these cases are asymptomatic, particularly in the early phase, but a third to half develop cortical expansion.[5,7] A significant number develop a secondary osteomyelitis, particularly in patients wearing prostheses. Ulceration occurs over these dense masses because of progressive alveolar resorption and pressure points over the expanding mass. Patients with secondary osteomyelitis manifest dull to marked pain, swelling, prevalent drainage from the sinus tracts, mucosal ulceration, and sequestra.[4,7]

Radiographs, at first glance, seem to demonstrate a pagetoid, cotton-wool appearance with multiple irregularly shaped radiopaque areas. On closer examination, well-defined radiolucent rims can be seen surrounding most of the radiopaque areas[6-8] (see Fig. 30-1). The radiopaque patterns vary in size but are usually large and may be multiple or diffuse and continuous throughout the tooth-bearing regions of the jaw (see Figs. 30-1 and 30-2). As with most odontogenic hard tissue lesions, FLCOD commences as a radiolucency and matures through the mixed stage into the radiopaque stage. Root clubbing with hypercementosis may also be seen.[7]

Serum chemistry levels are within normal limits in cases of FLCOD. Microscopically a dense avascular admixture of dense cementum or bone may be seen in varying proportions in a meager fibroblastic stroma.

Differential Diagnosis

The following conditions should be considered in a differential diagnosis list when considering FLCOD: multiple cementoosseous dysplasia, familial gigantiform cementomas,[2] and diffuse sclerosing osteomyelitis (DSO). Cases of multiple cementoosseous dysplasia are more common and have multiple small lesions of periapical cementoosseous dysplasia and focal cementoosseous dysplasia distributed throughout the tooth-bearing regions of the jaws. Contrary to cases of FLCOD, these lesions remain small and characteristically do not cause cortical expansion or become susceptible to osteomyelitis.

Familial gigantiform cementomas are rare and are occasionally familial. Both genders are affected, and patients are usually affected at an earlier age than they are with FLCOD.[2]

DSO usually involves only one segment of the jaws; the radiopaque part is diffuse, and its margins blend into normal bone at the periphery of the lesion. Clearly, it does not have the well-defined radiolucent margination that is common in FLCOD. Also, DSO does not show a predilection for black women.[9]

Classic cases of Paget's disease and osteopetrosis can be easily ruled out because of the involvement of additional bones of the skeleton and jaws.

Management

Patients with asymptomatic cases of FLCOD do not require treatment. The disease must be correctly identified and observed annually with radiographs. Every effort must be made to preserve the natural dentition, since patients with this disease exhibit poor healing and osteomyelitis may develop after tooth removal. For the same reason, biopsy or surgical intervention should be avoided.

Superimposed osteomyelitis should be treated by antibiotics, sequestrectomy, and excision of the sinus tract and the associated cementoosseous mass.[7]

PAGET'S DISEASE—MATURE STAGE

Paget's disease is a chronic disease of bone that may occur in three stages: (1) the early osteoclastic stage (generalized rarefaction); (2) the intermediate stage, which demonstrates osteoclastic and osteoblastic activities (a mixed radiolucent-radiopaque appearance); and (3) the mature stage, in which osteoblastic activity predominates (a generalized cotton-wool radiopacity).

The osteoclastic stage is described in Chapter 23 as a generalized rarefaction, and the intermediate stage is described in Chapter 25 as a mixed radiolucent-radiopaque image. The mature cotton-wool appearance is emphasized in this chapter.

Features

Dental problems become notable as osteoblastic activity creates expansion and progressive enlargement of the maxilla. The alveolar ridge is widened; the palate is flattened; and any teeth present undergo migration, tipping, possible loosening, and increased interproximal spacing. It is difficult for edentulous patients to wear removable prostheses, which must be periodically remade to accommodate alveolar expansion.

The radiographic appearance varies according to the stage of the disease. The osteoblastic phase eventually becomes predominant. Osteoblastic areas initially show as small radiopaque foci but coalesce as the disease matures into large radiopaque patches with few residual radiolucent areas (Figs. 30-3 to 30-5). This latter image is often referred to as the *cotton-wool appearance*.

In patients with jaw involvement, the skull is also affected; sometimes, osteolytic activity continues intermittently in these bones even after the predominant activity in the jaws has become osteoblastic. Dental radiographs of later stages of Paget's disease demonstrate proliferation of bone and hypercementosis of tooth roots, and the hypercementosis may become quite exaggerated. Frequently a loss of definite lamina dura around the teeth and, rarely, some root resorption occur. On occasion, local areas of the jaw continue to grow at an accelerated rate. Dentists must be alert to the oral changes because they may be the first clinicians to suspect a diagnosis of

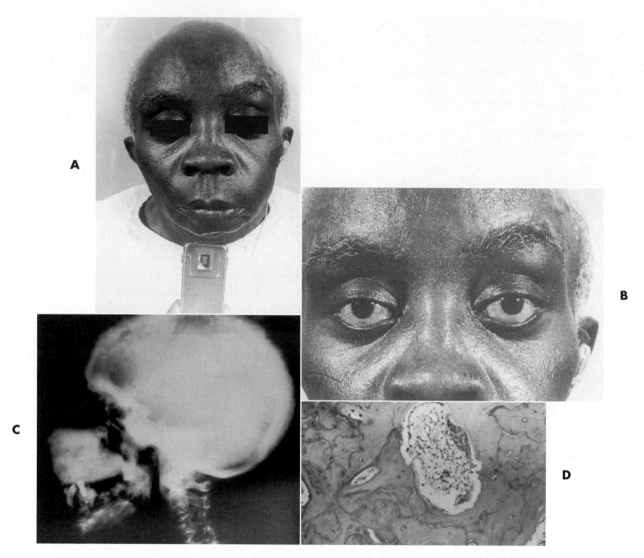

Fig. 30-3. Paget's disease. **A** and **B,** The enlarged skull and maxilla, the marked exophthalmos, and the hearing aid in the left ear are evident. **C,** Lateral radiograph reveals a dense, cotton-wool appearance throughout the skull and maxilla. **D,** Photomicrograph depicts the classic mosaic pattern within the bone, which resembles finger painting. The presence of osteoblasts and osteoclasts at the bone margins is evident.

Paget's disease.[10] Also, osteogenic sarcoma has an increased incidence in Paget's disease.

Serum alkaline phosphatase values are characteristically markedly elevated, whereas serum calcium and phosphorus levels are usually within normal limits.

The mature stage of Paget's disease produces some distinct microscopic features:

1. The bone is very dense with a few small fibrovascular spaces appearing between massive trabeculae that have resulted from the fusion of smaller trabeculae.
2. The classic mosaic pattern is usually present in the trabeculae and is produced by the many reversal lines that result from the increased resorption and apposition of bone.
3. Osteoblasts and some osteoclasts are seen rimming the trabeculae (see Fig. 30-3, *D*).

Differential Diagnosis

The differentiating aspects of generalized radiopacities of the jawbones are discussed in the section on differential diagnosis at the end of the chapter.

Management

The management of patients with Paget's disease is discussed in Chapters 23 and 25. Sofaer[11] discusses the special problems encountered with extractions in patients with Paget's disease.

OSTEOPETROSIS

Osteopetrosis (Albers-Schönberg disease, marble bone disease) is a name given to a group of diseases that affect the growth and remodeling of bone.[12] It is characterized by overgrowth and sclerosis of bone, with resultant thick-

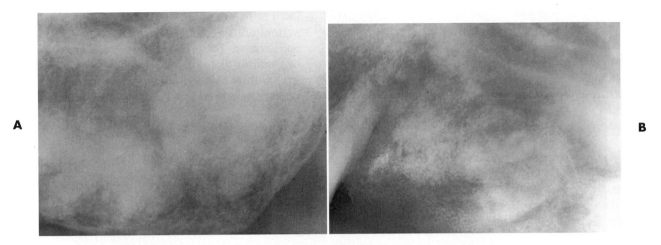

Fig. 30-4. Paget's disease. The cotton-wool appearance can be seen in the edentulous maxillary molar region (**A**) and in the canine and premolar regions (**B**). (Courtesy R. Goepp, Chicago.)

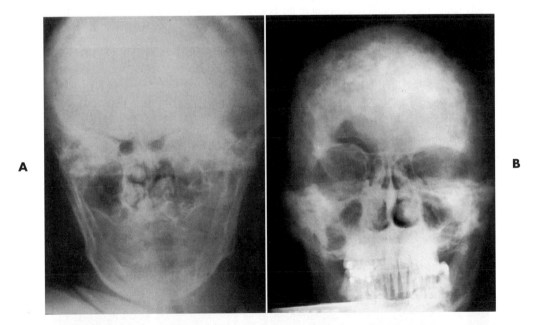

Fig. 30-5. Paget's disease in two patients. **A,** The dense, cotton-wool pattern is shown in the skull. The maxilla and mandible are not involved. **B,** The cotton-wool radiopacities can be seen throughout the maxilla, zygoma, and skull. The mandible is not involved. (**A** courtesy E. Palacios, Maywood, Ill; **B** courtesy O.H. Stuteville, deceased.)

ening of the bony cortices and narrowing of the marrow cavities throughout the skeleton. Osteopetrosis is an uncommon disease of unknown cause, although a failure of bone resorption related to defective osteoclasts is at the root of the problem[12,13] (Figs. 30-6 and 30-7). The resultant generalized radiopacity of the skeleton qualifies this disease for inclusion in this chapter. First described by Albers-Schönberg,[14] it is uncommon; Wong, Balkany, Reeves, et al[15] identified a total of 450 cases in 1978.

Features

Osteopetrosis is generally subdivided into two main types: the clinically benign, dominantly inherited form and the clinically malignant, recessively inherited form.[16]

Benign osteopetrosis usually develops later in life than the malignant form of the disease and is considerably less severe, a few cases not being diagnosed until middle age. Although the patient may sustain fractures after minor trauma, the marked symptoms of the malignant form are not characteristic of the benign disorder. Usually, benign osteopetrosis is discovered incidentally on routine radiographs. The serum chemistry levels characteristically show normal values in both forms of the disease.

The malignant (infantile) form of osteopetrosis is present at birth or develops in early childhood.[17] The disease is severe and debilitating, with no known survivors beyond the age of 20 years. Patients with malignant osteopetrosis have symptoms indicative of neurologic and

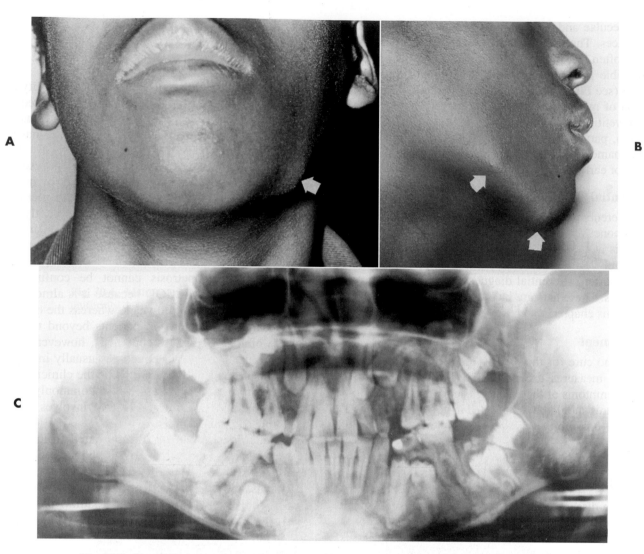

Fig. 30-9. Familial adenomatosis coli (Gardner's syndrome) in a young man. **A** and **B,** Facial views showing nodular enlargements *(arrows)* on the inferior aspect of the mandible caused by multiple osteomas. **C,** Panograph showing the diffuse and nodular radiopacities produced by multiple osteomas in the jaws. (Courtesy W. Heaton, Chicago.)

of the teeth, in combination with generalized radiopacities of several bones, is often considered pathognomonic, although hypercementosis is also seen in FLCOD.[7]

FLCOD has a strong predilection for black women over 30 years of age in the United States. The most salient features of this disease are that only the jaws are affected and radiographs of the jaws reveal radiopaque masses frequently rimmed by a radiolucent border. These two features are unique to FLCOD and clearly differentiate it from Paget's disease and osteopetrosis. The differential diagnosis of FLCOD is further developed with the discussion of this condition earlier in the chapter.

Normal variations in form and radiodensity of the jawbones must be considered in the differential diagnosis, and this aspect is discussed in detail in Chapter 23. Dense radiographic images of the jawbones may be seen in patients who have heavy jawbones or are overweight. However, such images may also be related to incorrectly exposed or processed radiographs.

The clinician should also bear in mind the rarer diseases that are capable of causing this condition, but a discussion of these is beyond the scope of this text.

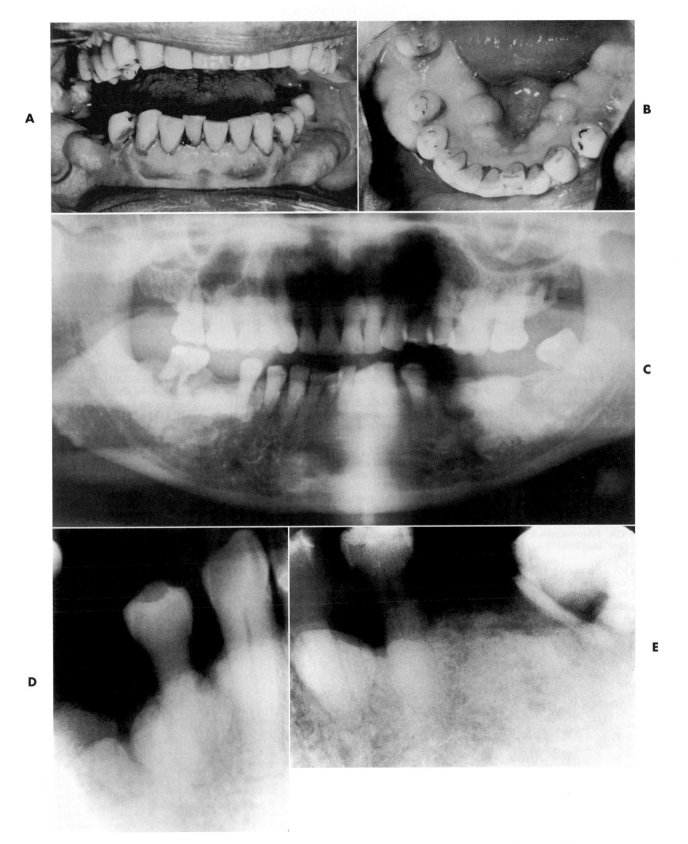

Fig. 30-10. Unusually large and numerous exostoses and tori in a 56-year-old man. **A** and **B,** Intraoral clinical views. **C** to **E,** Panographic and periapical radiographs showing the dense radiopaque pattern throughout the body of the mandible.

CHAPTER 31

Masses in the Neck

RAYMOND L. WARPEHA

The more common masses occurring in the neck, ranked in approximate order of frequency, follow:

ANATOMIC STRUCTURES
BENIGN LYMPHOID HYPERPLASIA
ACUTE LYMPHADENITIS
FIBROSED LYMPH NODES
SEBACEOUS CYSTS
SPACE ABSCESSES
SALIVARY GLAND INFLAMMATIONS
LIPOMAS
SALIVARY GLAND TUMORS
THYROID GLAND ENLARGEMENTS
BENIGN SYSTEMIC LYMPH NODE
 ENLARGEMENTS (INFECTIOUS
 MONONUCLEOSIS AND VIRAL
 DISEASES)
EPIDERMOID AND DERMOID CYSTS
METASTATIC TUMORS

THYROGLOSSAL CYSTS
CYSTIC HYGROMAS
LYMPHOMAS
BRANCHIAL CYSTS
RARITIES
 Actinomycosis[1]
 Benign lymphoepithelial disease
 Bulimia (bilateral parotid swelling)[2]
 Burkitt's lymphoma
 Carotid body tumor
 Cat-scratch disease
 Chronic obstructive pulmonary disease (bilateral parotid swelling)[3]
 Cutaneous emphysema
 Diabetes (parotid enlargement)
 Ectopic salivary gland tissue

Hydatid cyst[4]
Inflammatory pseudotumor[5]
Laryngocele
Ludwig's angina
Plunging ranula[6-9]
Mesenchymal tumors
Mikulicz' disease
Neural tumors
Primary tumors of mesenchymal tissue
Sarcoidosis
Subcutaneous emphysema
Temporomandibular joint masses (parotid region)[10]
Tuberculosis (scrofula)
Tuberculosis of parotid[11]
Wegener's granulomatosis[12]

In other chapters, lesions are discussed in the same order as they are listed. In this chapter, however, it was considered more useful to group the neck lesions according to the regions where they predominantly occur. Thus the discussion of pathologic masses of the neck is divided into the following segments:

1. Masses of nonspecific location
2. Masses in the submandibular region
3. Masses in the parotid region
4. Masses in the median-paramedian region
5. Masses in the lateral neck region

The identification of a particular mass in the neck involves a reasoning process that combines the information obtained from the medical history and the physical examination of the mass and then evaluates it in relation to the normal structures and their positions in the neck. In addition, further information from laboratory and radiographic studies may be required. After this information is analyzed, possible diagnoses can be listed and a clinical diagnosis made through the process of differential diagnosis. Although a clinical diagnosis might suffice in some instances, a definitive (microscopic) diagnosis is frequently required for proper treatment. For this determination, tissue for microscopy or material for culture is necessary. Obtaining tissue or tissue products for study may involve certain additional insult that when done ineptly may compromise therapy or perhaps even hinder the cure of a malignant neoplasm. For these reasons the most definitive step in diagnosis—microscopic study—may be reserved for final consideration.

PHYSICAL EXAMINATION AND ANATOMY OF THE NECK

Physical examination of a region involves inspection, palpation, percussion, and auscultation. Palpation plays the major role in the examination of neck masses. Although auscultation of bruits within blood vessels is a necessary part of a complete neck examination,[13] auscultation and percussion are seldom the focus of the clinician's evaluation of neck masses.

To detect subtle changes in the contour of the neck, the clinician must know the normal topography of this region. Good lighting and total exposure of the neck with the shoulders bared are necessary for proper visualization. Most visible neck masses cause asymmetries that rapidly attract the examiner's attention.

Certain normal skeletal and soft tissue structures of the neck are readily identified by palpation. Familiarity with the usual size, contour, consistency, and mobility of these structures is necessary to identify them readily and to distinguish the normal palpable masses from pathologic ones.

Skin and Subcutaneous Tissues Within the Neck

The investing cervical fascia is attached to the readily palpable lower border of the mandible, mastoid process, hyoid bone, and clavicles. It forms a heavy membrane over the deep structures of the neck, placing a screen between these structures and the examiner's fingers. The mobile skin and subcutaneous tissues are superficial to the investing fascia. Thus masses arising within this layer exhibit the mobility of the layer unless fibrosis or a malignancy has secondarily fixed the layer to deeper structures.

Specific Regions of the Neck and Their Palpable Anatomic Structures

Submandibular region The boundaries of the submandibular region are easily recognized. The lower border of the mandible from its angle to the canine region forms the superior margin, and the bellies of the digastric muscle constitute the anterior and posterior limits of the inferior border of the region (Fig. 31-1, *A*). The examiner can define the limits of this region by asking the patient to open the jaw against resistance (the examiner holding the jaw shut) while the examiner palpates the rising ridges of the digastric muscle.

The submandibular gland lies within this region on the extremely mobile mylohyoid muscle, which forms a hammock between the hyoid bone and the inner aspect of the mandibular body. Although most of the gland lies superficial to the mylohyoid muscle and consequently is in the neck, a small part insinuates itself around the free posterior border of the muscle and lies in the posterior floor of the mouth.

Merely palpating the gland externally gives only a vague impression of its dome. Bimanual palpation offers the greatest opportunity to feel the entire structure and is a mandatory step in any physical examination. The examiner accomplishes this by inserting two or three fingers into the patient's mouth to support the distensible mylohyoid muscle while palpating the submandibular gland externally with the fingers of the opposing hand (see Chapter 3).

The submandibular gland shares the submandibular region with numerous lymph nodes found within the areolar tissue of this region. These lymph nodes are not palpable in the normal state (Fig. 31-2).

Parotid region The parotid gland fills the "parotid region" (Fig. 31-1, *B*). This is the area bounded anteriorly by the posterior border of the ascending mandibular ramus and posteriorly by the external auditory canal, mastoid process, and upper portion of the sternocleidomastoid muscle. The gland overlaps the mandibular ramus and masseter muscle for a short distance beyond their posterior borders. Also, the inferior tip of the gland extends 1 to 2 cm below the projected line of the inferior border of the mandible (see Fig. 31-1, *B*).

The parotid gland is more difficult to palpate than the submandibular gland because the firm, adherent investing fascia normally prevents precise identification of the normal gland's margins. In addition, bimanual examination is difficult to perform because of the presence of the interposed pharyngeal structures and ramus and because of the gag reflex. In some cases, however, bimanual palpation of the parotid region is mandatory to establish certain clinical findings and may be accomplished by resorting to topical or general anesthesia.

Lymph nodes are found within and superficial to the parotid gland in the subcutaneous tissues of the preauricular area and at the lower pole of the gland (see Fig. 31-2). Consequently, pathoses of these structures must also be considered in the differential diagnosis of any mass in the parotid region.

Median-paramedian region The median-paramedian area is bounded superiorly by the lower border of the mandible and laterally by the attachments of the anterior bellies of the digastric muscles. The posterior boundary is delineated by the posterior extremities of the hyoid bone and the thyroid and cricoid cartilages. The medial parts of the clavicles and superior margin of the manubrium form the inferior boundaries of the region (Fig. 31-1, *C*).

The most important structure in the median-paramedian region is the butterfly-shaped thyroid gland, which has two lateral lobes connected by a narrow isthmus that crosses the trachea at a variable distance below the palpable ridge produced by the cricoid cartilage. Like the submandibular and parotid glands, the thyroid gland lies deep to the investing cervical fascia, and its features are partially masked from palpation. The lateral lobes of the gland, forming the greater part of its mass, are further concealed by the overlying infrahyoid strap muscles and the bulky sternocleidomastoid muscle. Thus the normal

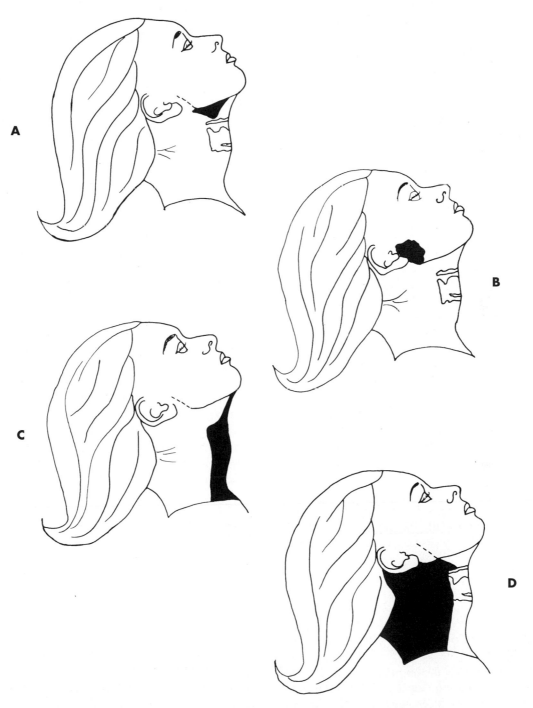

Fig. 31-1. **A,** Submandibular region. **B,** Parotid region. **C,** Median-paramedian region. **D,** Lateral region. See text for the description of the boundaries of each region.

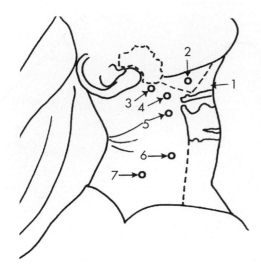

Fig. 31-2. Major cervical lymph node areas. *1,* Submental; *2,* submandibular; *3,* subparotid; *4,* subdigastric; *5,* bifurcation; *6,* juguloomohyoid; *7,* posterior triangle.

thyroid gland is not palpable in the usual sense but rather is recognized by a feeling of fullness to the touch. The left lobe frequently imparts a greater fullness because it is usually larger than the right.

A mass within or an enlargement of the lateral lobes of the thyroid gland is best appreciated by manipulation of the overlying sternocleidomastoid muscle. While one hand stabilizes the gland by insinuating the fingers behind the posterior border of that muscle, the palpating fingers of the opposite hand determine the features of the lateral lobe. The isthmus is palpated near the midline below the prominent, ringlike cricoid cartilage and is best felt during swallowing, since the gland is attached to the trachea and moves upward with this structure during deglutition. The presence of a mass in a lateral lobe is similarly verified by palpation while the patient swallows. In such a case the intrinsically attached mass moves with the thyroid gland.

The palpable hyoid bone and thyroid cartilages are also present within the median-paramedian region. The mobility of these structures requires bimanual fixation similar to that used in examining the submandibular and thyroid glands. The greater cornu of the hyoid bone and superior cornu of the thyroid cartilage are occasionally mistaken for stony-hard lymph nodes in the upper cervical chain, which would imply malignant metastasis. However, the two cornua are normal structures anterior to the cervical node chain, and they are identified by their presence bilaterally and their upward displacement during swallowing.

In the median-paramedian region, lymph nodes are found above the hyoid bone in the submental area and in front of the cricothyroid membrane. Normally these nodes are not palpable, and such masses in the neck are considered in the ensuing discussion.

Lateral region   The lateral neck region is the area posterior to the hyolaryngotracheal conduit, below the posterior belly of the digastric muscle and tip of the parotid gland, and it extends down to the clavicle (Fig. 31-1, *D*). It is crossed obliquely by the sternocleidomastoid muscle, which obliterates the detail of the central structures in this region.

The contents of this region include the large vessels and nerves of the neck just anterior to the bodies and transverse processes of the cervical vertebrae. The transverse processes of the first and seventh cervical vertebrae are vaguely palpable as immovable hard masses below the tip of the mastoid and in the supraclavicular area, respectively. They become more apparent in the thin and emaciated patient and are prominent in the postsurgical patient after radical neck dissection with removal of the sternocleidomastoid muscle and soft tissues of the lateral neck region.

The carotid pulse can be felt on the prominent bulge marking the carotid bifurcation. This structure lies below the posterior belly of the digastric muscle, level with the angle of the mandible, and is frequently mistaken for a pathologic mass by the unwary examiner. Just as the greater cornu of the hyoid bone, superior cornu of the thyroid cartilage, or transverse processes of the first or seventh cervical vertebra may be mistaken for disease, in the elderly patient, calcification within the arterial wall at the carotid bifurcation may be misinterpreted as a hard node of metastatic cancer. However, careful manipulation of the artery and determination of whether the carotid pulse can be detected through the hard mass identify the mass as part or not part of the artery.

The lateral neck region is the region of the neck with the greatest number of lymph nodes (see Fig. 31-2). It is also the most common site of lymph node metastases from head and neck cancer because the lymph from several of the common primary cancer sites drains first to nodes in this area. As in other regions, the normal lymph nodes of the lateral neck region are not palpable. Within the lateral region, the posterior triangle of the neck occupies the area between the posterior border of the sternocleidomastoid muscle and the anterior border of the trapezius muscle and contains lymph nodes that drain the scalp skin and posterolateral pharyngeal mucosa.

Lymph Nodes of the Neck

A capillary plexus of endothelial tubes is found below the epidermis and oral mucosa of the head and neck. It collects the fluid from the interstitial spaces for return to the large venous trunks at the base of the neck. Between a given capillary plexus and the veins are increasingly larger channels, the lymphatics, with one or more lymph nodes in their course. Within each of these lymph nodes the fluid must again pass capillary-sized channels before proceeding through to the efferent lymphatic channel.

The first lymph node encountered in a channel draining a particular submucosal or subepidermal lymph capillary plexus is called the *first-echelon node* because it is here that pathogenic organisms or free tumor cells within the lymph fluid meet their first resistance to travel.

The first-echelon nodes are also found in the preauricular (superficial to the parotid gland and investing fascia), postauricular, and suboccipital areas. With the submental and submandibular nodes, they form a collar around the face and scalp, filtering the drainage from the subepidermal lymph plexuses of the skin in this region.

GENERAL CHARACTERISTICS OF PATHOLOGIC MASSES

Before the discussion of specific masses by region, it is appropriate to review some of the characteristics of abnormal masses, since the presence or absence of certain features often directs the clinician to the correct disease or group of diseases. These characteristics are common to abnormal masses no matter where the masses are found in the body.

Degree of Tenderness

Tenderness usually indicates inflammation, infection, or both within the tissues affected. Benign or malignant tumors and cysts are usually nontender. Painful tumors are usually the result of frank invasion of a nerve, but pain may also reflect rapid growth and simple compression of sensory nerves. In other cases a secondary inflammatory process, abscess, or both within a tumor or cyst may be the cause of tenderness.

Consistency

Solid masses impart a feeling of firmness, whereas cysts and abscesses are soft to rubbery. Fluctuation may be masked by a surrounding zone of inflammation or fibrous tissue, or a fluid-filled mass may be situated so deep in the tissues that fluctuance is not demonstrable. Although other signs of the inflammatory process are generally present, whether an abscess is fluctuant depends on its stage of development.

In the early stage before a pool of pus forms, the swelling is due to inflammation only, so the mass is not fluctuant but is firm in consistency. Later, if a pool of pus does form, the swelling becomes fluctuant. Still later, in the regressing stage, the fluctuance disappears as the pus is eliminated.

Malignant tumors and their metastases to lymph nodes are frequently described as stony hard, although lymph nodes involved by lymphoma have a distinctly rubbery feeling (Fig. 31-3). Tuberculosis characteristically produces a caseation necrosis of several nodes, resulting in a matted type of mass.

Degree of Mobility

Each structure of the neck has its own range of motion when manipulated. A decrease in mobility may be associated with fixation of the structure to less mobile ones.

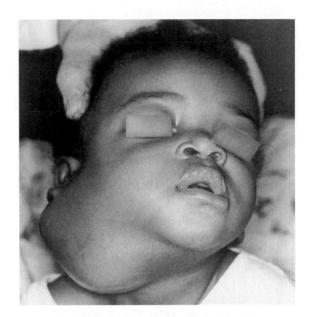

Fig. 31-3. Large lymphoma. This child had a rapidly growing, rubbery mass. (Courtesy O.H. Stuteville, deceased.)

Lymph nodes are ordinarily freely movable but become fixed in certain pathologic conditions. Usually, fixation of a node is the result of an inflammatory process that has penetrated the node's capsule and has caused fibrosis of the surrounding immovable structures. In cases of metastatic spread, the malignant cells may penetrate the capsule and invade the surrounding tissue.

PATHOLOGIC MASSES

Aside from masses originating in the skin, the majority of neck masses may be categorized into the following general types: (1) enlarged lymph nodes; (2) enlarged submandibular, parotid, and thyroid glands or masses within these glands; (3) congenital cysts of specific origin and location; and (4) derivatives of vessels and nerves in the lateral neck region. Other distinctive masses in the neck are also discussed in this chapter.

Masses of Nonspecific Location

Commonly occurring masses, although not specific to the neck region (e.g., the lipoma), are not classified or discussed here. Also, it is obvious that some masses are not peculiar to certain regions of the neck but may occur anywhere in the neck; these most frequently originate in the skin or lymph nodes and are referred to as *masses of nonspecific location.*

Enlarged lymph nodes Enlarged lymph nodes are by far the most common pathologic masses in the neck. The majority are the result of an acute or chronic response to an infectious organism (lymphadenitis), a resolution of the acute response in which the mass is still enlarged (benign lymphoid hyperplasia), the growth of a metastatic tumor, or a primary malignant neoplasm (lymphoma). Benign lymphoid hyperplasia is the most common.

Lymphadenitis is by definition an inflammation or infection of a lymph node, and it frequently occurs when an infection is present in the tissues drained by the particular node's pathway. Pathoses of this type may be classified as acute or chronic, solitary or multiple, local or disseminated, and specific or nonspecific.

As with the same process in other organs and tissues, the sequelae of a lymphadenitis depend on the modifying factors. If the adenitis is short lived, the node may subsequently return to practically normal size and architecture. If, on the other hand, the infection is acute, the node may become painful, necrotic, and liquefied and may lead to a space abscess.

In more chronic cases, permanent hyperplasia of the lymph node may result; such a pathosis is referred to as a *benign lymphoid hyperplasia*. In some instances of chronic lymphadenitis, scarring replaces the node architecture, so the enlarged node remains as a permanently fibrosed mass. Thus two distinct types of benign node enlargement can be found by clinical examination: (1) nontender and (2) tender or painful.

Nontender lymphoid hyperplasia. The majority of nontender, benign enlargements of the cervical lymph nodes are lesions of nontender lymphoid hyperplasia (Fig. 31-4). At least one or two such enlarged nodes are found during routine palpation of the neck of almost every patient examined. Nontender lymphoid hyperplasia represents persistent chronic lymphadenitis or a permanently enlarged node after an acute or chronic lymphadenitis.

FEATURES. The patient is usually unaware of the enlarged node but in some cases may recount the presence of a previous painful swelling in the region and perhaps identify the primary infection site. The nodes are solitary, discrete, asymptomatic, and usually freely movable. The submandibular, submental, and subdigastric groups are the nodes most frequently affected (see Fig. 31-4).

DIFFERENTIAL DIAGNOSIS. The nontender lymphoid hyperplasia is by far the most common pathologic mass in the neck. The painless nature of this benign enlargement differentiates it from the less frequently encountered acute lymphadenitis.

As a rule, nontender lymphoid hyperplasia can be differentiated from secondary carcinoma by the fact that the carcinoma may be stony hard and often fixed, whereas the lesion of hyperplasia is firm and usually freely movable. A complete head and neck examination and evaluation are necessary, however, before benign lymphoid hyperplasia can be made the final diagnosis because occasionally a metastatic tumor in an enlarged lymph node has a softer consistency.

MANAGEMENT. If the clinician has any doubt concerning the diagnosis, the patient should be reexamined at 2-week intervals to see whether the mass changes perceptibly. If doubt still exists, biopsy and microscopic study are advised. Biopsy, however, is withheld until a

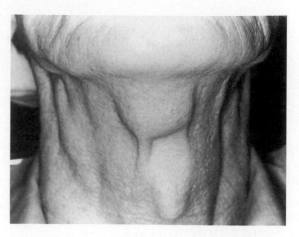

Fig. 31-4. Benign lymphoid hyperplasia. This unusually large example in the submental region was firm, nontender, and freely movable. (Courtesy S. Svalina, Palos Park, Ill.)

thorough upper aerodigestive tract examination is performed to identify a primary tumor.

Acute lymphadenitis. Acute lymphadenitis is the second most common pathologic cervical mass and the most common painful enlargement found in the neck. The primary infection may be in the oral cavity, nasal cavities, tonsils, or pharynx. Minor mucosal erosions or shallow ulcers frequently permit the entrance of sufficient bacteria to produce regional lymphadenitis. Depending on the location of the tooth (Fig. 31-5), a periapical abscess, periodontal abscess, or pericoronitis type of infection may cause painful, swollen nodes in the submental, submandibular, or subdigastric area (see Fig. 31-13, *C*). With tonsillar inflammation the subdigastric node is most commonly involved and thus has become known as the *tonsillar node*. Regression results in the node returning to normal and becoming nonpalpable, benign lymphoid hyperplasia, or fibrosed.

FEATURES. Acute lymphadenitis is usually tender on palpation. Single affected nodes are round, firm, and discrete and may be movable or fixed. Several nodes in one region may be involved, and in such cases an accompanying inflammation in the adjacent soft tissues causes a firm swelling that prevents palpation of the individual nodes (see Fig. 31-13, *C*). On microscopic examination the node is enlarged, has more numerous germinal centers, and contains acute inflammatory cells. Such a condition is termed a *nonspecific adenitis*. The architecture of nodes affected by a severe inflammation may be almost obliterated by the inflammatory process, even to the point of necrosis and liquefaction.

DIFFERENTIAL DIAGNOSIS. Acute lymphadenitis must be differentiated from infected cysts and Ludwig's angina.

Ludwig's angina is usually a nonpurulent hemolytic streptococcal infection of the floor of the mouth and submental and submandibular areas (see Fig. 5-8). The classic location of this entity, with the serosanguineous fluid obtained on incision, is almost pathognomonic.

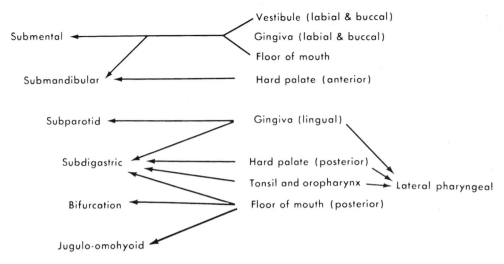

Fig. 31-5. Lymphatic drainage areas of the oral cavity (exclusive of the tongue) and pharynx showing first-echelon lymph nodes for various regions.

Infected cysts of the neck, except for the sebaceous type, which is very superficial, may be suspected in certain locations; in other words, branchial and thyroglossal cysts characteristically occur in the lateral neck and midline regions, respectively.

MANAGEMENT. In most cases, when the primary mucosal infection is eliminated, the secondary acute lymphadenitis soon regresses. Adequate doses of antibiotics specific to the organism involved are administered. Cases of generalized lymphadenitis in which lymph nodes are uniformly and symmetrically enlarged in all accessible areas, such as the axillae, groin, and neck, are not rare, and such a condition usually suggests a viremia or primary lymphoid disease. Thus in cases of multiple and bilateral nodes in the neck, a careful examination of other nodal areas and the spleen, as well as a complete history and physical examination, is necessary to determine whether the enlarged nodes in the neck are a manifestation of a local or a systemic disease.

Rare varieties of specific lymphadenitis. The majority of cases of cervical lymphadenitis result from primary infections by common bacteria or viruses. Microscopic examination does not show characteristics that relate to these common organisms, since only a nonspecific adenitis is seen. Specific diagnostic changes may occur in some rare diseases.[14]

The specific lesions within lymph nodes generated by tuberculosis, histoplasmosis, sarcoidosis, and infectious mononucleosis are similar to the lesions in other tissues infected by the organisms causing these diseases. Except for infectious mononucleosis, these are relatively uncommon in the neck, but in some cases, lymph node infection that initially appears to be nonspecific (Fig. 31-6) proves on biopsy and culture to be one of the specific infections.

Metastatic carcinoma to cervical nodes. The cervical lymph nodes are more frequently the site of metastatic carcinomas than of primary tumors (lymphomas). The

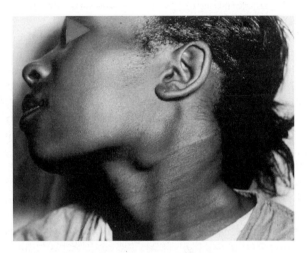

Fig. 31-6. Tuberculous adenitis. The nodular enlargement in the parotid region was tender and moderately soft on palpation. The patient also had pulmonary tuberculosis. (Courtesy O.H. Stuteville, deceased.)

majority are the result of metastatic spread from primary tumors in the head and neck, especially those in the oral and pharyngeal cavities (Plate J). In unusual cases, however, they represent secondary tumors from primary sites below the clavicles.

In addition, in squamous cell carcinoma of the larynx and vocal cords, tumors can metastasize to regional nodes. The first-echelon nodes for metastatic tumors occurring inferior to the oropharynx are located roughly opposite the primary tumor site in the jugular chain (Fig. 31-7).

Since squamous cell carcinoma constitutes the preponderance of primary malignancies of the head and neck (95% of all oral malignancies), it is by far the most common tumor spreading to the cervical nodes (see Fig. 31-9, *C*). Adenocarcinoma of the salivary glands, occasionally squamous cell carcinoma from the skin, and melanoma (see Fig. 31-9, *D*) are the tumors that next

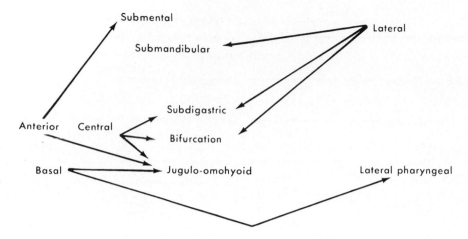

Fig. 31-7. Lymphatic drainage areas of the tongue showing first-echelon lymph nodes.

most commonly metastasize to the cervical nodes. Sarcoma characteristically spreads by the blood channels but on rare occasions involves a lymph node.

The lymphatic trunks draining the upper extremities and the rest of the body below the clavicles converge in the base of the lateral neck region, the supraclavicular area. Consequently, solitary metastatic nodes in this area are mostly from primary tumors in areas other than the head and neck, such as the breasts, lungs, and stomach. A complete history, physical examination, and specific laboratory studies usually reveal the primary tumor.

FEATURES. Metastatic tumors in lymph nodes are usually painless and thus are not detected by the patient until they reach considerable dimensions. The smaller nodes are usually detected on routine examination; they characteristically feel stony hard and are freely movable until the tumor cells penetrate the node capsule and invade the surrounding tissue. Then they become fixed, and the expanding tumor may amalgamate surrounding nodes into one larger, stony-hard, fixed mass. In the majority of cases the primary tumor is readily evident, especially if the primary site is in the oral cavity. Small tumors in the nasal cavities, nasopharynx, and larynx, however, may go undetected, the only evidence of their presence being the metastatic tumor. The submandibular and subdigastric nodes are the most frequent sites of early metastatic spread from primary tumors within the oral cavity.

DIFFERENTIAL DIAGNOSIS. The differential diagnosis of metastatic lymph node tumors is considered later in this chapter with the discussion of pathologic masses occurring in specific regions.

Small metastatic nodes may be confused with fibrosed nodes or nodes that have undergone nontender lymphoid hyperplasia because these entities are firm and may even be fixed to the surrounding tissue by fibrosis resulting from a previous infection. In such cases, however, the history relating to a significant infection in the region would probably direct the clinician to the working diagnosis of benign lymphoid hyperplasia.

Differentiating between a secondary tumor and a lymphoma is also necessary. A metastatic tumor is usually stony hard, whereas the lymphoma is more rubbery.

MANAGEMENT. Various combinations of resection, radiation, and chemotherapy are used, with inconsistent results. The prognosis for a patient with lymph node metastasis is guarded. To assess the efficacy of treatment and comparison of therapeutic results, a system of cancer staging was developed using the TNM system in which *T* represents the size and extent of the primary lesion, *N* represents the number and characteristics of lymph node involvement, and *M* represents the presence of distant metastasis. Cancers of the upper aerodigestive tract, skin, and organs of the head and neck are each staged with specific criteria.[15]

Lymphoma. Lymphoma is a neoplastic proliferation within the reticuloendothelial system that occurs as a primary tumor of lymph nodes but is not as common as a metastatic tumor.[16] There are several types of lymphoma, which vary in behavior and histopathology.[17] Current classifications reflect the behavior of the specific tumor.

Lymphomas may be solitary or multiple. Although it is generally accepted that they reflect a systemic disease, in about 10% of cases the initial finding is a mass in the neck.[17]

FEATURES. The nodes involved may be solitary or multiple and unilateral or bilateral; they are usually rubbery and may be a single discrete mass or several nodes joined together (see Fig. 31-3 and Plate J). In advanced cases the patient may be quite ill with fever, and the total and differential leukocyte counts may be markedly changed, indicating that the increased production of mononuclear cells has spilled over into the blood. Other node groups such as the axillae, groin, and mediastinum are frequently involved in these advanced cases.

DIFFERENTIAL DIAGNOSIS. Advanced and disseminated lymphomas (Hodgkin's disease) are readily differentiated from other tumors on a clinical basis.

Multiple and disseminated nodal involvement may also occur with certain viral diseases and in mononucleosis. In these diseases, however, the nodes are often tender and painful, and a Paul-Bunnell heterophil test is positive in infectious mononucleosis.

MANAGEMENT. Radiation and various chemotoxic drugs are used, with varying results, to treat patients who have malignant lymphoma and Hodgkin's disease. Because of the high cure rate in Hodgkin's disease, early diagnosis by biopsy is desirable.

Sebaceous cysts Sebaceous cysts occur in hair-bearing areas and are found in the neck with some regularity. They are superficial, dome-shaped masses and are usually detectable on visual examination (see Figs. 31-9, *B*, 31-10, *A*, 31-12, *C*, and 31-13, *B*).

FEATURES. Sebaceous cysts grow slowly and are painless unless secondarily infected. They range from a few millimeters to a few centimeters in diameter. The smaller cysts may have a dimple or enlarged pore on the surface. If situated in the anterior two thirds of the neck, they are movable over the deeper structures because masses arising within the dermis in this area have considerable mobility. The skin of the posterior neck region is more adherent to the underlying fascia, however, and cysts arising in the posterior third of the neck may appear to be fixed to the underlying structures.

Aspiration of a thick material from such a mass indicates a sebaceous cyst. Secondary infection is quite common and produces pain, induration, and fixation. Recurrent episodes of infection with periodic painful enlargement of the cyst and purulent drainage is a common sequence of events.

DIFFERENTIAL DIAGNOSIS. Unlike epidermoid and dermoid cysts, sebaceous cysts often are superficially located in the skin. Thus they usually cannot be moved independent of skin over the deeper structures. On the other hand, epidermoid cysts are deeper and freely movable unless involved with inflammation and resultant fibrosis.

Although numerous solid benign and malignant tumors of a primary and occasionally metastatic nature occur in the skin, their firm consistency differentiates them from a sebaceous cyst.

MANAGEMENT. Because of the simplicity of removal and the tendency toward secondary infection, excisional biopsy is recommended. This also identifies the occasional skin tumor that could be mistaken for a cyst on clinical examination. Suitable antibiotics should be administered if the sebaceous cyst is infected.

MASSES IN SPECIFIC REGIONS

The majority of pathologic masses in the neck occur in four regions: submandibular, parotid, median-paramedian, and lateral. Thus the masses are discussed here according to the region in which they occur.

Masses in the Submandibular Region

The majority of masses in the submandibular region originate in the lymph nodes or the submandibular salivary gland. The first step in diagnosis is to distinguish between the tissues of the submandibular gland and those of the nonsubmandibular gland using careful bimanual, intraoral, and extraoral palpation.

Masses separate from the submandibular gland A mass may be an enlarged lymph node if the clinician determines that it is not the submandibular salivary gland. In such a case, all possible sites in the mouth (Figs. 31-5 and 31-7), on the face, and in the nasal vestibule should be carefully examined to detect a source of infection or a primary tumor.

Tender nodes. If the node is tender, whether the constitutional signs of infection such as fever are present, and an obvious source of infection such as an abscessed tooth is found, the working diagnosis of lymphadenitis should be made. Such a case is treated with antibiotics, tooth extraction, or both. If no primary site of infection can be found, an antibiotic effective against staphylococcal and streptococcal infections should be administered and the patient frequently reexamined to determine whether the size and tenderness of the mass have changed.

If the tender mass subsides, it is assumed to have been an acute nonspecific nonsuppurative lymphadenitis. The specific adenitis of tuberculosis appears in rare cases as a tender mass in children. Such a mass does not respond to ordinary antibiotic treatment, and a general workup, including a skin test and chest radiograph, that confirms the presence of tuberculosis should alert the clinician to the possibility of tuberculous adenitis. An excisional biopsy establishes the diagnosis if the process is tuberculosis.

If the tender mass expands with or without softening and this change is accompanied by some reduction in pain and tenderness, the mass is assumed to be an abscess that is forming; incision and drainage are then indicated. In an adult a biopsy of the abscess wall should be performed during the drainage procedure if a primary infection is not found or if the usual signs of inflammation are minimal. This will allow the clinician to distinguish lymph node metastases from occult carcinomas, which may undergo necrosis and abscess formation.

A staphylococcal node abscess may be manifested in a fussy neonate or young child as a hard submandibular, submental, or suboccipital swelling (Fig. 31-8, *A*). A primary infection in the mouth or skin might not be obvious because the hardness of the swelling and the lack of constitutional symptoms suggest that the mass does not have an infectious origin. Usually the abscess matures after a few days, however, and the diagnosis becomes readily apparent.

A submandibular abscess may form by the direct extension of a preexisting infection or abscess in the mouth. This pathosis appears as a diffuse, tender, fluctuant swelling (see Fig. 31-8). The following sequence is typical in the formation of such an abscess:

1. A pericoronitis of a mandibular third molar develops with pus formation.
2. The pus extends into the pterygomandibular space, causing trismus.

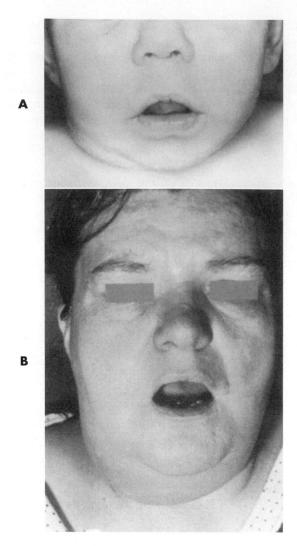

Fig. 31-8. A, Staphylococcal submandibular space abscess. This enlarging, hard, tender mass was present for 4 days in a fussy and mildly febrile child. No primary oral or skin infections were found. **B,** Submental and submandibular space abscess secondary to infected mandibular incisors.

3. From the pterygomandibular space the pus breaks through the connective tissue barrier around the anterior margin of the medial pterygoid muscle and gains access to the submandibular space.

4. When this happens, a space abscess is produced.

The history and physical findings of an abscess are diagnostic. Computed tomography is useful in the localization of head and neck space infections, since it can demonstrate abscess formation deep to muscle and bone and can differentiate between edema and pus formation.[18] Treatment consists of incision, drainage, and irrigation of the abscess and eradication of the primary infection.

Nontender nodes. The majority of nontender nodes in the submandibular region represent benign lymphoid hyperplasia or fibrosed nodes resulting from a previous oral infection. If a nontender node of short duration is detected, especially in a patient over 40 years of age, the clinician must be aware of the increased possibility that it may be a secondary malignant tumor.

Such a case requires a thorough physical and radiographic examination of the head and neck to detect a possible primary malignancy. When the primary tumor site is known and the expected site of nodal metastasis is positive, the primary lesion is resected with the neck dissection. In some institutions a combination of irradiation and surgical resection is used; in others, irradiation is the sole method of treatment.

When no primary tumor can be located but the clinician suspects that a submandibular mass may be malignant, an excisional biopsy of the mass should be performed. The patient is informed that the mass will be microscopically evaluated for malignancy during the biopsy procedure and that a neck dissection will be completed if the mass proves to be malignant. This policy seems justified, since a substantial increase in the cure rate has been observed when neck dissection is undertaken even though the primary site was not detected before removal of the lymph nodes. In over half of these patients, no primary site is ever discovered.[16]

Multiple nontender nodes occurring unilaterally in the neck without an overt primary cause should be managed the same as a single nontender node.

The occurrence of bilateral multiple nontender cervical nodes with or without generalized lymphadenopathy should prompt a complete medical examination for the detection of systemic disorders.

In the adult, excisional biopsy may be necessary for diagnosis, but it should await the results of other diagnostic tests, which might preclude the necessity for this step.

In the child, multiple enlarged bilateral neck nodes of inflammatory origin are common, whereas metastasizing neoplasms are rare. Conversely, lymphomas are more common than secondary tumors in children. Although biopsies of all asymptomatic nodes in children with multiple and bilateral cervical lymphadenopathy would not be feasible, any unusually large node in a child that shows progressive growth or is rubbery or stony hard should be excised and microscopically examined.

Masses within the submandibular gland If a mass is within the submandibular gland, the gland should be removed intact and examined histologically at the time of the surgery. A total excision of the gland is required because (1) a high proportion of submandibular tumors are malignant (50%) and (2) the most common tumor in this gland, the pleomorphic adenoma, does not have a restricting capsule (Fig. 31-9, *A*). Furthermore, a wide local resection of the surrounding tissues and occasionally a radical neck dissection at the time of the excisional biopsy may be necessary. A more complete discussion of salivary gland tumors appears elsewhere.[19-21]

Submandibular gland sialadenitis A painful enlargement of the submandibular gland (sialadenitis) may be produced by (1) an inflammation or infection of the gland

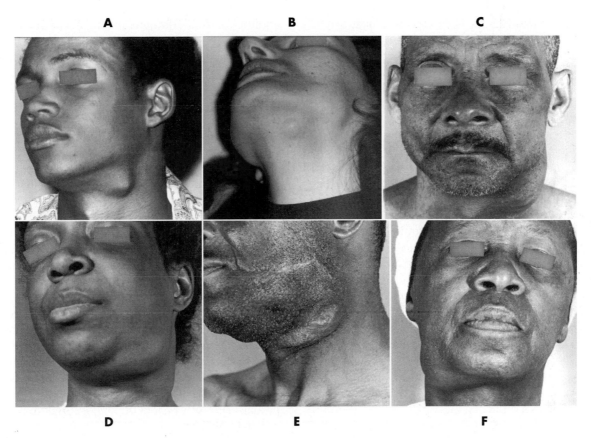

Fig. 31-9. Submandibular masses. **A,** Pleomorphic adenoma of the submandibular salivary gland. **B,** Sebaceous cyst. **C,** Metastatic squamous cell carcinoma to the submandibular and subdigastric nodes. The primary tumor was located in the left floor of the mouth. The mass was painless, firm, and fixed to the surrounding structures. **D,** Metastatic melanoma from a primary lesion on the palate. **E,** Actinomycosis. **F,** Tuberculous adenitis. (**A** courtesy E. Kasper, Maywood, Ill.)

caused by ductal occlusion and (2) an infection not preceded by ductal obstruction.

When the duct is obstructed, eating leads to pain and swelling in the gland because the secretions accumulate behind the obstruction. The pain and swelling tend to subside somewhat between meals and are minimal on waking in the morning. The clinician can determine that the duct is patent if milking the submandibular gland causes the expression of saliva at Wharton's papilla. The clinician may discover a sialolith in the submandibular duct by palpating the floor of the mouth bimanually. In approximately 90% of cases a sialolith is dense enough to show on a radiograph (see Figs. 28-14 and 28-15).

If the results of these examinations are equivocal, sialography with a radiopaque substance can be performed to show whether the duct is patent. The advantage of this procedure, however, must be weighed against the hazard of precipitating a retrograde infection. Also, the injection of the disclosing material into the inflamed gland causes the patient additional discomfort.

Obstruction of the duct may also have other causes such as changes in the floor of the mouth produced by a malignant tumor or postoperative scarring. Under these circumstances the obstructive process is frequently insidious; although the gland is enlarged and firm, tenderness is frequently not a feature.

Elimination of the obstruction by removal of the stone, tumor, or cicatrix is indicated. Complete removal of the gland may be necessary when much fibrosis is present in a chronic case or when the stone is near or within the gland.

Sialadenitis without prior ductal obstruction. Sialadenitis without prior ductal obstruction is caused by viral or bacterial infection.

Mumps is the type of viral sialadenitis most commonly occurring in childhood. Although primarily a disease of the parotid glands, it may also affect the submandibular glands. The diagnosis is usually made by confirming a history of contact with an infected person. When such information is lacking, the demonstration of mumps antibodies in the serum establishes the diagnosis.

Other viruses such as coxsackie A virus and echovirus may cause sialadenitis.[22,23] Although such a viral relationship has not been established in submandibular gland adenitis, such a cause might be considered in uncommon cases of enlarged tender unobstructed glands.

A suppurative sialadenitis is produced almost exclusively by a retrograde bacterial infection in patients with reduced salivary secretion. Such a reduction may be caused by dehydration or the use of parasympathetic blocking drugs and by partial occlusion of a major duct. The retrograde infection occurs because oral bacteria are able to ascend the duct to the gland in the absence of the duct-cleansing salivary flow.

Pus-producing sialadenitis seldom occurs in the major glands but is more common in the parotid gland. In the submandibular gland, it is usually associated with a ductal stone, and the clinical and radiographic examinations previously described should be completed. The use of sialography is contraindicated in suppurative sialadenitis.

Clinically the gland is firm and painful. Pressure over the gland causes the expression of pus from the opening of Wharton's duct if the duct is not completely obstructed. A specimen of pus should be collected and sent for culture and sensitivity tests so that an effective antibiotic may be administered. Systemic problems, as well as any local factors causing occlusion of the duct, should be eliminated. Occasionally a child or an adult has recurrent bouts of nonobstructive sialadenitis; such a condition is described as chronic recurrent sialadenitis.[22]

In rare instances a branchial cleft cyst may project into the submandibular region. Also a ranula of the sublingual gland may insinuate itself around the posterior border of the mylohyoid muscle and cause a cystlike mass in this region.[6-9] These entities must be considered when cystic masses are encountered in this region.

Involvement of the human immunodeficiency virus in the lymph nodes can present as parotid gland enlargement. Appropriate history and laboratory testing are necessary to confirm this diagnosis.

Masses in the Parotid Region

The masses common to the parotid region also occur in the submandibular region. This is to be expected, since the chief structures occupying both regions are the major salivary glands and the lymph nodes. Thus only lesions peculiar to the parotid region are detailed here. Concerning the masses previously discussed, only differences in emphasis are made.

When a mass is discovered in the parotid region, the clinician must first determine whether it is superficial or deep to the investing fascia of the salivary gland. The majority of masses superficial to the investing fascia are enlarged lymph nodes, whereas those masses within the gland are usually parotid masses or enlarged intraparotid nodes. Masses within the parotid gland are fixed beneath the confines of the investing fascia and capsule of the gland.

Enlarged masses superficial to the parotid fascia Various lymph nodes are present in the loose connective tissue superficial to the parotid gland and fascia. The preauricular node is found immediately anterior to the external auditory meatus. It is quite mobile unless fixed to the surrounding tissues as a result of penetrating pathoses.

An enlarged firm, tender, or painful mass that can be moved over the deeper structures in this superficial region is most likely an acute lymphadenitis resulting from a furuncle or another infection of the scalp, upper face, conjunctivae, or external auditory canal.

An infected congenital preauricular cyst or sebaceous cyst must also be considered because either may be found superficial to the parotid fascia (Fig. 31-10, *A*). The rubbery consistency and fluctuance of these masses help differentiate them from acute lymphadenitis. Also, erythema and edema of the overlying skin are more characteristic of an infected cyst than of an acute lymphadenitis.

Painless superficial masses are usually benign lymphoid hyperplasias, parotid tumors superficial to the gland, and preauricular or sebaceous cysts.

Lymph nodes in the preauricular area are seldom the site of a lymphoma or a metastatic carcinoma, which may originate from a primary carcinoma or a melanoma in the skin of the region drained.

Whether a mass located at the inferior tip of the parotid lobe is superficial to or within the parotid gland is frequently difficult to determine. In such an instance a primary site for possible tumors or inflammatory lesions is sought on the appropriate skin surfaces of the scalp and face or the mucosal surfaces of the oral cavity, pharynx, and nasal cavities. Because of the possibility that this mass may be a secondary or a salivary gland tumor, if the examination of the frozen section indicates that it is malignant, the mass should be excised and more extensive surgery completed at the same operation.

Masses within the parotid gland The majority of masses occurring within the parotid gland are salivary gland tumors. Approximately 70% of these are benign, most being benign mixed tumors that characteristically grow slowly and produce a noticeably firm swelling in the parotid area (see Fig. 31-10, *B*). Malignant mixed tumors (Plate I), on the other hand, usually grow more rapidly, may be stony hard, and may cause a unilateral paralysis of the muscles of facial expression. The types of salivary gland tumors are listed in Chapter 10. Although the clinician may develop an impression of whether the tumor is benign or malignant, the definitive diagnosis must be made by microscopic study in every case.

MANAGEMENT. Besides a parotid gland tumor, a mass within the parotid gland may be an enlarged node, a simple cyst, a cyst of the first and second branchial arches, or a hamartoma. Although the diagnosis of each of these entities is occasionally suspected on the basis of clinical features, the physical examination is not sufficiently definitive to rule out a tumor. Therefore biopsies must be performed on all masses detected within the parotid gland either by fine-needle aspiration or by excisional biopsy when the clinical examination is highly suspicious for a parotid neoplasm. Computed tomo-

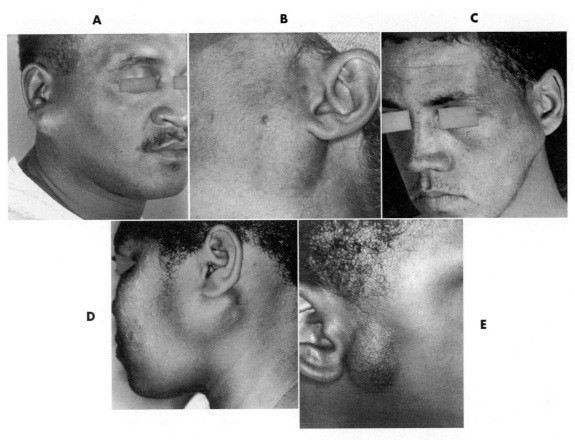

Fig. 31-10. Masses in the parotid region. **A,** Sebaceous cyst. **B,** Benign mixed tumor. The mass was firm and grew slowly. **C,** Malignant mixed tumor. This mass was firm and enlarged rapidly. **D,** Parotid space abscess resulting from a dental infection. **E,** Hemangioma. (**D** courtesy V. Barresi, DeKalb, Ill.)

graphic sialography and conventional sialography are helpful in the evaluation of parotid gland neoplasms.[24]

Excisional biopsy consists of removal of the superficial lobe of the gland, leaving the facial nerve intact. The complete lobe is sacrificed because the most common lesion, the pleomorphic adenoma, frequently penetrates its pseudocapsule and a high recurrence rate results if an attempt is made merely to enucleate the lesion.

When a mass extends into or originates in the deep parotid lobe,[25] the entire gland is removed for pathologic study. A malignant tumor that characteristically metastasizes to the cervical lymph nodes or that shows clinical evidence of metastasis may require resection of the cervical lymph nodes, in addition to removal of the primary lesion.

In rare instances, primary lesions arising in the mouth or oropharynx metastasize to the nodes within the parotid gland, so these regions should be examined carefully before the biopsy procedure. A wide variety of tumors are found within the parotid gland, and these are characterized in detail by others.[19-21]

Sialadenitis of the parotid gland

The information in the section on sialadenitis of the submandibular gland also applies to parotid sialadenitis (Fig. 31-11, *A*). The following points are peculiar to the parotid gland, however:

1. Salivary stones (calculi) in Stensen's duct occur less frequently than in Wharton's duct, and those that do develop are frequently poorly calcified and radiolucent.
2. Bimanual palpation of much of the duct is impossible because of the ramus of the mandible.
3. The greater susceptibility of the parotid gland to secondary infection[26] frequently prolongs the period of enlargement, pain, and tenderness, in contrast to the short symptomatic attacks characteristic of obstruction of the submandibular duct.
4. Scar tissue, intraductal tumor, and external ductal compression rarely cause obstruction of the parotid duct.

Bilateral parotid enlargement

An asymptomatic bilateral enlargement of the parotid glands caused by a benign lymphoepithelial lesion with or without enlargement of the submandibular and lacrimal glands has been classically referred to as *Mikulicz' disease* (Fig. 31-11, *B*). When a variety of systemic diseases such as lymphoma and sarcoidosis are associated with these findings, the symptom complex is termed *Mikulicz' syndrome.* The association of symptoms, including xerostomia, combined with conjunctivitis and connective tissue disease such as

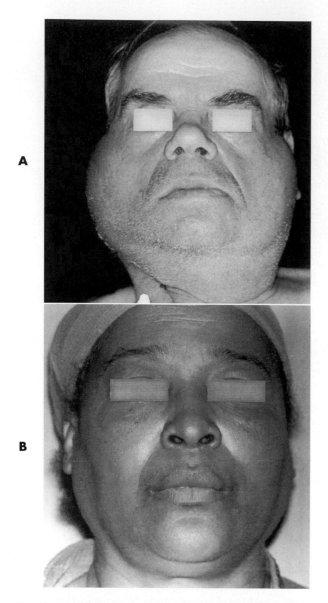

Fig. 31-11. Bilateral parotid swelling. **A,** Painful bilateral suppurative parotitis ("surgical mumps"). There was postoperative staphylococcal infection of the parenchyma of both glands. Pus could be expressed from Stensen's papillae. **B,** Mikulicz' disease. Note the bilateral parotid swelling, which was asymptomatic. (**A** courtesy O.H. Stuteville, deceased; **B** courtesy P. Akers, Chicago.)

rheumatoid arthritis is called *Sjögren's syndrome.* In all these disorders the parotid swelling may be bilateral or unilateral. Attempts have been made to interrelate this group of diseases, but the specific pathogenetic relationships remain unclear.

The identification of an asymptomatic parotid enlargement as one of these diseases depends on clinical and laboratory findings. The diagnosis of *Sjögren's syndrome* is strengthened by the demonstration of focal lymphocytic infiltrates in the labial minor salivary glands.

Bilateral parotid swelling has been noted in a variety of nutritional and metabolic disorders.[16] Enlargement be-

cause of alcohol is relatively common, whereas that caused by drugs (such as iodine and certain heavy metals) is infrequent but must be considered in the differential diagnosis of parotid swelling. Parotid enlargement is an early sign of bulimia in a significant number of cases[2] and has also been associated with chronic obstructive pulmonary disease.[3] Swelling of the major salivary glands may also occur after radiation (usually painful), and in Castleman's disease, nodular fasciitis, and polycystic disease of the parotid.

Masses in the Median-Paramedian Region

Pathoses of the thyroid gland and its developmental derivatives account for the majority of pathologic masses in the median-paramedian region.

Tender enlargement of the thyroid gland The thyroid gland may undergo inflammatory changes that produce an enlarged tender gland frequently accompanied by dysphagia and voice changes. Suppuration resulting from a bacterial infection is rare; if it occurs, treatment consists of antibiotics and surgical drainage.

A chronic nonsuppurative form of thyroiditis with persistent signs and symptoms of inflammation occurs. The cause of this type of thyroiditis appears to be an immunologic response to a viral infection. The thyroid glands of these patients usually show a decreased iodine uptake. Severity varies and, in milder cases, high doses of aspirin or acetaminophen have been successful. In severe cases, sustained high doses of fluocorticoids are necessary.[27]

Hashimoto's disease is a chronic disorder characterized by an enlarged, tender thyroid gland. The disease is thought to be caused by an autoimmune process in which the patient's thyroid gland is sensitive to its own thyroglobulin.[28,29] The diagnosis is made by laboratory means. When nodular glands are present in Hashimoto's disease, a complete biopsy may be necessary to rule out thyroid tumor. Treatment of the disease is controversial and ranges from the administration of thyroid hormone to surgical excision of the gland.

Nontender enlargement of the thyroid gland Simple goiter is the most common type of diffuse enlargement of the thyroid gland, having a variety of causes, such as familial enzyme defect and iodine deficiency. In some cases, multiple nodules accompany the goiter, and this condition presents a dilemma to the clinician, since the nodular architecture could be masking a tumor. Laboratory studies, including radioactive iodine uptake to evaluate thyroid function, are necessary in the diffusely enlarged or nodular glands. Treatment of the goiter may be medical or surgical, depending on the cause, symptoms, and nodularity.

Masses within the thyroid gland Benign and malignant tumors and cysts occur as masses within the thyroid gland.

If a mass is found within the thyroid gland (Fig. 31-12), it is excised with the lateral lobe of the gland. The excision is performed to determine whether the mass is malignant, and the involved lateral lobe is completely excised to prevent transection of a tumor during the removal of the mass.

An uncommon entity known as Riedel's thyroiditis develops as a fixed and hard mass, thus mimicking a malignant neoplasm. If the diagnosis of Riedel's thyroiditis is established, the treatment of choice is thyroid hormone, surgery being reserved for patients who require relief of tracheal and esophageal constriction.

When a thyroid mass is found, careful examination of the cervical lymph nodes is required to detect the infrequent occurrence of metastatic tumor. Furthermore, metastatic tumor from a primary lesion in the thyroid gland or the lower larynx may be present in an enlarged lymph node located on the cricothyroid membrane. Fineneedle aspiration biopsy has become a routine diagnostic procedure in the diagnosis of thyroid disease.

Thyroglossal cysts Cystic masses arising from remnants of the embryonic thyroglossal duct are found in the midline anywhere from the base of the tongue to the sternum (Fig. 31-13, *D*). The duct may persist in postnatal life as a draining tract or a cystic mass. A pathognomonic sign is the upward thrust of the mass when the patient protrudes the tongue, which demonstrates the connection of the thyroglossal duct and the tongue.

A thyroglossal cyst most commonly occurs below the hyoid bone and is usually readily visualized on clinical examination as a dome-shaped mass. These cysts may also be found submentally above the hyoid bone (see Fig. 31-13, *D*) and within the musculature of the tongue. On rare occasion, thyroid tumors develop in the walls of these cysts.[30] Treatment consists of total excision of the cyst and the entire tract to the base of the tongue.

Submental masses As stated in the preceding discussion, a thyroglossal cyst in a suprahyoid position is a submental mass.

Although it is uncommon, an epidermoid or dermoid cyst may occur in the submental area (Fig. 31-13, *E*), lying in the midline. Although it is fluctuant, its doughy consistency helps the clinician differentiate it from the more rubbery thyroglossal cyst. Excision of submental cystic masses of these two types with subsequent microscopic study establishes the diagnosis and is the recommended treatment.

Submental lymph nodes drain the regions of the lips and are subject to all the acute, chronic, inflammatory, and neoplastic changes described for nodes of the submandibular and parotid regions (Fig. 31-13, *A* and *C*). The differential diagnosis and management of submental lymph node pathoses are dictated by the same considerations as discussed for such conditions in the submandibular and parotid regions.

Masses in the Lateral Neck Region

Lymph nodes Most masses in the neck are enlarged lymph nodes extending along the linear path of the internal

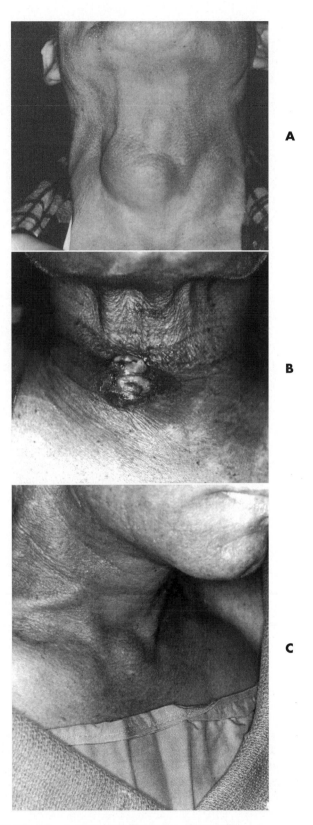

Fig. 31-12. Masses in the inferior aspect of the median-paramedian region. **A,** Benign adenoma of the thyroid gland. The mass was firm and smooth and arose from the right lobe of the gland. Swallowing caused the mass to be elevated. **B,** Anaplastic carcinoma of the thyroid gland. This mass was firm and fixed to the surrounding tissues. **C,** Sebaceous cyst. The cyst was just superficial to the isthmus of the thyroid gland.

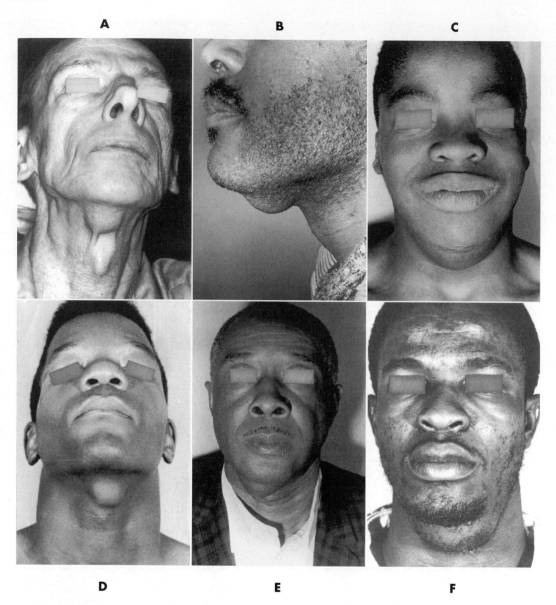

Fig. 31-13. Submental masses. **A,** Unusually large lymphoid hyperplasia. The mass was firm and freely movable. **B,** Sebaceous cyst. The mass was nontender, soft, fluctuant, and obviously attached to the skin. **C,** Diffuse submental acute lymphadenitis secondary to an infection of the lower lip. **D,** Thyroglossal cyst. This soft to rubbery, fluctuant mass was elevated as the patient protruded his tongue. **E,** Dermoid cyst. This mass was doughy, fluctuant, and freely movable. **F,** Plunging ranula. This unusual lesion was painless, soft, and fluctuant. (**A** courtesy S. Svalina, Palos Park, Ill; **B** courtesy P. Akers, Chicago.)

jugular vein from the angle of the mandible to the clavicle. The information concerning lymph nodes in other regions is especially pertinent to those in the lateral neck region, since the preponderance of cervical nodes occurs in this segment.

First-echelon nodes for the common cancer sites of the tongue, floor of the mouth, tonsil, and larynx are distributed along the jugular vein from the digastric to the omohyoid muscle (see Figs. 31-5 and 31-7). In cancer patients the alternate lymphatic chain of nodes residing along the course of the accessory nerve, posterior to the posterior border of the sternocleidomastoid muscle, must also be carefully examined for lymphadenopathy. Diagnostic and therapeutic measures for dealing with the masses presumed to be enlarged lymph nodes in the region follow the general principles detailed in the previous sections.

Masses displacing the upper region of the sternocleidomastoid muscle The normal structures lying deep to the upper section of the sternocleidomastoid muscle are lymph nodes that drain large submucosal plexuses, the carotid artery, the internal jugular vein, the vagus nerve, and the cervical sympathetic trunk.

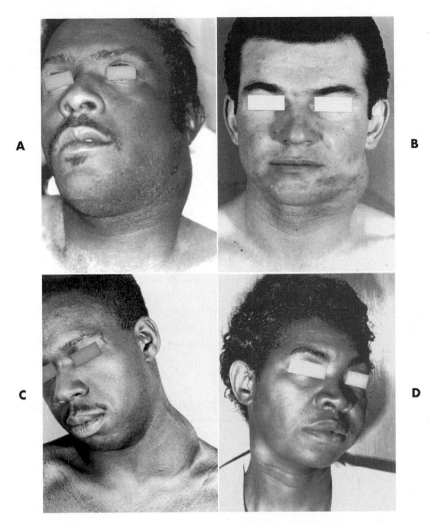

Fig. 31-14. Masses in the lateral neck. **A,** Metastatic squamous cell carcinoma in the subdigastric lymph nodes. This mass was stony hard and fixed. The primary tumor was located in the left side of the nasopharynx. **B,** Branchial cleft cyst. **C,** Cystic hygroma. **D,** Carotid body tumor. The mass was movable only in a lateral direction.

A bulging mass in this area may represent a metastatic carcinoma to the jugulodigastric and bifurcation nodes (Fig. 31-14, *A*), a branchial cyst of the second arch (Fig. 31-14, *B*), a carotid body tumor (Fig. 31-14, *D*), or a neurogenic tumor of the vagus nerve or of cervical sympathetic trunk origin.

Lymph node metastasis in this region is usually from a primary lesion at the base of the tongue or elsewhere in the oropharynx. As the mass enlarges, it displaces the superior aspect of the sternocleidomastoid muscle laterally. If necrosis occurs, the mass may become fluctuant and painful, causing the inexperienced clinician to misdiagnose it as a primary abscess; however, a clinical diagnosis of primary abscess should not be considered likely without a history of an antecedent oropharyngeal infection. To further ensure the detection of a possible malignancy in such a case, a biopsy should be performed at the time the mass is drained. If the primary tumor is discovered, the primary and secondary lesions are treated simultaneously.

Branchial cleft or lymphoepithelial cyst. Cystic masses in this area usually prove to be of branchial cleft origin. Branchial cleft cysts may occur at any level in the neck and frequently lie under the sternocleidomastoid muscle (see Fig. 31-14, *B*).

If a sinus is present, its opening usually occurs at the anterior border of the sternocleidomastoid muscle. If a cyst and sinus of the second branchial cleft are present, the tract leads to the tonsillar fossa. Complete excision of the cyst is the indicated treatment.

Frequently, microscopic lymph node follicles are seen in the walls of a branchial cyst. Secondarily infected cysts are often mistaken for abscesses,[31] and if these cysts are incised and drained, a cutaneous sinus usually persists.

Carotid body tumors and neurogenic tumors. Carotid body tumors and neurogenic tumors of cervical sympathetic origin commonly occur under the anterosuperior aspect of the sternocleidomastoid muscle as solid masses (see Fig. 31-14, *D*).

Because the masses are affixed to the nerves and vessels, they characteristically are mobile in a lateral direction but not in a vertical direction. Excision of these slow-growing and usually benign tumors is the required treatment, and the final diagnosis is made from the biopsy. For further details on these tumors, the reader is referred to the article by Batsakis.[19]

Miscellaneous masses of the lateral neck region

Panneck infection. When all or most of the potential spaces of the neck are abscessed, the patient is said to have a panneck infection (Fig. 31-15). In such a patient, two grave complications may develop: respiratory obstruction and spread of the infection to the mediastinum.

Much has been written about the grave complication of a dental or tonsillar infection reaching the mediastinum through the neck. Although fascial planes play a prominent role in the passage of pus from one potential space in the head and neck to another, it appears more likely that the transmission of infection from the upper neck to the mediastinum is through the areolar tissues in general. The virulence of the organism and the resistance of the patient are frequently more important considerations for the prognosis of the infection than the size or extent of the abscess.

This means that the patient with a panneck infection may be near death, even when the swelling is minimal (see Fig. 31-15, A). The gravity of the case is determined by the degree of systemic sepsis, which is reflected in the patient's vital signs. Radiographs of the neck and chest may provide clues as to the type of infection; for example, when a gas-forming organism such as *Bacteroides* is responsible for the infection, radiographs may reveal the presence of gas in the tissues.

The treatment for panneck infections is the wide surgical opening of all the planes at the base of the neck and drainage of the mediastinum when involved. Specific antibiotic therapy is unquestionably lifesaving in advanced infections.

Cystic hygroma. A cystic hygroma is a developmental benign cystic dilatation of lymphatic vessel aggregates that is seen at variable ages. The characteristically soft swelling may occur at any point in the neck from the base of the skull down to the mediastinum (see Fig. 31-14, *C*), and frequently, it enlarges at an alarming rate. The cystic mass may be solitary or multiple and may infiltrate into and around muscle and nerve, making excision extremely difficult and hazardous.

Few other entities occur in the child as soft, compressible masses of indistinct dimensions, so recognition of

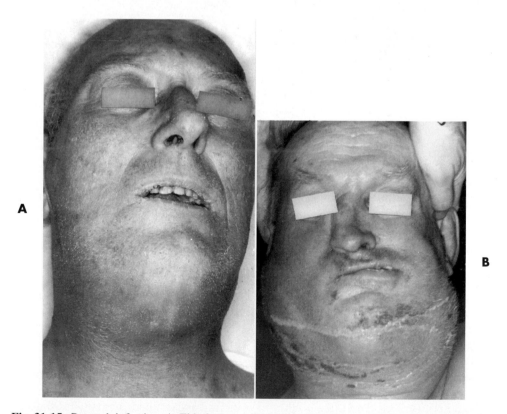

Fig. 31-15. Panneck infection. **A,** Elderly man with an infected left upper molar of 5 days' duration and only moderate upper neck swelling. The swelling subsequently became generalized. A chest radiograph showed gas in the mediastinum, and a culture of the region revealed *Bacteroides* organisms. The infection traveled from the upper neck into the mediastinum through the areolar connective tissues. **B,** Panneck infection of dental origin. The patient had severe diabetes. (Courtesy O.H. Stuteville, deceased.)

the cystic hygroma is seldom difficult. Also, fluid aspirated from the mass froths readily on agitation; this indicates a cystic hygroma because lymph fluid has a high fat content.

A cystic hygroma frequently occurs at an age when respiratory complications from the mass or from the surgical excision have a high mortality rate. Unfortunately, in the infant there is also danger of sudden enlargement, with obstruction of the airway. Thus management in the small child presents a dilemma: whether to remove the cystic hygroma to prevent a possible airway obstruction and risk death resulting from the surgery or to wait until the child is older and risk sudden enlargement in the interim with death by suffocation.

REFERENCES

1. Sa'do B, Yoshiura K, Yuasa K, et al: Multimodality imaging of cervicofacial actinomycosis, *Oral Surg* 76:772-782, 1993.
2. Vavrina J, Muller W, Gelbers JO: Enlargement of salivary glands in bulimia, *J Otolaryng Otol* 106:516-518, 1994.
3. Cook JN, Layton SA: Bilateral parotid swelling associated with chronic obstructive pulmonary disease: a case of pneumoparotid, *Oral Surg* 76:157-158, 1993.
4. Shuker S: Hydatid cyst in the maxillofacial region, *J Oral Maxillofac Surg* 52:1086-1089, 1994.
5. Inua M, Tagawa T, Mori A, et al: Inflammatory pseudotumor in the submandibular region: clinicopathologic study and review of the literature, *Oral Surg* 76:333-337, 1993.
6. Mizuno A, Yamaguchi K: The plunging ranula, *Int J Oral Maxillofac Surg* 22:113-115, 1993.
7. Langlois NE, Kolbe P: Plunging ranula: a case report and a literature review, *Human Path* 23:1306-1308, 1992.
8. Nathan H, Luchansky E: Sublingual gland herniation through the mylohyoid muscle, *Oral Surg* 59:21-23, 1985.
9. Tavill MA, Wetmore RF, Poje CP, Faro SH: Imaging case study of the month: plunging ranulas in children, *Ann Otol Rhinol Laryngol* 104:405-408, 1995.
10. Thompson K, Schwartz HC, Miles JW: Synovial chondromatosis of the temporomandibular joint presenting as a parotid mass: possibility of confusion with benign mixed tumor, *Oral Surg* 62:377-380, 1986.
11. Zheng JW, Zhang OH: Tuberculosis of the parotid gland: a report of 12 cases, *J Oral Maxillofac Surg* 53:849-851, 1995.
12. Lustman J, Segal N, Markitziv A: Salivary gland involvement in Wegener's granulomatosis: a case report and review of the literature, *Oral Surg* 77:254-259, 1994.
13. Oats CP, Wilson AW, Ward-Booth RP, Williams ED: Combined use of Doppler and conventional ultrasound for the diagnosis of vascular and other lesions in the head and neck, *Int J Oral Maxillofac Surg* 19:235-239, 1990.
14. Robbins SL: *Pathologic basis of disease,* ed 3, Philadelphia, 1984, WB Saunders.
15. Banks OH, Henson DE, Hulter RVP, Myers MH: *Manual for staging of cancer,* ed 3, Philadelphia, 1988, JB Lippincott.
16. Batsakis JG: *Tumors of the head and neck,* Baltimore, 1974, Williams & Wilkins.
17. Kissane JM: *Anderson's pathology,* vol 2, ed 10, St Louis, 1996, Mosby.
18. Hall MB, Arteaga DM: Use of computed tomography in the localization of head and neck space infections, *J Oral Maxillofac Surg* 43:978-980, 1985.
19. Batsakis JG: *Tumors of the head and neck,* ed 2, Baltimore, 1979, William & Wilkins.
20. Garnick MS, Hanna DC III: *Management of salivary gland lesions,* Baltimore, 1992, Williams & Wilkins.
21. Ellis GL, Auclair PL, Gnepp DR: *Surgical pathology of the salivary glands,* Philadelphia, 1991, WB Saunders.
22. Zollar LM, Mufson MA: Parotitis of non-mumps etiology, *Hosp Pract* 5:93-96, 1970.
23. Scully C: Viruses and salivary gland disease: are there associations? *Oral Surg* 66:179-183, 1988.
24. Hansson LG, Johansen CC, Biorklund A: CT sialography and conventional sialography in the evaluation of parotid gland neoplasms, *J Laryngol Otol* 102:163-168, 1988.
25. Carr RJ, Bowerman JE: A review of tumors of the deep lobe of the parotid salivary gland, *Br J Oral Maxillofac Surg* 24:155-168, 1986.
26. Fox PC: Bacterial infections of salivary glands, *Current Opin Dent* 1:414, 1991.
27. Rose LF, Kaye D: *Internal medicine for dentistry,* ed 2, St Louis, 1990, Mosby.
28. Morita S, Arima T, Matsuda M: Prevalence of nonthyroid specific antibodies in autoimmune thyroid disease, *J Clin Endocrin Metab* 80:1203-1206, 1995.
29. Davies TF, Amino N: A new classification for human autoimmune thyroid disease, *Thyroid* 3:331-333, 1993.
30. Van Der Wal JD, Wiener RHB, Allard SC, et al: Thyroglossal cysts in patients over 30 years of age, *Int J Oral Maxillofac Surg* 16:416-419, 1987.
31. Smyth AG, Ward-Booth RP: Lymphoepithelial cysts: a maxillofacial surgeon's perspective, *Br J Oral Maxillofacial Surg* 31:120-123, 1993.

CHAPTER 32

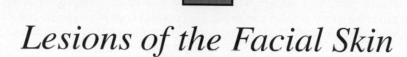

Lesions of the Facial Skin

JERALD L. JENSEN
RONALD J. BARR

The following cutaneous diseases are discussed:

PREMALIGNANT AND MALIGNANT
  EPIDERMAL LESIONS
  Actinic keratosis
  Squamous cell carcinoma
  Keratoacanthoma
  Basal cell carcinoma
BENIGN TUMORS OF EPIDERMAL
  APPENDAGES
  Trichoepithelioma
  Syringoma
  Dermal cylindroma
MISCELLANEOUS TUMORLIKE
  CONDITIONS
  Sebaceous hyperplasia
  Seborrheic keratosis
  Epidermoid cyst
TUMORS OF THE MELANOCYTIC
  SYSTEM
  Junctional nevus
  Intradermal nevus
  Compound nevus
  Blue nevus

Nevus of Ota
Malignant melanoma
VASCULAR TUMORS
  Juvenile hemangioma
  Nevus flammeus
  Pyogenic granuloma
  Nevus araneus
  Kaposi's sarcoma
  Angiosarcoma
MISCELLANEOUS TUMORS
CONNECTIVE TISSUE DISEASES
  Discoid lupus erythematosus
  Systemic lupus erythematosus
  Dermatomyositis
  Scleroderma
PAPULOSQUAMOUS DERMATITIDES
  Psoriasis
  Seborrheic dermatitis
CUTANEOUS REACTIONS TO ACTINIC
  RADIATION
  Photosensitivity dermatitis
  Phototoxic dermatitis

Photoallergic dermatitis
DRUG ERUPTIONS
  Dermatitis medicamentosa
  Dermatitis venenata
ACNE AND ACNEIFORM DERMATOSES
  Acne vulgaris
  Rosacea
  Rhinophyma
  Perioral dermatitis
DERMATOLOGIC INFECTIONS
  Bacterial infections
    Impetigo
    Sycosis barbae
    Erysipelas
  Viral infections
    Herpes zoster
    Viral warts
MISCELLANEOUS CONDITIONS
  Xanthelasma
  Amyloidosis

Every patient seeking consultation from a dentist should receive a thorough oral examination. As part of this examination, the dentist should look for and be able to recognize abnormalities of facial skin. The clinician should then be able to develop a reasonable differential diagnosis. If the lesion requires treatment, or if the diagnosis is in doubt, the patient should be referred to a dermatologist.

This chapter is not an encyclopedic work on diseases of facial skin. Rather, it includes diseases that the dentist is most likely to encounter in practice. A detailed discus-

sion of treatment is not presented because therapy should be provided by a physician trained in the management of diseases of the skin.

PREMALIGNANT AND MALIGNANT EPIDERMAL LESIONS
Actinic Keratosis

Actinic keratoses are precancerous lesions that typically arise on sun-exposed skin of light-complexioned individuals in response to solar irradiation.

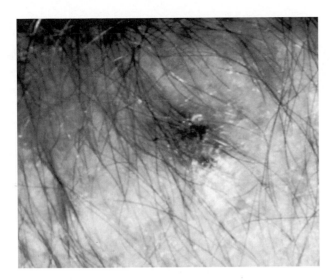

Fig. 32-1. Actinic keratosis. This lesion is a nonspecific, erythematous, slightly scaling or crusted, small plaque on the sun-damaged skin of the dorsal forearm. (Courtesy the Upjohn Co, Kalamazoo, Mich.)

Features The lesions are commonly multiple and most frequently involve the face, lower lip, back of the hands, forearms, neck, and bald scalp. Each lesion is round or irregular, scaly, and keratotic; varies from gray to deep brown; and measures 0.1 to 1 cm or more in diameter (Fig. 32-1). The keratotic scale is adherent and may be very thick, producing a cutaneous horn.[1]

The histopathologic appearance of actinic keratosis is characteristic. The epidermis reveals epithelial dysplasia with overlying parakeratosis that is responsible for the scale or horn seen clinically. The dermis exhibits solar elastosis, and frequently a chronic inflammatory infiltrate is present.

Untreated actinic keratoses slowly enlarge, and a small percentage of them (about 1 per 1000 per year) progress to squamous cell carcinoma (SCC).[2] Electrodessication, curettement, and cryotherapy with liquid nitrogen are effective forms of therapy. Studies suggest that the regular use of sunscreens prevent the development of actinic keratoses.[3]

Differential diagnosis Lesions that should be included in the differential diagnosis include seborrheic keratoses, arsenic keratoses, and SCCs. Seborrheic keratoses are greasy, elevated, brown or black lesions. Arsenic keratoses are seen mainly on the palms and soles, and SCCs have the features described previously.

Squamous Cell Carcinoma

Although SCC is less common than basal cell carcinoma (BCC), its incidence is increasing at an alarming rate.[4] Cumulative sun exposure is a major risk factor. Other risk factors include exposure to ionizing radiation, arsenic or industrial chemicals, viral infections, preexisting burns and scars, and immunosuppression.[4]

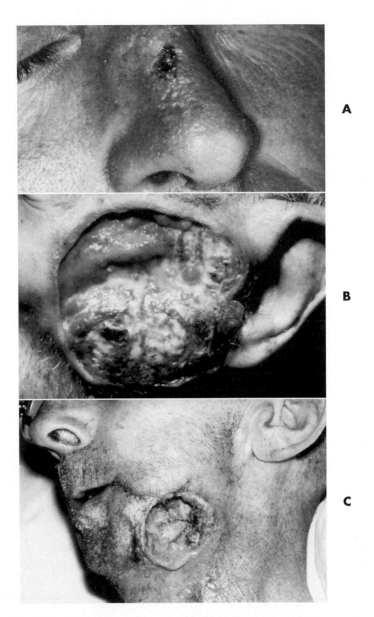

Fig. 32-2. SCC. These tumors of the skin of the face may clinically resemble BCC. **A,** Small lesion on the bridge of the nose in a male patient. **B,** Large, ulcerated, and necrotic lesion originating in the skin of the left cheek in an elderly man. **C,** Advanced lesion that originated in the buccal mucosa and has eroded through onto the face. (**A** Courtesy John Wright, Dallas; **B** Courtesy the Upjohn Co, Kalamazoo, Mich.)

Features SCC of the skin occurs most commonly on sun-exposed areas, especially the face; is more common in men; and increases with age. Tumors arising in actinic keratoses typically exhibit slow but progressive enlargement, ulceration, and increasing induration and have little or no tendency to metastasize.[5] When arising de novo (without evidence of a precursor lesion or insult), the tumor usually appears as a slowly enlarging, firm nodule and eventually develops an ulcer and central crust (Fig. 32-2 and Plate I). These neoplasms, in contrast to those arising in actinic keratoses, are biologically aggressive, with an estimated metastatic rate of around 8%.[5]

The treatment of choice for SCC depends on the location, size, and depth of penetration of the tumor. Curettement and electrodesiccation are effective for small lesions that are not deeply invasive. For large neoplasms, the most commonly used treatment modalities are primary resection, radiation therapy, and Mohs' micrographic surgery.[6]

Differential diagnosis The differential diagnosis includes BCC, keratoacanthoma, other skin tumors, and granulomas. A definitive diagnosis can be made on the basis of characteristic histologic features.

Keratoacanthoma

Keratoacanthoma is a benign, self-limited epithelial lesion that closely resembles SCC.[7] The lesion can be classified into a number of clinical types, including solitary, multiple, and eruptive.[8] Only the solitary type is considered here, since it is the most common.

Features Solitary keratoacanthomas occur primarily on exposed skin, especially on the central face, in patients over 45 years of age. The typical lesion begins as a firm, erythematous papule that rapidly enlarges over 2 to 8 weeks. The fully developed lesion typically reaches 1 to 2 cm in diameter and is firm, raised, dome shaped, and flesh colored or slightly pink. Its borders are rolled and firm. The center of the lesion exhibits a large keratotic plug that may drop out, leaving a dry crater (Fig. 32-3). After reaching its maximum size, the lesion remains static for approximately 2 to 8 weeks and then spontaneously regresses. During the period of regression, the mass gradually shrinks, the keratin plug is expelled, and the lesion heals, leaving a scar. The total duration of the lesion is usually 2 to 8 months.[9] Some of these lesions become large and aggressive, invading and destroying adjacent tissue.

Differential diagnosis The differential diagnosis includes SCC and BCC. Since distinguishing between keratoacanthoma and SCC is frequently difficult on clinical examination, and since the ultimate size and aggressiveness of keratoacanthoma cannot be predicted, early diagnosis is indicated. Surgical excision, intralesional injection of 5-fluorouracil, or radiation therapy may be indicated, depending on the size and location of the lesion.

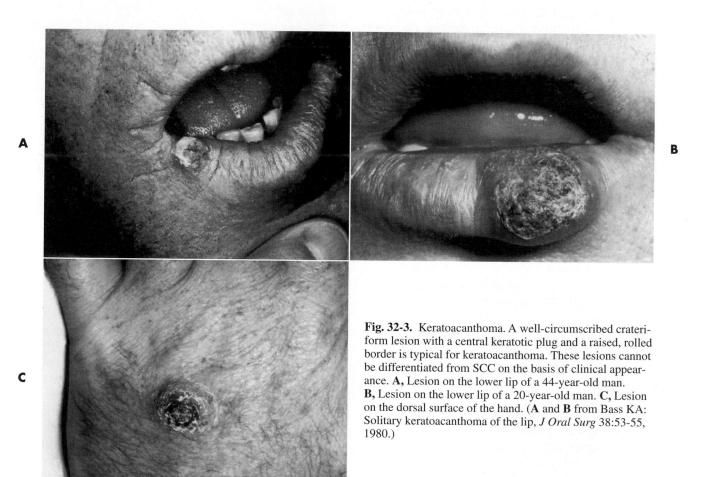

Fig. 32-3. Keratoacanthoma. A well-circumscribed crateriform lesion with a central keratotic plug and a raised, rolled border is typical for keratoacanthoma. These lesions cannot be differentiated from SCC on the basis of clinical appearance. **A,** Lesion on the lower lip of a 44-year-old man. **B,** Lesion on the lower lip of a 20-year-old man. **C,** Lesion on the dorsal surface of the hand. (**A** and **B** from Bass KA: Solitary keratoacanthoma of the lip, *J Oral Surg* 38:53-55, 1980.)

Basal Cell Carcinoma

BCC is a malignant epithelial tumor that usually arises from basal cells of the epidermis. It can be divided into the following types: nodular, superficial, morpheiform, fibroepithelial, and infundibulocystic. Nodular BCC is the most common type.[10] As with actinic keratoses and SCC, light-complexioned individuals have an increased risk of developing BCC, and as might be expected, the risk factors are similar for all three conditions.

BCC is more common in men and is uncommon before 40 years of age. Childhood onset occurs, however, in basal cell nevus syndrome (Fig. 32-4), in association with xeroderma pigmentosum, and rarely in otherwise normal children.[11]

Features Nodular BCCs are common on the face, and as a general rule, they occur above a line drawn from the tragus of the ear to the angle of the mouth. The early lesions are small, translucent papules that may be flesh colored, pale, or erythematous. They enlarge slowly and eventually exhibit a central depression and firm, elevated borders (Fig. 32-5 and Plate I). Occasionally, these tumors are heavily pigmented and may be mistaken for melanomas or other melanocytic lesions. If left untreated, BCCs eventually ulcerate and may result in extensive local tissue destruction. Although metastases may occur, they are uncommon.[12] However, when they do occur, approximately 67% originate from facial sites.[13]

Differential diagnosis The noduloulcerative BCC may be confused clinically with SCC, malignant melanoma, intradermal nevus, sebaceous gland hyperplasia, and adnexal carcinoma. Characteristic histologic features differentiate these lesions.

In general, the treatment for BCC is similar to that for SCC.

BENIGN TUMORS OF EPIDERMAL APPENDAGES

Trichoepithelioma

Trichoepitheliomas are benign neoplasms with follicular differentiation. They may be solitary and nonfamilial or familial and multiple.[10] The familial tumors begin to appear at puberty, mainly on the nasolabial folds, over the nose, and on the forehead, upper lip, and eyelids. The individual lesions are flesh-colored, firm papules that average 0.5 to 0.8 cm in diameter. The larger lesions may contain telangiectatic vessels on their surfaces and resemble BCCs.[10] Solitary, nonhereditary trichoepitheliomas usually occur in early adult life as nondescript, flesh-colored papules on the face[10] (Fig. 32-6).

Syringoma

Syringomas typically occur as multiple skin-colored or slightly yellowish, firm papules, 0.1 to 0.3 cm in diam-

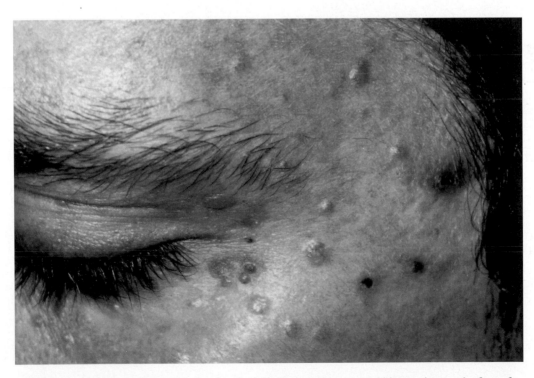

Fig. 32-4. Multiple small, nodular basal cell carcinomas and two crusted biopsy sites on the face of a young man with the basal cell nevus syndrome.

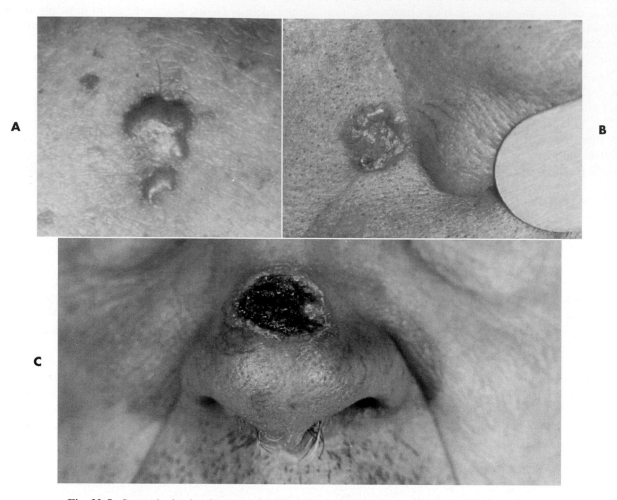

Fig. 32-5. Stages in the development of BCC. **A,** Typical early lesion characterized by bosselated, irregular nodule. **B,** Small, ulcerated lesion under the ala of the nose. **C,** Larger ulcerated lesion on the nose. In **B** and **C,** raised, rolled borders surround the ulcers. The borders are pearly in color and have fine telangiectasias. (**A** Courtesy the Upjohn Co, Kalamazoo, Mich.)

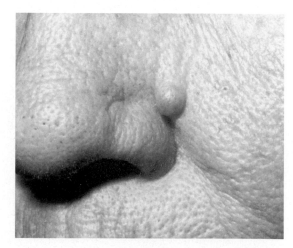

Fig. 32-6. Trichoepithelioma. This lesion presents as a flesh-colored, dome-shaped nodule immediately adjacent to the nose.

eter on the face (especially the eyelids), neck, and anterior chest (Fig. 32-7). These tumors usually appear during adolescence and occur primarily in women. Histochemical and electron microscopic observations suggest that syringoma is an adenoma of the eccrine ducts.[14,15]

As with multiple trichoepitheliomas, treatment is not indicated except for cosmetic reasons.

Cylindroma

Cylindromas are neoplasms thought to show apocrine differentiation by some authors and eccrine differentiation by others.[14] These tumors are more frequent in women and are solitary and nonhereditary in 90% of cases. In about 10%, the tumors are inherited in an autosomal dominant fashion with variable penetrance. The neoplasms are firm, smooth, dome shaped, pink, and movable, and they typically measure 0.3 cm to 3.0 cm. The lesions commonly occur on the face and scalp and may cover the scalp like a turban (Fig. 32-8), thus prompting the designation *turban tumor.* The tumors begin to appear in early adulthood and gradually increase in size and number throughout life. The association of multiple cylindromas, trichoepitheliomas, and spiradenomas is well known.[14] Also, the association of multiple cylindromas and membranous basal cell adenomas of the parotid gland has been reported.[16-18]

Individual cylindromas can be easily excised. However, removal of multiple lesions may require extensive skin grafting.

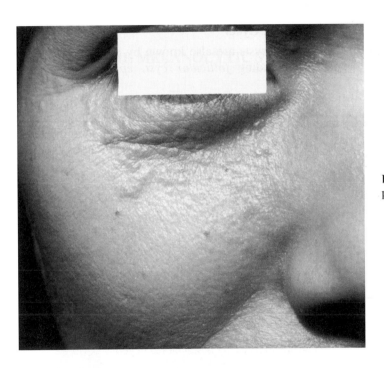

Fig. 32-7. Syringoma. Numerous small, flesh-colored papules are present on the upper and lower eyelid and cheek.

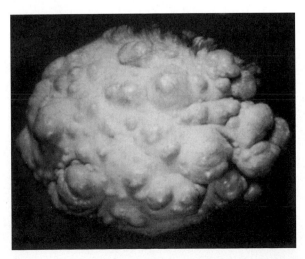

Fig. 32-8. Cylindroma. The multiple large, solitary, and confluent nodules replacing most of the scalp are responsible for this lesion being known as a *turban tumor.*

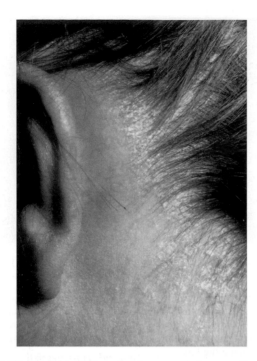

Fig. 32-25. Psoriasis. This patient has a well-circumscribed plaque with micaceous scales involving the scalp and nape of the neck.

dimpling of the nail plate is seen in at least 30% of cases.[41] The prevalence of arthritis is increased in patients with psoriasis.[42]

Differential diagnosis The differential diagnosis includes seborrheic dermatitis and atopic eczema.

Management The treatment of psoriasis consists of topical corticosteroids, tars, keratolytics, ultraviolet light, and in severe cases, methotrexate.

Seborrheic Dermatitis

Seborrheic dermatitis is a chronic inflammatory condition of the skin that cannot be cured; however, remissions of varying duration do occur.

Features Seborrheic dermatitis is frequently associated with an oily skin and has a predilection for the scalp, eyebrows, eyelids, nasolabial crease, lips, ears, sternal area, axillae, submammary folds, umbilicus, groin, and gluteal crease. The characteristic appearance is dry, moist, or greasy scales and pinkish-yellow patches of various sizes and shapes. The margins of the patches are indistinct. Mild involvement of the scalp is commonly known as *dandruff*. Chronic worry and loss of sleep frequently appear to aggravate this condition.

Seborrheic dermatitis is seen in association with certain other skin diseases (e.g., severe acne and psoriasis). It is also seen with certain general diseases such as Parkinson's disease and endocrine states with obesity[43] and AIDS.

Topical corticosteroids are effective in the treatment of seborrheic dermatitis.

CUTANEOUS REACTIONS TO ACTINIC RADIATION

Exposure to actinic radiation has a number of harmful effects in the skin. These include the sunburn reaction, photoaging, and carcinogenesis. Adverse cutaneous reactions may also occur after simultaneous exposure to chemicals and actinic radiation. These reactions are known as *phototoxic* and *photoallergic reactions.*

Phototoxic Reactions

A phototoxic reaction is a nonimmunologic reaction that develops within a few hours after the skin has been exposed to a photosensitizing agent and light of proper wavelength and intensity. This reaction usually occurs with the first exposure to the agent.[44]

Features The most common clinical finding is a sunburned appearance followed by hyperpigmentation. One well-known example of phototoxic dermatitis is berlock (berloque, perfume) dermatitis. In women, it is seen in areas where perfume is applied, such as the sides of the neck and behind the ears. In men, this type of dermatitis is most common on the bearded area where after-shave lotion is applied. Perfumes and after-shave lotions containing furocoumarin, bergamot oil, or related substances are chiefly responsible for this reaction.

Most systemic photosensitizers tend to produce phototoxic reactions. Frequent offenders are tetracyclines, sulfonamides, chlorothiazide, sulfonylureas, phenothiazines, griseofulvin, and halogenated salicylanilide.[1]

Photoallergic Dermatitis

The majority of cases of photoallergy develop after contact with photosensitizing chemicals. Such a reaction is known as a *photoallergic contact dermatitis.* These reactions occur only in sensitized persons and are out of proportion to the amount of exposure received. The most common etiologic chemicals are found in bar soaps and cosmetics.[45] The initial signs and symptoms are oozing, weeping, and crusting of the affected areas along with intense pruritus. The reaction begins 24 to 48 hours after combined chemical and light exposure.

Management Treatment of photoallergic dermatitis consists of the identification and elimination of the photosensitizing chemical or chemicals. In addition, broad-spectrum sunscreens and antimalarials may be of value.

DRUG ERUPTIONS (DERMATITIS MEDICAMENTOSA)

Drug eruptions are unintended reactions that occur after administration of diagnostic or therapeutic agents. Almost any drug administered systemically is capable of causing a dermatitis.

Features

Drug eruptions are often marked by a sudden onset, wide and symmetric dissemination, and pruritus. These eruptions may simulate a wide variety of cutaneous diseases.[46] The lesions may be maculopapular, erythematous, vesiculobullous, urticarial, and purpuric or pustular and may be accompanied by constitutional signs and symptoms. Fixed drug eruptions occur persistently at the same site each time the drug is given. They are often bullous and eczematous initially and later are hyperpigmented.

When trying to elicit a drug history from a patient, the clinician should remember that the patient may be unaware of exposure. For example, the offending agent may be used as a preservative or flavoring agent in food or may be an antibiotic present in milk or meat. Moreover, the patient may not mention the taking of vitamins or laxatives, either of which may be responsible for the eruption.

Contact Dermatitis

Contact dermatitis (dermatitis venenata) can be divided into two types: irritant contact dermatitis, which is caused by a nonallergic reaction, usually from exposure to an irritating substance, and allergic contact dermatitis, which is an acquired immunologic response to a substance that has come in contact with the skin.

Features Most allergic contact reactions and many irritant contact reactions are of the eczematous type; that is, the primary lesions exhibit any of the stages from erythema and swelling to oozing or vesiculation or both (Fig. 32-26). The secondary lesions exhibit crusting, excoriation, lichenification, and hyperpigmentation.

Certain substances commonly affect certain skin areas. Substances that commonly affect the face and neck are cosmetics, soaps, perfumes, hair sprays, fingernail polish (eyelids), hatbands (forehead), nickel (earlobes), and industrial oil. As expected, lesions of contact dermatitis begin in areas of contact, and the shape of the lesions reflects the localization of exposure.

Differential diagnosis The differential diagnosis includes seborrheic dermatitis, nummular eczematous dermatitis, lichen simplex chronicus, and other types of inflammatory lesions.

Management The therapy for drug eruptions consists of eliminating the offending agent and providing symptomatic and supportive measures.

ACNE AND ACNEIFORM DERMATOSES
Acne Vulgaris

Acne vulgaris is a chronic inflammatory disorder of pilosebaceous structures and is seen primarily in adolescents. The disorder is characterized by comedones, papules, pustules, nodules, and cysts, and it tends to occur in areas of the skin where sebaceous glands are well developed (Fig. 32-27), including the face, back, and upper arms.

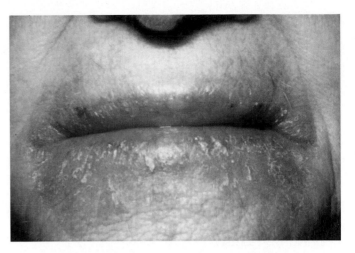

Fig. 32-26. Contact dermatitis. The extensive erythema, fissuring, and crusting involving both lips was caused by neomycin in a cream used for chapped lips. (Courtesy R.J. Herten, San Luis Obispo, Calif.)

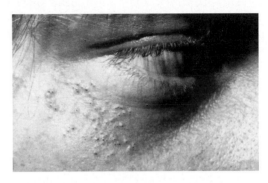

Fig. 32-27. Acne with comedones. The bulk of the lesions are small blackheads. There are a few inflammatory papules and pustules.

Acneiform eruptions may be produced by various drugs. The best-known examples are the corticosteroid hormones and the simple salts of iodine and bromine. Many oils, waxes, and chlorinated hydrocarbons produce acneiform eruptions when they come in contact with the skin. This type of acne is known as *occupational acne*.

Management The treatment of acne includes topical anticomedogenic agents and antibiotics, either topical or systemic.

Rosacea

Rosacea is a chronic acneiform disorder of the areas of the face capable of flush, especially the nose. The condition is seen most commonly in women between the ages of 20 and 60 years.

Features In the mildest form of the disease, there is slight erythema of the nose and cheeks. As the disease progresses, the lesions become red or purplish red with edema, papules, pustules, and telangiectasia.[47] Treatment consists of oral tetracycline; nonfluorinated, low-potency, topical steroids; and avoidance of factors that cause flushing. Fluorinated steroids may exacerbate the condition or even cause periorificial dermatitis.

Differential diagnosis The differential diagnosis includes lupus erythematosus, bromoderma, and iododerma.

Rhinophyma

Rhinophyma is a condition characterized by overgrowth of sebaceous glands and connective tissue of the distal half of the nose. This condition is seen almost exclusively in men over 40 years of age.[1]

Features The tip and wings of the nose are involved by large, lobulated, hyperemic masses that may become pendulous.

Perioral Dermatitis

Perioral dermatitis is a distinctive dermatitis confined symmetrically around the mouth with a clear zone between the vermilion border and the affected skin. It is seen primarily in young women and occasionally in men.[48,49]

Features The primary lesion is a pinhead-sized papule or papulovesicle, either flesh colored or red (Fig. 32-28). Eventually the papules are replaced by a more diffuse redness capped by a dry, fissured, yellowish-red scale. An uncomfortable burning sensation may be present.

The cause of perioral dermatitis is unknown, but sensitivity to sunlight, atopy, rosacea, demodicidosis, candidiasis, and the prolonged use of fluorinated corticosteroid creams and fluoride dentrifices have all been blamed.[50] In some patients, circumoral dermatitis and cheilitis have been caused by tartar-control toothpaste.[49]

Differential diagnosis The differential diagnosis includes acne vulgaris, seborrheic dermatitis, and contact dermatitis. The symmetric distribution around the mouth and the clear zone around the lips help differentiate perioral dermatitis from other entities.

Management The treatment consists of systemically administered tetracycline and elimination of the etiologic agent (e.g., fluorinated corticosteroids).

DERMATOLOGIC INFECTIONS

Bacterial Infections

Bacterial infections of the skin may be primary or secondary. Primary infections arise on normal skin, are initially caused by a single organism, and tend to have a characteristic appearance. Secondary infections occur on diseased skin. This discussion is limited to selected primary infections in which involvement of facial skin is a prominent feature.

Impetigo Impetigo is a highly communicable infection caused most commonly by group A streptococci. The disease occurs mostly in preschool children during the late summer and early fall. Poor hygiene, crowding, and minor trauma contribute to the spread of the infection. In the absence of complications the general health of affected individuals is excellent.

Features. The disease begins with small, reddish macules that soon develop into vesicles or bullae. The lesions are very superficial (subcorneal) in location and consequently have thin roofs that rupture easily, discharging a thin, straw-colored, seropurulent exudate. This exudate then dries to form a crust, which may become quite thick and has a "stuck-on" appearance. These golden-yellow crusts are the hallmark of impetigo (Fig. 32-29).

Individual lesions rarely exceed 1 to 2 cm in diameter. The face, especially around the mouth and nose, is the usual location; however, the lesions may occur anywhere.[51] If untreated, the disease may last for many weeks. Glomerulonephritis is an uncommon, but feared, complication of impetigo.

Differential diagnosis. The differential diagnosis includes contact dermatitis caused by poison ivy, tinea infections, and herpes simplex infections. The thick, yellow crusts with loose edges should differentiate impetigo from tinea and herpes simplex infections. Linear lesions are not characteristic of impetigo but are clearly seen in contact dermatitis resulting from poison ivy. Moreover, impetigo vesicles are more crusted and pustular.

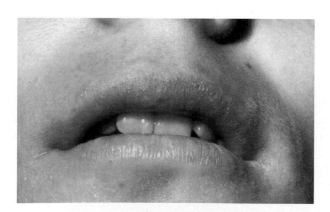

Fig. 32-28. Perioral dermatitis. Very subtle, slightly erythematous papules surround the mouth. There is a thin zone of uninvolved skin most noticeable along the lower lip.

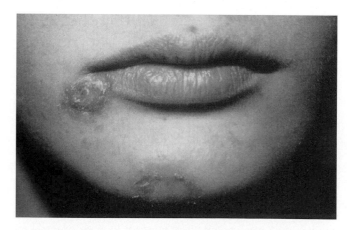

Fig. 32-29. Impetigo contagiosa. Both lesions are characterized by a honey-colored crust with some surrounding erythema.

Management. Treatment includes scrupulous cleansing of the area and antibiotic therapy.

Sycosis barbae Sycosis barbae, or barber's itch, is a deep, folliculitis of the beard.

Features. The primary lesion in sycosis barbae is a follicular pustule. Initially, there is erythema and a burning or an itchy sensation. Lesions commonly appear first on the upper lip near the nose. The pustules rupture after washing or shaving, leaving an erythematous area that is later the site of a new crop of pustules (Fig. 32-30). In this way the infection gradually spreads. The hairs of the involved follicles are usually not retarded in their growth and usually do not fall out; however, they may be readily epilated.[52]

Differential diagnosis. The differential diagnosis includes contact dermatitis, tinea of the beard, and ingrown hairs (pseudofolliculitis barbae). In contact dermatitis the involved areas are vesicular and crusted, and there are no follicular pustules. Tinea barbae is a slowly spreading, often annular, superficial fungal infection with broken hairs, and a deeper, nodular type of inflammation may be present. Moreover, tinea barbae rarely affects the upper lip. Pseudofolliculitis barbae manifests 1- to 3-mm papules at sites of ingrown hairs in black men. The anterior neckline and chin are the areas commonly affected. Bacterial and fungal culture studies should be performed and are helpful in the differential diagnosis. Most cases of sycosis barbae are caused by *Staphylococcus aureus.*

Management. Treatment consists of systemic and locally applied antibiotics. In addition, shaving should be light and infrequent, and a new razor blade should be used each day. Infected hairs should be manually epilated daily.

Erysipelas Erysipelas is an uncommon type of superficial cellulitis caused most commonly by group A streptococci.[53] A preexisting skin wound or pyoderma can frequently be found and is a predisposing condition. The upper respiratory tract is commonly the source of the organism.

Features. The basic lesion of erysipelas is a red, warm, raised, sharply circumscribed plaque that enlarges peripherally. Vesicles and bullae may form on the surface of the plaque. The process evolves rapidly, with constitutional signs and symptoms that include malaise, chills and fever, headache, vomiting, and joint pains. This disease most commonly involves the face, scalp, and area around the ear, but no area is exempt.[52] When the face is involved, the process may extend into the orbit and can be life threatening.

Untreated cases last for 2 to 3 weeks, but the response is rapid with antibiotic treatment. Recurrences are common and tend to be in the same location.

Differential diagnosis. Erysipelas may be confused with contact dermatitis and with angioneurotic edema, but fever is absent in these conditions. A butterfly pattern on the face may suggest lupus erythematosus, and ear involvement may suggest polychondritis; in addition, herpes zoster may mimic erysipelas.

Viral Infections

Herpes zoster Herpes zoster (shingles) and varicella (chickenpox) are caused by the same virus. Varicella is regarded as the primary manifestation of exposure to varicella-zoster virus. The virus is then thought to lie dormant in dorsal root ganglia to later recur as zoster.

Features. Herpes zoster is characterized by groups of vesicles or crusted lesions on an erythematous and edematous base situated unilaterally along the distribution of a spinal or cranial nerve (Fig. 32-31). The cranial nerves most frequently involved are the fifth and seventh. The lesions appear 1 to 7 days after onset of pain and hyperesthesia. New crops of vesicles can appear for 3 to 5 days and then dry and form crusts that take about 3 weeks to disappear. Severe lancinating pain is common but not invariable. Severe postherpetic neuralgia may occur, especially in older patients.

An increased incidence of herpes zoster in patients with lymphoma and leukemia has been recognized for

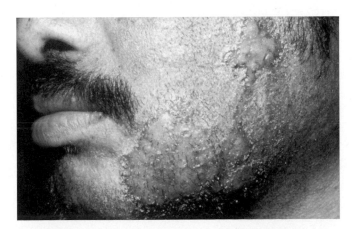

Fig. 32-30. Sycosis barbae. This patient has extensive weeping, crusted, purulent erythematous lesions involving the entire bearded area.

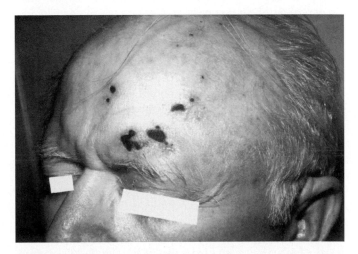

Fig. 32-31. Herpes zoster. Several hemorrhagic crusts with a few small, intact vesicles are present in the skin along the distribution of the ophthalmic branch of the trigeminal nerve. (Courtesy J.A. Klein, Long Beach, Calif.)

many years. However, Ragozzino, et al.[54] have shown that patients with herpes zoster are not at increased risk for the subsequent development of cancer. Their findings suggest that there is no need to search for an occult cancer or to increase surveillance for cancer after the diagnosis of herpes zoster is made.

Differential diagnosis. The unilateral distribution of painful, grouped vesicles in a dermatomal pattern is typical of herpes zoster. A simple and reliable way of confirming the diagnosis is to demonstrate giant cells with multiple nuclei and acidophilic intranuclear inclusions in stained (Giemsa or Wright's) cytologic smears of scrapings from the base of a vesicle.[55]

Intravenous and oral acyclovir in immunocompetent patients is associated with significant improvement in the rate of healing and the severity of the pain of herpes zoster.[56]

Viral warts Human papillomaviruses are small deoxyribonucleic acid viruses that cause a variety of proliferative lesions, including verruca vulgaris (common wart), verruca plana (flat wart), verruca plantaris (plantar wart), and condyloma acuminatum (venereal wart).

Features. At least 66 types of human papillomaviruses have been identified,[57] and certain types are associated with specific lesions. For example, common warts are associated with types 2 or 4, flat warts with type 3, plantar warts with type 2, and veneral warts with type 6. Predisposition to infections of human papillomavirus may reflect a select inherited immunodeficiency or an acquired immunodeficiency such as that accompanying immunosuppressive drug therapy.

Common warts are manifested as one or more irregularly shaped, vegetative, hyperkeratotic, tan to brown papillomas that can occur anywhere but have a predilection for the hands. A variant that occurs on the face is the filiform wart, which is characterized by longer, thinner projections, as the name implies. Flat warts are most common in children and frequently occur in large numbers on the face. They are flat, flesh-colored to tan, finely papillated papules, 0.2 to 0.5 cm in diameter (Fig. 32-32). Plantar warts are located on the soles, particularly the ball of the foot. They are usually endophytic and painful. Multiple plantar warts are referred to as *mosaic warts.* Venereal warts occur on the genitalia but have also been reported perianally, on the oral mucosa, and even on the laryngeal mucosa. They are elevated, keratotic, mulberry-like growths. All warts, particularly the common variety, may spread to traumatized skin. This is Koebner's phenomenon, which was discussed in the section on psoriasis. Although a rare event, malignant transformation can occur in some warts.[57,58]

Differential diagnosis. Usually the diagnosis is straightforward. Seborrheic keratosis or epithelial nevus may be confused with common warts. Biopsy is helpful because warts display cytopathic changes of human papillomavirus infection such as vacuolation, hypergranulosis, and even occasional intranuclear inclusions. Flat warts should be distinguished from multiple syringomas or trichoepitheliomas,

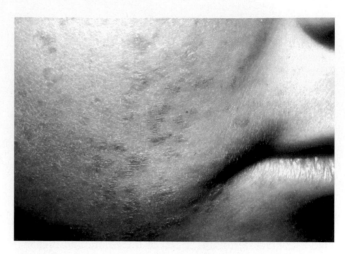

Fig. 32-32. Flat warts. Numerous individual and confluent, flesh-colored to slightly tan, flat-topped papules are typical.

venereal warts from condylomata lata (syphilitic warts), and plantar warts from calluses or clavi (corns). Paring down a plantar wart with a scalpel blade usually demonstrates punctate hemorrhage or punctate thrombi associated with multiple superficial capillaries. These are not present in calluses or clavi.

Management. The treatment of warts varies, and numerous remedies have been described. Common warts frequently respond to liquid nitrogen freezing or keratolytic agents, which usually contain salicylic acid and lactic acid. If possible, facial warts in children should not be treated; like most warts, they spontaneously resolve without scarring in 6 months to 2 years. If treatment is necessary, light liquid nitrogen freezing to a few lesions or the use of topical antiacne medication such as 2.5% to 5% benzoyl peroxide can be effective. Podophyllin is the treatment of choice for venereal warts, and plantar warts may be treated with salicylic acid plasters, liquid nitrogen freezing, or in selected cases, superficial x-ray therapy.

MISCELLANEOUS CONDITIONS
Xanthelasma

Xanthomas are tumors characterized by collections of lipid-laden macrophages. In many cases, these tumors occur in association with acquired or familial disorders, leading to hyperlipidemia. Xanthelasma is the most common type of xanthoma.

Features Xanthelasmas occur mainly on the upper eyelids but may also involve the lower eyelids (Fig. 32-33), especially the area of the inner canthus. The lesions are soft, chamois to light yellowish-gray, oblong plaques. They vary from 0.2 to 3.0 cm in length. The lesions are seen in adults and rarely in children and adolescents.

Individuals with xanthelasmas should have a workup for the presence of hyperlipidemia, since such an association is present in about 50% of cases.[59]

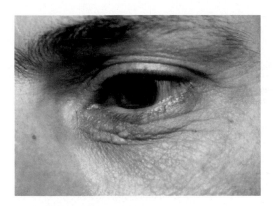

Fig. 32-33. Xanthelasma. Yellow plaques are present on the lower eyelids.

Management Treatment of individual lesions is probably best accomplished by surgical excision.

Amyloidosis

Primary amyloidosis is associated with cutaneous lesions in about 30% of cases.[60]

Features Amyloid infiltrates of the skin in primary amyloidosis are characteristically asymptomatic, translucent, waxy, amber papules that have the appearance of translucent vesicles. These papules coalesce to form plaques of various sizes. Amyloid deposition in blood vessels results in purpuric lesions and ecchymoses. The hemorrhagic lesions, as well as the papules and plaques, involve the periorbital areas (Fig. 32-34), the sides of the nose, and the regions around the mouth. In addition, these patients may have oral lesions.[61]

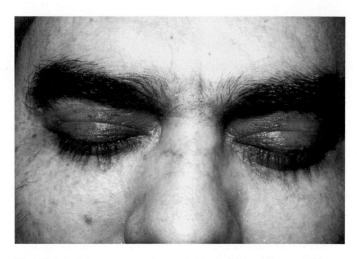

Fig. 32-34. Primary systemic amyloidosis. This patient exhibits the typical periorbital hemorrhage secondary to rupture of the blood vessels infiltrated by amyloid. A few small, infiltrative papules can be seen along the free margin of the upper eyelids.

Localized amyloidosis may occur in the skin. Amyloid also is occasionally deposited in the stroma of certain epithelial tumors. Cutaneous amyloid deposits are not seen in secondary amyloidosis.

The diagnosis of amyloidosis is established by demonstration of the characteristic emerald-green birefringence of tissue specimens stained with Congo red and examined by polarizing microscopy.

There is no specific therapy for primary amyloidosis.

REFERENCES

1. Domonkos AN, Arnold HL Jr, Odom RB: *Andrews' diseases of the skin: clinical dermatology,* Philadelphia, 1982, WB Saunders.
2. Sober AJ, Burstein JM: Precursors to skin cancer, *Cancer* 75:645-650, 1995.
3. Thompson SC, Jolley D, Marks R: Reduction of solar keratoses by regular sunscreen use, *N Engl J Med* 329:1147-1151, 1993.
4. Hacker SM, Flowers FP: Squamous cell carcinoma of the skin: will heightened awareness of risk factors slow its increase? *Postgrad Med* 93:115-121, 125-126, 1993.
5. Graham JH, Helwig EB: Premalignant cutaneous and mucocutaneous diseases. In Graham JH, Johnson WC, Helwig EB, editors: *Dermal pathology,* New York, 1972, Harper & Row.
6. Fleming ID, et al: Principles of management of basal and squamous cell carcinoma of the skin, *Cancer* 75:699-704, 1995.
7. Schwartz RA: Keratoacanthoma, *J Am Acad Dermatol* 30:1-19, 20-22, 1994.
8. Baer RL, Kopf A: Keratoacanthoma. In *Yearbook of dermatology,* Chicago, 1962-1963, Mosby.
9. Caro WA, Bronstein BR: Tumors of the skin. In Moschella SL, Hurley HJ Jr, editors: *Dermatology,* vol 2, Philadelphia, 1985, WB Saunders.
10. Ackerman AB, DeViragh PA, Chongchitnant N: *Neoplasms with follicular differentiation,* Baltimore, 1993, Lea & Febiger.
11. Milstone EB, Helwig EB: Basal cell carcinoma in children, *Arch Dermatol* 108:523-527, 1973.
12. Mikhail GR, et al: Metastatic basal cell carcinoma, *Arch Dermatol* 113:1261-1269, 1977.
13. Snow SN, et al: Metastatic basal cell carcinoma: report of five cases, *Cancer* 73:328-335, 1994.
14. Abenoza P, Ackerman AB: *Neoplasms with eccrine differentiation,* Baltimore, 1990, Lea & Febiger.
15. Hashimoto K, Gross BG, Lever WF: Syringoma: histochemical and electron microscopic studies, *J Invest Dermatol* 46:150-166, 1966.
16. Batsakis JG, Brannon RB: Dermal analogue tumors of major salivary glands, *J Laryngol Otol* 95:155-164, 1981.
17. Headington JT, et al: Membranous basal cell adenoma of parotid gland, dermal cylindromas and trichoepitheliomas, *Cancer* 39:2460-2469, 1977.
18. Reingold IM, Keasbey LE, Graham JH: Multicentric dermal-type cylindromas of the parotids in a patient with florid turban tumors, *Cancer* 40:1702-1710, 1977.
19. Steffen C, Ackerman AB: *Neoplasms of the skin with sebaceous differentiation,* Baltimore, 1994, Lea & Febiger.
20. Lindelof B, Sigurgeirsson B, Melander S: Seborrheic keratoses and cancer, *J Am Acad Dermatol* 26:947-950, 1992.
21. Gardner EJ: Follow-up of a family group exhibiting dominant inheritance for a syndrome including intestinal polyposis, osteomas, fibromas, and epidermal cysts. *Am J Hum Genet* 14:376-390, 1962.
22. Shaffer B: Pigmented nevi, *Arch Dermatol* 72:120-132, 1955.
23. Dubow BE, Ackerman AB: Melanoma in situ: the evolution of a concept, *Mod Pathol* 13:734-744, 1990.

24. Breslow A: Thickness, cross-sectional areas and depth of invasion in the prognosis of cutaneous melanoma, *Ann Surg* 172:902-908, 1970.

25. Sober AJ, Fitzpatrick TB, Mihm M: Primary melanoma of the skin: recognition and management, *J Am Acad Dermatol* 2:179-197, 1980.

26. Bowers RE, Graham EA, Tomlinson KA: The natural history of the strawberry nevus, *Arch Dermatol* 82:667-680, 1960.

27. Bluefarb SM: Sturge-Weber syndrome, *Arch Dermatol Syph* 59:531-541, 1949.

28. Mills SE, Cooper PH, Fechner RE: Lobular capillary hemangioma: the underlying lesion of pyogenic granuloma: a study of 73 cases from the oral and nasal mucous membranes, *Am J Surg Pathol* 4:471-479, 1980.

29. Taira JW, Hill TL, Everett MA: Lobular capillary hemangioma (pyogenic granuloma) with satellitosis, *J Am Acad Dermatol* 27:297-300, 1992.

30. Krigel RL, Friedman-Kien AE: Kaposi's sarcoma in AIDS: diagnosis and treatment. In DeVita VT, Hellmann S, Rosenberg SA, editors: *AIDS: etiology, diagnosis and treatment,* Philadelphia, 1988, JB Lippincott.

31. Axiotis CA, et al: AIDS-related angiomatosis, *Am J Dermatopathol* 11:177-181, 1989.

32. Northfelt DW: Treatment of Kaposi's sarcoma: current guidelines and future perspectives, *Drugs* 48:569-582, 1994.

33. Rosai J, et al: Angiosarcoma of the skin: a clinicopathologic and fine structural study, *Hum Pathol* 7:83-109, 1976.

34. Mark RJ, et al: Angiosarcoma of the head and neck: the UCLA experience, 1955 through 1990, *Arch Otolaryngol Head Neck Surg* 119:973-978, 1993.

35. Gilliam JN, Cohen SB, Sontheimer RD, Moschella SL: Connective tissue diseases. In Moschella SL, Hurley HJ Jr, editors: *Dermatology,* vol 2, Philadelphia, 1985, WB Saunders.

36. Lever WF, Schaumburg-Lever G: *Histopathology of the skin,* Philadelphia, 1983, JB Lippincott.

37. Estes D, Christian CL: The natural history of systemic lupus erythematosus by prospective analysis, *Medicine* 50:85-95, 1971.

38. Tan EM, et al: The 1982 revised criteria of systemic lupus erythematosus, *Arthritis Rheum* 25:1271-1277, 1982.

39. Callen JP: The value of malignancy evaluation in patients with dermatomyositis, *J Am Acad Dermatol* 6:253-259, 1982.

40. Weinstein GD, Van Scott EJ: Autoradiographic analysis of turnover times of normal and psoriatic epidermis, *J Invest Dermatol* 45:257-262, 1965.

41. Ramsay DL, Hurley HJ Jr: Papulosquamous eruptions and exfoliative dermatitis. In Moschella SL, Hurley HJ Jr, editors: *Dermatology,* vol 1, Philadelphia, 1985, WB Saunders.

42. Leczinsky CD: The incidence of arthropathy in a ten year series of psoriasis cases, *Acta Dermatol Venereol* 82:483-487, 1948.

43. Soloman LM: Eczema. In Moschella SL, Hurley HJ Jr, editors: *Dermatology,* vol 1, Philadelphia, 1985, WB Saunders.

44. Epstein JH: Phototoxicity and photoallergy in man, *J Am Acad Dermatol* 8:141-147, 1983.

45. Willis I: Photosensitivity. In Moschella SL, Pillsbury DM, Hurley HJ Jr, editors: *Dermatology,* vol 1, Philadelphia, 1974, WB Saunders.

46. VanArsdel PP Jr: Allergy and adverse drug reactions, *J Am Acad Dermatol* 6:833-845, 1982.

47. Tolman EL: Acne and acneiform dermatoses. In Moschella SL, Pillsbury DM, Hurley IIJ Jr, editors: *Dermatology,* vol 2, Philadelphia, 1985, WB Saunders.

48. Epstein S: Perioral dermatitis, *Cutis* 10:317-321, 1972.

49. Beacham BE, Kurgnasky D, Gould WM: Circumoral dermatitis caused by tartar control dentifrices, *J Am Acad Dermatol* 22:1029-1032, 1990.

50. Wells K, Brodell RT: Topical corticosteroid "addiction:" a cause of perioral dermatitis, *Postgrad Med* 93:225-230, 1993.

51. Dillon HC Jr: Impetigo contagiosa, *Am J Dis Child* 115:530-541, 1968.

52. Maibach HI, Aly R, Noble W: Bacterial infections of the skin. In Moschella SL, Hurley HJ Jr, editors: *Dermatology,* vol 1, Philadelphia, 1985, WB Saunders.

53. Schwartz MN, Weinberg AN: Infections due to gram-positive bacteria. In Fitzpatrick TB, et al, editors: *Dermatology in general medicine,* vol 2, New York, 1987, McGraw-Hill.

54. Ragozzino MW, et al: Risk of cancer after herpes zoster: a population based study, *N Engl J Med* 307:393-397, 1982.

55. Barr RJ, Herten RJ, Graham JH: Rapid method for Tzanck preparations, *JAMA* 237:1119-1120, 1977.

56. Wood MJ: A randomized trial of acyclovir for 7 days or 21 days with and without prednisolone for treatment of acute herpes zoster, *N Engl J Med* 330:896-900, 1994.

57. Laimins LA: The biology of human papillomaviruses: from warts to cancer, *Infect Agents Dis* 2:74-86, 1993.

58. Cirelli R, Tyring SK: Interferons in human papillomavirus infections, *Antiviral Res* 24:191-208, 1994.

59. Bergman R. The pathogenesis and clinical significance of xanthelasma palpebrarum, *J Am Acad Dermatol* 30:236-242, 1994.

60. Rubinow A, Cohen AS: Skin involvement in generalized amyloidosis, *Ann Intern Med* 88:781-785, 1978.

61. Schwartz HC, Olson DJ: Amyloidosis: a rational approach to diagnosis by intraoral biopsy, *Oral Surg* 39:837-843, 1975.

CHAPTER 33

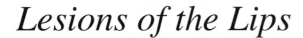

Lesions of the Lips

BRUCE F. BARKER

COLORED LESIONS
WHITE LESIONS
  Candidiasis
  Squamous cell papilloma
  Verruca vulgaris
  Condyloma
  Lichen planus
  Lichenoid drug eruption
  Actinic keratosis
  Squamous cell carcinoma
  Snuff dipper's lesion
  Cigarette smoker's lip
  Focal epithelial hyperplasia
RED LESIONS
  Hemangioma
  Sturge-Weber syndrome
  Thrombocytopenic purpura
  Rendu-Osler-Weber disease (hereditary
    hemorrhagic telangiectasia)
  Kaposi's sarcoma
  Contact allergy

BROWN LESIONS
  Nevus
  Labial melanotic macule
  Melanoma
  von Recklinghausen's disease
  Albright's syndrome
  Peutz-Jeghers syndrome
  Addison's disease
  Hemochromatosis
  Kaposi's sarcoma
YELLOW LESIONS
  Lipoma
  Fordyce's disease
ULCERATIVE LESIONS
TRAUMATIC ULCER
APHTHA
HERPES SIMPLEX VIRUS
ERYTHEMA MULTIFORME
KERATOACANTHOMA
SYPHILIS
ELEVATED LESIONS

FIBROMA (FIBROUS HYPERPLASIA)
MUCOCELE
ANGIOEDEMA
LIPOMA
SALIVARY GLAND TUMOR
MINOR SALIVARY GLAND CALCULUS
HEMANGIOMA
NASOLABIAL CYST
CONTACT ALLERGY
CHEILITIS GLANDULARIS
CHEILITIS GRANULOMATOSA
MELKERSSON-ROSENTHAL SYNDROME
SQUAMOUS CELL PAPILLOMA
DEVELOPMENTAL ABNORMALITIES
CLEFT LIP
DOUBLE LIP
LOWER LIP SINUS
COMMISSURAL PIT

A careful examination of the lips is often neglected by members of the medical and dental professions; yet the lips reveal a heterogeneous group of lesions ranging from congenital abnormalities to benign and malignant neoplasms. The lower lip, for instance, is a common site for squamous cell carcinoma; the early signs of the dysplastic changes are often present for years before the development of cancer. In addition, easily observed lip lesions may help the clinician recognize more obscure lesions of the skin and mucosa, as well as systemic diseases. It therefore behooves the clinician to perform a thorough examination of the lips.

This chapter describes the common lesions of lips and explores some uncommon conditions that may have manifestations on the lips.

The lesions are arranged in four categories: colored lesions, ulcerative lesions, elevated lesions, and develop-mental abnormalities. This chapter covers only a small number of the multitude of conditions that may appear on the lips, since almost any skin or mucous membrane disease and almost any soft tissue neoplasm may occur here.

COLORED LESIONS

WHITE LESIONS
Candidiasis

A classification of *Candidia* organisms can be found in Chapter 5. Angular cheilitis, also called perlèche, occurs only at the commissures as a white, red, or more often a red and white fissured lesion (Figs. 33-1 and 33-2). It is most often seen bilaterally, and the major predisposing factor is a

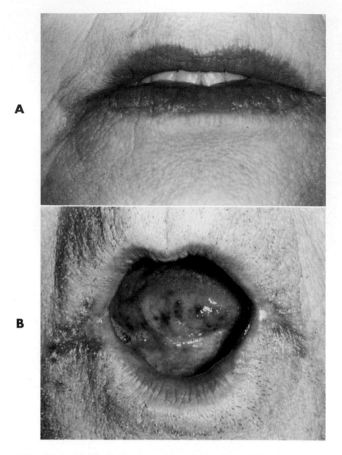

Fig. 33-1. Candidiasis as angular cheilosis. **A,** Lips in a more or less closed position in an elderly woman who has a loss in vertical dimension. **B,** Lips in an open position in an elderly man.

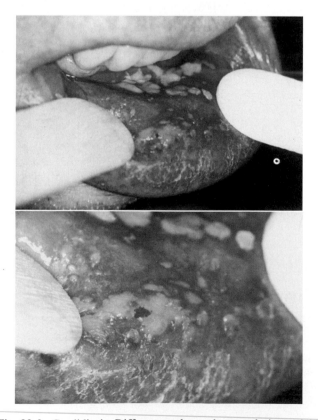

Fig. 33-2. Candidiasis. Diffuse pseudomembranous lesions of the lip and labial mucosa.

decreased vertical dimension usually caused by the nonuse of dentures or by chronic bone resorption under complete dentures. Vitamin B deficiencies, often blamed for this lesion, are a rare cause. Patients who drool or have lip-licking habits are at increased risk, as are those undergoing radiation therapy or chemotherapy. Other forms of candidiasis can also affect the labial mucosal surfaces (see Fig. 33-2).

A diffuse form of chronic candidiasis characterized by pain, swelling, erythema with focal ulcerations, and crusting is called cheilocandidiasis. It represents a secondary candidal infection superimposed on areas of trauma from mechanical or solar factors.[1]

Candida infections of the lip are successfully treated by appropriate antifungal medications such as nystatin, ketoconazole, fluconozole, or imidazole derivatives, unless the patient has underlying medical problems predisposing to fungal infections. Microbiologic studies of angular cheilitis also reveal the presence of *Staphylococcus aureus* in 60% of cases. Antibiotics may be necessary in these patients.[2-4] A detailed discussion of treatment of candidiasis is found in Chapter 5.

Squamous Cell Papilloma

The papilloma, a common, benign growth, may occur on the lips but is more frequently encountered within the oral cavity. The lesion is classically an exophytic papillary mass, either white or a normal mucosal color (Fig. 33-3). Papillomas occur as single lesions or more uncommonly as multiple lesions. They may be sessile or pedunculated and may occur at any age but are most common in adults. They are not premalignant but do not spontaneously regress. Surgical excision is the treatment of choice. Studies have identified human papillomavirus (HPV) in more than 50% of oral papillomas.[5] Viral subtypes HPV-6 and HPV-11 are

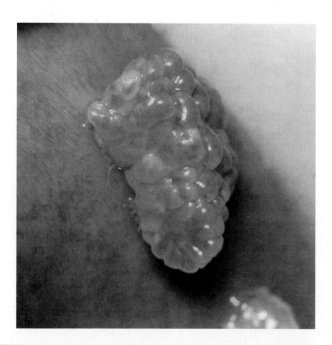

Fig. 33-3. Papilloma on the mucosal surface of the upper lip in a child who had multiple papillomas.

usually identified by in situ hybridization, polymerase chain reaction, or immunohistochemistry. Whether all squamous cell papillomas are of viral origin is unknown. ***Differential diagnosis*** On clinical examination the papilloma is almost identical to verruca vulgaris, condyloma acuminatum, condyloma latum, and even an early verrucous or papillary squamous cell carcinoma. Microscopic evaluation should be performed on all papillomas removed.

Verruca Vulgaris

Verruca vulgaris is the common wart of the skin; however, it may also occur in the oral cavity, often the result of self-inoculation. Its cause is HPV-2, HPV-4, or HPV-40.[5-7] Identification of HPV is necessary for a definitive diagnosis. Verruca vulgaris should be suspected when multiple papillary, wartlike lesions are found on the oral mucosa of children, especially those with verrucae on their hands. Surgery is the treatment of choice; however, some may spontaneously regress.

Condyloma

Condylomas are divided into two types: condyloma acuminatum (Fig. 33-4) of viral origin (HPV-6, HPV-11, HPV-16 and HPV-18) and condyloma latum, which is a lesion of secondary syphilis.[8,9] Both may be sexually transmitted and may occur on the lips. Diagnosis is determined by an accurate history and microscopic evaluation.

Carcinoma

Verrucous or exophytic squamous cell carcinoma may appear identical to papillomas. Most papillomas do not exceed 1 cm, whereas carcinomas have unlimited growth potential. Again, a biopsy is the only sure way to establish an accurate diagnosis.

Other Considerations

Multiple papillomatous lesions should be differentiated from those in Cowden syndrome (multiple hamartoma and neoplasia syndrome), Goltz-Gorlin syndrome (focal dermal hypoplasia), or focal epithelial hyperplasia (Heck's disease).

Lichen Planus

Lichen planus, previously discussed in Chapters 6 and 8, may also involve the labial mucosa. The lip lesions usually exhibit the typically white striations (erroneously referred to as *striae of Wickham*), which are usually asymptomatic (Fig. 33-5). The lesions may become erosive, red, and painful. If suspect lesions are noted on the lips, the patient should be examined for intraoral lesions or skin

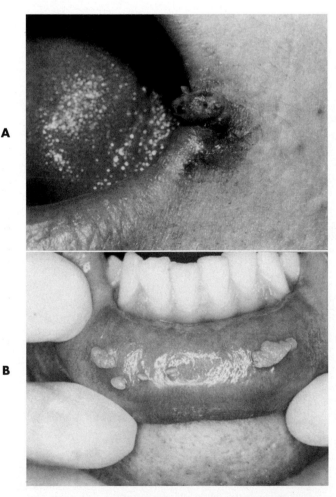

Fig. 33-4. Condyloma acuminatum. **A,** Exophytic lesion at the commissure. **B,** Multiple lesions on the mucosal surface of the lower lip. (**A** courtesy Robert Hiatt, Kansas City, Mo; **B** courtesy Steven Smith, Chicago.)

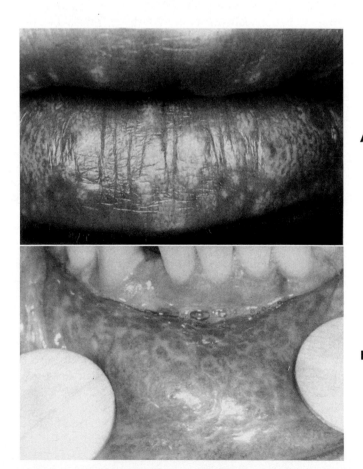

Fig. 33-5. Lichen planus. White reticular type of lesions on the vermilion border in **A** and on the mucosal surface of the lower lip in **B**. (**A** courtesy Matt Hourigan, deceased.)

lesions, especially on the arms or legs, which help confirm the diagnosis.

Differential diagnosis The conditions that must be differentiated from lichen planus are lichenoid drug eruption, lupus erythematosus, graft-versus-host disease, and actinic keratosis. Lupus may appear identical to lichen planus, complete with striae (Fig. 33-6); however, it more commonly occurs as a red area. Biopsy with immunofluorescence studies is usually diagnostic.

Lichenoid drug eruptions may also appear clinically and are histologically identical to lichen planus (see Fig. 33-6). Many drugs and chemicals may cause these reactions, but the most common appears to be nonsteroidal antiinflammatories, thiazide diuretics, methyldopa, phenothiazines, and gold salts.[10] If the offending medications or chemicals can be identified and removed, the lesions may disappear in 3 to 4 weeks. Months may be required in other cases. Lichenoid reactions to many dental materials have been reported the most commonly implicated being mercury in dental amalgams. Lesions may disappear after removal of the restorations.[11-12]

Actinic keratosis can be differentiated by the lack of other skin or mucosal lesions; also, striae should not be present. Biopsy, however, is the sure way to a correct diagnosis.

The clinical lesions of graft-versus-host disease may be identical to lichen planus. A history of an allogenic bone marrow transplant should differentiate the two conditions.[13]

Actinic Keratosis

Actinic keratosis (solar keratosis) is a premalignant lesion of the skin, including the vermilion border of the lower lip. Excessive exposure to ultraviolet radiation is responsible for the dysplastic epithelial changes.[14] Collagen and elastic fibers of the underlying connective tissue are also broken down by the same process, leading to a smudged microscopic appearance, often referred to as *basophilic degeneration.* Usually, long-term exposure to sunlight is necessary to induce dysplastic changes; however, as with other skin cancers, fair-complexioned persons are at greater risk. These changes are most often encountered in adults whose occupations require extensive outside work, such as farmers, sailors, painters, and construction workers. "Sun worshippers," as would be expected, are not immune.

The typical early lesions are filmy white, but with continued exposure the tissues may become slightly elevated, crusted, or red and ulcerated (Fig. 33-7). Lesions may be localized or involve the entire lip. Sunscreen lip balm or shading of the lips by protective hats may prevent progression to squamous cell carcinoma.

Differential diagnosis No reliable method is available to distinguish actinic changes from severe dysplasia or carcinoma. Therefore periodic biopsies may be necessary. If severe dysplasia or early carcinoma is detected, it is most

often treated by local excision or, if more diffuse, by a vermilionectomy.

Advanced carcinoma must be treated with more extensive surgery or radiation therapy. Actinic changes must also be differentiated from lichen planus, lichenoid drug reaction, lupus erythematosus, and chronic lip biting.

Squamous Cell Carcinoma (Epidermoid Carcinoma)

The vermilion border of the lower lip is a common location of squamous cell carcinoma, which typically develops in preexisting actinic cheilitis.[15-17]

The clinical appearance varies considerably, depending on the stage.[18] Early lesions may be subtle and identical to actinic keratosis; however, crusting, flaking, and ulceration remain as more serious prognostic factors (Plate I). An advanced lesion is usually an indurated mass with a cratered, crusted, central area (Fig. 33-8). The incidence of squamous cell carcinoma of the lower lip is highest in men with histories of chronic exposure to excessive ultraviolet radiation. Earlier studies supported a strong association with pipe smoking; however, this has

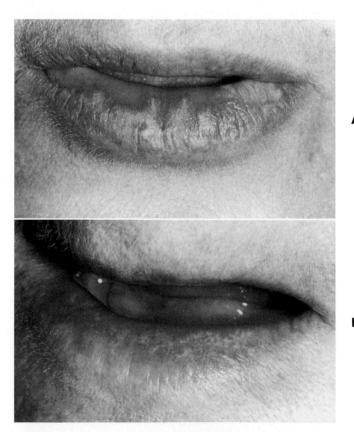

A

B

Fig. 33-6. A, Discoid lesion on the vermilion border of a patient with systemic lupus erythematosus. This appearance is similar to that seen in keratotic types of lichen planus and lichenoid drug reactions. **B,** Lichenoid drug reaction to an antihypertensive drug in an elderly woman. The white reticular pattern is identical to that seen in lichen planus.

been overshadowed by actinic damage in more recent studies. Women have been less affected, possibly because of the use of lipstick and less occupational exposure to sunlight.

The treatment of choice is surgery or radiation therapy. Both are very effective in controlling early lesions. As in advanced actinic keratoses, vermilionectomy is widely used with excellent cosmetic effects. The 5-year survival rate for patients with well-differentiated lesions that have not metastasized is above 90%. Large cratered or indurated lesions may require more extensive surgery, radiation therapy, or both. Metastases are uncommon but must be ruled out by a thorough neck examination. Prophylactic neck dissections are not usually indicated.

Differential diagnosis Because early lesions may look like persistent chapped lips or asymptomatic actinic keratosis, a biopsy is absolutely necessary for diagnosis. Most advanced cratered lesions must be differentiated from keratoacanthoma. Basal cell carcinomas may appear identical on clinical examination, but most clinicians agree that these arise only on the skin surface and extend to the mucosa.

Smokeless Tobacco Lesion

Areas of the labial mucosa that come in direct contact with smokeless tobacco products may develop hyperkeratosis, dysplasia, and squamous cell or verrucous carcinoma (Fig. 33-9). (A previous discussion is in Chapter 8.) This habit is of great concern to public health officials because of the increasing numbers of youth who are becoming addicted to smokeless tobacco and the future potential for oral cancers.

Cigarette Smoker's Lip

Cigarette smoker's lip is a localized, usually well-defined, flat or slightly elevated lesion of the lips that corresponds to the area where the patient holds cigarettes. The lesion usually begins as a reddened area but becomes more white with time (Fig. 33-10). This lesion was first reported by Berry and Landwerlen[19] and is usually seen in neuropsychiatric patients as a result of thermal injury. A high percentage of patients also had burns on their fingers corresponding to where they held their cigarettes. This should be a diagnostic clue. Another aid is that the lesions are confined to the mucosal aspect of the lip and almost never cross the vermilion border. It is postulated

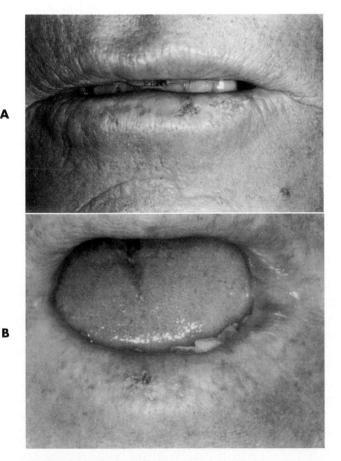

Fig. 33-7. Actinic keratosis. Indistinct vermilion border, filmy white areas, and crusting. (**A** courtesy Brian Brungardt, Topeka, Kan; **B** courtesy Matt Hourigan, deceased.)

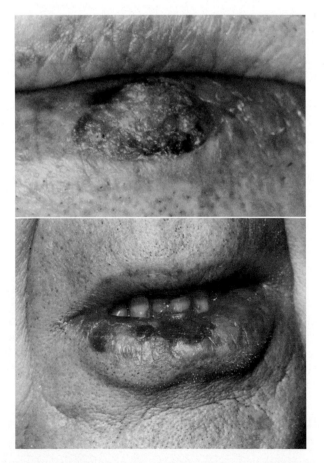

Fig. 33-8. Squamous cell carcinoma. **A,** Solitary squamous cell carcinoma of the lower lip. **B,** Numerous eroded and ulcerated lesions that would not heal.

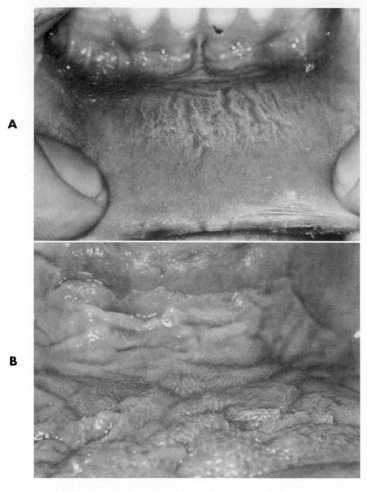

Fig. 33-9. Typical white, corrugated appearance of smokeless tobacco user lesion.

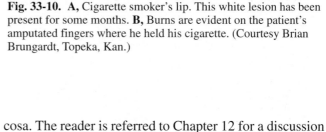

Fig. 33-10. A, Cigarette smoker's lip. This white lesion has been present for some months. **B,** Burns are evident on the patient's amputated fingers where he held his cigarette. (Courtesy Brian Brungardt, Topeka, Kan.)

that the patient's psychiatric medications increase their pain threshold, thereby allowing the tissues to be burned. Lesions may involve one or both lips. Malignant transformation has not been reported despite years of smoking by some patients.

Focal Epithelial Hyperplasia

Focal epithelial hyperplasia (Heck's disease), although relatively rare in whites, is common in Native Americans and Innuits. It is characterized by multiple slightly raised papules that may become papillary.[20] They typically occur in children and are of normal mucosal color. The lesions are induced by HPV-13 and possibly HPV-32.[21] Spontaneous regression has been reported.

BROWN AND RED LESIONS
Melanocytic Nevus and Melanoma

The melanocytic nevus (mole), a benign neuroectodermal lesion, and melanoma, a malignant neoplasm of melanocytic origin, may occasionally occur on the labial mu-

cosa. The reader is referred to Chapter 12 for a discussion of these lesions.

Labial Melanotic Macule

First described by Weathers, Corio, Crawford, et al[22] and later reviewed by Kaugers, Heise, and Riley[23] a labial melanotic macule usually occurs as a single brownish-black, sharply circumscribed lesion of the lower lip (Fig. 33-11). The macules are found most frequently toward the midline in patients with fair complexions and have been detected most frequently in people between the ages of 30 and 45. Histologically, there is increased melanin deposition in the basilar epithelium similar to ephelis (freckle). In contrast to the ephelis, the labial melanotic macule is not associated with exposure to sunlight. No treatment is necessary for the labial melanotic macule; however, if there is any question about the exact nature of the lesion, an excisional biopsy is indicated.

Differential diagnosis Differential diagnosis of pigmented lesions is presented in Chapter 12 in the discussion of the oral melanotic macule.

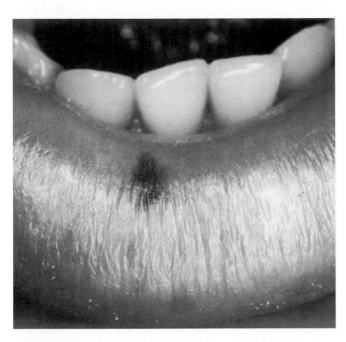

Fig. 33-11. Labial melanotic macule. (Courtesy Matt Hourigan, deceased.)

Hemangioma

The hemangioma is a benign proliferation of blood vessels that occurs in the head and neck region in more than 50% of cases. On histologic study, they are usually divided into cavernous (large vessels) and capillary (small vessels). Most are congenital or occur at a young age and show limited growth potential. Some lesions undergo spontaneous regression, which leads many to believe that hemangiomas are not true neoplasms but rather hamartomas. To support the claim of neoplastic potential in hemangiomas, one can point to those lesions that exhibit unlimited growth with extensive involvement of soft tissues and bone. Some even lead to fatal hemorrhage.

On clinical examination, hemangiomas appear as flat or elevated, red or bluish lesions, which usually blanch under pressure (Fig. 33-12). The lips, buccal mucosa, tongue, and palate are common oral locations. The borders of the lesions are not usually well demarcated; therefore what appears to be a small, superficial lesion may have its bulk beneath the surface. Large lesions often pulsate.

Small lesions are usually successfully treated with surgery, but such procedures should not be attempted before careful evaluation of the extent of the tumor. Other forms of therapy include radiation, sclerosing agents, cryotherapy, embolization with various materials, and laser therapy.

Differential diagnosis Hemangiomas must be differentiated by histologic examination from other vascular lesions such as Kaposi's sarcoma, hemangioendothelioma, hemangiopericytoma, angiosarcoma, arteriovenous malformation, pyogenic granuloma, and varices. Mucoceles may also be a consideration, but they fail to blanch under

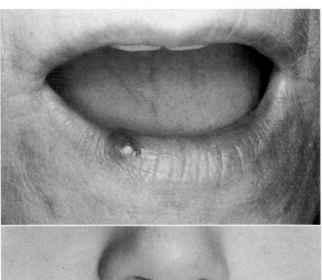

A

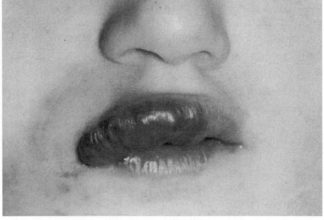

B

Fig. 33-12. Hemangioma. **A,** Small, nodular lesion on vermilion border of the lower lip. **B,** Large, diffuse lesion of the upper lip in a child. (**B** courtesy James Lowe, Kansas City, Mo.)

pressure, which should eliminate them from consideration in most cases.

Multiple Pigmentations

Several conditions include pigmentation of the lips as a partial expression of the disease. These conditions include the following:

1. Peutz-Jeghers syndrome
2. Addison's disease
3. Sturge-Weber syndrome
4. Rendu-Osler-Weber disease (hereditary hemorrhagic telangiectasia)
5. Thrombocytopenic purpura
6. Kaposi's sarcoma
7. von Recklinghausen's disease (neurofibromatosis)
8. Albright's syndrome
9. Hemochromatosis

Multiple brown or black lesions may occur with Peutz-Jeghers syndrome, von Recklinghausen's disease, Addison's disease, Albright's syndrome, and hemochromatosis. Almost all of these may present with multiple macular lesions; however, Addison's disease and hemochromatosis may have a more diffuse pigmentation.

The diagnosis depends on the other manifestations of these conditions rather than biopsy of the lip lesions. A biopsy can determine whether the pigmentation is melanin, which is of little help, since all these lesions have melanin deposition. Hemochromatosis exhibits iron deposits in the tissues, as well as melanin. Albright's syndrome, von Recklinghausen's disease, and hemochromatosis are discussed in Chapter 12.

Peutz-Jeghers syndrome The major manifestations of Peutz-Jeghers syndrome (hereditary intestinal polyposis) are the intestinal polyps that may be found throughout the intestinal tract but most commonly in the ileum. The syndrome is inherited as an autosomal dominant trait; however, sporadic individual cases have been reported. The hamartomatous polyps only rarely have malignant transformation. Despite the benign nature of the polyps, significant morbidity is caused by obstruction and intussusception.

The oral manifestation of this syndrome is melanocytic pigmentation of the oral mucosa, especially of the lips and perioral skin (Fig. 33-13, *C*). These macular lesions appear at birth or soon after and are usually multiple. Most are small, less than 0.5 cm in diameter, and asymptomatic. The lesions are of clinical significance only as a diagnostic clue to the more serious intestinal problems.

Addison's disease Addison's disease is caused by adrenal cortical insufficiency and is characterized by melanin pigmentation of the skin and mucous membranes (Fig. 33-13, *E*), anemia, diarrhea, nausea, vomiting, lethargy, and hypotension. Discussion of the pathophysiology of Addison's disease is beyond the scope of this text.

The pigmentation of the lips is usually multifocal but may be diffuse. Pigmentations have been observed on the buccal mucosa, gingiva, and tongue, as well as the lips. These pigmentations may be the first manifestation of Addison's disease. A biopsy is not diagnostic.

Sturge-Weber syndrome Sturge-Weber syndrome (vascular ectasia) consists of telangiectases that most commonly occur in the head and neck region, following the distribution of the trigeminal nerve and venous angiomas in the leptomeninges. It is much easier to remember the manifestations of this disease by using the descriptive name, *encephalotrigeminal angiomatosis,* rather than the eponym. The disease is congenital and is therefore initially diagnosed at birth. Extensive angiomas in the leptomeninges may cause neurologic manifestations, including seizures. Hemangioma-like lesions may occur throughout the oral cavity, including the lips (Fig. 31-13, *A*). Dentists should be cautious of performing surgery in such areas, since significant bleeding may occur. Patients may seek dental care for the gingival enlargement associated with the anticonvulsant drugs used to control the associated seizures.

Rendu-Osler-Weber disease Rendu-Osler-Weber disease is probably better known in medicine as *hereditary hemorrhagic telangiectasia.* This is an inherited autosomal dominant condition characterized by multiple small aneurysmal telangiectases of the skin and mucosa. Bleeding from the lesions is common and is often one of the symptoms that brings attention to the disease. Lesions appear to increase in number with age. In the oral region the lips are one of the most frequently involved locations (Fig. 33-13, *D*). There is no treatment, and if bleeding occurs, it may be difficult to control. The hereditary nature of the disease is important in making a diagnosis.

Idiopathic thrombocytopenic purpura Thrombocytopenia is a reduction in the number of circulating platelets. When counts fall below 50,000/mm^3, spontaneous bleeding may develop. There are many causes of thrombocytopenia, but "idiopathic" thrombocytopenic purpura indicates an autoimmune disease characterized by antibody-mediated destruction of platelets. Significant bleeding may result from petechial or ecchymotic lesions (Fig. 33-13, *F*). Splenectomy or systemic steroids are often curative; however, some cases spontaneously regress.

ITP must be differentiated from secondary immune thrombocytopenia associated with drug therapy, systemic lupus erythematosus, and viral infections, including HIV.

Kaposi's sarcoma Kaposi's sarcoma may occur on the labial mucosa as single or multiple lesions particularly in individuals who test positive for the human immunodeficiency virus. Lesions may be relatively flat (plaque stage) or raised (nodular stage). A biopsy is necessary for a definitive diagnosis. A more complete discussion of Kaposi's sarcoma is found in Chapter 36.

ULCERATIVE LESIONS

Ulcers of the lip are common. Some are manifestations of a specific disease, whereas others are consequences of a particular treatment or injury. Traumatic lesions are far more common.

TRAUMATIC ULCERS

Traumatic ulcers are commonly found on the lips (Fig. 33-14). Many occur in accidents or altercations, are self-inflicted (facticial), or are caused by health care professionals (iatrogenic). The lower lip is most commonly involved. An extensive discussion of traumatic ulcers is found in Chapter 11.

APHTHAE

Aphthae (canker sores, recurrent aphthous stomatitis) are discussed more completely in Chapter 11, but they deserve attention here because of their common occurrence on the lips. Aphthae occur as a single ulcer or multiple ulcers of the mucosal surface of the lips. They do not occur on the skin. This is in contrast to recurrent herpes labialis, which is often found on the vermilion border or skin surface of the lips. Aphthae of the lip are similar in appearance and behavior to other intraoral

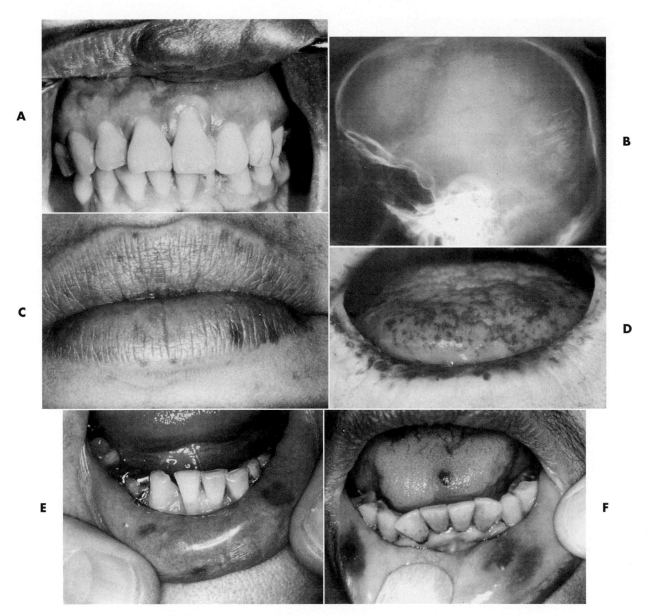

Fig. 33-13. Multiple pigmentation of the lips. **A** and **B,** Sturge-Weber syndrome. **A** shows nevus flammeus of the left side of the upper lip and gingiva. **B** is a lateral radiograph of the skull showing calicfied cranial blood vessels as radiopaque "tram-line tacks." **C,** Peutz-Jeghers syndrome. Many pigmented macules are present on the upper and lower lips. **D,** Rendu-Osler-Weber syndrome. Multiple small, red macules represent dilated end capillaries. **E,** Three pigmented macules on the lower lip resulting from Addison's disease. **F,** Multiple ecchymotic areas of a patient with thrombocytopenia. (**D** courtesy John Bellome, Kansas City, Mo; **E** courtesy Steven Smith, Chicago.)

locations (Fig. 33-15). They are recurrent, with the intervals between episodes varying from weeks to years. Most ulcers heal within 2 weeks. Healing may be accelerated with the topical application of a corticosteroid, although systemic prednisone may be necessary for large or persistent lesions.

Differential Diagnosis

Aphthae are most commonly confused with herpes labialis. Herpes begins as groups of vesicles on the vermilion border or skin, whereas aphthae begin as reddish mucosal macules that undergo ulceration without vesiculation. Differentiation from other diseases and traumatic ulcers is best accomplished by a history of recurrent lesions. In the absence of this history, a biopsy should be performed if healing does not begin within 2 weeks.

HERPES SIMPLEX VIRUS

A discussion of herpesvirus infections may be found in Chapters 6, 11 and 36. The discussion here is limited to herpetic lesions found on the lips.

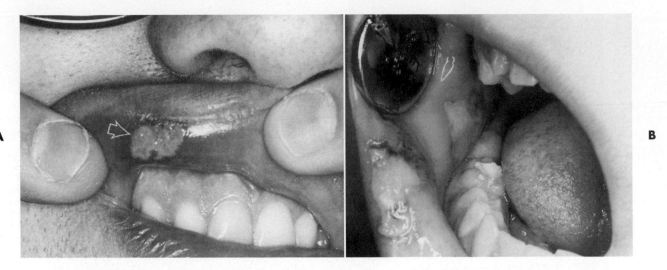

Fig. 33-14. Traumatic ulcer. **A,** A blow to the lip of the patient resulted in a painful ulcer with ragged borders. **B,** Multiple ulcerations from cheek and lip biting occurred during mandibular block anesthesia. (**B** courtesy James Lowe, Kansas City, Kan.)

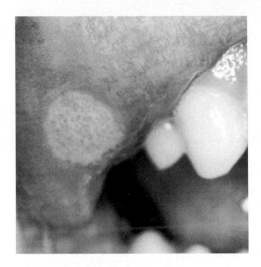

Fig. 33-15. Large aphthous ulcer on the mucosal surface of the upper lip.

Herpes Labialis

Herpes labialis (fever blister) is a recurrent or secondary manifestation of herpes simplex virus (HSV). These lesions occur only in patients who have had primary infections and have developed antibodies to HSV. Many factors appear to reactivate HSV and cause recurrent lesions. Sunlight and trauma are major factors; however, fever, hormonal influence, and emotional stress are also implicated.

Lesions are most commonly located on the vermilion border of the lip, with involvement of the skin and mucosa. Patients often have a tingling or burning sensation before developing multiple small vesicles that are usually in small groups. These vesicles ulcerate quickly and then are covered by a crust (Figs. 33-16 and 33-17). The lesions heal without scarring in 7 to 10 days.

Management Management is discussed in Chapters 6, 11, and 36.

ERYTHEMA MULTIFORME

Erythema multiforme (Stevens-Johnson syndrome) may involve the skin and all areas of the oral mucosa, with the lips being a classic location. The disease is characterized by rapid development of lesions with the skin showing the typical target, iris, or bull's-eye lesions. Mucous membrane lesions are usually multiple red macules, papules, vesicles, or bullae that ulcerate or rupture quickly, leaving raw, painful lesions. These are discussed in Chapter 6. The lips are often extensively involved and crusted (Fig. 33-18 and Plate C). Most patients have mucous membrane and skin lesions; however, occasionally only oral lesions are present.[24,25]

Erythema multiforme is thought to be an immunologic mediated disease or hypersensitivity reaction. In approximately half the cases, precipitating factors such as medications or preceding infections can be identified. Antibiotics, barbiturates, and analgesics are prime offenders. HSV infections, histoplasmosis, and *Mycoplasma pneumoniae* infections may be precipitating factors, with most new research supporting a strong relationship to HSV. HSV-specific deoxyribonucleic acid is often present in biopsies of tissue from patients with erythema multiforme.[26]

There are several severe forms of erythema multiforme, including Stevens-Johnson syndrome and toxic epidermal necrolysis. Both are usually triggered by a drug rather than a prior infection. Stevens-Johnson syndrome involves the skin, oral mucosa, eyes, and genitalia. Toxic epidermal necrolysis causes extensive sloughing of the skin and mucous membranes and may be fatal.[27]

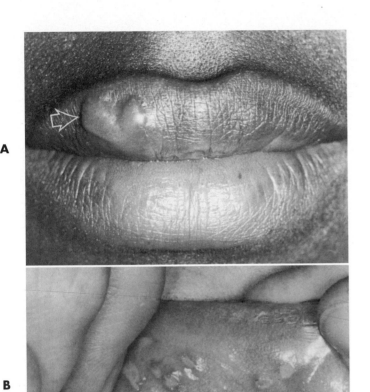

A

B

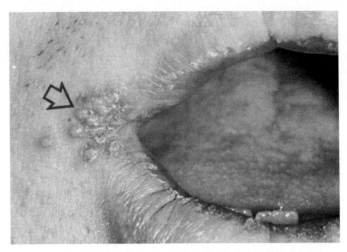

Fig. 33-17. Recurrent herpes. Multiple smaller vesicles at the commissure.

Fig. 33-16. Recurrent herpes. **A,** Two large vesicles on the upper lip. A tingling sensation accompanied their formation. **B,** Recurrent herpes on the mucosa of the upper lip showing the characteristic clustering of small, discrete ulcers. (**B** courtesy of A.C.W.H. Hutchinson Collection, Northwestern University Dental School, Chicago.)

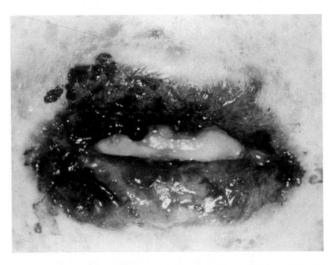

Fig. 33-18. Erythema multiforme. These lesions developed in the child after antibiotic therapy for an ear infection. Skin lesions were also present.

Lesions of erythema multiforme usually heal spontaneously in several weeks, although some cases may persist longer. Recurrences are common unless precipitating factors can be identified and avoided.

There is no specific treatment or cure, but precipitating factors should be identified. When no etiologic factors are found, analgesics and anesthetics are palliative. Corticosteroid therapy is controversial.

Differential Diagnosis

Many diseases, including recurrent aphthous, Behçet's syndrome, Reiter's syndrome, pemphigus, pemphigoid, and herpetic stomatitis, can be confused with erythema multiforme. Herpetic stomatitis may be quite similar to erythema multiforme but can usually be differentiated by initial gingival involvement, lack of iris skin lesions, positive viral culture, and no history of previous episodes. Aphthae and Behçet's and Reiter's syndromes do not have vesicles or bullous mucosal lesions as features.

KERATOACANTHOMA

Keratoacanthoma (self-healing carcinoma) is best known by dermatologists, since the majority of cases occur on sun-exposed tissues of the face. Oral lesions are rare, with the lips being the most common site.[28] It resembles a squamous cell carcinoma on both clinical and microscopic examinations but is a benign lesion. It is a lesion of adults, predominantly older men. The lesion begins as a sometimes painful nodule that rapidly increases in size and develops a central crater (Fig. 33-19). After reaching maximal growth, which rarely exceeds 1.5 cm in diameter, the lesion begins to regress and heals. The entire process may take 3 to 4 months; however, some lesions have been reported to last as long as several years. Because of the close clinical and histologic resemblance to squamous cell carcinoma, the keratoacanthoma should be treated by surgical excision.[29]

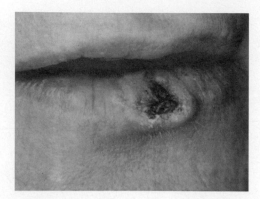

Fig. 33-19. Keratoacanthoma of the lower lip in a 38-year-old man showing the typical appearance of the central keratin plug in a central depression surrounded by smooth, rolled borders. This lesion is clinically indistinguishable from squamous cell carcinoma. (From Bass KD: Solitary keratoacanthoma of the lip, *J Oral Surg* 38:53-55, 1980.)

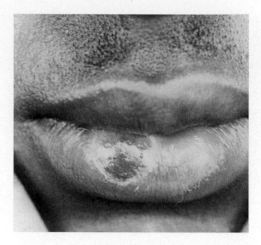

Fig. 33-20. Syphilitic chancre of the lower lip in a young man. (Courtesy Matt Hourigan, deceased.)

The cause of the keratoacanthoma is unknown; however, considerations include viruses and chemical carcinogens.

Differential Diagnosis

The most important consideration is squamous cell carcinoma. Keratoacanthoma usually shows a more rapid initial growth than squamous cell carcinoma; however, this is not a reliable criterion. Biopsy is necessary for a diagnosis.

SYPHILIS

The primary lesion of syphilis occurs at the site of inoculation. This site is most commonly on the genitalia; however, the oral cavity and especially the lips are possible locations. The initial lesion or chancre usually begins as a papule at approximately 3 weeks after contact with the spirochete *Treponema pallidum*. The papule eventually ulcerates, leaving a lesion similar to an aphthous or traumatic ulcer (Fig. 33-20). The chancre heals spontaneously within several months and is highly contagious during this period. Regional lymphadenopathy may also be present.

The classic lesions of secondary syphilis in the oral cavity, called *mucous patches,* are single or multiple plaques that are gray or white and that overlie an ulcerated base. These patches represent macerated papules, which because of the moisture are covered with a soft, boggy membrane. They are teeming with organisms and are highly contagious. Secondary lesions of syphilis usually develop approximately 6 weeks after initial contact; however, the time is greatly variable. Serologic tests for syphilis are usually positive during the secondary stages of syphilis, in contrast to the results obtained in primary syphilis. Macular or papular skin lesions usually accompany the mucous patches.

Condyloma latum is another lesion of secondary syphilis that may occur on the lip. This papular, wartlike lesion may be red or white. It could easily be confused with a papilloma, verruca vulgaris, or condyloma acuminatum. These three lesions usually have individual, elevated, fingerlike processes, whereas syphilis is more likely to be lobulated.

Treatment of primary or secondary syphilis is with the appropriate antibiotic, usually penicillin.

Differential Diagnosis

Chancres may be difficult to distinguish from other, more innocuous lesions, since the results of the serologic study are usually normal. Dark-field microscopy is not recommended for the examination of intraoral lesions because of the presence of other intraoral spirochetes; however, the lesions located on the vermilion border can be examined in this manner. It is probable that many chancres go undiagnosed or are cured unknowingly with antibiotic therapy.

Positive serologic findings may aid in the diagnosis of mucous patches and condyloma latum. The presence of accompanying skin lesions is also helpful. Mucous patches might also be confused with candidiasis.

ELEVATED LESIONS

NODULAR FIBROUS HYPERPLASIA

A true fibrous neoplasm of the oral mucosa is an extremely rare entity, and the ensuing discussion deals with the extremely common nodular fibrous hyperplasia, which is often erroneously called a *fibroma (traumatic or irritation fibroma)*. This nodular lesion of normal color is the most common soft tissue lesion encountered in the oral cavity and occurs commonly on the lips (Fig. 33-21). Since the lesion is a fibrous hyperplasia, usually initiated by trauma such as lip biting, it is not a true neoplasm and

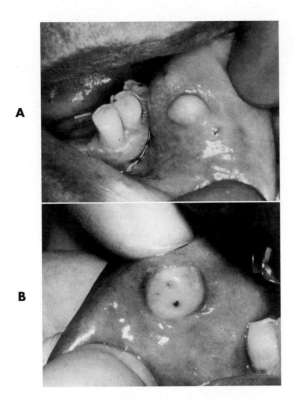

Fig. 33-21. Typical lesions of fibrous hyperplasia of the lower lip. These lesions are associated with chronic lip biting in both cases.

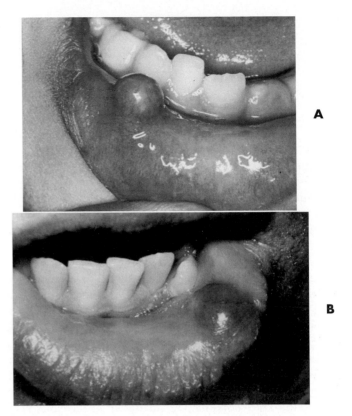

Fig. 33-22. Mucoceles of the lower lip in two patients.

has limited growth potential, rarely exceeding 1 or 2 cm in diameter. The lesion typically grows slowly and varies in consistency from very soft to firm. The reader is referred to Chapter 10 for further discussion.

Although occasional fibrous hyperplasias may regress or disappear when the offending irritant is eliminated, most must be surgically removed. Recurrence is rare.

Differential Diagnosis

All soft tissue tumors, mucoceles, and salivary gland tumors must be ruled out. Multiple recurrences or variations in size favor mucocele; however, a biopsy with histologic evaluation is the only way to obtain a definitive diagnosis.

MUCOCELE

Approximately 75% of all mucoceles (mucus escape phenomenon) occur on the lower lip; however, this lesion may develop in any location where minor salivary glands exist. Most mucoceles occur as the result of the severance of a minor salivary gland duct, with resultant escape of mucous secretions into the surrounding tissues. Occlusion or partial obstruction of a duct can also result in a marked dilatation of that duct. This is termed a *mucous retention cyst,* since the mucus-filled cavity is lined with epithelium (in contrast to mucoceles, which have no epithelial lining).

Some type of trauma, such as lip biting, is the usual cause of mucoceles. Since this type of trauma most commonly occurs on the lower lip, the upper lip is an infrequent location. A fluctuation in size is characteristic of mucoceles. Multiple fluctuations may occur as the mucin is phagocytosed, carried off, and replaced by newly secreted mucin.

Mucoceles appear suddenly and reach maximum size within several days. The typical lesion appears as an elevated vesicular or bullous lesion, which often has a slightly bluish or translucent appearance (Fig. 33-22). However, if the lesions are situated more deeply in the tissues, they may be of normal color. The lesion is soft on palpation and often fluctuant. The treatment of choice is surgical excision, including excision of the glands from which the mucin is escaping. Recurrence of the mucocele is possible despite surgery, since adjacent salivary gland ducts may be severed during the surgical procedure.

Differential Diagnosis

The sudden appearance and the fluctuation in size is almost diagnostic of the mucocele; however, biopsy is necessary for a definitive diagnosis. Lesions that may be confused with mucoceles include neurofibroma, lipoma, salivary gland tumors, varix, vascular tumors, and nodular fibrous hyperplasia. Vascular lesions should blanch under pressure, which aids in the differential diagnosis. Salivary gland tumors, such as mucoepidermoid carcinoma, may appear identical; consequently, all tissue excised during surgery should be submitted for microscopic study.

ANGIOEDEMA

Angioedema (angioneurotic edema) often involves the lips and is characterized by a sudden, diffuse swelling. The swelling, although edematous, is usually somewhat firm and nonpitting (Fig. 33-23). Any tissue may be involved, and multiple lesions have also been reported. Usually, only one lip is involved; however, the whole face occasionally may be swollen. Of special concern is swelling of areas such as the tongue, uvula, and larynx, which may lead to respiratory distress.[30]

Angioedema is currently divided into two types: hereditary and nonhereditary. The latter is more common; unfortunately, in more than 70% of cases the cause is unknown. Food and drugs are the most common causes, resulting in an immunoglobulin E–mediated hypersensitivity with mast cell degranulation. Angiotensin-converting enzyme (ACE) inhibitor medications may also precipitate angioedema via pathways not mediated by immunoglobulin E. The uncommon hereditary form fits into the complement-mediated group and results from a quantitative or functional defect of $\overline{C1}$ inhibitor.[31] This type of angioedema is inherited as an autosomal dominant trait.

In all types of angioedema the clinical manifestations are similar. In some cases the swelling may last only several hours, but in others, it may last as long as 3 days. Accompanying generalized urticaria may be present in approximately 50% of cases. Recurrence is common, and the intervals are greatly variable, probably depending on exposure to the precipitating factors.

After clinical swellings develop, the standard drug of choice for treatment has been the antihistamines, although they are not effective when ACE inhibitors are the cause. Obviously, for the nonhereditary type the offending allergen should be identified if possible and eliminated. Hereditary angioedema is often precipitated by trauma; dental extractions frequently are implicated. Since not all trauma can be eliminated, several types of drugs have been effective as prophylactics. Antifibrinolytic agents, such as ϵ-aminocaproic acid, are one type, whereas the other agents are androgens, such as danazol.[30,32,33]

Differential Diagnosis

Infections, sarcoidosis, Melkersson-Rosenthal syndrome, cheilitis glandularis, and cheilitis granulomatosa are the conditions likely to be confused with angioedema. The sudden onset and a history of recurrent episodes are major differentiating features. The diffuse character of the swelling should also help rule out smaller, well-demarcated mucoceles.

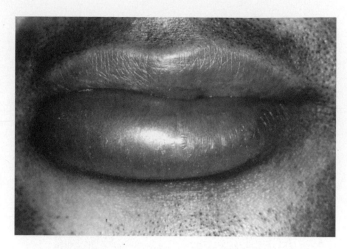

Fig. 33-23. Angioedema. The swelling developed quickly and was present for only 2 hours before this photograph was taken.

LIPOMA

Lipoma is a rather rare lesion of the oral cavity, but it occasionally occurs on the mucosal aspect of the lips.[34] It is a neoplasm composed of mature adipose tissue. It may occur as a sessile or pedunculated mass covered by atrophic epithelium with the underlying adipose tissue often giving the lesion a yellowish appearance. Lipomas are soft and sometimes almost fluctuant to palpation; therefore they are often confused on clinical examination with cystic lesions or mucoceles. Excisional biopsy is the treatment of choice. Recurrence is rare.

Differential Diagnosis

Soft traumatic fibromas and mucoceles are the most common lesions to be confused with a lipoma. Variation in size may indicate a mucocele, but a biopsy is necessary to distinguish a lipoma from a traumatic fibroma. Other soft tissue neoplasms and salivary gland tumors are usually more firm on palpation. Malignant tumors of adipose tissue (liposarcomas) may also appear yellowish and must be ruled out.

SALIVARY GLAND TUMORS

As discussed in Chapter 10, tumors of the minor salivary glands occur most commonly on the palate, buccal mucosa, and tongue. Occurrence on the lips appears to account for approximately 5% of these tumors, with most occurring on the upper lip. There is little difference in the clinical appearance of benign and malignant salivary gland tumors that occur on the lips.

Salivary gland tumors appear as soft or firm masses, with most having a nodular, exophytic component (Fig. 33-24). Ulceration of the nodular mass may occur, but the presence of the ulcer gives no clues as to the tumor's benign or malignant nature. Those that are soft on palpation usually have large cystic cavities and an abundance of

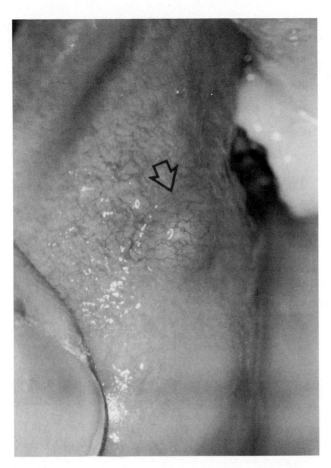

Fig. 33-24. Benign mixed tumor on the labial mucosa near the commissure.

mucin. The more solid tumors, both benign and malignant (especially benign mixed tumors with large amounts of bone and cartilage), are firm on palpation.

One salivary gland tumor, canalicular adenoma, deserves special mention in relation to its frequent location on the upper lip. Almost 75% of canalicular adenomas occur on or near the upper lip, and the majority are near the midline.[35]

Most salivary gland tumors grow slowly and often exist for years before treatment is sought. Rapid growth or a sudden change in growth is more consistent with malignant tumors or benign tumors that have undergone malignant change. Since there is no good method of clinically differentiating salivary gland tumors from other soft tissue tumors, cysts, or reactive lesions of the lip, biopsy is mandatory for diagnosis.

MINOR SALIVARY GLAND CALCULI

Sialolithiasis of the major salivary glands is a well-known entity; however, similar mineralizations may occur in ducts of minor glands and are thought to be more common than reported in the literature. They occur primarily in the upper lip of patients in the fifth to seventh decades. Most

appear as firm to hard, movable submucosal nodules (see Fig. 28-25). The lesions vary from 3 to 15 mm in diameter; the majority are less than 5 mm. Etiologic factors include unusual morphologic features of the involved duct and local trauma.[36,37] Excisional biopsy is the treatment of choice, since on clinical examination alone a submucosal nodule could represent a variety of soft tissue tumors. This entity is discussed further in Chapter 27.

NASOLABIAL CYST

The nasolabial cyst (nasoalveolar cyst) is a nonodontogenic developmental cyst found in the upper lip or soft tissues of the face inferior to the nose in the nasolabial fold. It is thought to be derived from epithelial remnants of the nasolacrimal duct or from entrapment of epithelial rests during the fusion of the globular portion of the medial nasal process and the maxillary process. Therefore the cyst lies entirely within soft tissue and exhibits no radiographic abnormalities. It appears to be slightly more common in female patients, with no preference for right or left sides. Occasionally, it is found bilaterally.

On clinical examination the cyst appears as a fullness of the nasal vestibule. If it enlarges inferiorly, it may appear to originate in the lip, whereas in other instances, it may appear as a swelling in the floor of the nose. The cyst is usually asymptomatic and rarely recurs after surgical removal. On histologic study the lining epithelium may range from cuboidal to squamous to respiratory.

Differential Diagnosis

In the lip, this lesion must be distinguished from lesions of pulpal origin (e.g., periapical cyst, granuloma, or abscess). Vitality tests of adjacent teeth help in the differential diagnosis. Radiographs should also aid in ruling out pulp-related or odontogenic cysts. Epidermal inclusion cysts, sebaceous cysts, and salivary gland tumors must be ruled out by biopsy.

CONTACT ALLERGY

The labial mucosa is commonly affected by the numerous agents associated with contact allergies of skin and mucosa. Foods, dentifrices, mouthwashes, chewing gum, candies, flavoring agents (especially mint and cinnamon), dental impression material, cosmetics, and metals are possible causes. Clinically, there may be a diffuse erythema, with or without swelling, vesicles, tissue sloughing, or thickened hyperkeratotic areas. Some reactions may mimic lichen planus (lichenoid reaction).[38-41] The condition called *plasma cell cheilitis* probably represents a contact allergy. Treatment involves identification of the suspected allergen. Withdrawal visually results in rapid improvement. Topical or systemic steroid may be used to alleviate symptoms.

Candidiasis and facticial injury (exfoliative cheilitis) should be ruled out.[42]

CHEILITIS GLANDULARIS

Cheilitis glandularis is a relatively rare inflammatory disease primarily affecting the lower lip. In the early stages the mucosal surface reveals numerous dilated salivary duct orifices surrounded by a red macular area. Patients occasionally note a mucous secretion at the orifice of the ducts. As the condition progresses, the labial glands may become enlarged, which may cause the lip to become everted (Fig. 33-25). There may be a superficial inflammatory process or a deep-seated infection. These variations have caused authors to divide this disease into three types: simple, superficial suppurative (Baelz disease), and deep suppurative (cheilitis glandularis apostematosa). The latter two may cause the lip to become crusted and ulcerated with resultant scarring. The condition occurs most commonly in white men; occasionally cases are reported in children, blacks, and women.

Although the cause is not completely understood, chronic exposure to the sun or severe weather may induce inflammation of the labial salivary glands.[43] Other proposed etiologic factors include bacteria, tobacco, poor oral hygiene, hereditary factors, and even emotional disturbances. Cases of squamous cell carcinoma arising in cheilitis glandularis have been reported. Because of the potential for malignant transformation, surgical stripping or vermilionectomy is the recommended treatment in advanced cases.[44,45]

Differential diagnosis includes angioedema, sarcoidosis, and cheilitis granulomatosa.

CHEILITIS GRANULOMATOSA AND MELKERSSON-ROSENTHAL SYNDROME

Cheilitis granulomatosa (Miescher's syndrome) is characterized by a diffuse, soft swelling that develops slowly and may persist for months or years. It is seen most commonly on the lower lip, which is usually of normal color and is asymptomatic (Fig. 33-26). Cheilitis granulomatosa may occur alone or in association with facial paralysis and fissured (plicated) tongue. This is referred to as *Melkersson-Rosenthal syndrome.*[46] Worsaae and Pindborg[47] have included gingival enlargement as an occasional occurrence.[48]

Histologic examination reveals the presence of noncaseating granulomas complete with Langhans' giant cells. It has been impossible to identify any specific organism or to demonstrate a relationship to sarcoidosis, which it resembles histologically. Radiation therapy, corticosteroids, and surgery have been used as treatments, with limited success.[49] Some studies have shown that elimination of infections, such as periodontitis, may reduce the swelling or cause it to disappear.[50]

The differential diagnosis includes angioedema and sarcoidosis. Angioedema usually appears more suddenly and possibly has a history of repeated episodes. Sarcoidosis may be excluded by the absence of any of its other manifestations or by a negative Kveim test. Crohn's disease may also have oral involvement and cause granulomatous cheilitis. The absence of gastrointestinal symptoms usually rules out Crohn's disease.

DEVELOPMENTAL ABNORMALITIES

CLEFT LIP

Cleft lip is a relatively common defect that occurs in approximately 1 in 655 to 1200 births. The cleft is limited to the upper lip, where it represents failure of complete fusion of the maxillary, lateral nasal, and medial nasal processes. Animal studies have shown inadequate mesodermal penetration in the areas of the clefts, which results in destruction of the overlying ectoderm.

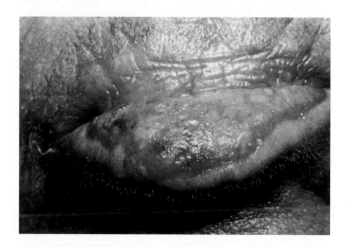

Fig. 33-25. Cheilitis glandularis. The elderly patient had persistent swelling and drainage of the lower lip.

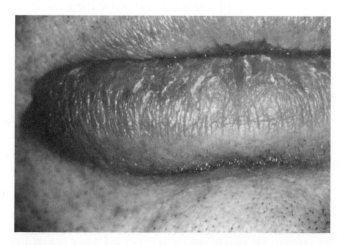

Fig. 33-26. Cheilitis granulomatosa. This patient had persistent swelling of the lower lip for 1 month. Biopsy revealed granuloma formation.

Clefts may be unilateral or bilateral (Fig. 33-27). Unilateral clefts are more common and have a predisposition for the left side. They are also slightly more common in male patients. Cleft lips occur more frequently in association with cleft palate than alone. When the clefts extend through the lip and nostril and toward the palate, they are termed *complete.* Incomplete clefts do not extend into the nostril. Complete clefts are more common in the unilateral and bilateral types.

The cause of clefts of the lip and palate remains unknown; however, heredity is probably the most important factor. No single gene has been identified, and most researchers believe that the defect is polygenic; however, hereditary factors do not usually act alone and are influenced by a number of environmental factors.[51] Voluminous papers have incriminated nutritional deficiencies, certain drugs, excessive cortisone (both intrinsic or extrinsic), and local factors such as decreased blood flow or infections. A discussion of these factors is beyond the scope of this chapter.

Treatment is complex, especially in complete clefts with palatine involvement. Such cases are usually managed by a team of specialists from dentistry, plastic surgery, speech therapy, and psychology. Incomplete cleft lips are usually corrected surgically; surgery often begins as soon as the baby has regained original birth weight.

DOUBLE LIP

Double lip (Ascher's syndrome) is a developmental abnormality usually seen on the upper lip; however, both lips may be involved (Fig. 33-28). It consists of redundant tissue and is of no serious consequence other than cosmetic considerations. It may occur alone or in association with other oral clefts.[52]

Ascher's syndrome includes a double lip associated with thyroid enlargement and drooping of the upper eyelid (blepharochalasis).

LOWER LIP SINUSES

Lower lip sinuses (lip pits, commissural pits, and fistulas) are congenital or developmental defects that occur as singular anomalies or more often with cleft lip or palate. These entities are also discussed in Chapter 13. The defects appear as unilateral depressions or more frequently as bilateral depressions or grooves. They are found at the vermilion border of the lower lip (lip pits) or at the commissures (commissural pits) (Fig. 33-29). The upper lip is infrequently affected. The pits or sinuses are thought to represent embryonic remnants of sulci and fissures. Autosomal dominant transmission has been reported in some studies.[53] The sinuses or pits end as blind tracts and usually require no surgical intervention. The commissural pits are more common than lip pits, occurring in 10% to 20% of the population.[51]

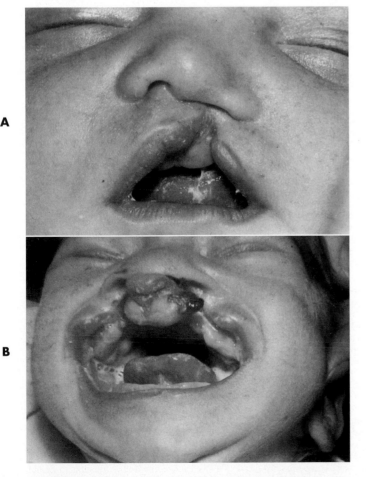

Fig. 33-27. Cleft lip. **A,** Unilateral incomplete cleft. **B,** Bilateral complete clefts. (**A** courtesy James Lowe, Kansas City, Mo; **B** courtesy Matt Hourigan, deceased.)

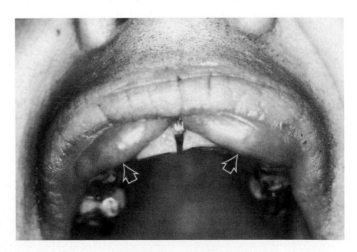

Fig. 33-28. Double lip.

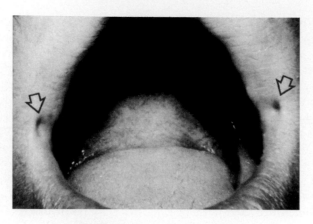

Fig. 33-29. Commissural lip pits.

REFERENCES

1. Reade PC, Rich AM, Hay KD, et al: Cheilocandidosis: a possible clinical entity, *Br Dent J* 152:305-308, 1982.
2. Allen CM: Diagnosing and managing oral candidiasis, *J Am Dent Assoc* 123:77-82, 1992.
3. Fotos PG, Vincent SD, Hellstein JW: Oral candidosis: clinical, historical and therapeutic features of 100 cases, *Oral Surg* 74:41-49, 1992.
4. Ohman SC, Dahlén G, Möller A, et al: Angular cheilitis: a clinical and microbiologic study, *J Oral Pathol* 15:213-217, 1986.
5. Miller CS, White DK, Royse DD: In situ hybridization analysis of human papilloma virus in orofacial lesions using a consensus biotinylated probe, *Am J Dermatopathol* 15:256-259, 1993.
6. Adler-Storthz K, Newland JR, Tessin BA, et al: Identification of human papillomavirus types in oral verruca vulgaris, *J Oral Pathol* 15:230-233, 1986.
7. Green TL, Eversole LR, Leider AS: Oral and labial verruca vulgaris: clinical histologic and immunohistochemical evaluation, *Oral Surg* 62:410-416, 1986.
8. Zunt SL, Tomich CE: Oral condyloma acuminatum, *J Dermatol Surg Oncol* 15:591-594, 1989.
9. Barone, R, Ficarra G, Gaglioti D, et al: Prevalence of oral lesions among HIV-infected intravenous drug abusers and other risk groups, *Oral Surg* 69:169-173, 1990.
10. Lamey D-J, McCartan BE, Mac Donald DG, Mackie RM: Basal cell cytoplasmic autoantibodies in oral lichenoid reactions, *Oral Surg* 79:44-49, 1995.
11. Burrows D: Hypersensitivity to mercury, nickel and chromium in relation to dental materials, *Int Dent J* 36:30-34, 1986.
12. Stenman E, Bergman M: Hypersensitivity reaction to dental materials in a referred group of patients, *Scand J Dent Res* 97:30-34, 1986.
13. Schubert MN, Sullivan KM: Recognition incidence and management of oral graft-versus-host disease, *NCI Mongr* 9:135-143, 1990.

14. Picascia DD, Robinson JK: Actinic cheilitis: a review of the etiology, differential diagnosis and treatment, *J Am Acad Dermatol* 17:255-264, 1987.
15. Lindquist C, Teppo L: Epidemiological evaluation of sunlight as a risk factor of lip cancer, *Br J Cancer* 37:983-989, 1978.
16. Pukkala E., Soderholm AL, Lindquist C: Cancers of the lip and oropharynx in different social and occupational groups in Finland, *Oral Oncol Eur J Cancer* 30B:209-215, 1994.
17. Douglass CW, Gammon MD: Reassessing the epidemiology of lip cancer, *Oral Surg* 57:631-642, 1984.
18. La Riviere W, Pickett AB: Clinical criteria in diagnosis of early squamous cell carcinoma of the lower lip, *J Am Dent Assoc* 99:972-977, 1979.
19. Berry HH, Landwerlen JR: Cigarette smoker's lip lesion in psychiatric patients, *J Am Dent Assoc* 86:657-662, 1973.
20. Archard HO, Heck JW, Stanley HR: Focal epithelial hyperplasia: an unusual oral mucosal lesion found in Indian children, *Oral Surg* 20:201-212, 1965.
21. Carlos R, Sedano HO: Multifocal papilloma virus epithelial hyperplasia, *Oral Surg* 77:631-635, 1994.
22. Weathers DR, Corio RL, Crawford BE, et al: The labial melanotic macule, *Oral Surg* 42:196-205, 1976.
23. Kaugars GE, Heise AP, Riley WT: Oral melanotic macules: a review of 353 cases, *Oral Surg* 76:59-61. 1993.
24. Lozada F, Silverman S Jr: Erythema multiforme: clinical characteristics and natural history in fifty patients, *Oral Surg* 46:628-636, 1978.
25. Schofield JK, Tatnall FM, Leigh IM: Recurrent erythema multiforme: clinical features in a large series of patients, *Br J Dermatol* 128:542-555, 1993.
26. Aslanzadeh J, Helm KF, Espy MJ, et al: Defection of HSV-specific DNA in biopsy tissue of patients with erythema multiforme by polymerase chain reaction, *Br J Dermatol* 126:19-23, 1992.

27. Bastuji-Garin S, Rzany B, Stern RS, et al: Clinical classification of cases of toxic epidermal necrolysis, Stevens-Johnson syndrome, and erythema multiforme, *Arch Dermatol* 129:92-96, 1993.
28. Eversole LR, Leider AS, Alexander G: Intraoral and labial keratoacanthoma, *Oral Surg* 54:663-667, 1982.
29. Schwartz RA: Keratoacanthoma, *J Am Acad Dermatol* 30:1-19, 1994.
30. Greaves M, Lawlor F: Angioedema: manifestations and management, *J Am Acad Dermatol* 25:155-165, 1991.
31. Angostoni A, Cicardi M: Hereditary and acquired Cī-inhibitor deficiency in 235 patients, *Medicine* 71:206-215, 1992.
32. Atkinson JC, Frank MM: Oral manifestation and dental management of patients with hereditary angioedema, *J Oral Pathol Med* 20:139-142, 1991.
33. Rodgers GK, Galos RS, Johnson JT: Hereditary angioedema: case report and review of management, *Orolaryngol Head Neck Surg* 104:394-398, 1991.
34. Zussman KM, Correll RW, Schott TR: Large nonpainful swelling of the lower lip, *J Am Dent Assoc* 117:849-850, 1988.
35. Ellis GL, Auclair PL, Gnepp DR: *Surgical pathology of the salivary glands*, Philadelphia, 1991, WB Saunders.
36. Jensen JL, Howell FV, Rick GM, Correll RW:Minor salivary gland calculi: a clinicopathologic study of forty-seven new cases, *Oral Surg* 47:44-50, 1979.
37. Anneroth G, Hansen LS: Minor salivary gland calculi: a clinical and histopathological study of forty-nine cases, *Int J Oral Surg* 12:80-89, 1983.
38. Van Loon LAJ, Bos JD, Davidson CL: Clinical evaluation of fifty-six patients referred with symptoms tentatively related to allergic contact stomatitis, *Oral Surg* 7:572-575, 1992.
39. Burrows D: Hypersensitivity to mercury, nickel and chromium in relation to dental materials, *Int Dent J* 36:30-33, 1986.

40. Miller RL, Gould AR, Bernstein ML: Cinnamon-induced stomatitis venenata: clinical and characteristic histologic features, *Oral Surg* 73:708-716, 1992.

41. Dunlap CL, Vincent SK, Barker BF: Allergic reaction to orthodontic wire: report of case, *J Am Dent Assoc* 118:449-450, 1989.

42. Reade PC, Sim R: Exfoliative cheilitis: a factitious disorder? *Int J Oral Maxillofac Surg* 15:313-317, 1986.

43. Swerlick RA, Cooper PH: Cheilitis glandularis: a re-evaluation, *J Am Acad Dermatol* 10:466-472, 1984.

44. Oliver ID, Pickett AB: Cheilitis glandularis, *Oral Surg* 49:526-529, 1980.

45. Lederman DA: Suppurative stomatitis glandularis, *Oral Surg* 78:319-322, 1994.

46. Greene RM, Rogers RS III: Melkersson-Rosenthal syndrome: a review of 36 patients, *J Am Acad Dermatol* 21:1263-1270, 1989.

47. Worsaae N, Pindborg JJ: Granulomatous gingival manifestations of Melkersson-Rosanthal syndrome, *Oral Surg* 49:131-138, 1980.

48. Bataineh AB, Pillai KG, Mansour M, Al-Khail AA: An unusual case of the Melkersson-Rosenthal syndrome, *Oral Surg* 80:289-292, 1995.

49. Williams PM, Greenberg MS: Management of cheilitis granulomatosa, *Oral Surg* 72:436-439, 1991.

50. Worsaae, N, Christensen KC, Schidt M, Reibel J: Melkersson-Rosenthal syndrome and cheilitis granulomatosa, *Oral Surg* 54:404-413, 1982.

51. Gorlin RJ, Cohen MM Jr, Levin LS: *Syndromes of the head and neck,* ed 3, New York, 1990, Oxford University Press.

52. Kenny KF, Hreha JP, Dent CD: Bilateral redundant mucosal tissue of the upper lip, *J Am Dent Assoc* 120:193-194, 1990.

53. Vélez A: Congenital lower lip pits (Van der Woude syndrome), *J Am Acad Dermatol* 32:520-521, 1995.

CHAPTER 34

Intraoral Lesions by Anatomic Region

DANNY R. SAWYER
NORMAN K. WOOD

One of the purposes of this textbook is to teach the student and fledgling clinician how to arrive at a logical differential diagnosis when a lesion or condition is encountered in everyday practice. The text has done this, in part, by helping the reader arrange knowledge of lesions by grouping disease entities according to clinical or radiographic appearance. This chapter, in addition to those that discuss the lip, face, and neck, attempts to aid the student and clinician in arriving at a sound differential diagnosis by considering that certain lesions have a predilection for specific anatomic sites. This approach has been found to be helpful in the past and has been incorporated in other textbooks. In listing lesions by anatomic sites, an attempt has been made to rank lesions according to frequency. On occasion, this may be objectionable to some experts in the various fields of dentistry, and certainly no inerrant authority is being claimed. In developing the list of lesions by areas according to frequency, many sources, including other textbooks, journal articles, computer-determined statistical rankings, and several authorities, have been consulted. The lists are not exhaustive, and the very rare lesions are listed only as rarities. Very common lesions may be seen more often by the dental clinician than by the oral pathologist who bases observations of the frequency of lesions primarily on a biopsy service. In addition, those in a referral practice will view a skewed frequency, generally seeing more difficult cases than the general practitioner. Further, the frequency of specific lesions is known to vary from one geographic location to another.

With this in mind, this chapter presents first a brief listing and discussion of the normal anatomic structures of the several oral regions. This is followed by a brief list of the more common lesions of the anatomic locations. The intraoral environment has been divided into the following anatomic locations:

1. Labial and buccal mucosa and vestibule
2. Gingiva and alveolar mucosa
3. Palate (hard and soft)
4. Oropharynx (fauces, pharynx, and retromolar region)
5. Tongue (dorsal and lateral surfaces)
6. Tongue (ventral surface)
7. Floor of the mouth

LABIAL AND BUCCAL MUCOSA AND VESTIBULE
Anatomic Structures

1. Frenum attachments—midline and lateral (labial and vestibular mucosa)
2. Stensen's (parotid) papilla (buccal mucosa)
3. Linea alba (buccal mucosa)
4. Fordyce's granules (labial and buccal mucosa)

Normally the texture of the labial mucosa is smooth, soft, and resilient. The color of this mucosa is normally pink to brown, depending on the presence of racial pigmentation. This area is well endowed with vascularity and minor salivary glands. This labial mucosa is commonly traumatized. Thus because of the rich minor salivary gland component, mucoceles are seen with some degree of frequency. Cheek biting or chewing is also rather common. These last two statements are apropos because the student and fledgling clinician must keep in mind what structures are contained in the mucosa of the area of a lesion, as well as the patient's habits, since they may relate to a lesion presented for diagnosis. The texture of the buccal mucosa is similar to that of the labial mucosa, being soft and smooth to granular. It may feel granular because of the rich supply of sebaceous glands and minor salivary glands in this mucosa. The buccal fat pad may appear prominent, especially in young patients. In whites the color of the buccal mucosa is normally pink, but in persons of the dark-skinned races, it may appear blue to bluish-gray. In blacks, there may be a patchy distribution to the pigmentation, and the coloration may be more brown to black than blue to bluish-gray. The oral mucous membrane of the vestibule is thin, and the many small vascular channels are easily observed. The more common lesions of the labial and buccal mucosa and vestibule follow; detailed discussions of them are found elsewhere in the text.

Common Lesions

1. Fordyce's granule (may be considered a normal variation)
2. Leukoedema (may be considered a normal variation)
3. Cheek biting or chewing
4. Recurrent aphthous ulcer
5. Traumatic ulcer
6. Inflammatory hyperplastic lesion (pyogenic granuloma, fibrous hyperplasia, epulis fissuratum of denture wearers)
7. Leukoplakia and snuff dipper's lesion, erythroleukoplakia, or erythroplakia
8. Lichen planus
9. Mucous retention phenomenon (mucocele)
10. Varix
11. Draining sinus of periapical abscess
12. Amalgam tattoo
13. Aspirin burn
14. Hemangioma
15. Squamous cell carcinoma
16. Salivary gland neoplasm
17. White sponge nevus
18. Traumatic neuroma
19. Benign mesenchymal lesion
20. Rarities

GINGIVA AND ALVEOLAR MUCOSA
Anatomic Structures

1. Retrocuspid papillae
2. Frenum attachments

The oral mucous membrane continues from the vestibular sulcus over the tooth-supporting bone. This portion of the oral mucosa may be divided into (1) the alveolar mucosa, which is the zone adjacent to the vestibule, and (2) the zone adjacent to the teeth, which is the gingiva. The gingiva may be subdivided into the attached gingiva and the free gingiva. The surface of the attached gingiva is generally stippled in healthy patients, although the degree of stippling varies. The free gingival margins and borders of the interdental papillae are smooth. The alveolar mucosa is more delicate in texture, more mobile, and darker red than the gingiva because it has a greater vascular supply and because the covering epithelium is nonkeratinized. The alveolar mucosa, unlike the stippled gingival mucosa, is smooth. The normal color of the attached and free gingivae is pink and white, but again, darker pigmentation may be observed in persons of the dark-skinned races. Normally, no minor salivary glands are present in the gingiva. Consequently the clinician would rank a salivary gland lesion of the gingiva low in the list of likely diagnoses.

Common Lesions

1. Gingivitis
   a. Localized (localized with periodontitis)
      (1) Related to poor oral hygiene
          (a) Microorganisms
          (b) Calculus
          (c) Food impaction
      (2) Related to restorations or appliances
      (3) Related to mouth-breathing
      (4) Related to tooth alignment
      (5) Related to drugs or chemicals
   b. Generalized (generalized with periodontitis)
      (1) Nonspecific (related to poor oral hygiene and plaque)
      (2) Acute necrotizing ulcerative gingivitis
      (3) Related to nutrition (scurvy)
      (4) Related to drugs (phenytoin [Dilantin])
      (5) Hormonal (pregnancy, diabetes, endocrine dysfunctions)
      (6) Related to allergy
      (7) Hereditary (fibromatosis gingivae, although not always hereditary)
      (8) Related to psychotic phenomenon
      (9) Specific granulomatous disease
      (10) Neoplastic (leukemia)
      (11) Desquamative gingivitis and vesiculobullous diseases
2. Torus and exostosis
3. Amalgam tattoo
4. Recurrent herpes
5. Inflammatory hyperplasia (pyogenic granuloma, fibrous hyperplasia or fibroma, peripheral giant cell granuloma)
6. Periodontal abscess
7. Periapical abscess
8. Parulis
9. Eruption cyst, dental lamina cyst, or gingival cyst
10. Leukoplakia, erythroleukoplakia, or erythroplakia
11. Squamous cell carcinoma
12. Congenital epulis
13. Rarities

PALATE (HARD AND SOFT)
Anatomic Structures

1. Palatine midline raphe
2. Palatine papilla
3. Ruga
4. Fovea palatinae
5. Small nodules of tonsillar tissue

The mucous membrane covering the anterior hard palate is orthokeratinized and firmly attached to the underlying bone. On the posterior hard palate lateral to the raphe, the submucosa contains numerous nerves, blood vessels, and mucous salivary glands. Thus the majority of minor salivary gland tumors arise here. These areas may be soft on palpation because of the presence of fat and mucous glands. The hard palate is normally light pink but may be bluish-gray. The soft palate begins posterior to an imaginary line running laterally near the fovea palatinae, which are openings for the common ducts of groups of minor salivary glands in this region. The soft palate extends posteriorly into a thick pendant of mucous membrane known as the *uvula*. This mucosa of the soft palate is thin and nonkeratinized. The mucosa is quite vascular and may give a slightly darker red color to the soft palate than seen in the hard palate. There is considerable fat tissue in the soft palate, and if this tissue is prominent, the mucosa may become pale yellow. The texture is generally smooth but punctuated by the openings from numerous salivary glands. Again, as with the posterior lateral aspect of the hard palate, these mucous salivary glands may lead to occasional salivary gland tumors.

Common Lesions

1. Torus
2. Draining sinus from periapical abscess
3. Traumatic ulcer
4. Nicotine stomatitis
5. Candidiasis
6. Inflammatory papillary hyperplasia
7. Herpes (hard palate)
8. Recurrent aphthous ulcer (soft palate)
9. Minor salivary gland tumor (posterior hard palate and soft palate)
10. Cleft palate or bifid uvula
11. Leukoplakia, speckled leukoplakia, or erythroplakia
12. Squamous cell carcinoma (soft palate)
13. Oroantral fistula
14. Median anterior maxillary cyst
15. Median palatine cyst
16. Exophytic bony lesions of the hard palate
17. Benign mesenchymal tumor
18. Necrotizing sialometaplasia
19. Atypical lymphoproliferative disease
20. Rarities

OROPHARYNX (FAUCES, PHARYNX, AND RETROMOLAR REGION)
Anatomic Structures

1. Retromolar pad
2. Pterygomandibular raphe
3. Tonsillar pillars
    a. Palatoglossal arch—anterior
    b. Palatopharyngeal arch—posterior
4. Tonsillar fossa
5. Posterior wall of pharynx
6. Waldeyer's tonsillar ring (adenoids, nasopharyngeal tonsils, pharyngeal bands, palatine tonsils, and lingual tonsils)

The oropharynx and fauces show remarkable variation in size and form. The amount of lymphoid tissue in Waldeyer's tonsillar ring and the size of this tissue varies among people and from time to time in the same person. Lymphoid tissue not only enlarges in response to problems such as infections, but also tends to gradually decrease in size with age. The mucosal surface of this area is normally soft, moist, and smooth, with small elevations that represent the scattered aggregates of lymphoid tissue seen in this location. The mucosa is normally bright pink because of the prominent vascularity. Vascular dilatation may give the mucosa a red appearance.

Common Lesions

1. Nonspecific viral inflammatory disease
2. Nonspecific bacterial inflammatory disease
3. Enlarged tonsils
4. Recurrent aphthous ulcer
5. Traumatic ulcer
6. Inflammatory fibrous hyperplasia or fibroma
7. Leukoplakia, speckled leukoplakia, or erythroplakia
8. Squamous cell carcinoma
9. Herpes
10. Herpangina
11. Pemphigus or other dermatologic disorders
12. Rarities

TONGUE (DORSAL AND LATERAL SURFACES)
Anatomic Structures

1. Fungiform papillae
2. Filiform papillae
3. Foliate papillae
4. Circumvallate papillae
5. Median sulcus
6. Terminal sulcus
7. Lingual tonsil tissue

The dorsal surface of the tongue has an oral mucous membrane that is thick and keratinized and that contains papillae, some of which bear taste buds. Mucous and serous glands are present, as is lymphoid tissue (lingual tonsil). Posteriorly there is rich innervation, and vascularity is prominent throughout the surface. The dorsal surface is fairly uniform in appearance, soft, and pinkish, and it shows little or no variation among races. The lateral border of the tongue usually shows a rather sharp contrast in texture and color to the dorsal and ventral surfaces. The color is normally a deeper red on the lateral aspect than on the dorsal surface.

Common Lesions

1. Geographic lesion
2. Fissured lesion
3. Traumatic ulcer
4. Recurrent aphthous ulcer
5. Inflammatory hyperplasia
6. Hemangioma
7. Leukoplakia, speckled leukoplakia, or erythroplakia
8. Median rhomboid glossitis—Candidal infection
9. Lichen planus
10. Herpes
11. Hyperplastic lingual tonsil
12. Hairy tongue
13. Bald tongue—vitamin, iron deficiency
14. Squamous cell carcinoma (lateral border)
15. Granular cell myoblastoma
16. Neurofibromatosis
17. Syphilis
18. Macroglossia—amyloid, hypothyroidism, angioneurotic edema
19. Lingual thyroid nodule
20. Rarities

TONGUE (VENTRAL SURFACE)
Anatomic Structure

1. Lingual frenum

The mucous membrane of the ventral surface of the tongue is thin and smooth. It is closely adherent to the musculature of the tongue. The normal color varies from red to pink. On this lingual surface the veins may be large and prominent, imparting a bluish color to the ventral surface.

Common Lesions

1. Lingual varix
2. Ankyloglossia
3. Traumatic ulcer
4. Leukoplakia, speckled leukoplakia, or erythroplakia
5. Squamous cell carcinoma
6. Benign mesenchymal tumor
7. Mucous retention phenomenon
8. Rarities

FLOOR OF THE MOUTH
Anatomic Structures

1. Sublingual folds or ridges (Sublingual glands and ducts of the submandibular glands cause these elevations.)
2. Sublingual caruncles (These papillae contain openings for the flow of saliva from Wharton's duct.)
3. Openings from the ducts of numerous minor salivary glands
4. Genial tubercles
5. Mylohyoid ridge

The oral mucosa of the floor of the mouth is nonkeratinized, soft, and smooth. The mucosa is normally pink in this location. Racial differences are nonexistent to minimal. The degrees of vascularity and prominence vary.

Common Lesions

1. Traumatic ulcer
2. Recurrent aphthous ulcer
3. Abscess
4. Leukoplakia, speckled leukoplakia, or erythroplakia
5. Mucous retention phenomenon (ranula)
6. Squamous cell carcinoma
7. Sialolithiasis and sialadenitis
8. Dermoid cyst
9. Salivary gland tumor
10. Lymphoepithelial cyst
11. Ludwig's angina
12. Rarities

PART V

ADDITIONAL SUBJECTS

CHAPTER 35

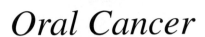

Oral Cancer

NORMAN K. WOOD
DANNY R. SAWYER

EPIDEMIOLOGY

Oral cancer is a serious problem in many countries. Not only does it account for significant mortality, but it is also responsible for extensive disfigurement, loss of function, behavioral changes, and financial and sociologic hardship. Frustration abounds because the cure rate is dismally low for such an accessible tumor. Oral cancer accounts for 2% of all human malignancies.[1]

Cure Rates

Approximately 29,490 new cases will be found and 8260 people will die of oral cancer in the United States in 1996.[1] Theoretically, 5-year survival rates (cure rates) would be 100% for promptly and properly treated precancers (preinvasion) such as carcinoma in situ. Five-year cure rates overall, for regional cases, for regional metastasis, and for distant involvement are 52%, 81%, 42%, and 18%, respectively.[1] These results are dismal, considering the fact that squamous cell carcinomas occur in the surface epithelium of the oral cavity and thus produce early, visible changes.

Reasons for Delayed Detection and Treatment

1. The public is generally unaware of oral cancer and its risk factors.
2. Approximately 50% of the public does not have routine dental or oral examinations and care.
3. Most early oral cancers are symptomless.
4. In the cancers that do produce symptoms, the symptoms are common to those produced by common dental diseases.
5. A significant number of oral clinicians may not perform a thorough systematic oral, face, and neck examination.
6. A significant number of oral clinicians are not able to recognize premalignant lesions or early oral cancer.
7. Unnecessary delays occur among lesion detection, diagnosis, and treatment.
8. Some practitioners treat oral cancer only occasionally. This usually means that the treatment received by the patient is inferior to that rendered by a practitioner who treats oral cancer on a regular basis.

ETIOLOGY

It is believed that the etiology of oral cancer is multifactorial and that the process is a multiple, stepwise one.[2] Clearly, change or damage to genetic material renders deoxyribonucleic acid and its associated processes unstable. Studies indicate that viruses such as herpes simplex and papillomavirus may play a role in this process.[2] The role of carcinogen promoters such as tobacco and alcohol have been well established.

Risk Factors

The following risk factors are recognized:
1. Smoking of cigarettes, cigars, and pipes
2. Use of smokeless tobacco: snuff and chewing tobacco
3. Drinking of 3 ounces or more of ethanol per day
4. Smoking and ethanol (highest risk)
5. Betel nut
6. Age over 40 years
7. High accumulation of x-irradiation over the years
8. Previous history of oral cancer
9. Infection with human immunodeficiency virus and other immunosuppression conditions
10. Ethnic or family history[3]
11. Certain oral sites (high-risk oval) (Fig. 35-1)
12. Mouthrinse with a significant alcohol content?
13. Chronic mechanical irritation?
14. Poor oral hygiene?[4]
15. Candidal infection?

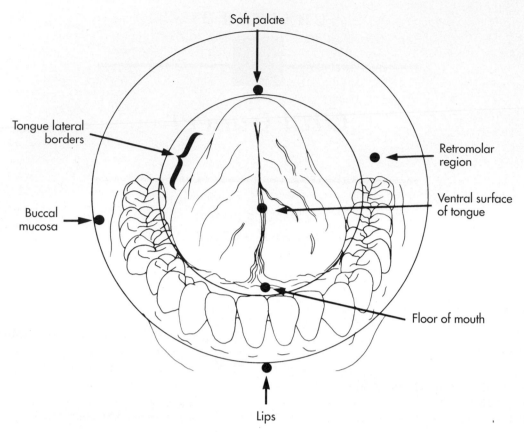

Fig. 35-1. High-risk oval identifies the most frequent sites of oral squamous cell carcinoma. (From Sawyer DR, Wood NK: Oral cancer: etiology, recognition and management, *Dent Clin North Am* 36(4):919–944, 1992.)

Smoking and ethanol The combination of smoking and alcohol provides a significantly higher risk than the use of each agent alone.[5-8] The retromolar region is the most common site associated with tobacco smoking, and it is followed by the floor of the mouth. The floor of the mouth is the most common site related to ethanol disuse.[9] Moller has related the significant increase in oral cancer in Denmark to the increasing level of alcohol consumption.[10]

Smokeless tobacco Smokeless tobacco is an addictive substance that produces many of the harmful effects of smoking tobacco. It damages the tissues of the mouth, produces serious systemic effects, and causes oral cancer.[11] Intraorally, it causes abrasion, staining of the teeth, bad breath, lessening of taste, unsightly expectorate, gingivitis, serious gingival recession, periodontitis, premalignant lesions, and oral and pharyngeal cancer. The oral lesions seen in smokeless tobacco use may be white lesions, red and white plaques, or raised white or red or white lesions. These may be precancerous, in situ carcinomas, squamous cell carcinomas, or verrucous carcinomas, predominantly occurring at the mucosal location where the quid is placed. Smokeless tobacco produces field cancerization,[12] as does tobacco smoke and alcohol. The latency period is longer, and changes are more gradual in comparing malignant change in smokeless tobacco

use and that in smoking.[13,14] Smokeless tobacco use has about half the risk of oral cancer than smoking does.[15] Nevertheless smokeless tobacco is no substitute for smoking. It is also important to recognize that malignancy can develop quickly through use of smokeless tobacco in individuals (even young people) who are very susceptible to cancer.[16]

Age Oral cancer has a much greater incidence in individuals over 40 years of age. From 1% to 3% of squamous cell carcinomas occur in patients under 40 years of age in the United States.[17] This percentage may be increasing.[17,18] At the other end of the spectrum, there is an increased incidence in elderly people who are on bed rest.[4]

Gender In this century the incidence of squamous cell carcinoma has favored male over female patients by 4 to 1. Recently, this has fallen to an approximate ratio of 2 to 1 or less.[18,19] There may be a concomitant decrease in male patients with an increase in female patients.[18] However, the male to female ratios vary from site to site in the oral cavity.[18] For instance, carcinoma of the gingiva or alveolus is 1.5 times as frequent in female patients.[21] There appears to be an increase in the incidence of carcinoma of the tongue in women, as well.[20] The increased incidence of cancer in female patients may relate to factors in addition to increased smoking and drinking.[20]

High-risk sites Fig 35-1 depicts the high-risk oval of the oral cavity. Basically the oral soft tissues that contact a donut placed over the raised tongue represent the high frequency sites of squamous cell carcinoma: lower lip, floor of the mouth, ventral surface and lateral borders of the tongue, retromolar regions, and soft palate. Tumors of the tongue and floor of the mouth are the most common site by far,[5,9] and the soft palate is next.[7] The clinician needs to examine these sites carefully and thoroughly during the systematic clinical examination.

Mouthrinses Several studies have raised concerns about the possible carcinogenic properties of mouthrinses with significant alcohol content.[22,23] According to the results of a survey by Blot, Winn, McLauglin, et al,[24] there is an increased risk for oral and oropharyngeal carcinoma with regular use of such mouthwashes. Risks were raised by 40% for male and 60% for female patients.[24] Although no cause-and-effect relationship has been firmly established, it seems prudent to exercise caution in advocating the use of mouthrinses with a high alcohol content.[25]

Field Cancerization

The concept of field cancerization was introduced first in 1953,[26] has proved true clinically, and has been verified by using cytologic markers in buccal smears.[27] This concept relates to the fact that whole oral surfaces and sometimes adjacent surfaces have been repeatedly exposed to carcinogens. As a result, several primary tumors may commence on these surfaces, usually in a sequential manner.[28] A second primary incidence is between 5.2% and 23%.[28-30] One study indicated that 30% of patients who continued tobacco use had a secondary tumor.[28] Therefore posttreatment examinations must include a check for new primary tumors, as well as for recurrences, and this includes examintion of the entire aerodigestive tract in high-risk patients.[31]

Premalignant Lesions and Predisposing Conditions

Some oral lesions show a propensity to become cancerous as time progresses. Some predisposing systemic conditions increase the risk of oral cancer.

Premalignant lesions

1. Erythroplakia (It has the highest risk of being or becoming malignant.) (Plate G)
2. Speckled leukoplakia and erythroleukoplakia (Plate G) (The red component is actually erythroplakia.)
3. Leukoplakia (homogeneous type) (Plate G) Possibly 1% to 7% of pure homogeneous types become malignant. These homogeneous white lesions may take on a red component with time and as such would be reclassified as the second lesion in the differential diagnosis, which would thus be assigned a markedly higher suspicion index. Mashberg, Morrissey, and Garfinkel[32] report that 95.8% of early asymptomatic squamous

cell carcinomas have erythroplakic components and that approximately 64% have white components.
4. Lichenoid dysplasia?[33,34]
5. Proliferative verrucous leukoplakia (Plate G)[35,36]
6. Candidal infection?

Predisposing conditions

1. Submucous fibrosis (common in India)
2. Immune deficiency states (e.g., acquired immunodeficiency syndrome)
3. Dyskeratosis congenita
4. Syphilitic glossitis (rare in industrialized countries)
5. Ethnic and familial history of oral cancer[3]
6. Atrophic erosive or bullous lichen planus
7. Diets low in fresh vegetables, fruits, and grains?

Symptoms and Signs of Oral Cancer

Cancerous lesions do not produce unique symptoms. The majority are asymptomatic in the early stages. Malignancies that have symptoms actually mimic the symptoms of lesions produced by common oral diseases. The box below details a list of these symptoms.

Signs A complete head, neck, and oral examination for oral cancer must be performed for each new patient and for patients during recall appointments. This examination can be performed in 60 seconds and easily becomes a habit. The box on p. 590, left, lists the clinical appearances of oral cancer. Acquaintance with these appearances is mandatory so that the appropriate suspicion index might be assigned when a precancerous or cancerous lesion is detected. Prompt recognition of the small

---

SYMPTOMS OF ORAL CANCER

- Lump or swelling
- Rough spot
- Crust
- Pain or tenderness
- Bleeding
- Change in bite
- Loose tooth or teeth
- Malfitting denture
- Neck lump or swelling
- Restriction of the tongue
- Change in jaw movement
- Dysgeusia (change in taste)
- Change in sensation (hyperesthesia, paresthesia, or anesthesia)
- Paresis or paralysis
- Diplopia
- Chronic cough
- Speech change
- Voice change
- Dysphagia (difficulty in swallowing)
- Symptoms of distant primary tumor

CLINICAL APPEARANCES OF ORAL CANCER (PLATES G TO J)

- Patch or plaque
  - Red (see Chapter 5)
  - Red and white (see Chapter 9)
  - White (see Chapter 8)
- Exophytic (rough) surface
  - Red (see Chapter 5)
  - White (see Chapter 8)
  - Pink (see Chapter 10)
  - Multicolored (see Chapter 10)
  - Ulcerated (see Chapter 10)
  - Nonulcerated (see Chapter 10)
- Ulcer (see Chapter 11)
- Crust (see Chapter 33)
- Bluish, brownish, or black lesion (see Chapter 12)
- Bleb

RADIOGRAPHIC APPEARANCE OF ORAL CANCER

- Radiolucency with ragged and vague borders (see Chapter 21)
- Bandlike widening of the periodontal ligament (see Chapter 21)
- Combined radiolucent-radiopaque lesion with a vague pattern (see Chapter 25)
- Radiopacity with vague borders (see Chapter 27)
- Sunburst appearance from the border of the bone, possibly combined with changes in the first three appearances (see Chapters 25 and 28)
- Onionskin appearance from the border of the bone, possibly combined with changes in the first three appearances (see Chapters 25 and 28)

---

early lesion gives the best opportunity for early treatment and the greatest chance for a cure. Large, advanced cancers are usually recognized readily.

Radiographic appearances Squamous cell carcinomas located close to the jawbones are prone to invade bone, and radiographs of the region reveal bony changes as soon as enough mineral change has occurred. Primary tumors of bone and metastatic tumors to bone have bony changes as well. Many of these changes are highly suggestive of malignancy. However, a few examples of slow-growing tumors or those that have been moderated by chemotherapy or x-irradiation may have smoothly contoured, well-defined margins and thus look more benign. The box above, right, contains a list of the radiographic appearances that malignancies can produce in bone. None of these is diagnostic, since other pathologic conditions can share these appearances.

Types of Intraoral Malignancies

The types of intraoral malignancies are listed with a quasiranking in the box on p. 591, left. Squamous cell carcinoma is the most common primary tumor by far in the older population, whereas Kaposi's sarcoma is the most frequent in individuals who have tested positive for the human immunodeficiency virus.

Perioral Malignancies

Dental clinicians must be aware and knowledgeable about perioral tumors (see box on p. 591, right, and Plates I and J). Primary oral carcinomas, such as squamous cell carcinoma, minor salivary gland tumors, and melanoma metastasizing to cervical lymph nodes, represent the most common malignancies in the neck. Cancers of the parotid and submaxillary salivary glands are the next most common. Lymphomas and tumors of the thyroid gland rank next. Basal cell carcinoma is the most common malignancy of

the face, and the majority occur superior to a line drawn from the tragus to the angle of the mouth.

Cancers of the maxillary sinus occur in an anatomic region intimately related to the oral cavity, so the dental clinician may be the first to identify their manifestations. This is particularly true when the tumor intrudes into the oral cavity, but the clinician should be alert to other questionable manifestations. Squamous cell carcinoma is the most common malignancy of the maxillary sinus, followed by adenocarcinoma.

Markers for Premalignant Lesions

The diagnosis of malignancy in individual cases is made by the pathologist observing certain pathognomonic cellular changes in the tissue. Likewise, certain examples of premalignant lesions show these changes within the stratified squamous epithelium lining the oral mucosa. Such findings prompt a recommendation to remove these premalignant lesions before they invade the underlying lamina propria and become frankly malignant. Many researchers have attempted to discover microscopic "indicators" or "markers" that would indicate leukoplakic lesions with a propensity to advance to frank malignancy if not treated.[36-41] A reliable early marker would be very helpful in identifying these lesions so that they could be promptly and aggressively eliminated.

Detection of Lesions

Early detection, prompt referral and treatment give the best chance for a cure. A systematic history and proper cancer screening examinations for all new patients, as well as all patients during periodic examinations, is the only way to ensure early detection. Some recommend the use of toluidine blue rinse to ensure that all small red lesions are found (see Chapter 2).

Exfoliative cytologic study works well for identifying erythroplakias (red plaques) and necrotic white candidal

TYPES OF INTRAORAL MALIGNANCIES

- Primary
  - Squamous cell carcinoma (90% to 95%)
  - Malignant salivary gland tumor
  - Mesenchymal, osteogenic sarcoma, chondrosarcoma, and others
  - Melanoma
  - Verrucous carcinoma
- Systemic
  - Metastatic carcinoma
  - Multiple myeloma
- Lymphoma and leukemia
- Kaposi's sarcoma

PERIORAL MALIGNANCIES

- Cervical lymph node metastasis
- Salivary cancers of the parotid and submandibular glands
- Basal cell carcinoma of the face
- Malignancy of the maxillary sinus

lesions but is not of use for keratotic white lesions or lesions situated beneath the epithelial surface.[42]

Excisional biopsy is the best diagnostic procedure for suspicious lesions and avoids the seeding of cells beyond the area of malignant involvement, which may occur with incisional biopsy of superficial lesions. For large lesions in which incisional biopsy is indicated, a large biopsy that includes the deep, invading margins would be taken if possible because squamous cell carcinomas are often composed of heterogeneous cell populations.[43]

Histopathology

Intraoral squamous cell carcinomas vary microscopically in degree of malignancy from low grade with excellent differentiation to anaplastic, high grade with poor or no differentiation. Varying degrees of anaplasia (malignancy) may be present in the same tumor.[43]

Lymph Node Metastasis

Intraoral carcinomas, melanomas, and some salivary malignancies spread to the regional cervical lymph nodes, of which the submaxillary, superficial, and deep cervical nodes are the most commonly affected. In some cases, contralateral nodes may be involved. Unfortunately, computed tomography and even physical examination under anesthesia for the presence of neck metastasis are poor diagnostic tools except with bulky metastatic deposits.[44] The following factors help in predicting whether lesions are likely to metastasize: poorly differentiated tumors,[45,46] poorly differentiated cells at deep invading margins of the tumor,[43,47-49] and lesions located in the posterior third of the tongue and oropharynx.[50] Possibly grading of deoxyribonucleic acid[51-53] and diminished desmosomal glycoprotein may be helpful.[54]

T1 and T2 lesions (see tumor classification, p. 592) in 60% of cases present with no clinical symptoms of neck lesions; however, 30% of these show tumor on elective neck dissection.[55] Deeper infiltrating tumors, staged as T3 and T4, have a high propensity for neck metastasis.[56]

Tumors of the tongue, followed in descending order by the floor of the mouth, lower gingiva, buccal mucosa, maxillary gingiva, hard palate, and lips, have the highest incidence of neck metastasis.

Distant metastasis Papac[57] reports that 30.7% of 169 patients with advanced cancers of the head and neck have distant metastasis. The most frequent organs involved, ranked in decreasing order are: lung, bone, liver, gastrointestinal tract, brain, skin, and kidney.[57] Some 74% of the metastases are found in patients who had T3 to T4 lesions; the remainder are from patients with T2 lesions.[57] Sun, Gin, Yu, and Wang[58] indicate that of 103 metastatic lung lesions from oral and maxillofacial tumors, 62% are salivary tumors, only 12% are squamous cell carcinomas, and 7.8% are melanomas. Computed tomography promotes accurate detection of pulmonary metastases in comparison with conventional chest radiographs.[59]

Early Detection

Early detection depends on high numbers of the population presenting for periodic systemic examinations of the oral cavity, head, and neck by informed and concerned clinicians. Early detection and treatment of oral cancer are mandatory for a high cure rate. Unfortunately, valuable time is lost in accomplishing both targets. The magnitude of the problem is highlighted by the following statistics. The average time delay between patients' first symptoms and a professional examination is 4 to 9 months.[60] The average time delay between detection and initiation of treatment is 5 to 6 months.[60] Another study indicates that the physician is better than the dentist at diagnosis and referral.[61] The ability to assign a high index of suspicion is a prerequisite for early diagnosis and referral.[62]

Triage of Lesions

The box on p. 592, left, gives definitive indications regarding the triage for detected lesions. If the low suspicion index lesion has not disappeared or responded significantly to treatment within 2 weeks, its suspicion index should be promptly upgraded. Moderate- and high-suspicion lesions call for immediate referral to a clinician or tumor board competent to manage oral cancer. The referring clinician must follow up to ensure that the patient keeps the appointment, to learn the final diagnosis, and to

---

TRIAGE OF LESIONS

- Low suspicion index: treat and follow to observe disappearance within 2 weeks; upgrade if appropriate
- Moderate suspicion index: refer immediately
- High suspicion index: refer immediately

---

be ready to help coordinate oral and dental care before, during, and after cancer treatment.

Management

Oral cancer team Oral cancer is best managed through a board or team. Such a team might consist of a dental hygienist, dentist, dental specialist, oncologists (surgeon, radiation specialist, chemotherapist), nutritionist, psychiatrist or psychologist, and social worker.

Tumor classification First, the lesion is staged using the TNM system.[62] The TNM classification has been used for many years and is described in the box at right. Microscopic evaluation of the degree of anaplasia at the deep invading borders is used to supplement this system.[46-48]

The location or site of the lesions is factored in to render a composite formula of *STNMP*, in which *S* means "site" and *P* means "histodifferentiation."[63] Prognosis on the basis of site deteriorates as the site moves posteriorly in the oral cavity.[51]

In addition to providing the team with information that contributes to a more accurate prognosis of an individual lesion, clinical staging provides a systematic basis for selecting the most appropriate mode of treatment.

Modes of treatment The modes of treatment of oral cancer, the various surgical modalities, and the chemotherapeutic agents used in oral cancer are located in the boxes on p. 593.

Treatment decisions The tumor board may decide that the particular lesion should be treated by surgical excision[65] with possibly a complete or partial neck dissection,[56,66] by presurgical or postsurgical radiation,[67-69] by radiation alone,[70,71] by chemotherapy,[72,73] or by a combination of these procedures.[74,75]

It is generally agreed that complete surgical excision of T1 and most T2 lesions without metastasis is the treatment of choice if the patient is a good surgical risk. Interstitial radiotherapy remains a viable alternative for these tumors.[76] Larger T2, T3, and T4 lesions are generally managed with a combined approach.[74,75] Computer-aided individual prognosis is a software package available to aid in anticipating results in individual cases.[77] The 5-year survival rate for patients with T1 and T2 lesions that show no clinical evidence of metastasis is approximately 81%, whereas that of patients with carcinomas that have metastasized regionally is approximately

---

TNM CLASSIFICATION

The T (primary tumor) categories are as follows:
- T1—Greatest diameter of primary tumor is 2 cm or less
- T2—Greatest diameter of primary tumor is more than 2 cm but no more than 4 cm
- T3—Greatest diameter of primary tumor is more than 4 cm
- T4—Massive tumor of more than 4 cm involves adjacent structures

The N (cervical lymph node) categories are as follows:
- N0—No clinically positive nodes
- N1—Single clinically positive homolateral node 3 cm or less in diameter
- N2—Single clinically positive homolateral node more than 3 cm but no more than 6 cm in diameter or multiple clinically positive homolateral nodes, none more than 6 cm in diameter
- N3—Massive homolateral node(s), bilateral nodes, or contralateral node(s)

The M (distant metastasis) categories are as follows:
- M0—No (known) distant metastasis
- M1—Distant metastasis present: specify site(s)

From Baker HW: Staging of cancer of the head and neck, oral cavity, pharynx, larynx and paranasal sinuses, *CA* 33(3):130-133, 1983.

42%. The overall 5-year survival rate for all oral cancer patients is approximately 52%.[1]

Coordinated patient care The members of the oral cancer team must work together in coordinating each aspect of patient care so that all the patient's needs are met. The dental hygienist and dentist play a major role in ensuring that preventive measures are in place before, during, and after cancer treatment to minimize the effects or complications of cancer treatment and to ensure optimal oral health[78] (see box on p. 593).

Prevention

Prevention is a top priority in oral cancer because of the high morbidity and low cure rates. The cancer societies and the dental community play important roles in this activity, but efforts need to be significantly increased. At the grass-roots and community levels, dental personnel must make individuals aware of the risks of oral cancer and encourage them to (1) discontinue *all* use of tobacco products, (2) lower their intake of alcoholic beverages to minimal amounts, and (3) visit health practitioners for periodic screening. Healthy diets should be recommended: high in fresh vegetables, fruits, and grains, with animal fat intake reduced to minimum. Good oral hygiene should be encouraged, and those with full dentures should be reminded that they need periodic examinations just like everyone

MODES OF CANCER TREATMENT

- Surgery
- Irradiation (external or interstitial)
- Chemotherapy (seldom used alone)
- Immunotherapy (in clinical trials)[64]
- Combinations of all of these

CHEMOTHERAPEUTIC AGENTS

- 5-Fluorouracil
- Cisplatin
- Methotrexate
- Cyclophosphamide
- Vinblastine
- Doxorubicin (Adriamycin)
- Bleomycin

SURGICAL MODALITIES FOR ORAL CANCER

- Blade
- Laser
- Electrosurgery
- Cryosurgery

MAJOR COMPLICATIONS OF ORAL CANCER TREATMENT

- Surgical defects with loss of esthetics and function
- Xerostomia and mucositis
- Radiation caries and dental infection
- Soft tissue infections (bacterial, viral, and fungal)
- Osteoradionecrosis

else. Mouthrinses with moderate to high alcohol content should be avoided. The local dental and dental hygiene societies can take the lead in this activity, or it may fall to the individual practitioners. This message can be given through speeches at local clubs or schools, or in radio and television spots. Newspaper columns can be dedicated to educating the public.

Every member of the dental office should be involved in patient education. Signs around the office, pamphlets, video tapes, and advice while conversing with patients are effective ways of informing the individual about the risks of oral cancer.

Dental practitioners are entirely responsible for obtaining and maintaining a comprehensive grasp of oral cancer. Those who are unaware of the signs and symptoms of oral cancer must take refresher courses. A continuing education course on oral cancer should be required every 5 years for relicensure. Licensed denturists should be subject to these same regulations.

Chemoprevention is being tried on leukoplakia in the form of topical bleomycin.[79] Systemically administered antioxidants such as retinoic acid, β-carotene, and vitamins C and E, have been administered in attempts to cause regression of leukoplakia.[80-82] However, recent findings indicate that chronic β-carotine users who smoke significantly increase their risk of lung cancer.[83] Further studies are needed to clarify these issues, and because results are inconclusive, excision remains the treatment of choice.[84]

The dental community has a responsibility for education, early detection, diagnosis, and referral of oral cancer to confreres competent in the treatment of oral cancer. Meeting these responsibilities generates a much higher cure rate and a marked reduction in the morbidity and mortality rates.

REFERENCES

1. American Cancer Society: *Cancer facts and figures,* Atlanta, 1996, The Society.
2. Scully C: Oncogenes, tumor suppressors and viruses in oral squamous cell carcinoma, *J Oral Pathol Med* 22:337-347, 1993.
3. Gorsky M, Littner, MM, Sukman Y, Begleiter A: The prevalence of oral cancer in relation to the ethnic origin of Israeli Jews, *Oral Surg* 78:408-411, 1994.
4. Natsume N, Suzaki T, Kawai T: Prevalence of oral cancer in bedridden elderly, *J Oral Maxillofac Surg* 53:864-865, 1995 (letter to the editor).
5. Llewelyn J, Mitchell R: Smoking, alcohol and oral cancer in South East Scotland: a 10-year experience, *Br J Oral Maxillofac Surg* 32:146-152, 1994.
6. Feldman J, Hazan M, Nagarajan M, et al: A case-control investigation of alcohol, tobacco and diet in head and neck cancer, *Prev Med* 4:444-463, 1975.
7. Mashberg A, Meyers H: Anatomical site and size of 222 early asymptomatic oral squamous cell carcinomas, *Cancer* 37:2149-2157, 1976.
8. Blot WJ, McLaughlin JK, Winn DM, et al: Smoking and drinking in relation to oral and pharyngeal cancer, *Cancer Res* 48:382-387, 1988.
9. Jovanovic A, Schulten EAJM, Kostense PJ, et al: Tobacco and alcohol related to the anatomical site of oral squamous cell carcinoma, *J Oral Pathol Med* 22:459-462, 1993.
10. Moller H: Changing incidence of cancer of the tongue, oral cavity, and pharynx in Denmark, *J Oral Pathol Med* 18:224-229, 1989.

11. Winn DM, Blot WJ, Shy CM, et al: Snuff dipping and oral cancer among women in the Southern United States, *N Engl J Med* 304:745-749, 1981.

12. Wray A, McGuirt WF: Smokeless tobacco usage associated with oral carcinoma: incidence, treatment, outcome, *Arch Otolaryngol Head Neck Surg* 119(9):929-933, 1993.

13. Grady D, Greene J, Daniels T, et al: Oral mucosal lesions found in smokeless tobacco users, *J Am Dent Assoc* 121:117-123, 1990.

14. Main J, Lecavalier D: Smokeless tobacco and oral disease: a review, *J Can Dent Assoc* 54:586-591, 1988.

15. Vigneswaran N, Tilashalski K, Rodu B, Cole P: Tobacco use and cancer: a reappraisal, *Oral Surg* 80:178-182, 1995.

16. Wood NK: Smokeless tobacco and oral cancer: summary, *Ill Dent J* 57:334-336, 1988.

17. Burzynski NJ, Flynn MB, Faller NM, Ragsdale TL: Squamous cell carcinoma of the upper aerodigestive tract in patients 40 years of age and younger, *Oral Surg* 74:404-408, 1992.

18. Krutchkoff DJ, Chen J, Eisenberg EE, Katz RV: Oral cancer: a survey of 566 cases from the University of Connecticut Oral Pathology Biopsy Service, 1975-1986, *Oral Surg* 70:192-198, 1990.

19. Boring C, Squires T, Tong T: Cancer statistics, 1992, *CA* 42:19-38, 1992.

20. Worall SF: Oral cancer incidence between 1971 and 1989, *Br J Oral Maxillofac Surg* 33:195-197, 1995 (letter to the editor).

21. Barasch A, Gota A, Krutchkoff DJ, Eisenberg E: Squamous cell carcinoma of the gingiva: a case analysis, *Oral Surg* 80:183-187, 1995.

22. Weaver A, Fleming SM, Smith DB: Mouthwash and oral cancer: carcinogenic or coincidence? *J Oral Surg* 37:250-253, 1979.

23. Bernstein ML: Oral mucosal white lesions associated with excessive use of Listerine mouthwash, *Oral Surg* 46:781-785, 1978.

24. Winn DM, Blot WJ, McLauglin JK, et al: Mouthwash and oral conditions in the risk of oral and pharyngeal cancer, *Cancer Res* 51:3044-3047, 1991.

25. Gagari E, Kabani S: Adverse effects of mouthwash use: a review, *Oral Surg* 80:432-439, 1995.

26. Slaughter DP, Southwick HW, Smejkal W: Field cancerization in oral stratified squamous epithelium, *Cancer* 6:963-968, 1953.

27. Ogden GR, Cowpe JG, Green MW: Evidence of field change in oral cancer, *Br J Oral Maxillofac Surg* 28:390-392, 1990.

28. Silverman S, Greenspan D, Gorsky M: Tobacco usage in patients with head and neck carcinomas: a follow-up study on habit changes and second primary oral/pharyngeal cancers, *J Am Dent Assoc* 106:33-35, 1983.

29. Eckardt A: Clinical impact of synchronous and metachronous malignancies in patients with oral cancer, *Int J Oral Maxillofac* 22:282-284, 1993.

30. Ildstad ST, Bigelow ME, Remensynder JP: Intraoral cancer at Massachusetts General Hospital: squamous cell carcinoma of the floor of the mouth, *Ann Surg* 197:34-41, 1983.

31. Hays GL, Lippman SM, Flaitz CM, et al: Co-carcinogenesis and field cancerization: oral lesions offer first signs, *J Am Dent Assoc* 126:47-51, 1995.

32. Mashberg A, Morrissey JB, Garfinkel L: A study of the appearance of early asymptomatic oral squamous cell carcinoma, *Cancer* 32:1436-1445, 1973.

33. Eisenberg E, Krutchkoff DJ: Lichenoid lesions of oral mucosa: diagnostic criteria and their importance in the alleged relationship to oral cancer, *Oral Surg* 73:699-704, 1992.

34. Lovas JGL, Harsanyi BB, Elbeneidy AK: Oral lichenoid dysplasia: a clinical pathologic analysis, *Oral Surg* 68:57-63, 1989.

35. Hansen LS, Olson JA, Silverman S: Proliferative verrucous leukoplakia: a long-term study of thirty patients, *Oral Surg* 60:285-298, 1985.

36. Kahn MA, Dockter ME, Hermann-Petrin JM: Proliferative verrucous leukoplakia: four cases with flow cytometric analysis, *Oral Surg* 78:469-475, 1994.

37. Scully C, Burkhardt A: Tissue markers of potentially malignant oral epithelial lesions, *J Oral Pathol Med* 22:246-256, 1993.

38. Girod SC, Krueger G, Pape H-D: p^{53} ki^{67} expression in preneoplastic and neoplastic lesions of the oral mucosa, *Int J Oral Maxillofac Surg* 22:285-288, 1993.

39. Vigneswaron N, Peters KP, Hornstein OP, Haneke E: Comparison of cytokeratin, filaggrin and involucrin profiles in oral leukoplakias and squamous carcinomas, *J Oral Pathol Med* 18:377-390, 1989.

40. Warnakulasuriya KAAS, Johnson NW: Expression of p^{53} mutant nuclear phosphoprotein in oral carcinoma and potentially malignant oral lesions, *J Oral Pathol Med* 21:404-408, 1992.

41. Lumerman H, Freedman P, Kerpel S: Oral epithelial dysplasia and the development of invasive squamous cell carcinoma, *Oral Surg* 79:321-329, 1995.

42. Bernstein ML, Miller RL: Oral exfoliative cytology, *J Am Dent Assoc* 96:625-629, 1978.

43. Byrne M, Koppany HS, Lilleng R, et al: New malignancy grading is a better prognostic indicator than Broders grading in oral squamous cell carcinomas, *J Oral Pathol Med* 18:432-437, 1989.

44. Woolgar JA, Beirne JC, Vaughan ED, et al: Correlation of histopathologic findings with clinical and radiologic assessments of cervical lymph-node metastasis in oral cancer, *Int J Oral Maxillofac Surg* 24:30-37, 1995.

45. Shear M, Hawkins DM, Farr HW: The prediction of lymph node metastasis from oral squamous cell carcinoma, *Cancer* 37(4):1901-1907, 1976.

46. Bouquot JE, Weiland LH, Kurland LT: Leukoplakia and carcinoma in situ synchronously associated with invasive oral/oral pharyngeal carcinoma in Rochester, Min, 1935-1984, *Oral Surg* 65:199-207, 1988.

47. Bryne M: Prognostic value of various molecular and cellular features in oral squamous cell carcinomas: a review, *J Oral Pathol Med* 20:413-420, 1991.

48. Anneroth G, Batsakis J, Luna M: Review of the literature and a recommended system of malignancy grading in oral squamous cell carcinomas, *Scand J Dent Res* 95:229-249, 1987.

49. Shingaki S, Suzuki I, Nakajima T, Kawasaki T: Evaluation of histopathologic parameters in predicting cervical lymph node metastasis of oral and oropharyngeal carcinomas, *Oral Surg* 66:683-688, 1988.

50. Urist MM, O'Brien CJ, Soorg SJ, et al: Squamous cell carcinoma of the buccal mucosa: analysis of prognostic factors, *Am J Surg* 154:411-414, 1987.

51. Chatelain R, Hoffmeister B, Harle F, et al: DNA grading of oral squamous carcinomas: a preliminary report, *Int J Oral Maxillofac Surg* 18:43-46, 1989.

52. Saito T, Sato J, Satoh A, et al: Flow cytometric analysis of nuclear DNA content in tongue squamous cell carcinoma: relation to cervical lymph node metastasis, *Int J Oral Maxillofac Surg* 23:28-31, 1994.

53. Chen R-B, Katsuya S, Nomura T, Nakajima T: Flow cytometric analysis of squamous cell carcinomas of the oral cavity in relation to lymph node metastasis, *J Oral Maxillofac Surg* 52:397-401, 1993.

54. Harada T, Shinohara M, Nakamura S, et al: Immunohistochemical detection of desmosomes in oral squamous cell carcinoma: correlation with differentiation, mode of invasion, and metastatic potential, *Int J Oral Maxillofac Surg* 21:346-349, 1992.

55. Shah JP, Andersen PE: Evolving role of modifications in neck dissection for oral squamous cell carcinoma, *Br J Oral Maxillofac Surg* 33:3-8, 1995.

56. Crissman JD, Gluckman J, Whitley J, Quentelle D: Squamous cell carcinoma of the floor of the mouth, *Head Neck Surg* 3:2-7, 1980.

57. Papac RJ: Distant metastasis from head and neck cancer, *Cancer* 53:342-345, 1984.

58. Sun D-X, Jin Y-W, Yu Q, Wang P-Z: A radiologic study of pulmonary metastasis originating from oral and maxillofacial tumors, *Oral Surg* 73:633-637, 1992.

59. Sun D-X, Luo J-C, Liu D-H, et al: Computed tomography of pulmonary metastases from oral and maxillofacial tumors, *Oral Surg* 79:255-261, 1995.

60. Bruun JP: Time lapse by diagnosis of oral cancer, *Oral Surg* 42:139-149, 1976.

61. Schnetler JFC: Oral cancer diagnosis and delays in referral, *Br J Oral Maxillofac Surg* 30:210-213, 1992.

62. Baker HW: Staging of cancer of the head and neck: oral cavity, pharynx, larynx and paranasal sinuses, *CA* 33(3):130-133, 1983.

63. Langdon JD, Rapidis AD, Harvey PW, Patel MF: STNP: a new classification for oral cancer, *Br J Oral Surg* 15:49-54, 1977.

64. Fukazawa H, Ohashi Y, Sekiyama S, et al: Multidisciplinary treatment of head and neck cancer using BCG, OK-432 and GE-132 as biologic response modifiers, *Head Neck* 16:30-38, 1994.

65. Strong E: Surgical management of oral cancer, *Dent Clin North Am* 34:185-203, 1990.

66. Bier J, Schlums D, Metelmann H, et al: A comparison of radical and conservative neck dissection, *Int J Oral Maxillofac Surg* 22:102-107, 1993.

67. Nair MK, Sankaranarayanan R, Padmanabhan TK: Evaluation of the role of radiotherapy in the management of carcinoma of the buccal mucosa, *Cancer* 61:1326-1331, 1988.

68. Ampil F, Datta R, Shockley W: Adjuvant postoperative external beam radiotherapy in head and neck cancer, *J Oral Maxillofac Surg* 46:569-573, 1988.

69. Vikram B, Farr HW: Adjuvant radiation therapy in locally advanced head and neck cancer, *CA* 33(3):134-138, 1983.

70. Wang CC, Kelly J, August M, Donoff B: Early carcinoma of the oral cavity: a conservative approach with radiation therapy, *J Oral Maxillofac Surg* 53:687-690, 1995.

71. Parsai E, Ayyangar K, Bowman D, et al: 3D reconstruction of Ir-92 implant dosimetry for irradiating gingival carcinoma on the mandibular alveolar ridge, *Oral Surg* 79:787-792, 1995.

72. Bier J: Chemotherapy for squamous cell carcinomas of the head and neck: a reappraisal, *Int J Oral Maxillofac Surg* 19:232-234, 1990.

73. Amrein P: Current chemotherapy of head and neck cancer, *J Oral Maxillofac Surg* 49:864-870, 1991.

74. Olasz L, Szabo I, Horvath A: A combined treatment for advanced oral cavity cancers, *Cancer* 62:1267-1274, 1988.

75. Mohr CH, Bohndorf W, Carstens J, et al: Preoperative radiotherapy and radical surgery in comparison with radical surgery alone, *Int J Oral Maxillofac Surg* 23:140-148, 1994.

76. Podd TJ, Carton ATM, Barrie R, et al: Treatment of oral cancers using iridium[192] interstitial irradiation, *Br J Oral Maxillofac Surg* 32:207-213, 1994.

77. Platz H, Fries R, Hudec M: Computer-aided individual prognosis of squamous cell carcinomas of the lips, oral cavity and oropharynx, *Int J Oral Maxillofac Surg* 21:150-155, 1992.

78. National Institutes of Health: Consensus Development Conference statement: oral complications of cancer therapies: diagnosis, prevention and treatment, 7(7):17-19, 1989.

79. Epstein JB, Wong FLW, Millner A, Le ND: Topical bleomycin treatment of oral leukoplakia: a randomized double-blind clinical trial, *Head Neck* 16:539-544, 1994.

80. Hong WK, Endiocott J, Itri LM, et al: 13-*cis*-retinoic acid in the treatment of oral leukoplakia, *N Engl J Med* 315:1501-1505, 1986.

81. Lippman SM, Batsakis JG, Toth BB, et al: Comparison of low-dose isotretinoin with beta carotene to prevent oral carcinogenesis, *N Engl J Med* 328(1):15-20, 1993.

82. Kaugers GE, Silverman S Jr, Lovas GL, et al: A clinical trial of antioxidant supplements in the treatment of oral leukoplakia, *Oral Surg* 78:462-468, 1994.

83. Heinonen OP, Huttunen JK, Albanes D, et al: The effect of vitamin E and beta carotene on the incidence of lung cancer and other cancers in male smokers, *N Engl J Med* 330(15):1029-1035, 1994.

84. Kaugers G, Silverman S: The use of 13-*cis*-retinoic acid in the treatment of oral leukoplakia: short term observation, *Oral Surg* 79:264-265, 1995, (letter to the editor).

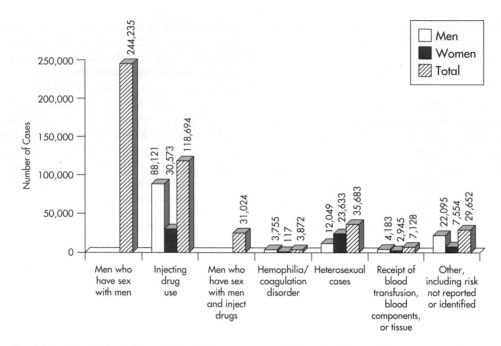

Fig. 36-1. Distribution of reported AIDS cases among adults and adolescents by exposure category as of Sept. 15, 1995. Please note that there are 4 people whose gender is unknown.

cells/µL or a CD4[+] T-cell percentage of total lymphocytes of less than 14. In addition, three clinical conditions have more recently been added to the AIDS surveillance case definition, bringing the total to 26. The three additions are pulmonary tuberculosis, recurrent pneumonia, and invasive cervical cancer.

Although the significance of the CD4[+] T-cell count should not be diminished, there have been patients with low CD4[+] T-cell counts and the symptoms of AIDS but without evidence of HIV infection.[27] This syndrome is being called *idiopathic CD4[+] T-lymphocytopenia.*[27]

COURSE OF THE DISEASE

After exposure and introduction of HIV into body tissues, a window period of 6 to 9 weeks ensues before the patient's blood becomes HIV-positive. During the latter part of the window period, the patient's serum tests positive to HIV antibody. HIV reaches high levels in the blood shortly after conversion but soon dips to low levels until late-stage disease.[7] Patients are extremely contagious during this first 60-day period. Using PCR assays, researchers have shown that high levels of HIV replication occur in lymph nodes and other lymphoid tissue such as the adenoids and tonsils.[28] This represents fivefold to tenfold greater frequency of infected cells in lymphoid tissue than in infected blood.[28] Clearly, lymph nodes serve as a major reservoir for infectious virus.[28]

A significant segment of early infected cases show no overt clinical illness at the beginning. However, 53% to 92.3% experience some influenza-like symptoms (higher in homosexual HIV seroconverters), whereas a smaller percentage (5% to 34%) experience acute retroviral syndrome.[29] Again, this percentage is probably higher in sexually transmitted infections than in IV drug users.[29] Acute retroviral syndrome is a mononucleosis-like syndrome with onset around the time of seroconversion.[29] Symptoms may include fever, night sweats, fatigue, weakness, sore throat, skin rash, weight loss, diarrhea, infection with herpes simplex virus, visual disorders, and generalized lymphadenopathy.[29]

The clinical manifestations disappear after about 4 to 6 weeks. These patients, along with those experiencing mild or no symptoms, continue on a mostly asymptomatic course until they develop AIDS 3 to 10 years later (average, 5 years). Patients who develop acute retroviral syndrome show several times more rapid progression to AIDS.[29] Median survival rates for adults generally are 11 months from the development of AIDS to death, whereas children have 62 months.[30]

A battle continues between HIV and the immune system from the time of exposure or invasion until the clinically quiet period. (It is thought that HIV attacks and destroys CD4 cells directly.) HIV multiplies prodigiously, and the immune system responds very well. Millions to billions of viruses and CD4 cells are destroyed daily.[28] It appears that the number of HIV and CD4 cells is somewhat depleted, but the immune response has beaten back HIV. Unfortunately, a few mutant strains of HIV survive and replicate swiftly during a brief recognition-delay period on the part of the immune system. However, the immune system soon prepares to fight against the mutant strain. This process probably repeats itself for several years, but gradually the continual development of mutants

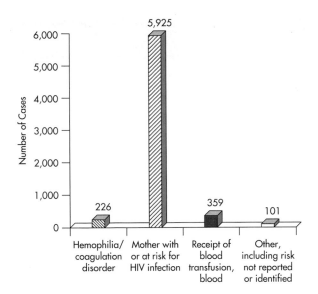

Fig. 36-2. Distribution of reported AIDS cases among children by exposure category as of Sept. 15, 1995. The term *children* refers to people under age 13 at time of diagnosis.

causes the manifestations of AIDS.[28,31] In this scenario, AIDS occurs because of the ability of HIV to readily undergo mutation rather than because of a primary failure on the part of the immune system. Accompanying this chronic course are high levels of CD4[+] cells in the blood and low levels of viral load in the blood. At this point CD4[+] cell levels begin to definitively decrease, symptoms ensue, and the viral load increases in the blood. CD4[+] cell total counts of less than 200/100 ml usually accompany severe symptoms of AIDS. Although there is some fluctuation of CD4[+] cell counts over the asymptomatic years, CD4[+] counts are considered to be dependable clinical prognostic markers in HIV infection.[32] Just recently, Mellors et al[33] reported that baseline blood viral load powerfully predicted survival, whereas CD4[+] counts did not.

Other schools of thought believe that HIV must affect the decrease in CD4 cells through indirect means.[34] In this case the binding of HIV to CD4 cells confuses the counting and genesis mechanism of the immune system, and increased proptosis (programmed cell death) of CD4 cells may occur as a result; perhaps, death of bystander CD4 cells occur.[34] Another theory suggests that lowered levels of CD4 blood cells occur as a result of a maldistribution caused by a sequestration of CD4 cells in damaged lymphoid tissue.[34] Yet another theory considers that HIV attacks the thymus gland (where CD4 cells are produced) to such a degree that there is a shutdown of CD4 cells, causing AIDS.[34]

Neither gender nor pregnancy appears to influence the course of HIV infection,[35] however, the occurrence of acute retroviral syndrome speeds up conversion to AIDS by a factor of 3.[29] Transmission by receptive anal intercourse[9] and transfusion products speeds the development of AIDS as well. Perinatal cases progress at a much slower pace than in adult cases.[30] Also, infection with HIV-2 alone shows a slower progression to AIDS than infection with HIV-1 or a dual infection with HIV-1 and HIV-2.[3]

Nonprogressors represent a small cohort of infected individuals who have not developed symptoms of AIDS, even after 12 to 15 years from seroconversion.[3] Nonprogressors have remarkably low levels of HIV in the blood and better neutralizing antibody responses, and viral isolates are attenuated for replicative ability.[3]

Patients progressing to early AIDS or AIDS-related complex experience some manifestations of full-blown AIDS. Details are summarized in *Morbidity and Mortality Weekly Report*[26] and include *Pneumocystis carinii* pneumonia, tuberculosis, diarrhea, many oral and cutaneous infections and tumors,[36] and permanent neurological defects (50% to 60% of cases[37]). A smaller percentage of transient neurologic defects has been observed as well.[38] The cause of death in full-blown AIDS may be difficult to attribute to a single cause. The most common serious events are: *P. carinii* pneumonia (45%), *Mycobacterium avium complex* (25%), wasting syndrome (25%), bacterial pneumonia (24%), cytomegaloviral infection (23%), and candidiasis (esophageal or pulmonary) (22%).[39] Significant gender and ethnic differences are found.[39]

ORAL MANIFESTATIONS OF AIDS

Characteristic oral infections represent some of the earliest manifestations of HIV infection, and some of these may be of prognostic significance in the development of AIDS. Some produce very serious discomfort and morbidity. The box on p. 600 presents a classification of oral lesions associated with HIV infection. Specific oral lesions and concurrent different oral lesions are indications of severe immunosuppression.[40,41] The predictive values of lesions indicating severe suppression, ranked with the highest are first, major aphthous ulcer, necrotic (ulcerative) periodontitis, Kaposi's sarcoma, long-standing herpes simplex infection, hairy leukoplakia, and xerostomia.[40]

Oral candidiasis and hairy leukoplakia are the most common lesions and thus the best prognosticators of the development of AIDS.[42,43] Some 48% of HIV-positive patients with candidiasis and 10% of those with hairy leukoplakia on initial examination were diagnosed with having AIDS within 1 year.[36] This holds true for any clinical subtype of candidiasis.[44] However, the frequency of incidence of lesions vary according to mode of transmission and between children and adults. For instance, homosexual and bisexual male AIDS patients are 20 times more likely to develop Kaposi's sarcoma than heterosexuals, IV drug users, or young children.[45] Fewer blacks and Hispanics than whites experience Kaposi's sarcoma.[39] Candidiasis is frequent in perinatal AIDS.[46] Apparently, white lesions of the tongue (including hairy leukoplakia) followed by candidiasis and noncandidal red lesions were the most common lesions in HIV-positive male homosexuals, whereas

CLASSIFICATION OF ORAL LESIONS ASSOCIATED WITH HIV INFECTION*

Lesions strongly associated with HIV infection

- Candidiasis
  - Erythematous
  - Pseudomembranous
- Hairy leukoplakia
- Kaposi's sarcoma
- Non-Hodgkin's lymphoma
- Periodontal disease
  - Linear gingival erythema
  - Necrotizing (ulcerative) gingivitis
  - Necrotizing (ulcerative) periodontitis

Lesions less commonly associated with HIV infection

- Bacterial infections
  - *Mycobacterium avium-intracellulare*
  - *Mycobacterium tuberculosis*
- Melanotic hyperpigmentation
- Necrotizing (ulcerative) stomatitis
- Salivary gland disease
  - Xerostomia
  - Unilateral or bilateral swelling of major glands
- Thrombocytopenic purpura
- Ulceration (not otherwise specified)
- Viral infections
  - Herpes simplex
  - Human papillomavirus
    - Condyloma acuminatum
    - Focal epithelial hyperplasia
    - Verruca vulgaris

- Varicella-zoster virus
  - Herpes zoster
  - Varicella

Lesions seen in HIV infection

- Bacterial infections
  - *Actinomyces israelii*
  - *Escherichia coli*
  - *Klebsiella pneumoniae*
- Cat-scratch disease
- Drug reactions
  - Erythema multiforme
  - Lichenoid reaction
  - Toxic epidermolysis
  - Ulcerative reaction
- Epithelioid (bacillary) angiomatosis
- Fungal infections
  - *Cryptococcus neoformans*
  - *Geotrichum candidum*
  - *Histoplasma capsulatum*
  - Mucoraceae
  - *Aspergillus flavus*
- Neurologic disturbances
  - Facial palsy
  - Trigeminal neuralgia
- Recurrent aphthous stomatitis
- Viral infections
  - Cytomegalovirus
  - Molluscum contagiosum

*Modified from Williams et al: Classification and diagnostic criteria for oral lesions in HIV infection, *J Oral Pathol Med* 22:289-91, 1993.

candidiasis followed by gingival marginal erythema were most common in HIV-positive IV drug users.[47] Approximately 40% of HIV-positive adults have some type of oral lesions,[41,42] whereas almost 30% of perinatal HIV-positive children experience oral lesions.[46] Almost all AIDS patients (90% to almost 100%) have oral lesions at some time during the course of HIV infection.[36,41] In the following section, oral lesions are discussed in order of frequency in the HIV-positive and AIDS population.

Cervical Lymphadenopathy

Although not in the oral cavity per se, the cervical lymph node groups must be systematically palpated during each patient examination. Almost all normal adults have enlarged cervical nodes, usually in the submandibular space; these enlarged nodes represent benign lymphoid hyperplasia.

One of the earliest signs of HIV infection is the development of generalized tender lymphadenopathy (Fig. 36-3) in as high as 70% of cases.[48] Other sources indicate a much higher percentage.[49] Although any and all regional groups may be involved, the head and neck region is the initial location in most cases.[49] Generalized tender lymphadenopathy that is present for longer than 3 months and involves two or more extrainguinal sites is classed as persistent generalized lymphadenopathy.[48] In most instances, the lymph node swelling is related to the intensity of the infection-host battle and activated immune response. Lymphoma should be ruled out if a mass becomes especially prominent.[48]

Candidiasis

Candidiasis is discussed at length in Chapter 5. Described as being "a disease of the diseased," it represents the most common opportunistic oral fungal infection in HIV-positive individuals (Fig. 36-4).[50] *Candida* organisms have been shown by culture to be present in the oral cavities more often in these patients than in normal patients: 75% to 93.4% vs 57.4% to 68%.[51,52] On average, the HIV-infected individual has a higher oral candidal load as well.[53] Some 52% of HIV-infected individuals have candidal lesions in the early stages of infection.[52]

The majority of lesions are caused by *Candida albicans,* but other candidal species seem to be increasing, apparently

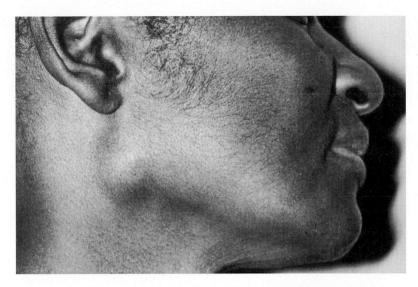

Fig. 36-3. Tender cervical lymphadenopathy in a patient with AIDS.

CLINICAL TYPES OF CANDIDIASIS

- Pseudomembranous/necrotic
- Atrophic or erythematous
- Hyperplastic
- Mucocutaneous
- Median rhomboid glossitis

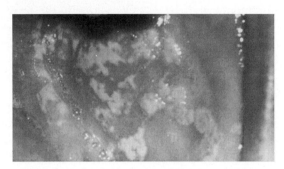

Fig. 36-4. Pseudomembranous candidiasis in an HIV-positive patient. (Courtesy J. Epstein, Vancouver, British Columbia, Canada.)

as a result of increased exposure to antifungal agents[36,49] and the development of resistant strains.[49,54-56]

All five clinical types of candidiasis (see Chapter 5) occur in HIV-infected individuals (see box above) (Fig. 36-4, Plate E). No clinical form of candidiasis appears to be a more serious prognosticator for the development of AIDS than another clinical form.[44] HIV-related candidiasis is less likely to develop in patients with dentures.[50]

The treatment of candidiasis is discussed generally in Chapter 5. Treatment of HIV oral candidiasis raises special concerns because this yeast infection frequently recurs, it may become a deep-seated systemic infection, or lesions may become continuous when AIDS occurs. Such an extensive course highly favors the development of drug-resistant strains. In this vein, researchers suggest delaying the use of fluconazole to treat lesions or to maintain prophylaxis until advanced HIV disease, severe immunodeficiency, and severe oral candidiasis are present.[56-58] It would seem preferable then to commence with nystatin pastilles for oral candidal lesions in the earlier stages of HIV infection and, when cases become unresponsive, to switch to the imidazole troches (clotrimazole [Mycelex]) then on to imidazole parenteral tablets (ketoconazole [Nizoral]) if necessary, combining the use of troches and oral parenteral tablets. Triazoles and polyenes (nystatin, amphotericin B) to-

gether may not be effective because triazoles induce changes in the fungal membrane, which interferes with polyene binding.[55] Itraconazole, a newer antifungal triazole, can be inserted into the regimen when resistance is encountered.[55,56]

Fluconazole (Diflucan), parenteral tablets or IV administration, can then be used when lesions do not respond to these agents.[56-58] When lesions fail to respond to fluconazole, amphotericin B can be used intravenously for refractory cases; the clinician must weigh the very significant toxic effects of the drug against the seriousness of advanced systemic candidal infection. Gentian violet painted on the lesions and chlorhexidine mouthrinse can be effective prophylactically and also as useful supplemental treatment.[55]

Fungal culture and sensitivity tests with antifungegrams are helpful in identifying *Candida* and carious species, as well as microbe susceptibility, but the latter tests are not always clinically reliable.[56,58]

Hairy Leukoplakia

It appears that the Epstein-Barr virus is the causative agent in hairy leukoplakia.[49,59-62] Hairy leukoplakia is

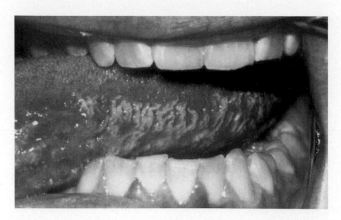

Fig. 36-5. Hairy leukoplakia on the lateral border of the tongue in a patient with AIDS. (Courtesy J. Epstein, Vancouver, British Columbia, Canada.)

seen in approximately 25% of adults with HIV[49,63] but is rare in children with HIV.[64] Occasionally the lesions of hairy leukoplakia are seen in other immunosuppressive diseases,[65-67] and a case has been reported in Behçet's syndrome.[68] In some instances, it can represent an isolated innocuous Epstein-Barr virus infection in the absence of immunosuppression.[69,70]

Clinically, hairy leukoplakia is an adherent asymptomatic white patch most often located on the lateral border of the tongue (Fig. 36-5, Plate E) and may extend on to the dorsal and ventral surfaces. The lesions on the tongue may be smooth or corrugated. Occasionally, lesions are located on the buccal mucosa. Microscopically the surface is composed of hyperparakeratin; corrugations and often thin tufts ("hairs") may be seen projecting from the surface. The epithelium is hyperplastic, and "balloon" cells are prominent in the prickle cell layer.

The definitive diagnosis is established by identifying the Epstein-Barr virus using exfoliative cytology with electron microscopy,[62,71] as well as in situ hybridization and the PCR.[72]

It is important to complete a differential diagnosis because several lesions, such as hyperplastic candidiasis, leukoplakia, lichen planus, white sponge nevus, severe leukoedema,[73] and proliferative verrucous leukoplakia, may mimic hairy leukoplakia. The persistence of lesions after local antifungal therapy is highly suggestive of hairy leukoplakia.[74]

Treatment is unnecessary; the condition disappears perhaps temporarily when zidovudine, acyclovir, or ganciclovir is administered.[49] A single topical application of podophyllum resin, 25% solution, induces a short-term resolution with minimal side effects.[75]

AIDS-Associated Gingival and Periodontal Disease

Conventional gingivitis and adult periodontitis are observed in HIV infection. Their clinical appearance may be exaggerated or altered because of the underlying immunosuppression, although recent reports indicate that periodontal health in these patients may be better than previously reported.[76] Specific forms of gingival and periodontal disease are associated with HIV infection. These forms include gingivitis with band-shaped and/or punctate erythema, acute necrotizing gingivitis, rapidly progressive periodontitis, periodontitis with soft tissue loss and irregular bone destruction, acute necrotizing periodontitis, and acute necrotizing stomatitis.[49,76-81]

Gingivitis with band-shaped and/or punctate erythema or diffuse erythema is very painful and is often associated with spontaneous bleeding on probing (Figs. 36-6 and 36-7 and Plate E). It does not appear to be associated with plaque, and no ulceration is present. The prevalence in reports of HIV-infected individuals varies from 4% to 49%.[76] The lesions most frequently occur in all quadrants, but sometimes they are limited to one or two teeth. The differential diagnosis includes atrophic or erosive lichen planus, mucous membrane pemphigoid, *G. candidum* infection, plasma cell gingivitis (hypersensitivity reactions), and thrombocytopenia.[76]

Microscopically an increased number of blood vessels but no inflammatory infiltrate has been seen.[79] There is evidence that *C. albicans* may play an etiologic role.[76] The microbiology of this type of gingivitis is as follows: *C. albicans, Porphyromonas gingivalis, Prevotella intermedia, Actinobacillus actinomycetemcomitans, Fusobacterium nucleatum,* and *Campylobacter rectus.*[76] This is consistent with that found in conventional periodontitis and different from that of conventional gingivitis (see Fig. 36-7). The removal of plaque and hard deposits and the institution of good oral home care are advised but usually do not improve this type of gingivitis, even when supplemented with povidone iodine irrigation 3 to 5 times daily.[80] Povidone iodine does relieve the considerable pain, however.[80] The condition shows significant improvement with the use of 0.12% chlorhexidine gluconate rinse twice daily for 3 months. Successful treatment of oral candidiasis seems to produce regression of the gingivitis.[76]

Acute necrotizing gingivitis of HIV infection is similar to conventional acute necrotizing gingivitis but is usually more intense, with fiery red and swollen gingiva and marginal necrosis covered with fibrous slough, resulting in the loss of interdental papillae.[76] The anterior gingiva is most commonly affected (Fig. 36-8, Plate E). Lesions are limited to the gingiva only. Some studies report a prevalence similar to that found in HIV-negative patients (1.8%), whereas others reported a prevalence of 5% to 11.2%.[76] Treatment is similar to that for the conventional condition: debridement by use of oxygenating rinses, prophylaxis, scaling, and optional administration of penicillin or metronidazole, depending on severity of the case. Chlorhexidine rinses are also helpful.

Some researchers indicate that they have not seen unique HIV-associated periodontics in their patients,[77] but others report positive findings.[76] HIV-associated peri-

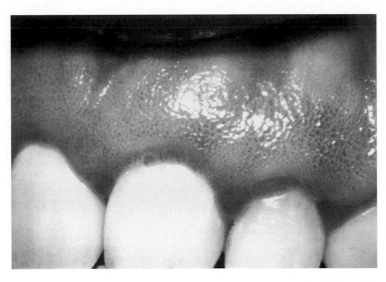

Fig. 36-6. HIV-associated gingivitis. Note the erythematous band along the free margin of the gingiva and the punctate erythema distributed over the gingival surface. (From Glick M: *Dental management of patients with HIV,* Carol Stream, Ill, 1994, Quintessence.)

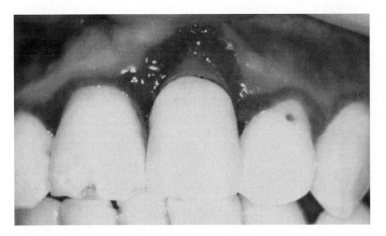

Fig. 36-7. HIV-associated gingivitis and periodontitis. Note erythematous band along the gingival margin and the periodontal defect. (Courtesy M. Glick, Philadelphia.)

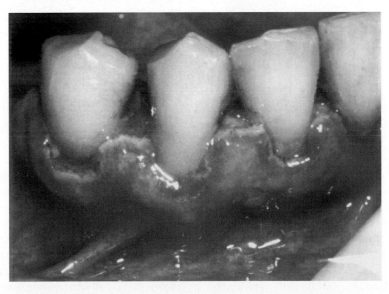

Fig. 36-8. HIV-associated acute necrotizing gingivitis. (Courtesy J. Guggenheimer, Pittsburgh.)

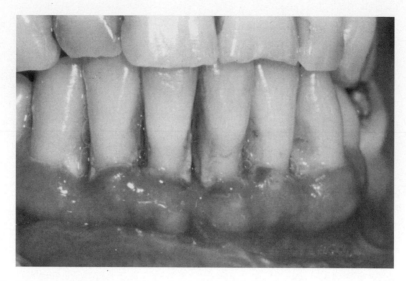

Fig. 36-9. HIV-associated periodontitis in the mandibular incisor region. (Courtesy J. Guggenheimer, Pittsburgh.)

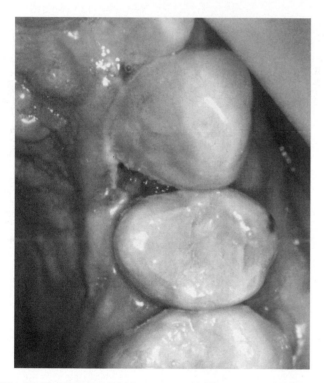

Fig. 36-10. HIV-associated acute necrotizing periodontitis. Note the necrosis of the lingual interdental papillae. The underlying bone is exposed in the lesion between the canine and premolar. (Courtesy M. Glick, Philadelphia.)

odontitis may follow HIV-associated gingivitis, but there may be a wide variation in features (Fig. 36-9). Rapidly progressive periodontitis is associated with poor oral hygiene and resembles conventional periodontitis but has a more rapid course. The reported prevalence varies widely (5% to 69%)[76] but may be higher in IV drug users.[76] Another type observed is periodontitis with soft tissue loss and irregular bone destruction, often seen in clean mouths.[76] Good oral home care and frequent preventive dental care are mandatory.

Acute necrotizing periodontitis is seen in approximately 1.8% of nonhomosexual HIV-infected men and in 8.4% of HIV-infected homosexuals.[78] The disease is characterized by localized ulcerations, necrosis of gingival tissue (Fig. 36-10) and exposure of underlying alveolar bone (Plate E).[78] Rapid resorption of alveolar bone and sequestration results.[78] Deep-seated severe pain and spontaneous bleeding are usually present.[78] *C. albicans* may contribute to the development of this lesion.[81] HIV-infected individuals with acute necrotizing periodontitis are 20.8 times more likely to have CD4[+] cell counts below 200 cells/mm^3 than their HIV-seropositive counterparts. A cumulative probability of death within 24 months of such a diagnosis has been reported.[78] This condition appears to be a predictable marker for deterioration of immune-response and disease progression.[78] The disease responds to local tissue debridement, metronidazole (1 g/day in four doses for 5 days), and rinses with chlorhexidine gluconate 0.12%.[78]

Acute necrotizing stomatitis of periodontal origin is characterized by rapid and extensive destruction of the gingiva into adjacent mucosa and bone[50,76] (Fig. 36-11) and may be life threatening.[76] Treatment is similar to that used for acute necrotizing periodontitis.[76]

Kaposi's Sarcoma

Kaposi's sarcoma is a multicentric endothelial neoplasm that represents the most common tumor found in HIV-positive individuals. Although a cause has not been established, it is believed to result from immunosuppression and a sexually transmissible infectious agent.[45,82] Possible agents may be a new human herpesvirus[45] or human papillomavirus.[82] Before AIDS, Kaposi's sarcoma was seen rarely, mostly in Mediterranean men over 50 years of age or

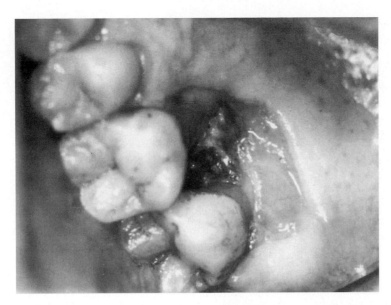

Fig. 36-11. HIV-associated acute necrotizing stomatitis of periodontal origin. (Courtesy M. Glick, Philadelphia.)

endemically in certain regions of Africa.[83] Currently, 12% to 25% of homosexual and bisexual men have this condition.[36,84] It is seen in only 2% of women with HIV infection, generally those sexually active with bisexual men.[36] Kaposi's sarcoma also occurs in patients with drug-induced immunosuppression[81] and in non-HIV patients who are sexually active.[84] HIV patients with this lesion also have oral lesions in 50% to 65% of cases.[83-85] Kaposi's sarcoma involves the skin, oral mucosa, lymph nodes, gastrointestinal tract, lung, liver, spleen,[84] and rarely bone,[83] but virtually can be found in every tissue and organ.[84]

Intraoral Kaposi's sarcoma is found most frequently in the palate,[84,85] gingiva, and tongue[84] (Fig. 36-12, Plate F). The early lesion appears as a reddish, bluish, or purple macule that later becomes nodular[84] and may reach a large size with surface ulceration and necrosis. Less superficial lesions may be colorless. Differential diagnosis lists include all reddish, bluish, purple, brownish, or black lesions (see Chapters 6 and 12), as well as multiple-lesion conditions such as bacillary angiomatosis and multiple hemangiomas.[40] A definitive diagnosis is based on biopsy. Two clinicopathologic types of oral Kaposi's sarcoma have been identified[86]: macular, small spindle cell lesions and nodular, infiltrative vascular lesions.

Treatment is indicated for cosmetic and functional reasons and for cumbersome lesions that have necrotic and ulcerative areas. Although chemotherapy can often control the multiple lesions, great care must be exercised in further suppressing the immune response in patients who may have very significant suppression already. Radiation therapy gives excellent reduction of oral Kaposi's sarcoma but may produce serious mucositis.[84] Fractionated dosages over a prolonged period minimize these complications. Surgical removal or debulking may improve

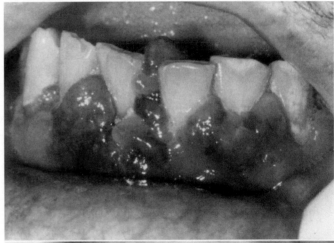

A

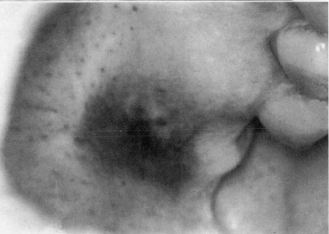

B

Fig. 36-12. Kaposi's sarcoma. **A,** Gingiva. **B,** Palate. (**A** courtesy J. Guggenheimer, Pittsburgh; **B** courtesy S. Fischman, Buffalo, NY.)

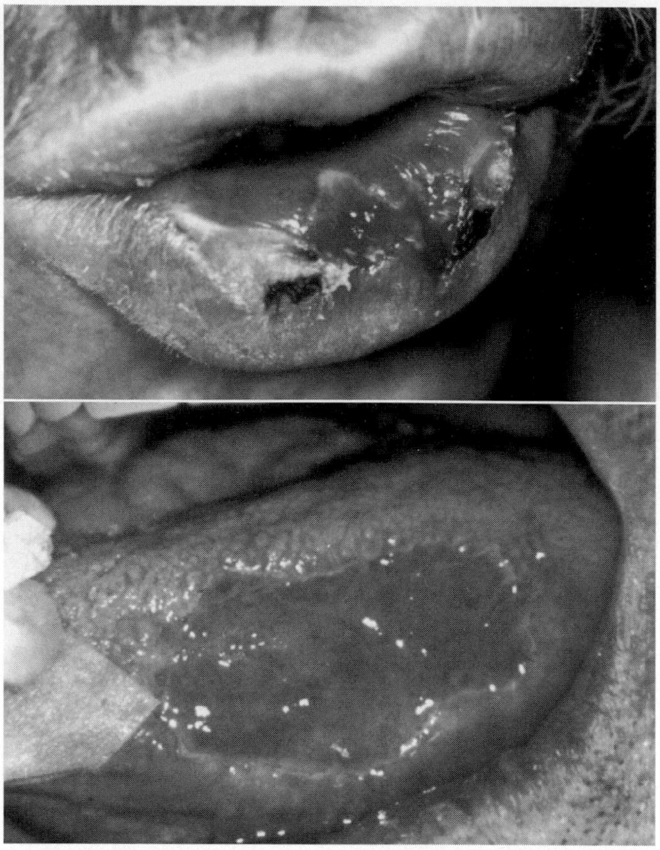

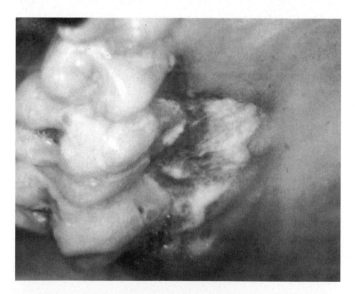

Fig. 36-13. HIV-associated herpes simplex. **A,** Lower lip. **B,** Lateral border of the tongue. (**A** courtesy J. Guggenheimer, Pittsburgh; **B,** courtesy M. Glick, Philadelphia.)

Fig. 36-14. HIV-associated herpes zoster. (Courtesy M. Glick Philadelphia.)

function and esthetics and allow better oral home care; a carbon-dioxide laser can be used also. Intralesional injection of vinblastine gives good results.[87,88] Injection of a sclerosing agent into the lesions has been reported to work well.[89]

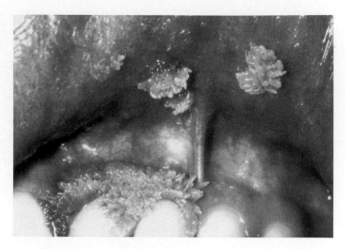

Fig. 36-15. HIV-associated condyloma acuminatum. Multiple lesions on the gingiva and vestibule. (Courtesy J. Guggenheimer, Pittsburgh.)

Many other oral lesions or conditions occur in HIV infection, some with a higher prevalence than in non-HIV individuals: viruses[90] such as herpes simplex[90-92] (Fig. 36-13, Plate F) and herpes zoster[36,93] (Fig. 36-14); condyloma acuminatum[36,94] (Fig. 36-15); increased pigmentation;[36,92] perioral molluscum contagiosum (Plate F);[95] bacterial glossitis; tuberculosis;[96-98] cytomegalovirus[99,100] (Fig. 36-16, Plate F); recurrent aphthous ulcers[101,102] (Fig. 36-17, Plate F); major aphthous ulcers[103,104] (Plate F); non-Hodgkin's lymphoma;[105] swelling of major salivary glands;[106-108] rare fungal infections;[109,110] sexually transmitted diseases; thrombocytopenia; lichenoid lesions;[111] squamous cell carcinoma;[112] xerostomia; and cancrum oris.[113] Several lesions may occur in combination.[114]

TREATMENT OF HIV INFECTION AND PROGNOSIS

Despite education, much research, and many treatment advances, infection with HIV and deaths from AIDS continue to increase worldwide. Education of the public about the nature of the disease, modes of transmission, and prevention has made some inroads. The campaign calling for safe-sex practices has met with some success among the American homosexual community, whereas the advice to IV drug users concerning reusing and sharing needles has yielded mixed results. Prevention is paramount, since drug regimens may slow the disease somewhat or delay the onset of severe symptoms; AIDS is almost invariably fatal.[115]

Recent research, which indicates that the immune system responds very well to the virus for many years until emerging mutant viruses (probably drug resistant) finally wear it down, tends to focus on the virus itself.[28,31] Combined drug therapy is the current trend, since good results have been shown in early trials.[3,116]

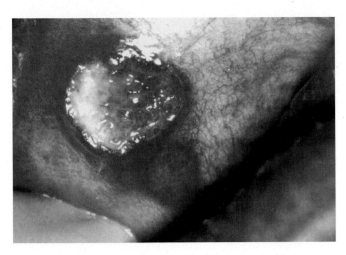

Fig. 36-16. HIV-associated cytomegaloviral lesions. (Courtesy M. Glick, Philadelphia.)

For instance, protease inhibitors in combination with reverse transcriptase inhibitors such as zidovudine (AZT), ZDV or didanosine (ddI), and zalcitabine (ddC) seem to delay the onset of drug-resistant strains. The treatment of and prophylactic measures for opportunistic infections are used with the main regimen and are tailored to individual cases. Current antiretroviral drugs produce moderately severe side effects, and early clinical benefits disappear with the emergence of drug-resistant viruses.[3] New directions in clinical research include protease inhibitors (such as ritonavir [Abbott] and indinavir [Merck]), combination antiretroviral drug therapy, gene therapy,[117] and immunomodulating agents.[3] Early studies indicate that patients receiving ritonavir or indinavir show markedly decreased viral loads, especially in those patients receiving drug combinations.[33] Nonprogressors are being studied intensively to learn why they are resistant to AIDS.

Vaccines

Development of a safe and effective HIV-1 vaccine has become an international priority, but formidable basic problems exist.[19] Unfortunately, there is no appropriate animal model for vaccine testing. Simian immunodeficiency virus infects primates such as the Rhesus monkey, but the disease differs markedly from HIV-1. The chimpanzee is the only animal that can be readily infected with HIV, but to date, manifestations of AIDS have not been produced.[118]

Another serious problem is the great number of genotypic variations of HIV-1 that have developed in vivo.[23,118] This generates a considerable variety of envelope protein sequences in HIV-infected patients. The first vaccines were based on single-envelope proteins, so full protection in clinical trials was not achieved.[118] Perhaps greater success will occur with a "cocktail" vaccine that includes multiple-envelope sequences from several distinct strains of HIV viruses.[118]

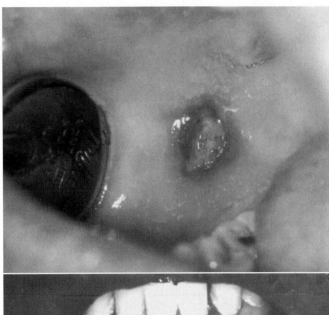

A

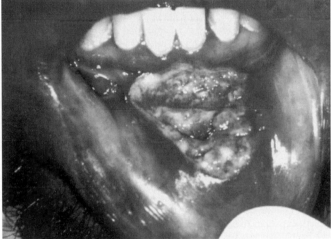

B

Fig. 36-17. HIV-associated recurrent aphthous ulcers: **A,** Minor, **B,** Major. (**A** from Glick M: *Dental management of patients with HIV,* Carol Stream, Ill, 1994, Quintessence; **B** courtesy M. Glick, Philadelphia.)

RISK OF HIV TRANSMISSION TO AND FROM THE DENTAL COMMUNITY

The risk of HIV transmission to dental health care workers is extremely small when proper dental management and universal precautions are practiced.[119] Although HIV has been identified in saliva, it appears that the levels are low.[1] Also, a protein, secretory leukocyte protease inhibitor, attaches to white blood cells and protects them from infection.[120] As of Sept. 30, 1993, 11,604 health care workers had AIDS. Among those for whom a specific occupation was identified, 309 were dental workers; of these, 234 have died.[121] Many of the 309 were in high-risk groups.[121] Needle-stick injuries and open wounds account for most of the cases of occupational exposure.

The possibility of transmission of blood-borne infections from dental health care workers to patients is very small. The facts surrounding the case of alleged transmission of HIV infection to five patients by a HIV-infected dentist in Florida have not been firmly established, so it is not clear whether the dentist transmitted the infection. Currently most states and provinces have established expert panels to determine the limitations of practice of HIV-infected health care workers.

Dental Management

Most of the dental care required by HIV patients can and should be provided in dental offices. Dental work that requires the services of a specialist may be referred to such professionals. Some cases may require hospitalization because of the patient's serious medical status.

REFERENCES

1. Liuzzi G, Bagnarelli P, Chirianni A, et al: Quantitation of HIV-1 genome copy number in semen and saliva, *AIDS* 9:651-653, 1995.
2. Toniolo A, Serra C, Conaldi PG, et al: Productive HIV-1 infection of normal human mammary epithelial cells, *AIDS* 9:859-866, 1995.
3. Chang L-Ji, Chen Y-MA, Chou C-CA: HIV 10 years later: where do we stand now? (Paper presented at the Tenth International Meeting, Yokohama, Japan, Aug 8, 1994) *J Biomed Sci* 2:1-11, 1995.
4. Sorvillo F, Kerndt P, Cheng K-J, et al: Emerging patterns of HIV transmission: the value of alternative surveillance methods, *AIDS* 9:625-629, 1995.
5. Porter SR, Scully C: HIV: the surgeon's perspective. I. Update of pathogenesis, epidemiology and management and risk of nosocomial transmission, *Br J Oral Maxillofac Surg* 32:222-230, 1994.
6. Centers for Disease Control: Heterosexually acquired AIDS: United States, 1993, *MMWR* 43:155-160, 1994.
7. Centers for Disease Control: Update: AIDS among women: United States, 1994, *MMWR* 44:81-84, 1995.
8. N'Gbichi J-M, De Cock KM, Batter V, et al: HIV status of female sex partners of men reactive to HIV-1, HIV-2 or both viruses in Abidjan, Côte d'Ivoire, *AIDS* 9:951-954, 1995.
9. Phair J, Jacobson L, Detels R, et al: AIDS occurring within 5 years of infection with HIV type 1: the multicenter AIDS Cohort Study, *J Acquir Immune Defic Syndr* 5:490-496, 1992.
10. Ghys PD, Diallo MO, Ettiègne-Traoté V, et al: Dual seroreactivity to HIV-1 and HIV-2 in female sex workers in Abidjan, Côte d'Ivoire, *AIDS* 9:855-958, 1995.
11. Center for Disease Control: Update: HIV-2 infection among blood and plasma donors: United States, June 1992–June 1995, *MMWR* 44:603-606,1995.
12. Tamalet C, Simon F, Dhiver C, et al: Autologous neutralizing antibodies and viral load in HIV-2 infected individuals, *AIDS* 9:90-91, 1995.
13. Albert J, Fiore J, Fenyo EM, et al: Biological phenotype of HIV-1 and transmission, *AIDS* 9:822-823, 1995.
14. Centers for Disease Control: Testing for antibodies to human immunodeficiency virus type 2 in the United States, *MMWR* 41(RR-12):1-8, 1992.

15. Imagawa DT, et al: Human immunodeficiency virus type I infection in homosexual men who remain seronegative for prolonged periods, *N Engl J Med* 320:1458-1462, 1989.
16. Food and Drug Administration: Recommendations for donor screening with a licensed test for HIV-1 antigen (memorandum to all registered blood and plasma establishments), Rockville, Md, 1992, US Department of Health and Human Services, Public Health Service, Food and Drug Administration, Center for Biologies Evaluation and Research.
17. Urquia M, Rodriguez-Archilla A, Gonzales-Moles MA, Ceballos A: Detection of anti-HIV antibodies in saliva, *J Oral Pathol Med* 22:153-156, 1993.
18. Frerichs RR, Eskes N, Htoon MT: Validity of three saliva assays for HIV antibodies, *J Acquir Immune Defic Syndr* 7:522-524, 1994.
19. Smith AJ, Walker DM: The origins of human immunodeficiency viruses: an update, *J Oral Pathol Med* 21:145-149, 1992.
20. Centers for Disease Control: World AIDS Day: December 1, 1994, *MMWR* 43:825, 1994.
21. Merson, M: *Global status of the HIV/AIDS epidemic and the response.* Lecture 7 presented at the Tenth Annual Conference on AIDS, Yokohama, Japan, Aug 8, 1994.
22. Centers for Disease Control: AIDS among racial/ethnic minorities: United States, 1993, *MMWR* 43:645-655, 1994.
23. Centers for Disease Control: Update: trends in AIDS among men who have sex with men: United States, 1989-1994, *MMWR* 44:401-404, 1995.
24. Centers for Disease Control: Update: Acquired Immunodeficiency Syndrome: United States, 1994, *MMWR* 44:64-66, 1995.
25. Kalish ML, Baldwin A, Raktham S, et al: The evolving molecular epidemiology of HIV-1 envelope subtypes in injecting drug users in Bangkok, Thailand: implications for HIV vaccine trials, *AIDS* 9:851-857, 1995.
26. Centers for Disease Control: 1993 revised classification system for HIV infection and expanded surveillance case definition for AIDS among adolescents and adults, *MMWR* 41(RR-17):1-10, 1992.
27. Smith DK, Neal JJ, Holmberg SD: Unexplained opportunistic infections and CD4+ T-lymphocytopenia without HIV infection: an investigation of cases in the United States, *N Engl J Med* 328:373-379, 1993.

28. Burroughs Welcome: New perspectives on HIV pathogenesis: viral replication is continuous throughout the course of disease, *AIDS* 9(7), 1995.
29. Dorrucci M, Rezza G, Vlahov D, et al: Clinical characteristics and prognostic values of acute retroviral syndrome among injecting drug users, *AIDS* 9:597-604, 1995.
30. Turner BJ, Eppes S, McKee LJ: A population based comparison of the clinical course of children and adults with AIDS, *AIDS* 9:65-72, 1995.
31. Nowak MA, McMichael AJ: How HIV defeats the immune system, *Sci Am* 273:58-65, 1995.
32. Savin CA, Mocroft A, Phillips AN: The use of CD4 counts as prognostic markers in HIV infection, *AIDS* 9:1205, 1995.
33. Cohen J: AIDS: research results on new AIDS drugs bring cautious optimism, *Science* 271:755-756, 1996.
34. Cohen J: AIDS research: researchers air alternative virus on how HIV kills cells, *Science* 269:1044-1045, 1995.
35. Brettle RP, Raab GM, Ross A, et al: HIV infection in women: immunologic markers and the influence of pregnancy, *AIDS* 9:1177-1184, 1995.
36. Jewell ME, Sweet DE: Oral and dermatologic manifestations of HIV infection, *Postgrad Med* 96:105-116, 1995.
37. Ficarra G: Oral lesions of iatrogenic and undefined etiology and neurologic disorders associated with HIV infection, *Oral Surg* 73:201-211, 1992.
38. Bailey GG, Mandal BK: Recurrent transient neurological deficits in advanced HIV infection, *AIDS* 9:709-712, 1995.
39. Chan ISF, Neaton JD, Saravolatz LD, et al: Frequencies of opportunistic diseases prior to death among HIV-infected persons, *AIDS* 9:1145-1151, 1995.
40. Glick M, Muzyka BC, Lurie D, Salkin LM: Oral manifestations associated with HIV-related disease as markers for immune suppression and AIDS, *Oral Surg* 77:344-349, 1994.
41. Barone R, Ficarra G, Gagliotti D, et al: Prevalence of oral lesions among HIV-infected intravenous drug abusers and other risk groups, *Oral Surg* 69:169-173, 1990.
42. Moniaci D, Greco D, Flecchi G, et al: Epidemiology, clinical features and prognostic value of HIV-1 related oral lesions, *J Oral Pathol Med* 19:477-481, 1990.

43. Gillespie G, Mariño R: Oral manifestations of HIV infection: a Panamerican perspective, *J Oral Pathol Med* 22:2-7, 1993.
44. Nielsen H, Bentsen KD, Højtred L, et al: Oral candidiasis and immune status of HIV-infected patients, *J Oral Pathol Med* 23:140-143, 1994.
45. Chang Y, Cesarman E, Pessin MS, et al: Identification of herpes virus–like DNA sequences in AIDS-associated Kaposi's sarcoma, *Science* 266:1868-1869, 1994.
46. Moniaci D, Cavallari M, Greco D, et al: Oral lesions in children born to HIV-1 positive women, *J Oral Pathol Med* 22:8-11, 1993.
47. Lamster IB, Begg MD, Mitchell-Lewis D, et al: Oral manifestations of HIV infection in homosexual men and intravenous drug users, *Oral Surg* 78:163-174, 1994.
48. Neville BW, Damm DD, Allen CM, Bouquot JE: *Oral and maxillofacial pathology,* Philadelphia, 1994, WB Saunders.
49. Porter S, Scully C: HIV: The surgeon's perspective. II. Diagnosis and management of non-malignant oral manifestations, *Br J Oral Maxillofac Surg* 32:231-240, 1994.
50. McCarthy GM: Host factors associated with HIV-related oral candidiasis: a review, *Oral Surg* 73:181-186, 1992.
51. Hester C, Hauman J, Medsci B, et al: Oral carriage of *Candida* in healthy and HIV-seropositive persons, *Oral Surg* 76:570-572, 1993.
52. Felix DH, Wray D: The prevalence of oral candidiasis in HIV-infected individuals and dental attenders in Edinburgh, *J Oral Pathol Med* 22:418-420, 1993.
53. Tylenda CA, Larsen J, Yeh C-K, et al: High levels of oral yeasts in early HIV-1 infection, *J Oral Pathol Med* 18:520-524, 1989.
54. Fetter A, Partisoni M, Koenig H, et al: Asymptomatic Candida carriage in HIV-infection: frequency and predisposing factors, *J Oral Pathol Med* 22:57-59, 1993.
55. Greenspan D: Treatment of oral candidiasis in HIV infection, *Oral Surg* 78:211-215, 1994.
56. Powderly WG: Resistant candidiasis, *AIDS Res Hum Retroviruses* 10:925-929, 1994.
57. Dios PD, Hermida AO, Alvarez CM, et al: Correspondence: fluconazole-resistant oral candidiasis in HIV-infected patients, *AIDS* 9:809-824, 1995.
58. Dios PD, Alvarez JA, Feijoo JF, Ferreiro MC: Fluconazole response patterns in HIV-infected patients with oropharyngeal candidiasis, *Oral Surg* 79:170-174, 1995.
59. Corso B, Eversole LR, Hutt-Fletcher L: Hairy leukoplakia: Epstein-Barr virus receptors on oral keratinocyte plasma membranes, *Oral Surg* 67:416-421, 1989.
60. Mabruk MJEMF: Detection of Epstein-Barr virus DNA in tongue tissues from AIDS autopsies without clinical evidence of oral hairy leukoplakia, *J Oral Pathol Med* 24:109-112, 1995.
61. Felix DH, Jalal H, Cubie HA, et al: Detection of Epstein-Barr virus and human papillomavirus type 16 DNA in hairy leukoplakia by *in situ* hybridization and the polymerase chain reaction, *J Oral Pathol Med* 22:277-281, 1993.

62. Epstein JB, Fatahzadeh M, Matisic J, Anderson G: Exfoliative cytology and election microscopy in the diagnosis of hairy leukoplakia, *Oral Surg* 79:564-569, 1995.
63. Reichart PA, Langford A, Gelderblom HR, et al: Oral hairy leukoplakia: observations in 95 cases and review of the literature, *J Oral Pathol Med* 18:410-415, 1989.
64. Laskaris G, Laskaris M, Theudoridou M: Oral hairy leukoplakia in a child with AIDS, *Oral Surg* 79:570-571, 1995.
65. Greenspan D, Greenspan JS: Oral manifestations of human immunodeficiency virus infection, *Dent Clin North Am* 37:21-32, 1993.
66. Syrjänen LP, Happonen R-P, Niemela M: Oral hairy leukoplakia is not a spcific sign of HIV-infection but related to immunosuppression in general, *J Oral Pathol Med* 18:28-31, 1989.
67. King GN, Healy CM, Glover MT, et al: Prevalence and risk factors associated with leukoplakia, hairy leukoplakia, erythematous candidiasis and gingival hyperplasia in renal transplant patients, *Oral Surg* 78:718-726, 1994.
68. Schiødt M, Nørgaard T, Greenspan JS: Oral hairy leukoplakia in an HIV-negative woman with Behçet's syndrome, *Oral Surg* 79:53-56, 1995.
69. Lozada-Nur F, Robinson J, Regezi JA: Oral hairy leukoplakia in nonimmunosuppressed patients: report of four cases, *Oral Surg* 78:599-602, 1994.
70. Eisenberg E, Krutchkoff D, Yamase H: Incidental oral hairy leukoplakia in immunocompetent persons: report of two cases, *Oral Surg* 74:332-333, 1992.
71. Kratochvil FJ, Riordan GP, Auclair PL, et al: Diagnosis of oral hairy leukoplakia by ultrastructural examination of exfoliative cytologic specimens, *Oral Surg* 70:613-618, 1990.
72. Mabruk MJEMF, Flint SK, Toner M, et al: In situ hybridization and the polymerase chain reaction (PCR) in the analysis of biopsies and exfoliative cytology specimens of oral hairy leukoplakia, *J Oral Pathol Med* 23:302-308, 1994.
73. Green T, Greenspan J, Greenspan D, DeSouza Y: Oral lesions mimicking hairy leukoplakia: a diagnostic dilemma, *Oral Surg* 67:422-426, 1989.
74. Schulten EAJM, Snijders PJF, Ten Kate RW, et al: Oral hairy leukoplakia in HIV infection: a diagnostic pitfall, *Oral Surg* 71:32-37, 1991.
75. Gowdey G, Lee RK, Carpenter WM: Treatment of HIV-related hairy leukoplakia with podophyllum resin 25% solution, *Oral Surg* 79:64-67, 1995.
76. Holmstrup P, Westergaard J: Periodontal diseases in HIV-infected patients, *J Clin Periodontal* 21:270-280, 1994.
77. Riley C, London JP, Burmeister JA: Periodontal health in 200 HIV-positive patients, *J Oral Pathol Med* 21:124-127, 1992.
78. Glick M, Muzyka BC, Salkin LM, Lurie D: Necrotizing ulcerative periodontitis: a marker for immune deterioration and a predictor for the diagnosis of AIDS, *J Periodontal* 65:393-397, 1994.

79. Glick M, Pliskin ME, Weiss RC: The clinical and histologic appearance of HIV-associated gingivitis, *Oral Surg* 69:395-398, 1990.
80. Winkler JR, Robertson PB: Periodontal disease associated with HIV infection, *Oral Surg* 73:145-150, 1992.
81. Odden K, Schenck K, Koppang HS, Hurlen B: Candidal infection of the gingiva in HIV-infected persons, *J Oral Pathol Med* 23:178-183, 1994.
82. Peterman TA, Joffe HW, Berol V: Epidemiologic clues to the etiology of Kaposi's sarcoma, *AIDS* 7:605-611, 1993.
83. Nichols CM, Flaitz CM, Hicks MS: Primary intraosseous Kaposi's sarcoma of the maxilla in human immunodeficiency virus infection: review of the literature and report of a case, *J Oral Maxillofac Surg* 53:325-329, 1995.
84. Porter S, Scully C: HIV: The surgeon's perspective. III. Diagnosis and management of malignant neoplasms, *Br J Oral Maxillofac Surg* 32:241-247, 1994.
85. Ramires-Amador V, González M, De la Rosa E, et al: Oral findings in Mexican AIDS patients with cancer, *J Oral Pathol Med* 22:87-91, 1993.
86. Regezi JA, MacPhail LA, Daniels TE, et al: Oral Kaposi's sarcoma: a 10-year retrospective histopathologic study, *J Oral Pathol Med* 22:292-297, 1993.
87. Nichols CM, Flaitz CM, Hicks MJ: Treating Kaposi's lesions in the HIV-infected patient, *J Am Dent Assoc* 124:78-84, 1993.
88. Epstein JB: Treatment of oral Kaposi's sarcoma with intralesional vinblastine, *Cancer* 71:1722-1730, 1993.
89. Lucatorto FM, Sapp JP: Treatment of oral Kaposi's sarcoma with a sclerosing agent in AIDS patients, *Oral Surg* 75:192-198, 1993.
90. Eversole LR: Viral infections of the head and neck among HIV-seropositive patients, *Oral Surg* 73:155-163, 1992.
91. Peterson DE, Greenspan D, Squier CA: Oral infections in the immunocompromised host, *J Oral Pathol Med* 21:193-198, 1992.
92. Veenstra J, Krol A, Rienke ME, et al: Herpes zoster immunological deterioration and disease progression in HIV-1 infection, *AIDS* 9:1153-1158, 1995.
93. Ficarra G, Shillitoe EJ, Adler-Storthz K, et al: Oral melanotic macules in patients infected with human immunodeficiency virus, *Oral Surg* 70:748-755, 1990.
94. Flaitz CM, Nichols CM, Hicks MJ, Adler-Storthz K: *Oral human papillomavirus infection in HIV-seropositive males: diagnostic and therapeutic management.* Paper presented at the meeting of American Academy of Oral Pathology, Portland, Maine, May 14-19, 1993.
95. Ficarra G, Cortés S, Rubino I, Romagnoli P: Facial and perioral molluscum contagiosum in patients with HIV infection: a report of eight cases, *Oral Surg* 78:621-626, 1994.
96. Shearer BG: MDR: TB: another challenge from the microbial world, *J Am Dent Assoc* 125:43-49, 1994.
97. Centers for Disease Control: Co-incidence of HIV/AIDS and tuberculosis, Chicago, 1982-1993, *MMWR* 44(11):227-231, 1995.

98. Kassim S, Sassan-Morokro M, Ackah A, et al: Two-year follow-up of persons with HIV-1– and HIV-2–associated pulmonary tuberculosis treated with short-course chemotherapy in West Africa, *AIDS* 9:1185-1191, 1995.

99. Jacobson MA: Current management of cytomegalovirus disease in patients with AIDS, *AIDS Res Hum Retroviruses* 10:917-918, 1994.

100. Greenberg MS, Dubin G, Stewart JCB, et al: Relationship of oral disease to the presence of cytomegalovirus DNA in the saliva of AIDS patients, *Oral Surg* 79:175-179, 1995.

101. MacPhail LA, Greenspan D, Greenspan JS: Recurrent aphthous ulcers in association with HIV infection, *Oral Surg* 73:283-288, 1992.

102. Regezi JA, MacPhail LA, Richards DW, Greenspan JS: A study of macrophages, macrophage-related cells and endothelial adhesion molecules in recurrent aphthous ulcers in HIV-positive patients, *J Dent Res* 72:1549-1553, 1993.

103. Phelan JA, Eisig S, Freedman PD, et al: Major aphthous-like ulcers in patients with AIDS, *Oral Surg* 71:68-72, 1991.

104. Muzyka BC, Glick M: Major aphthous ulcers in patients with HIV disease, *Oral Surg* 77:116-120, 1994.

105. Gowdey G, Lipsey LR, Lee R, et al: Gingival mass in a patient with HIV infection, *Oral Surg* 79:7-9, 1995.

106. Schiødt M, Dodd CL, Greenspan D, et al: Natural history of HIV-associated salivary gland disease, *Oral Surg* 74:324-331, 1992.

107. Fox PC: Salivary gland involvement in HIV-1 infection, *Oral Surg* 73:168-170, 1992.

108. Mandel L, Reich R: HIV parotid gland lymphoepithelial cysts: review and case reports, *Oral Surg* 74:273-278, 1992.

109. Chinn H, Chernoff DN, Migliorati CA, et al: Oral histoplasmosis in HIV-infected patients, a report of two cases, *Oral Surg* 79:10-14, 1995.

110. Samaranayake LP: Oral mycosis in HIV infection, *Oral Surg* 73:171-180, 1992.

111. Ficarra G, Flaitz CM, Gaglioti D, et al: White lichenoid lesions of the buccal mucosa in patients with HIV infection, *Oral Surg* 76:460-466, 1993.

112. Flaitz CM, Nichols CM, Adler-Stortz K, Hicks MJ: Intraoral squamous cell carcinoma in human immunodeficiency virus infection: a clinicopathologic study, *Oral Surg* 80:55-62, 1995.

113. Barrios TJ, Aria AA, Brahney C: Cancrum oris in an HIV-positive patient, *J Oral Maxillofac Surg* 53:851-855, 1995.

114. Jones AG, Migliorati CA, Baughman RA: The simultaneous occurrence of oral herpes simplex virus, cytomegalovirus and histoplasmosis in an HIV-infected patient, *Oral Surg* 74:334-339, 1992.

115. Goldschmidt RH, Dong BJ: Current report: HIV, treatment of AIDS and HIV related conditions, 1995, *J Am Board Fam Pract* 8:139-162, 1995.

116. Johnson VA: Combination therapy: more effective control of HIV type 1? *AIDS Res Hum Retroviruses* 10:907-912, 1994.

117. Pomerantz RJ, Trono D: Genetic therapies for HIV infections: promise for the future, *AIDS* 9:985-993, 1995.

118. Rencher SD, Slobod KS, Dawson DH, et al: Does the key to a successful HIV type 1 vaccine lie among the envelope sequences of infected individuals? *AIDS Res Hum Retroviruses* 11:1131-1133, 1995.

119. Centers for Disease Control: Recommended infection-control practices for Dentistry, *MMWR* 41:1-12, 1993.

120. Mc Neely TB, Dealy M, Dripps DJ, et al: Secretory leukocyte protease inhibitor: a human salivary protein exhibiting anti–human immunodeficiency virus 1 activity in vitro, *J Clin Invest* 96:456-464, 1995.

121. Centers for Disease Control: Investigations of patients who have been treated by HIV-infected health-care workers: United States, *MMWR* 42:329-331, 1993.

CHAPTER 37

Viral Hepatitis

JAMES F. LEHNERT

NORMAN K. WOOD

Viral hepatitis is of particular concern to the dental practitioner because of the potential for infection of the dentist and dental staff. Dentists in the United States are approximately 3 to 5 times (oral and maxillofacial surgeons approximately 6 times) more likely to be exposed to hepatitis B virus than the general population.[1] There are also reports of dentists transmitting hepatitis B to patients.[2] Consequently, the practitioner must fully understand the epidemiologic and clinical courses of the various types of viral hepatitis so that each patient who gives a positive history of hepatitis A, B, C, D, E, F,[3,4] or G[3,4] can be fully assessed.

ACUTE VIRAL HEPATITIS

The majority of symptomatic cases of viral hepatitis fit into a classic pattern, which is described here as acute viral hepatitis. However, the range of clinical manifestations, laboratory findings, histopathologic changes, and sequelae of acute viral hepatitis is broad. Most cases resolve completely within 4 months after the onset of symptoms, but some end in fulminant disease, and others progress to chronic hepatitis. This sequela may lead to cirrhosis or predispose the patient to primary hepatocellular carcinoma. For every clinically apparent case of acute viral hepatitis, several subclinical cases remain undetected.

Symptoms and Signs

After exposure to viral hepatitis, a variable incubation period ensues before the onset of symptoms, depending on the infecting agent: for hepatitis A it ranges from 2 to 6 weeks, for hepatitis B from 1 to 6 months, for hepatitis C probably 6 to 8 weeks,[4] and for hepatitis D from 3 to 7 weeks.[4]

The onset of nonspecific symptoms marks the beginning of the prodromal or preicteric phase. These symp-toms are often described as systemic, influenza-like complaints and may include malaise, nausea, vomiting, anorexia, myalgia, and right upper quadrant pain. In some patients, there is a serum sickness–like reaction with fever, skin rash, and arthralgia; this reaction is more likely to occur with hepatitis B. The prodromal phase may last only a few days or as long as 2 weeks.

The icteric phase starts with the appearance of jaundice. The degree of jaundice varies with the severity of the disease but is usually moderate in acute viral hepatitis. Other symptoms include darkening of the urine and whitish stools. Physical findings at this time may include jaundice; an enlarged, tender liver; and splenomegaly. Usually, some of the nonspecific symptoms start to resolve, and the patient begins to feel better within a couple of weeks after the onset of jaundice.[5] The icteric phase lasts about 4 to 6 weeks.

The disappearance of jaundice marks the beginning of the convalescent or recovery phase. The signs and symptoms of the prodromal and icteric phases gradually disappear, and abnormal laboratory findings (discussed in the next section) return to normal levels. Complete recovery usually occurs within 4 months after the onset of jaundice.

Laboratory Tests

Several laboratory tests are available to aid in the diagnosis of acute viral hepatitis and to monitor hepatic dysfunction during the course of the disease. The abnormal laboratory findings reflect injury to the hepatocytes by the ongoing inflammatory process.

Bilirubin is a breakdown product of hemoglobin that is metabolized in the liver and excreted in the bile. The plasma bilirubin level, which is normally less than 1 mg/100 ml, is elevated. Jaundice, or yellowish staining of tissues, occurs when the plasma bilirubin level exceeds 3 mg/100 ml.

Liver function tests of particular concern are the serum transaminases. Alanine transaminase (ALT, formerly serum glutamate-pyruvate transaminase) and aspartate transaminase (AST, formerly serum glutamic-oxaloacetic transaminase) are specific, sensitive indicators of hepatocyte injury. In acute viral hepatitis, their levels are usually elevated to 10 times normal. Other liver enzymes that may show elevations include γ-glutamyl transpeptidase, alkaline phosphatase, and lactate dehydrogenase.

The prothrombin time, a measurement of the extrinsic coagulation pathway, may be slightly prolonged in acute viral hepatitis. A significantly prolonged prothrombin time (greater than 20 seconds) indicates severe liver disease with extensive hepatocellular injury.

The white blood cell count may show leukopenia and leukocytosis, possibly with atypical lymphocytes.

Tests to identify the specific serum antigens and/or antibodies associated with hepatitis A, B, C, D, and E are available. These tests are usually necessary to indicate the type of viral hepatitis; they may also be used to exclude any of these viruses as etiologic agents of acute hepatitis. There is also a serologic test (polymerase chain reaction) to identify hepatitis B virus deoxyribonucleic acid (DNA) and hepatitis C virus ribonucleic acid (RNA), but this technique is not routinely available.[6]

HEPATITIS A
Epidemiology

Hepatitis A (infectious hepatitis) is caused by an RNA virus known as the *hepatitis A virus (HAV)*. Transmission occurs via the fecal-oral route, usually through contaminated food or water.[7] Thus hepatitis A is often associated with poor personal hygiene or overcrowded living conditions and occurs 2 to 3 times more frequently within the lower social classes.[8] It may also result from homosexual practices, intravenous drug use, and blood transfusions.[4]

Although this disease may occur at any age, it is common in children, particularly those of primary and nursery school age.[9] Hepatitis A may occur as localized outbreaks or epidemics, and it accounts for approximately 20% to 30% of sporadic cases (i.e., no known exposure) of viral hepatitis.

Hepatitis A is usually a mild, self-limiting disease that spontaneously resolves within a month. In some cases the clinical course is so mild and nonspecific that the patient does not seek medical treatment, so the disease goes undiagnosed. Overall the mortality for type A disease is very low. The antibody response to HAV infection confers lasting immunity. There are no chronic carriers or chronic disease states associated with hepatitis A.

Serology

The average incubation period for hepatitis A is 4 weeks. Late in the incubation period, hepatitis A antigen (HA Ag) appears in the stool but usually disappears by the time, or shortly after, jaundice develops. During this time, the disease is highly contagious. Serum ALT and AST levels rise rapidly during the prodromal phase, peaking in the early icteric phase, and then decline, returning to normal in the early convalescent phase. Although HAV is usually not detectable in the serum, shortly after the appearance of clinical symptoms, there is a rising titer of hepatitis A antibody (anti-HAV). The anti-HAV initially consists mainly of immunoglobulin M (IgM), but after approximately 6 months it is replaced by immunoglobulin G (IgG). Thus the presence of anti-HAV IgM indicates acute HAV infection. Fig. 37-1 illustrates these changes.

HEPATITIS B
Epidemiology

Hepatitis B (serum hepatitis) is caused by a DNA virus known as the *hepatitis B virus (HBV)*. The major mode of

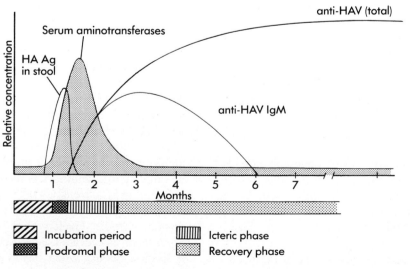

Fig. 37-1. Serologic changes in acute hepatitis A.

transmission of HBV is the parenteral route (e.g., blood, blood products, and contaminated needles). However, it can also be transmitted through close personal contact, since HBV can be found in the saliva, semen, and vaginal secretions of an infected individual.[7,10] The three principal modes of transmission are "percutaneous (injection drug use, blood or body fluid exposures among health care workers), sexual, and between siblings and other household contacts."[7] Heterosexual transmission with multiple partners now accounts for more cases than transmission via drug users and homosexuals. Transmission through blood transfusion is now rare in industrialized countries.[7] It is interesting that of dental school patients who tested positive for hepatitis B surface antigen (HBsAg), 2.8% reacted positively for the antibodies for human immunodeficiency virus type 1. This is compared with 0.4% of Americans who test positive for human immunodeficiency virus.[11]

HBV has three distinct antigens that elicit the production of corresponding antibodies in the infected individual. These antigen-antibody systems serve several purposes: (1) to establish or exclude the diagnosis of HBV as the etiologic agent; (2) to aid in determining whether the disease process is acute or chronic; (3) to serve as a prognostic indicator; and (4) to indicate a relative degree of infectivity.

HBsAg (Australia antigen) is derived from the outer coating of the complete HBV, the Dane particle. The presence of HBsAg indicates intact HBV or incomplete viral particles composed of HBsAg in the serum. Any individual whose test results are positive for HBsAg should be considered potentially infectious. Hepatitis B surface antibody (anti-HBs) is produced in response to HBsAg. The presence of serum anti-HBs thus indicates prior HBV infection. Hepatitis B core antigen (HBcAg) is derived from the inner core of the complete HBV. HBcAg is not detectable in the serum. However, antibodies to HBcAg (anti-HBc) are, and they consist of IgM and IgG subclasses (IgM initially, IgG later). Thus the presence of anti-HBc IgM is an indication of acute infection. The third antigen-antibody system associated with HBV infection is hepatitis B e antigen (HBeAg) and its antibody (anti-HBe). The HBeAg is thought to be related to the core antigen. The presence of HBeAg is associated with high viral activity and indicates active liver disease and increased potential for infectivity. HBeAg is always found in association with HBsAg. During acute type B disease, the seroconversion of HBeAg to anti-HBe usually signals the onset of resolution of the disease (this seroconversion does not occur when acute hepatitis progresses to chronic active hepatitis).

The onset of symptoms in acute hepatitis B is usually more insidious than in type A disease. However, the course of the disease in type B is usually more severe and prolonged, and fatalities are in the range of 3%.[5,12] Anti-HBs confers lifelong immunity to HBV infection.

Inapparent and Chronic Hepatitis

Two important features of hepatitis B should be mentioned. Up to this point, acute, symptomatic viral hepatitis has been considered. However, approximately 50% of the cases of hepatitis B are asymptomatic throughout their course. Thus despite a negative history for viral hepatitis or jaundice, an individual may be infectious during the subacute state associated with inapparent type B disease.

Second, as many as 10% of adults with hepatitis B, inapparent or symptomatic, later have the chronic carrier state or chronic hepatitis. Both sequelae are characterized by the persistence of serum HBsAg (for more than 6 months) with variable degrees of infectivity. The chronic HBsAg carrier is asymptomatic and has no clinical or biochemical evidence of liver disease. In addition to HBsAg, other antibodies associated with the HBV may be present. The chronic HBsAg carrier state may last for years, decades, or a lifetime. Chronic HBV infection is characterized by continued, mild to moderate symptoms and abnormal laboratory findings (e.g., elevated serum ALT and AST levels). Depending on the infection's severity, physical findings may be present. The HBsAg is accompanied by anti-HBc; anti-HBc is more likely present in chronic persistent hepatitis and HBeAg in chronic active hepatitis. Chronic persistent hepatitis and chronic active hepatitis are two major histologic variants of chronic type B disease. The former is more common than the latter, but a liver biopsy is often necessary to make the diagnosis. Chronic persistent hepatitis has a benign course with mild symptoms and only slightly elevated ALT and AST levels. It has a good prognosis and rarely progresses to chronic active hepatitis or cirrhosis. Chronic persistent hepatitis may eventually resolve, continue on indefinitely, or revert to the chronic HBsAg carrier state. Chronic active hepatitis, on the other hand, is a progressive, destructive inflammatory disease with fibrosis, which proceeds at a variable rate and may result in cirrhosis and possibly end-stage liver disease. Chronic active hepatitis may last for months or years, or it may revert to chronic persistent hepatitis.

Delta Hepatitis/Hepatitis D

A potential complication of HBV infection is the development of delta hepatitis (hepatitis D). Delta hepatitis is caused by the hepatitis delta virus (HDV), a defective RNA agent that requires the presence of HBsAg to replicate.[7,13] The development of screening tests for the delta antigen (HDAg) and its associated antibody (anti-HDV) has contributed to a better understanding of delta hepatitis. Acute delta hepatitis can occur as a coinfection with acute hepatitis B or a superinfection (i.e., an infection superimposed on the chronic HBsAg carrier state or chronic hepatitis B). The seroprevalence of anti-HDV among HBV-infected injected drug users ranges from 20% to 50%.[7] The combined effects of HBV infection and acute delta hepatitis are associated with fulminant

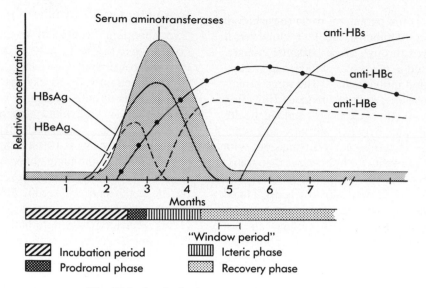

Fig. 37-2. Serologic changes in acute hepatitis B.

hepatitis 10 times more frequently than with HBV infection alone[4] and results in an increased mortality rate. This may be associated with severe, progressive liver disease.[13] Recovery from hepatitis B, with loss of HBsAg, also signals recovery from delta hepatitis. Individuals with anti-HBs are also immune to HDV infection.

Serology

Acute hepatitis B The average incubation period for HBV infection is 75 days. Approximately 4 to 6 weeks before the onset of symptoms, HBsAg appears in the serum, followed by HBeAg, and their titers begin to rise. Shortly thereafter the serum ALT and AST levels start to increase. Late in the incubation period, anti-HBc appears and rises in titer. Usually the HBsAg titer and the serum ALT and AST levels continue to climb through the prodromal phase and peak in the early icteric phase. HBeAg titers peak earlier and begin to fall, with seroconversion to anti-HBe occurring around the height of clinical symptoms. During the icteric phase, levels of HBsAg and serum ALT and AST begin to decrease. Generally, HBsAg is no longer detectable in the serum within 4 months after the appearance of symptoms. In the convalescent phase, liver enzyme levels return to normal, and seroconversion from HBsAg to anti-HBs occurs. During this seroconversion, there is a variable period of time after HBsAg is no longer detectable before the appearance of anti-HBs. This time is referred to as the *window period* (Fig. 37-2).

In inapparent hepatitis B, HBsAg and HBeAg may appear in the serum for a short time. Serum ALT and AST levels are mildly elevated but soon return to normal. High titers of anti-HBs and variable titers of anti-HBc and anti-HBe develop.

Chronic HBsAg carrier state In the chronic HBsAg carrier state, the serologic changes seen in acute hepatitis B are similar except for the persistence of HBsAg; therefore

there is no anti-HBs. Liver enzyme levels are normal, and the patient has no symptoms. Fig. 37-3 illustrates these changes.

Chronic active hepatitis B. In chronic active hepatitis B, HBsAg fails to seroconvert to anti-HBs in chronic active hepatitis, and HBcAg continues to be present. Anti-HBc rises to high titers. Serum ALT and AST levels remain elevated, though usually less than 10 times normal.[5] Mild to moderate symptoms may exist. These findings change as liver disease progresses. Fig. 37-4 illustrates these changes.

TYPE C HEPATITIS
Epidemiology and Clinical Features

Hepatitis C was formerly known as *blood-borne non-A, non-B hepatitis.* An RNA virus causes this disease and has been coded as *hepatitis C virus.*[7,14,15] At least four different strains of the hepatitis C virus have been identified in different countries.[16] The principal mode of transmission for HCV is the parenteral route.[7,14] Currently, 90% to 95% of the cases of posttransfusion hepatitis are hepatitis C. Type C disease thus occurs frequently in many of the same groups as hepatitis B: recipients of blood or blood products, patients on renal dialysis, certain health care professionals, and intravenous drug users. Hepatitis C also accounts for about 20% of sporadic cases of acute viral hepatitis, and in many of these cases, there is no history of parenteral exposure. As in hepatitis B, another route is through sexual contact. Male homosexuals and sexual partners of individuals with hepatitis C appear to be at increased risk for infection,[17,18] but the incidence is low. An outbreak of hepatitis C associated with intravenous administration of immune globulin occurred in the United States between October 1993 and June 1994, but a new step in the processing of immune globulin has eliminated this problem.[19] Other modes of person-to-person transmission are not clear; in-

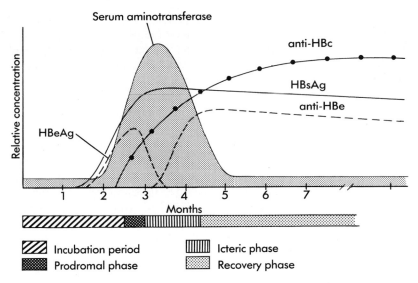

Fig. 37-3. Serologic changes in the chronic HBsAg carrier state.

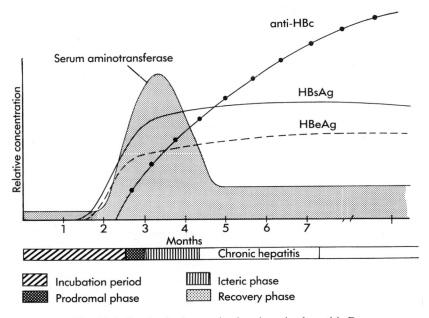

Fig. 37-4. Serologic changes in chronic active hepatitis B.

trafamilial spread of hepatitis from an individual with type C disease can infrequently occur.[7] A more thorough understanding of the epidemiology of hepatitis C will come with the information learned from screening and confirmative blood tests.

The clinical features of acute hepatitis C are usually less severe than those of hepatitis A or hepatitis B. After the incubation period (which averages 6 to 8 weeks for post-transfusion hepatitis),[4,19] acute hepatitis C often has insidious prodromal and icteric phases. Symptoms and physical finding, if present, are usually mild. Symptomatic disease with jaundice may occur in 25% of all cases.[4,20] Serum ALT and AST levels are elevated but are usually lower than in hepatitis B. These biochemical abnormalities have been associated with viremia and suggest that the patient is potentially infectious throughout the period of enzyme ele-

vation.[21] Spontaneous resolution usually occurs within 10 to 12 weeks after the onset of symptoms.

The long-term complications of this disease are more common than in HBV. From 50% to 60% develop chronic hepatitis and remain carriers for life. Half of these develop progressive cirrhosis.[20]

First- and second-generation serologic antibody tests are available for identification of HCV infections. These include enzyme immunoassays (EIA-1 and EIA-2) and recombinant immunoblot assays (RIBA-1 and RIBA-2).[6,14,22,23] Unfortunately, because of problems with sensitivity or selectivity, none is diagnostic by itself; a second type of test must confirm the diagnosis. The polymerase chain reaction test is specific for HCV RNA and can positively identify HCV infection, but this test is complicated and not routinely available.[6,22]

HEPATITIS E

The virus(es) formerly recognized as causing enterically transmitted non-A, non-B hepatitis has been isolated and coded as hepatitis E virus (HEV), an RNA virus. Transmission commonly occurs through fecally contaminated drinking water, and outbreaks have occurred in developing countries[3,4,24] in Africa, Asia, and Latin America.[4] Epidemics have not occurred in Canada and the United States, and only occasionally cases have been seen in the United States.[7]

The disease usually follows a benign pattern like HAV, with a mortality rate of 1% to 2%, which increases to 20% to 40% in pregnant women.[3,4] Serologic tests such as EIA and polymerase chain reaction assays of RNA are now available for HEV.[4]

HEPATITIS F AND G

There is some evidence of the existence of other unidentified hepatitis viruses, perhaps other enterically transmitted non-A, non-B agents, and these have been arbitrarily assigned as F and G.[3,4]

• • •

Table 37-1 summarizes the epidemiologies of hepatitis A, B, and C.

MEDICAL MANAGEMENT

Most patients with acute viral hepatitis are treated at home. Medical management includes bed rest (as necessary), instructions to prevent further spread of the disease, an adequate diet, and treatment of symptoms (e.g., an antiemetic to prevent vomiting). Corticosteroids are contraindicated in treatment of acute viral hepatitis because they may predispose the patient to relapse or progression to chronic hepatitis.[25] Prednisone, azathioprine, and interferon are used in the treatment of chronic active hepatitis.

Patients with severe disease, those who cannot care for themselves, or those who cannot maintain adequate oral intake may require hospitalization. Again, treatment is primarily supportive and palliative. For the majority of cases of acute viral hepatitis, complete recovery usually occurs within 3 to 4 months after the onset of symptoms.

Chronic persistent hepatitis requires no specific therapy, since it is a relatively benign disease with a good prognosis. Chronic active hepatitis may be treated with interferon-α,[4] after a short primary dose of prednisone in select cases.[26] Interferon-α, interferon-β, and ribavirin are used with some success in HCV infection.[4,27]

PROPHYLAXIS AND THE HEPATITIS VACCINES

Hepatitis prophylaxis is often initiated after exposure to viral hepatitis through contact (e.g., household, sexual, or close personal contact), accidental needle stick, or transfusion with contaminated blood products. Preexposure prophylaxis may also be warranted before traveling to an area where viral hepatitis is endemic.

Table 37-1   Summary of epidemiologies of acute viral hepatitis

	Hepatitis A	Hepatitis B	Hepatitis C
Agent	HAV	HBV	RNA virus
Antigens	HA Ag	HBsAg, HBcAg, HBeAg	
Antibodies	anti-HAV	anti-HBs, anti-HBc, anti-HBe	anti-HCV
Modes of transmission	Fecal-oral	Primarily parenteral but also by contact	Primarily parenteral and probably by contact
Incubation period	2 to 6 weeks	1 to 6 months	2 weeks to 6 months
Clinical course	Symptomatic or inapparent	Approximately 50% inapparent	As many as 75% inapparent
Mortality	Rare	1% to 3%	1% to 2%
Asymptomatic carrier state	No	0.1% to 0.2% of the population	Possibly as high as 3% to 7% of the population
Chronic hepatitis	No	5% to 10%	40% to 60% after transfusion; <10% of sporadic cases
Postexposure prophylaxis	IG usually effective	HBIG, occasionally IG	IG may be effective
Preexposure prophylaxis (vaccine) available	Yes	Yes	No

IG, Immune globulin; *HBIG,* hepatitis B immune globulin.

Individuals exposed to HAV are protected against hepatitis A (more than 90% of the time) by receiving immune globulin within 2 weeks after exposure. Immune globulin contains anti-HAV and appears to act by conferring temporary, passive immunity or by a passive-active mechanism. In the latter, immune globulin antibodies prevent clinical disease, but a subclinical or inapparent infection occurs and results in autogenous anti-HAV production and lifelong immunity. Newly approved inactivated hepatitis A vaccine, Havrix,* is now available in the United States for preexposure prophylaxis.[28] The vaccine regimen for adults consists of two intramuscular injections, the second 6 to 12 months after the first.[28] The vaccine may also be used with immune globulin for postexposure prophylaxis.[28]

Postexposure prophylaxis after accidental contact or inoculation with HBsAg-positive products in a susceptible individual (i.e., unvaccinated person whose test for anti-HBs is negative) consists of hepatitis B immune globulin (HBIG) and the hepatitis B vaccine. HBIG contains high titers of anti-HBs and confers temporary, passive immunity. The single dose of HBIG should be given as soon as possible after exposure, preferably within 24 hours but no later than 7 days after exposure. The first dose of the hepatitis B vaccine should be given at a separate site within 7 days after exposure; the schedule for the remaining doses is unchanged (the immunization regimen is discussed later in this section). The vaccine stimulates production of autogenous anti-HBs, thus enhancing or initiating an active immune response against HBsAg. Individuals not given the hepatitis B vaccine should receive a second dose of HBIG 1 month after the first. However, the use of only HBIG or the hepatitis B vaccine for postexposure prophylaxis is not as effective in preventing HBV infection as is their combined use.[28]

In other instances, when the relative risk for HBV infection is lower or unlikely, postexposure prophylaxis may require only HBIG (after sexual exposure) or the hepatitis B vaccine. Immune globulin has been recommended in postexposure prophylaxis for type C hepatitis,[25] but this recommendation appears to be an empirical judgment at this time.

The first hepatitis B vaccine (Heptavax-B†), licensed in 1981, is a highly purified, noninfectious preparation of HBsAg, which is derived from the pooled plasma of HBsAg-positive carriers. Numerous reports document the safety and efficacy of Heptavax-B.[4] However, plasma-derived hepatitis B vaccine is no longer produced in this country, although it is still available for those who need it. Recombivax HB† and Energex-B,* second-generation hepatitis B vaccines, contain recombinant HBsAg produced by yeast cells. Immunogenicity and safety are comparable with those of Heptavax-B but may be associated with the production of lower levels of anti-HBs in a recipient.[29] The immunization regimen for healthy adults using either vaccine consists of three intramuscular injections, with the second and third doses given at 1 and 6 months, respectively, after the initial dose.[4] Since the titer of anti-HBs initially produced in response to the vaccine varies (with some nonresponders) and decreases over time, 3-month postvaccine tests should be conducted and booster shots given depending on titers.[12]

Preexposure prophylaxis with the hepatitis B vaccine is recommended for dentists and auxiliary personnel, the highest-risk health care workers.[12] However, if prior exposure to HBV is equivocal, a screening test for anti-HBs should be performed to establish the need for the vaccine.

---

*SmithKline Beecham, Philadelphia.

†Merck Sharp & Dohme, West Point, Pa.

Table 37-2   Interpretation of serologic profiles seen in viral hepatitis

		Test results				
HBsAg	anti-HBs	anti-HBc	HBeAg	anti-HBe	anti-HAV	Comments
−					+IgM	Acute or recent hepatitis A
+						Acute or chronic hepatitis B
+		+IgM	+			Acute hepatitis B
−	−	+IgM		+		Window period after acute hepatitis B
+		+IgG		+		Asymptomatic chronic HBsAg carrier or, possibly, chronic type B hepatitis
+		+IgG	+			Chronic hepatitis B
	+	+IgG		+/−		Recovery from hepatitis B
	+	−		−		Prior immunization with hepatitis B vaccine or, possibly, long after hepatitis B infection
−		−			−	Possible type non-A, non-B hepatitis
					+IgG	Past HAV infection

Test not ordered.

DENTAL IMPLICATIONS

Dental practitioners must take every precaution to protect themselves and their staffs from viral hepatitis. A comprehensive medical history is important for identifying patients with histories of viral hepatitis or may elicit symptoms of acute disease. Furthermore, understanding the epidemiologic factors can aid in determining the type of viral hepatitis that the patient had (e.g., perhaps a localized outbreak, associated with intravenous drug abuse at summer camp, or perhaps the viral hepatitis followed multiple blood transfusions). However, the comprehensive medical history has limitations. As one study reported, 50% of the detected HBsAg carriers gave no history of ever having hepatitis, 58% of the patients who gave a history of hepatitis A actually had hepatitis B, and only 56% of the patients who gave a history of hepatitis B had serologic evidence of type B disease.[30] Therefore a positive history of hepatitis usually requires consultation with the patient's physician to determine the type and rule out a chronic carrier or disease state (not applicable with hepatitis A). If a history of hepatitis B is suspected and the patient's medical records are not available, a screening test for HBsAg should be ordered (Table 37-2).

Regional examination of the sclera and oral mucosa, particularly the lingual frenum, may reveal mild jaundice in a patient with an unremarkable past medical history and nonspecific symptoms of malaise, anorexia, weight loss, and fever. If acute viral hepatitis is suspected, no elective dental treatment should be performed until after medical consultation and resolution of the acute disease state.

The dental practitioner should be aware of the various groups considered at high risk for the different types of viral hepatitis. These groups are listed in the box at left.

Close communication between dentist and physician is essential for the patient with chronic hepatitis and cirrhosis. Potential complications include altered drug metabolism, anemia, bleeding abnormalities secondary to deficiency of clotting factors or thrombocytopenia, circulatory changes, and ascites. Antibiotic prophylaxis may be required for patients with vascular and surgical shunts.

During dental treatment of a patient with acute or chronic viral hepatitis, universal precautions must be used. Gloves, mask, and protective eyeglasses are mandatory. Aerosol production should be minimized by using a slow-speed handpiece as much as possible, working under a rubber dam, using high-speed evacuation, and judiciously using the air syringe. Strict aseptic technique is essential and should include sterilization of all instruments and handpieces, thorough postoperative disinfection, use of disposable smocks and drapes, and proper disposal of contaminated materials. Scheduling these patients late in the day eliminates the immediate use of the equipment by another patient. Other considerations include obtaining a preoperative prothrombin time before dental surgery (a platelet count may also be necessary if splenomegaly is a complicating factor), modifying the chair position to the sitting or semireclining position for patients with ascites, and avoiding the use of drugs metabolized by the liver.

REFERENCES

1. West DJ: The risk of hepatitis B infection among health professionals in the United States: a review, *Am J Med Sci* 287:26-33, 1984.

2. Ahtone J, Goodman RA: Hepatitis B and dental personnel: transmission to patients and prevention issues, *J Am Dent Assoc* 106:219-222, 1983.

3. The A to F of viral hepatitis, *Lancet* 336:1158-1160, 1990 (editorial).

4. Porter S, Scully C, Samaranayake L: Viral hepatitis: current concepts for dental practice, *Oral Surg* 78:682-695, 1994.

5. Hoofnagle JH: *Perspective on viral hepatitis: type A and B viral hepatitis,* Abbott Park, Ill, 1981, Abbott Laboratories Diagnostic Division.

6. Nakatsuji Y, Matsumoto A, Tannates E, et al: Detection of chronic hepatitis C virus infection by four diagnostic systems, *Hepatology* 16:300-305, 1992.

7. Shapiro CN: Transmission of hepatitis viruses, *Ann Intern Med* 120:82-84, 1994 (editorial).

8. Szmuness W, Dienstag JL, Purcell RH, et al: Distribution of antibody to hepatitis A antigen in urban adult populations, *N Engl J Med* 295:755-759, 1976.

9. Balistreri WF: Viral hepatitis, *Pediatr Clin North Am* 35(3):637-669, 1988.

10. Bernstein LM, Koff RS, Siegel ER, et al: The hepatitis knowledge base (short form), *Ann Intern Med* 93:183 222, 1980.

11. Cade JE, Boozer CH, Lancaster DM, Lundgren G: HIV-1 antibody positive hepatitis B surface antigen serum in dental school patient population, *Oral Surg* 78:670-672, 1994.

12. Davis GR, Porra M: The need for post-vaccination serology and the timing of booster vaccinations against hepatitis B in dental health care workers, *Aust Dent J* 39:238-241, 1994.

13. Rizzetto M, Ferruccio B, Verme G: Hepatitis delta virus infection of the liver: progress in virology, pathobiology, and diagnosis, *Semin Liver Dis* 8(4):350-356, 1988.

14. Berry MA, Herrera JL: Diagnosis and treatment of chronic viral hepatitis, *Comp Ther* 20:16-19, 1994.

15. Weis K: Hepatitis C: what a dentist should know, *J Can Dent Assoc* 61:537-540, 1995.

16. Takada N, Takase S, Takada A, Date T: Differences in the hepatitis C virus genotypes in different countries, *J Hepatol* 17:277-283, 1993.

17. Osmond DH, Charlebois E, Sheppard HW, et al: Comparison of risk factors for hepatitis C and hepatitis B virus infection in homosexual men, *J Infect Dis* 167:66-71, 1993.

18. Bresters D, Mauser-Bunschoten EP, Reesink HW, et al: Sexual transmission of hepatitis C virus, *Lancet* 342:210-211, 1993.

19. Centers for Disease Control: Epidemiologic notes and reports: outbreak of hepatitis C associated with intravenous immunoglobulin administration—United States, October 1993–June 1994, *MMWR* 43(28):505-509, 1994.

20. Epstein JB, Sherlock CH: Hepatitis C: rapid progress in medicine and implications for dentistry, *J Can Dent Assoc* 60:323-329, 1994.

21. Czaja AJ: Hepatitis and the dentist, *J Am Dent Assoc* 108:286-287, 1984.

22. Silva AE, Hosein B, Boyle RW, et al: Diagnosis of chronic hepatitis C: comparison of immunoassays and the polymerase chain reaction, *Am J Gastroenterol* 89:493-496, 1994.

23. Chaudhary RK, Maclean C: Detection of antibody to hepatitis C virus by second-generation enzyme immunoassay, *J Clin Pathol* 99:702-704, 1993.

24. Krawczynski K: Hepatitis E, *Hepatology* 17:932-941, 1993.

25. Orland MJ, Saltman RJ: *Manual of medical therapeutics,* Boston, 1986, Little, Brown.

26. Perrillo RP: The management of chronic hepatitis B, *Am J Med* 96(suppl 1A):34-39, 1994.

27. Davis GL: Interferon treatment of chronic hepatitis C, Amer J Med, 96(suppl 1A):41-46, 1994.

28. Centers for Disease Control: Licensure of inactivated hepatitis A vaccine and recommendations for use among international travelers, *MMWR* 43(29):559-560, 1995.

29. Centers for Disease Control: Update on hepatitis B prevention, *MMWR* 36:353-360, 1987.

30. Goebel WM: Reliability of the medical history in identifying patients likely to place dentists at an increased hepatitis risk, *J Am Dent Assoc* 98:907-913, 1979.

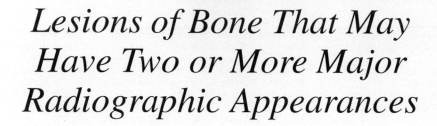

Lesions of Bone That May Have Two or More Major Radiographic Appearances

	Completely radiolucent	Radiolucent and radiopaque	Completely radiopaque
Adenomatoid odontogenic tumor	Yes	Yes	No
Ameloblastoma and variants	Yes	Yes	No
Calcifying epithelial odontogenic tumor	Yes	Yes	No
Cementoblastoma	Yes	Yes	Yes
Chondroma	Yes	Yes	No
Chondrosarcoma	Yes	Yes	No
Ewing's sarcoma	Yes	Yes	No
Fibroosseous lesions of periodontal ligament origin	Yes	Yes	Yes
Fibrous dysplasia	Yes	Yes	Yes
Giant cell granuloma	Yes	Yes	No
Hemangioma	Yes	Yes	No
Lymphosarcoma	Yes	Yes	No
Metastatic carcinoma	Yes	Yes	Yes
Odontogenic fibroma	Yes	Yes	No
Odontoma	Yes	Yes	Yes
Osteitis	Yes	Yes	Yes
Osteoblastoma	Yes	Yes	Yes
Osteomyelitis	Yes	Yes	Yes
Osteosarcoma	Yes	Yes	Yes
Paget's disease	Yes	Yes	Yes
Postsurgical bone defect	Yes	Yes	Yes
Proliferative periostitis	Yes	Yes	Yes
Reticulum cell sarcoma	Yes	Yes	No
Subperiosteal hematoma	Yes	Yes	Yes
Teeth	Yes	Yes	Yes

APPENDIX B

Normal Values for Laboratory Tests

I. Hematologic blood values (whole blood [EDTA])
   A. Red blood cell values
      1. Red blood cell count
         a. Male—4.5 to 6.0 million/mm^3
         b. Female—4.0 to 5.5 million/mm^3
         c. During pregnancy—greater than 3.6 million/mm^3
      2. Hemoglobin (Hbg) content
         a. Male—13.5 to 17.5 g/100 ml
         b. Female—12 to 16 g/100 ml
      3. Packed cell volume (PCV), or hematocrit
         a. Male—41% to 53%
         b. Female—36% to 46%
      4. Mean corpuscular volume (MCV)
         a. Male—82.2 to 100.6 μg^3
         b. Female—81.9 to 100.7 μg^3
      5. Mean corpuscular hemoglobin (MCH) content
         a. Male—28.4 to 32.0 pg
         b. Female—28.3 to 32.1 pg
      6. Mean corpuscular hemoglobin concentration (MCHC)
         a. Male—32.7% to 35.1% (g/100 ml)
         b. Female—32.5% to 34.7% (g/100 ml)
   B. White blood cell values
      1. White blood cell count
         a. Infants—6000 to 17,500/mm^3 (first day of life—9400 to 34,000 mm^3)
         b. Adolescents—4500 to 13,500/mm^3
         c. Adults—4500 to 11,000/mm^3
      2. Differential white blood cell count
         a. Neutrophils—35% to 73%; 1680 to 7884/mm^3
         b. Lymphocytes—23% to 33%; 1500 to 3000/mm^3
         c. Monocytes—2% to 6%; 100 to 900/mm^3
         d. Eosinophils—1% to 3%; 50 to 450/mm^3
         e. Basophils—0% to 1%; 50 to 200/mm^3
   C. Bleeding and clotting abnormalities
      1. Platelets (whole blood [EDTA])—150,000-400,000/mm^3
      2. (Ivy) bleeding time (blood from the skin)—2 to 7 min
      3. (Lee-White) clotting time (whole blood [no anticoagulant])—5 to 8 min
      4. Prothrombin time (one stage) (whole blood [no citrate])—12 to 14 sec
      5. Partial thromboplastin time (whole blood [no citrate])—25 to 30 sec
      6. Fibrinogen (whole blood [no citrate])—200 to 400 mg/100 ml
      7. Specific factor analysis (plasma [no citrate])
         a. Factor II assay—60% to 150% of normal, or 0.5 to 1.5 U/ml
         b. Factor V assay—60% to 150% of normal, or 0.5 to 2.0 U/ml
         c. Factor VII assay—65% to 135% of normal, or 60 to 135 AU
         d. Factor VIII assay—60% to 2145% of normal, or 60 to 145 AU
         e. Factor IX assay—60% to 140% of normal, or 60 to 140 AU
         f. Factor X assay—60% to 130% of normal, or 60 to 130 AU
      8. Prothrombin consumption test (whole blood [no anticoagulant])—greater than 30 sec
      9. Thrombin time (whole blood [no citrate])—control time (9 to 10 sec) ≠ 2 sec

Prepared by Paul W. Goaz. Compiled from Wyngarden JB, Smith LH Jr: *Cecil text book of medicine*, ed 18, vol 2, Philadelphia, 1988, WB Saunders; Ravel R: *Clinical laboratory medicine: clinical application of laboratory data*, Chicago, 1989, Mosby; Halsted JA, Halsted CH: *The laboratory in clinical medicine*, ed 2, Philadelphia, 1981, WB Saunders.

II. Serum enzymes (serum)
  A. Serum glutamic-oxaloacetic transaminase—15 to 40 U/L
  B. Serum glutamic pyruvic transaminase—15 to 35 U/L
  C. Lactate dehydrogenase—45 to 90 U/L
  D. Creatine phosphokinase—0 to 170 U/L
  E. Alkaline phosphatase
    1. Male—62 to 176 U/L
    2. Female—56 to 155 U/L
  F. Acid phosphatase
    1. Male—0.01 to 0.56 U/L
    2. Female—0.13 to 0.63 U/L
  G. Amylase—80 to 180 (Somogyi) U/dl
  H. Lipase
    1. Under 60 years of age—10 to 150 U/L
    2. Over 60 years of age—18 to 180 U/L
  I. Leucine aminopeptidase—8 to 200 (Goldbarg-Rutenbuirg) U/ml
  J. Cholinesterase—0.65 to 1.00 pH units or more per hour
III. Blood chemistry (serum)
  A. Calcium (total)—8.4 to 10.2 mg/100 ml
  B. Phosphorus—2.7 to 4.5 mg/100 ml
  C. Glucose
    1. Under 60 years of age—70 to 105 mg/100 ml
    2. Over 60 years of age—81 to115 mg/100 ml
  D. Blood urea nitrogen—7 to 18 mg/100 ml
  E. Uric acid
    1. Male—3.5 to 7.2 mg/100 ml
    2. Female—2.6 to 6.0 mg/100 ml
  F. Cholesterol (plasma [no citrate] or serum) (EDTA)
    1. 20 to 29 years of age
      a. Male—Greater than 194 mg/100 ml
      b. Female—Greater than 184 mg/100 ml
    2. 30 to 39 years of age
      a. Male—Greater than 218 mg/100 ml
      b. Female—Greater than 202 mg/100 ml
    3. 40 to 49 years of age
      a. Male—Greater than 231 mg/100 ml
      b. Female—Greater than 223 mg/100 ml
    4. Over 50 years of age
      a. Male—Greater than 230 mg/100 ml
      b. Female—Greater than 252 mg/100 ml
  G. Protein (total)—6 to 8.4 g/100 ml
    1. Albumin—3.5 to 5.0 g/100 ml
    2. Globulin—2.3 to 3.5 g/100 ml
  H. Bilirubin (total)—0.5 to 1.2 mg/100 ml
    1. Conjugated (direct)—Up to 0.2 mg/100 ml
    2. Unconjugated (indirect)—0.1 to 1.0 mg/100 ml
IV. Serum electrolytes and blood gas
  A. Sodium—136 to 146 mEq/L
  B. Potassium—3.5 to 5.1 mEq/L
  C. Chloride—98 to 106 mEq/L
  D. Bicarbonate—18 to 23 mEq/L
  E. Oxygen pressure (PCO_2) (whole blood, arterial [heparin])—83 to 100 mm Hg
  F. Carbon dioxide pressure (PCO_2) (whole blood, arterial [heparin])—95 to 100 mm Hg
  G. pH (whole blood, arterial [heparin])—7.35 to 7.45
V. Urinalysis (random sample)
  A. pH—4.7 to 8.0 (mean, 6.3)
  B. Specific gravity—1.016 to 1.022
  C. Protein—40 to 150 mg/24 hr (2 to 8 mg/100 ml)
  D. Ketones—Negative
  E. Bilirubin—0.02 mg/100 ml
  F. Blood—Negative
  G. Erythrocytes—0 to 1/high-power field
  H. Leukocytes—0 to 5/high-power field

Index

A

Abscess
  alveolar, 170, **211-212**
    chronic, 357
    chronic draining, 211-212
  dentoalveolar, 211-212
    chronic and acute, 259-263
    pulpoperiapical radiolucency, 259-263
    sinus draining chronic, 217, 218
  palatine space, 152
    from maxillary molar, 145
    midpalatine cyst *versus,* 326
  periodontal, 262
  radiolucency with ragged and poorly defined borders and, 356-379
  sinus draining, 38
  staphylococcal node, 529-530
  superficial, 226
Accessory tonsillar tissue, 133, 135
Acetaminophen, red lesions with necrotic component and, 128
Acid phosphatase, 622
Acne vulgaris, 555
Acneiform dermatoses, 555-556
Acquired immunodeficiency syndrome, 596-610
  associated gingival and periodontal disease, 602-604
  candidiasis and, 600-601
  cervical lymphadenopathy, 600
  course of disease, 598-599
  demography and epidemiology, 98, 597, 599
  hairy leukoplakia, 601-602
  human immunodeficiency virus, 596-597
  Kaposi's sarcoma, 604-606
  oral manifestations, 599-606
  risk of transmission to and from dental community, 607-608
  surveillance classification, 597-598
  treatment and prognosis, 606-607
  viral types, 596-597
Actinic keratosis, 540-541, 564, 565
Actinic radiation, cutaneous reactions to, 554
Actinomycosis
  aspiration in, 24
  consistency of, 31
Acute lymphonodular pharyngitis, 226-227
Acute necrotic ulcerative gingivitis, 171, Plate E
  in human immunodeficiency virus infection, 602-604
  red lesions with necrotic component, 128-129
  sloughing, pseudomembranous, necrotic white lesion, 121-122
Acute necrotizing stomatitis, 604, 605
Acyclovir, 75
Addison's disease, 203, 206, 568
Adenitis, tuberculous, 527

Adenoameloblastoma, *see* Adenomatoid odontogenic tumor
Adenocarcinoma of minor salivary gland origin, 366
Adenocystic carcinoma, 366
Adenoid cystic carcinoma, 20, 272, 273, Plate I
Adenoid hyperplasia of minor salivary glands, 153
Adenoma
  canalicular, 575
  papillary cyst, 35
  pleomorphic, 31, 33
Adenomatoid hyperplasia, 158
Adenomatoid odontogenic tumor, 289
  mixed radiolucent-radiopaque, 426-428
  multiple major radiographic appearances, 620
  pericoronal radiolucency, 280, 289, 290
Adipose tissue, 29
Adrenocorticotropic hormone, 206
Age
  development of differential diagnosis, 42, 43, 44
  oral cancer and, 588
Airway shadow, 240, 242
Ala of nose, 455, 468
Alanine aminotransferase, 612
Albers-Schönberg disease, 512-515
Albright's syndrome, 203, 204, 439, 486
Alcohol, oral cancer and, 588
Alkaline phosphatase
  normal lab values, 622
  in Paget's disease, 512
Allergic contact dermatitis, 555
Allergic macule, 65, 66
Allergic mucositis, 129
Allergy, multiple ulcerations in, 86
Alveolar abscess, 170
  chronic, 357
  chronic draining, 211-212
Alveolar crest, 305, 450
Alveolar mucosa
  amalgam tattoo, 186
  intraoral lesions of, 581
Alveolar process, 450, 451
Alveolar ridge
  lymphangioma of, 195
  verrucous carcinoma, 113
Alveolus, idiopathic osteosclerosis, 480
Amalgam tattoo, 186-187
  melanotic macule *versus,* 192
  nevus *versus,* 201
Amelanotic melanoma, 68, 148, 155, 156
Ameloblastic carcinoma, 339
Ameloblastic fibroma, 280, 290-291, 292

Ameloblastic fibroodontoma, 428, 429
Ameloblastic odontoma, 349, 446
Ameloblastoma, 176, 274, **283-285, 337-340**
 desmoplastic, 445
 ill-defined, ragged radiolucency, 371
 interradicular radiolucency, 300, 301, 302
 mixed radiolucent-radiopaque, 445
 multilocular radiolucency, 337-340, 349, 353
 multiple major radiographic appearances, 620
 multiple separate, cystlike radiolucency, 389
 odontogenic keratocyst *versus,* 320
 pericoronal radiolucency, 280, 289
 pseudomultilocular radiolucency, 334
 solitary cystlike radiolucency, 311, 321, 322
 unicystic, pericoronal radiolucency, 285-288
Amoxicillin, 262
Amphotericin B, 62, 63
Amputation neuroma, 31, 154, 155
Amylase, 622
Amyloidosis, 159, 559
Anatomic radiolucencies, 238-251
 interradicular, 296-298, 299
 mandibular, 239-244
 airway shadow, 240, 242
 anterior buccal mandibular depression, 244
 cortical plate mandibular defects, 244
 lingual foramen, 240, 241
 mandibular canal, 239-240
 mandibular foramen, 239
 medial sigmoid depression, 242, 243
 mental foramen, 240, 241
 mental fossa, 242, 243
 midline symphysis, 242, 243
 pseudocyst of condyle, 244
 submandibular fossa, 240, 242
 maxillary, 245-248
 greater palatine foramen, 247
 incisive foramen, incisive canal, and superior foramina of incisive
 canal, 245, 246
 intermaxillary suture, 245
 maxillary sinus, 246-247, 248
 nares, 246
 nasal cavity, 245
 nasolacrimal duct or canal, 246, 247
 multilocular, 334, 335
 periapical, 253-254
 solitary cystlike, not necessarily contacting teeth, 310-312
 structures common to both jaws, 248-250
 developing tooth crypt, 249, 250
 marrow space, 248-249
 nutrient canal, 249, 250
 periodontal ligament space, 248
 pulp chamber and root canal, 248
Anatomic radiopacities, 449-456
 anterior nasal spine, 451, 452
 bone, 450, 451
 coronoid process, 453
 external oblique ridge, 454
 false periapical, 467, 468
 genial tubercles, 454, 455
 maxillary tuberosity, 453
 mental ridge, 454
 mineralized tissue shadows, 456
 mylohyoid ridge, 454
 nasal septum and boundaries of nasal fossae, 450-451, 452
 pterygoid plates and pterygoid hamulus, 453
 soft tissue shadows, 455, 456

Anatomic radiopacities—cont'd
 teeth, 449-450
 walls and floor of maxillary sinus, 451, 452
 zygomatic process of maxilla and zygomatic bone, 451-453
Anemia
 Cooley, 401-402
 generalized rarefactions, 400-405
 glossitis in, 94
 hemolytic
 hereditary, 400-405
 sickle cell anemia and, 403-404
 thalassemia and, 401-402
Anesthesia, 41
Aneurysm
 consistency of, 31
 in oral cavity, 185
Aneurysmal bone cyst, 331, **343-346**
Aneurysm-like lesion, 37
Angina
 Ludwig's, 54-55, 56, 526, Plate B
Angioedema of lip, 574
Angiolith, 474
Angiosarcoma, facial, 551
Angular cheilitis, 64-65
Angular cheilosis, 180, 561-562
Annulus migrans, 90
Anterior buccal mandibular depression, 244
Anterior lingual mandibular bone concavity, 276
Anterior lingual mandibular bone defects, 318
Anterior nasal spine, 451, 452
Anterior palatine foramen, 245, 246
Antibiotics
 in dentoalveolar abscess, 262
 in syphilis, 174
Antibody
 in benign mucous membrane pemphigoid, 81
 in lupus erythematosus, 87
 in pemphigus, 82
Antigen
 Australia, 613
 CD4 surface, 596
 in migratory glossitis, 90
Antinuclear antibody, 87
Antral polyp, 142
Antrolith, 473-474, 496
 false periapical radiolucency and, 473
ANUG; *see* Acute necrotic ulcerative gingivitis
Aphthous stomatitis, 72-73
Aphthous ulcer, Plate B, Plate F
 human immunodeficiency virus-associated, 607
 of lip, 568-569, 570
 recurrent, 165-167
 red lesions with necrotic component, 128
Argyria, 207
Arterial calcification, 475
Arteriovenous malformation, 352
 multilocular radiolucency and, 348-349
Ascher's syndrome, 577
Aspartate aminotransferase, 612
Aspirate, 23-24
Aspiration, 20-23
Aspirin, red lesions with necrotic component, 128
Atrophic candidiasis
 multiple ulcerations in, 80
 recurrent aphthous stomatitis *versus,* 73
Atrophic lichen planus, Plate C
Atypical gingivostomatitis, 85

Auriculotemporal syndrome, 221
Auscultation, 38
Australia antigen, 613
Azathioprine, 80
AZT; *see* Zidovudine

B

Bacterial infection
    cutaneous facial lesions, 556-557
    sialadenitis, 532
Bad taste as chief complaint, 41
Baelz disease, 576
Barber's itch, 557
Basal cell carcinoma, 543, 544, Plate I
Basal cell nevus syndrome, 202, **382-384**
    well-defined radiolucency of, 382-384
Basement membrane antibody, 81
Basophilic degeneration, 564
Basophils, normal lab values, 621
Behçet syndrome
    multiple ulcerations in, 72-73
    recurrent oral ulcers in, 170
Benign lymphoid hyperplasia, 526
Benign mucous membrane pemphigoid, 177, Plate C
    immunofluorescence findings, 77
    multiple ulcerations in, 80-81
Benign tumor
    of epidermal appendages, 543-545
    mesenchymal, 154-155
    nonodontogenic
        interradicular radiolucency, 306
        solitary cystlike radiolucency, 311
        solitary cystlike radiolucency not necessarily contacting teeth, 329-330
    of soft tissue, 31
Bicarbonate, serum, 622
Bilirubin
    blood chemistry, 622
    urinalysis, 622
    viral hepatitis and, 611
Biopsy, 10-11
    in intraoral squamous cell carcinoma, 591
    in lichen planus, 75
    in lupus erythematosus, 87-88
    of neck mass, 530
    needle, 24
    in osseous lesion, 235
    of parotid gland tumor, 533
    in verrucous carcinoma, 115
Black as clinical feature, 18
Black conditions, 182-208
    Addison's disease, 206
    Albright's syndrome, 203, 204
    amalgam tattoo, 186-187
    argyria, 207
    black hairy tongue, 196-197
    chloasma gravidarum, 205-206
    cyanosis, 205
    giant cell granuloma, 195-196
    heavy metal lines, 203-204
    hemangioma, 190-192
    hematoma, 189-190
    hemochromatosis, 206-207
    Kaposi's sarcoma, 204, 205
    lymphangioma, 197
    melanoma, 197-200
    melanoplakia, 183-184
    mucocele, 193-194

Black conditions—cont'd
    mucous-producing salivary gland tumors, 202
    nevus, 200-202
    oral melanotic macule, 192-193
    petechia and ecchymosis, 187-189
    pigmented fibrous hyperplasia, 197
    ranula, 194
    rarities, 204-205
    smoker's mucosal melanosis, 184-185
    superficial cyst, 194-195
    varicosity, 185-186
    von Recklinghausen's disease, 202-203
Black hairy tongue, 196-197
Bleeding
    as chief complaint, 40
    clotting abnormalities, 621
    in vascular malformations and central hemangioma of bone, 348
Bleomycin, 115
Blood chemistry, 622
Blood urea nitrogen, 622
Blood-borne non-A, non-B hepatitis, 614
Blue as clinical feature, 18-19
Blue nevus, 201, 548
Bluish conditions, 182-208
    Addison's disease, 206
    Albright's syndrome, 203, 204
    amalgam tattoo, 186-187
    argyria, 207
    black hairy tongue, 196-197
    chloasma gravidarum, 205-206
    cyanosis, 205
    giant cell granuloma, 195-196
    heavy metal lines, 203-204
    hemangioma, 190-192
    hematoma, 189-190
    hemochromatosis, 206-207
    Kaposi's sarcoma, 204, 205
    lymphangioma, 197
    melanoma, 197-200
    melanoplakia, 183-184
    mucocele, 193-194
    mucous-producing salivary gland tumors, 202
    nevus, 200-202
    oral melanotic macule, 192-193
    petechia and ecchymosis, 187-189
    pigmented fibrous hyperplasia, 197
    ranula, 194
    rarities, 204-205
    smoker's mucosal melanosis, 184-185
    superficial cyst, 194-195
    varicosity, 185-186
    von Recklinghausen's disease, 202-203
Bone
    anatomic radiopacity, 450, 451
    central hemangioma of, 348-349
    consistency, 30
    diagram of, 15, 17
    healing, 434
    homeostasis of, 392-393
    lymphoma of, 438, 446
    normal variations of radiodensity, 393
    sclerosing and sclerosed conditions, 457-458
    surgical defect in, 263, 264
Bone cyst
    aneurysmal, 331, 343-346
    traumatic, 270-271, 300
        interradicular radiolucency, 300

Bone cyst—cont'd
  traumatic—cont'd
    periapical radiolucency, 270-271
    pseudomultilocular radiolucency, 334
    solitary cystlike radiolucency, 311
    solitary cystlike radiolucency not necessarily contacting teeth, 314-315, 316
Bone density
  normal variations, 393
  in osteopetrosis, 514-515
  in osteoporosis, 397
Bone destruction
  in osteomyelitis, 265
  in radicular cyst, 259
  radiographic considerations, 255
Bone eburnation, 460
Bone marrow defect
  focal osteoporotic, 321-322
  solitary radiolucency with ragged and poorly defined borders, 360
Bone marrow space, 248-249
  interradicular radiolucency, 298
  multilocular radiolucency, 334, 335
  multiple, 381
  solitary cystlike radiolucency, 310
Bone resorption
  in condensing or sclerosing osteitis, 459
  in multiple myeloma, 384
Bone scintigraphy, 360
Bone whorls, 460
Bony hard consistency, 28
Bony lesions, 233-518
  age and, 44
  anatomic radiolucencies, 238-251
    mandibular, 239-244
    maxillary, 245-248
    multiple separate, well-defined, 380-381
    structures common to both jaws, 248-250
  anatomic radiopacities, 449-456
    anterior nasal spine, 451, 452
    bone, 450, 451
    coronoid process, 453
    external oblique ridge, 454
    genial tubercles, 454, 455
    maxillary tuberosity, 453
    mental ridge, 454
    mineralized tissue shadows, 456
    mylohyoid ridge, 454
    nasal septum and boundaries of nasal fossae, 450-451, 452
    pterygoid plates and pterygoid hamulus, 453
    soft tissue shadows, 455, 456
    teeth, 449-450
    walls and floor of maxillary sinus, 451, 452
    zygomatic process of maxilla and zygomatic bone, 451-453
  gender and, 45
  generalized radiopacities, 508-518
    differential diagnosis, 515-516
    florid cementoosseous dysplasia, 509-511, 515-516
    osteopetrosis, 512-515
    Paget's disease, 511-512, 513, 515-516
    rarities, 515, 516, 517, 518
  generalized rarefactions, 392-413
    differential diagnosis, 409-412
    hereditary hemolytic anemia, 400-405
    homeostasis of bone, 392-393
    hyperparathyroidism, 393-397
    Langerhans' cell disease, 407
    leukemia, 405-406

Bony lesions—cont'd
  generalized rarefactions—cont'd
    multiple myeloma, 408
    normal variations in bone radiodensity, 393
    osteomalacia, 399-400
    osteoporosis, 397-399
    Paget's disease, 407-408
    rarities, 409, 410, 411
  interradicular radiolucencies, 296-308
    anatomic, 296-298, 299
    benign nonodontogenic tumors and tumorlike conditions, 306
    furcation involvement, 299
    globulomaxillary cyst, 300-301, 303, 304
    incisive canal cyst, 303-305
    lateral periodontal cyst, 305-306
    lateral radicular cyst, 299, 300
    malignancies, 305
    median mandibular cyst, 306-307
    odontogenic tumors, 300, 301, 302
    periodontal pockets, 298, 299
    primordial cyst, 300
    rarities, 307
    traumatic bone cyst, 300
  jawbone and regional predilection, 46
  mixed radiolucent-radiopaque associated with teeth, 415-432
    adenomatoid odontogenic tumor, 426-428
    ameloblastic fibroodontoma, 428, 429
    calcifying crown of developing tooth, 415-416
    calcifying epithelial odontogenic tumor, 428-431
    calcifying odontogenic neoplasm, 428, 429
    cementoossifying fibroma, 420-423
    odontoma, 423-426
    periapical cementoosseous dysplasia, 418-420
    rare periapical mixed lesions, 421, 422, 423
    rarefying and condensing osteitis, 417-418
    rarities, 431
    tooth root with rarefying osteitis, 416-417
  mixed radiolucent-radiopaque not necessarily contacting teeth, 433-448
    cementoossifying fibroma, 440, 441, 447
    chondroma and chondrosarcoma, 444-445, 447
    chronic osteomyelitis, 434, 435-436, 447
    desmoplastic ameloblastoma, 445
    fibrous dysplasia, 437-439, 447
    focal cementoosseous dysplasia, 437
    healing surgical site, 434-435
    ossifying subperiosteal hematoma, 445, 447
    osteoblastic metastatic carcinoma, 442-444, 447
    osteogenic sarcoma, 440-442, 447
    osteoradionecrosis, 436, 447
    Paget's disease, 439-440, 447
    rarities, 445-447
  multilocular radiolucencies, 333-355
    ameloblastoma, 337-340
    anatomic patterns, 334, 335
    aneurysmal bone cyst, 343-346
    central giant cell granuloma, 340, 341
    cherubism, 340-342
    differential diagnosis, 353, 354
    giant cell lesion of hyperparathyroidism, 340, 341
    metastatic tumor to jaw, 346-347
    multilocular cyst, 334-337
    odontogenic keratocyst, 343, 345
    odontogenic myxoma, 342-343, 344
    rarities, 349-352
    vascular malformations and central hemangioma of bone, 348-349
  multiple separate, well-defined radiolucencies, 380-391
    anatomic variations, 380-381

Bony lesions—cont'd
  multiple separate, well-defined radiolucencies—cont'd
    basal cell nevus syndrome, 382-384
    Langerhans' cell disease, 386-389
    metastatic carcinoma, 386
    multiple cysts or granulomas, 381-382
    multiple myeloma, 384-386
    rarities, 389-391
  multiple separate radiopacities, 500-508
    cleidocranial dysplasia, 506-507
    embedded or impacted teeth, 505-506
    hypercementosis, 504
    idiopathic osteosclerosis, 504
    mature periapical or focal cementoosseous dysplasia, 503-504
    periapical condensing osteitis, 504, 505
    rarities, 507, 508
    retained roots, 501, 502
    socket sclerosis, 501-503
    tori and exostoses, 500-501
  periapical radiolucencies, 252-278
    anatomic patterns, 253-254
    dentigerous cyst, 266, 267
    malignant tumors, 272-276
    nonradicular cysts, 271-272
    periapical cementoosseous dysplasia, 266-269
    periodontal disease, 269-270
    pulpoperiapical, 253-265; *see also* Pulpoperiapical radiolucencies
    pulpoperiapical disease and hyperplasia of maxillary sinus lining, 265-266
    rarities, 274, 275, 276
  periapical radiopacities, 457-476
    anatomic structures, 467, 468
    condensing or sclerosing osteitis, 459-460
    ectopic calcifications, 470-475
    foreign bodies, 465-466, 469-470
    hypercementosis, 466-467
    idiopathic osteosclerosis, 458-459, 460-463
    impacted teeth, supernumerary teeth, and compound odontomas, 467-469
    mature periapical cementoosseous dysplasia or focal cementoosseous dysplasia, 463-465
    mucosal cyst of maxillary sinus, 470
    rarities, 467, 475
    retained root tips, 469
    sclerosing and sclerosed condition, 457-458
    sclerosing osteitis, 458-459
    tori, exostoses, and peripheral osteomas, 469
    unerupted succedaneous teeth, 465
  pericoronal radiolucencies, 279-295
    adenomatoid odontogenic tumor, 289, 290
    ameloblastic fibroma, 290-291, 292
    ameloblastoma, 289
    calcifying odontogenic cyst, 289-290, 291
    dentigerous cyst, 283-285
    differential diagnosis, 292-294
    pericoronal or follicular space, 279-283
    rarities, 291, 293, 294
    unicystic ameloblastoma, 285-288
  radiography guidelines, 235-237
  solitary cystlike radiolucency not necessarily contacting teeth, 309-332
    ameloblastoma, 321, 322
    anatomic patterns, 310-312
    benign nonodontogenic tumor, 329-330
    central giant cell granuloma or lesion, 323-325
    early stage of cementoossifying fibroma, 328-329
    focal cementoosseous dysplasia, 326
    focal osteoporotic bone marrow defect of jaw, 321-322

Bony lesions—cont'd
  solitary cystlike radiolucency not necessarily contacting teeth—cont'd
    giant cell lesion of hyperparathyroidism, 325-326
    incisive canal cyst, 326, 327
    lingual mandibular bone defect, 315-318
    midpalatine cyst, 326-328
    odontogenic keratocyst, 318-320
    postextraction socket, 312, 313
    primordial cyst, 321
    rarities, 330, 331
    residual cyst, 312-314
    surgical defect, 322-323
    traumatic bone cyst, 314-315, 316
  solitary radiolucency with ragged and poorly defined borders, 356-379
    chondrosarcoma, 368-372
    chronic osteitis, 357
    chronic osteomyelitis, 358-360
    differential diagnosis, 374-378
    fibrous dysplasia, 363-365
    hematopoietic bone marrow defect, 360
    malignant minor salivary gland tumors, 366-367
    metastatic tumors to jaw, 365
    osteogenic sarcoma-osteolytic type, 367-368, 369
    rarities, 371, 372-373
    squamous cell carcinoma, 360-363
  solitary radiopacities not necessarily contacting teeth, 477-499
    condensing or sclerosing osteitis, 481-483
    diffuse sclerosing osteomyelitis, 487-488, 489
    fibrous dysplasia, 484-486
    focal sclerosing osteomyelitis, 486-487
    idiopathic osteosclerosis, 480-481, 482
    mature complex odontoma, 492-493
    mature focal cementoosseous dysplasia, 483-484
    ossifying subperiosteal hematoma, 493
    projected radiopacities, 493-498
    proliferative periostitis, 488-492
    retained roots, 479-480, 481
    tori, exostoses, and peripheral osteomas, 477-478, 479
    unerupted, impacted, and supernumerary teeth, 478-479
Borders of mass, 26-27
Botryoid cyst, 336
Brachial cleft cyst, 532, 537
Bronchogenic carcinoma, 365
Bronze diabetes, 206-207
Brown as clinical feature, 18-19
Brown giant cell lesion, 390, 396
Brownish, bluish, or black conditions, 182-208
  Addison's disease, 206
  Albright's syndrome, 203, 204
  amalgam tattoo, 186-187
  argyria, 207
  black hairy tongue, 196-197
  chloasma gravidarum, 205-206
  cyanosis, 205
  giant cell granuloma, 195-196
  heavy metal lines, 203-204
  hemangioma, 190-192
  hematoma, 189-190
  hemochromatosis, 206-207
  Kaposi's sarcoma, 204, 205
  of lip, 566-568, 569
  lymphangioma, 197
  melanoma, 197-200
  melanoplakia, 183-184
  mucocele, 193-194
  mucus-producing salivary gland tumors, 202

Brownish, bluish, or black conditions—cont'd
nevus, 200-202
oral melanotic macule, 192-193
petechia and ecchymosis, 187-189
pigmented fibrous hyperplasia, 197
ranula, 194
rarities, 204-205
smoker's mucosal melanosis, 184-185
superficial cyst, 194-195
varicosity, 185-186
von Recklinghausen's disease, 202-203
Buccal cyst, 307
Buccal fat pads, 133
Buccal mucosa
amalgam tattoo, 186
erythematous macules, 51
exophytic intramucosal nevus on, 201
Fordyce's granules, 225
hairy leukoplakia, 602
intraoral lesions of, 580-581
leukoedema, 97
lichen planus, 107
linea alba, 98
oral lipoma, 227
recurrent intraoral herpes simplex lesion, 167, 168-169
smoker's melanosis on, 185
verrucous carcinoma, 113
Bullet in cheek, 494
Bullous lichen planus, 22, Plate C
Bullous pemphigoid
benign mucous membrane pemphigoid *versus,* 81
immunofluorescence findings, 77
surface of, 22
Burkitt's lymphoma, 352, 410
Burning sensation as chief complaint, 40
Burns, red lesions with necrotic component, 128

C

Cafe-au-lait spots, 202, 203
Calcification
age and, 44
arterial, 497
basal cell nevus syndrome and, 383
cervical nodes, 474, 475, 496
crown of developing tooth, 415-416
ectopic, 470-475
epithelial odontogenic tumor, 428
hyperparathyroidism and, 394
odontogenic cyst/neoplasm, 428
submandibular lymph node, 472
Calcifying epithelial odontogenic tumor, 426
mixed radiolucent-radiopaque, 428-431
multiple major radiographic appearances, 620
Calcium
blood chemistry, 622
osteomalacia and, 399
parathyroid hormone and, 393
Calculus of salivary gland, 471-472, 473, 575
Canalicular adenoma, 575
Cancellous bone, 450
Cancer, oral; *see* **Oral cancer**
Candida albicans, 141
Candidiasis, 60-63, Plate A, Plate D
in acquired immunodeficiency syndrome, 599, 600-601
atrophic
multiple ulcerations in, 80
solitary red lesion in, 63

Candidiasis—cont'd
denture stomatitis, 63-64
diagnostic procedure, 61
erythematous, 63, 80
erythroplakia *versus,* 59
etiology and pathogenesis, 60-61
features, 61
keratotic white lesion in, 115
leukoplakia *versus,* 102
of lip, 561-562
management, 62-63
median rhomboid glossitis and, 92-93
nicotine stomatitis *versus,* 57, 58-59
red and white lesions, 128
sloughing, pseudomembranous, necrotic white lesion, 122-124
solitary red lesion, 60-65
treatment, 62-63
Canker, 568-569, 570
Capillary hemangioma, Plate A
emptiability of, 37
varicosity *versus,* 185-186
Carbon dioxide partial pressure, 622
Carcinoma in situ, 57-59, 100
Caries, pulp polyp and, 142
Carotenemia, 230
Carotid body tumor, 537-538
Carotid pulse, 524
Cartilage
consistency, 30
diagram of, 15, 17
Cavernous hemangioma, 191
salivary gland tumor *versus,* 153
varicosity *versus,* 185-186
Caviar tongue, 185, 186
CD4 cell, human immunodeficiency virus and, 598-599
CD4 surface antigen, 596
Cellulitis, 54-55, 56
Cementoblastoma, 269, 276, 422
multiple major radiographic appearances, 620
periapical idiopathic osteosclerosis *versus,* 463
periapical radiopacity, 467
Cementoosseous dysplasia
florid, 509-511, 515-516
focal, 269, **437**
condensing or sclerosing osteitis *versus,* 459-460
mature complex odontoma *versus,* 492
mixed radiolucent-radiopaque, 437
multiple separate radiopacities, 503-504
periapical idiopathic osteosclerosis *versus,* 462
periapical radiopacity, 463-465
solitary cystlike radiolucency not necessarily contacting teeth, 326
solitary radiopacity not necessarily contacting teeth, 483-484
multiple radiolucent jaw lesions in, 390
periapical, 266-269
condensing or sclerosing osteitis *versus,* 459
immature, 266-269, 418
mature, 463-465
mature complex odontoma *versus,* 492
mixed radiolucent-radiopaque, 418-420
multiple separate radiopacities, 503-504
periapical granuloma *versus,* 257
periapical idiopathic osteosclerosis *versus,* 462
periapical radiopacity, 463-465
retained root tip *versus,* 417
traumatic bone cyst *versus,* 270-271
Cementoossifying fibroma, 269, 294, **328-329,** 431
exostosis *versus,* 479

Cementoossifying fibroma—cont'd
  mixed radiolucent-radiopaque, 420-423, 440, 441, 447
  periapical cementoosseous dysplasia *versus,* 420
  solitary cystlike radiolucency, 311
  solitary cystlike radiolucency not necessarily contacting teeth, 328-329
Cementum, 30, 449-450
Centers for Disease Control and Prevention, 597-598
Central cavernous hemangioma, 316
Central exophytic lesion, 144-146, 147
Central giant cell granuloma
  multilocular radiolucency, 340, 341, 353
  solitary cystlike radiolucency, 311
  solitary cystlike radiolucency not necessarily contacting teeth, 323-325
Central hemangioma of bone, 348-349, 353
Cervical fascia, 522
Cervical nodes
  calcified, 496, 507
  lymphadenopathy in human immunodeficiency virus infection, 600, 601
  metastatic carcinoma to, 527-528
Chancre, 172-174, Plate B
  of lower lip, 572
  syphilitic, 172-174
Cheek chewing, Plate D
  leukoplakia *versus,* 103
  red and white lesions in, 128
  white sponge nevus *versus,* 116, 117
Cheesy consistency, 28
Cheilitis
  angular, 64-65
  plasma cell, 575
Cheilitis glandularis, 576
Cheilitis granulomatosa, 576
Chemical burn
  candidiasis *versus,* 124
  red lesions with necrotic component, 128
  sloughing, pseudomembranous, necrotic white lesion, 120-121
Chemical erythematous macule, 55-57
Chemotherapy
  in Kaposi's sarcoma, 605
  in verrucous carcinoma, 115
Chemotherapy mucositis
  multiple ulcerations, 84
  red lesions with necrotic component, 129
Cherubism, 340-342
  basal cell nevus syndrome *versus,* 384
  multilocular radiolucencies, 353
Chewing tobacco, 104
Chickenpox, 557
Chief complaint, 40-41
Child
  acquired immunodeficiency syndrome, 599
  bony or calcified lesions, 44
  Langerhans' cell disease, 387-388
  osteopetrosis, 513
  soft tissue lesions, 43
Chloasma gravidarum, 205-206
Chlorhexidine
  for candidiasis, 62
  in chemotherapy mucositis, 84
  in recurrent aphthous ulcer, 166
Chloride, serum, 622
Cholesteatoma, 287
Cholesterol, 622
Cholesterol clefts, 23
Cholinesterase, 622
Chondroma
  consistency of, 31

Chondroma—cont'd
  mixed radiolucent-radiopaque, 444-445, 447
  multiple major radiographic appearances, 620
Chondrosarcoma, 176, 273, **368-370,** Plate J
  consistency of, 31, 33
  mixed radiolucent-radiopaque, 444-445, 447
  multiple major radiographic appearances, 620
  periapical idiopathic osteosclerosis *versus,* 463
  radiolucent-radiopaque image, 438
  retained root tip *versus,* 416
  solitary ill-defined radiolucency, 377
  solitary radiolucency with ragged and poorly defined borders, 368-372
Chronic active hepatitis B, 614, 615
Chronic osteitis, 357
Chronic osteomyelitis
  mixed radiolucent-radiopaque, 434, 435-436, 447
  solitary radiolucency with ragged and poorly defined borders, 358-360
Chronic ulcerative stomatitis, 84
Cicatricial pemphigoid, 77
Cigarette smoker's lip, 565-566
Cinnamon reaction, Plate D
Civatte's body, 76
Cleft lip, 576-577
Cleft palate, 215
Cleidocranial dysplasia, 284, **506-507**
Clinical impression, 45-46
Clotrimazole, 62, 601
Cocaine lesion, Plate B
Codman's triangles, 441
Color as clinical feature, 16
Commissural pit, 210, 577, 578
Common venereal wart, 145
Common wart, 558
Complex odontoma, 423
  periapical idiopathic osteosclerosis *versus,* 463
  periapical radiopacity, 467
  solitary radiopacity not necessarily contacting teeth, 492-493
Compound odontoma, 467-469
Compound-complex odontoma, 423
Computed tomography, 7, 8
  of head and neck space infections, 530
  of parotid gland tumor, 532-533
Computer-assisted imaging, 6-9, 10-11
Condensing or sclerosing osteitis, 458
  multiple separate radiopacities, 504, 505
  periapical radiopacity, 459-460
  solitary radiopacity not necessarily contacting teeth, 481-483
Condyle pseudocyst, 244
Condyloma acuminatum, 145, 146, 563, Plate F
  exophytic small cell carcinoma *versus,* 148
  human immunodeficiency virus-associated, 606
  keratotic white lesion in, 111, 112
  of lip, 563
  red exophytic squamous cell carcinoma *versus,* 60
  red inflammatory hyperplasia lesion *versus,* 54
Condyloma latum, 22, 563
Cone cut, 473-474
Congenital aural sinus, 219-220
Connective tissue, 15, 29
Connective tissue diseases, 551-553
Consistency
  of neck mass, 525
  of surrounding tissue, 27
  of tissue, 28, 29-31, 32-33
Consultation, 12
Contact dermatitis
  erysipelas *versus,* 557

Contact dermatitis—cont'd
  erythroplakia *versus,* 59
  facial manifestations, 555
  lip manifestations, 575
  photoallergic, 554
  single red lesions, 65, 66
Contours as clinical feature, 16
Cooley's anemia, 401-403
Corium, 17
Coronoid process, 453
Corroborative data in radiographic evaluation, 235
Cortical hyperostosis, infantile, 515
Cortical plate, 450
Cortical plate mandibular defects, 244
Corticosteroids
  in benign mucous membrane pemphigoid, 81
  in erythema multiforme, 80
  in major recurrent aphthous ulcer, 169-170
  in pemphigus, 83
Cortisol, 399
Cortisone, 399
Cotton-wool appearance, 511, 513
Country of origin in development of differential diagnosis, 42
Coxsackie A virus, 226, 531
Cranial sutures, 391
Craniofacial fibrous dysplasia, 363
Creatine phosphokinase, 622
Cretinism, 505
Cryosurgery in mucocele, 194
Cryotherapy in hemangioma, 191
Curettement
  of benign nonodontogenic tumor, 330
  bone, 236
  of cementoossifying fibroma, 329
  in giant cell granuloma, 325
  of odontogenic keratocyst, 320
Cushing's syndrome, 398-399
Cutaneous facial lesions, 540-560
  acne and acneiform dermatoses, 555-556
  amyloidosis, 559
  bacterial infections, 556-557
  benign tumors of epidermal appendages, 5430545
  connective tissue diseases, 551-553
  drug eruptions, 554-555
  melanocytic tumors, 547-548, 549
  papulosquamous dermatitides, 553-554
  premalignant and malignant epidermal, 540-543, 544
  reactions to actinic radiation, 554
  tumorlike conditions, 546-547
  vascular tumors, 548-551
  viral infections, 557-558
  xanthelasma, 558-559
Cyanoacrylate, 166
Cyanosis, 205
Cylindroma, 545
Cyst
  acute lymphadenitis *versus,* 526
  aspirate of, 23
  brachial cleft, 532, 537
  consistency of, 30-31
  dentigerous, 145, 266, 267
    interradicular radiolucency, 300
    multilocular, 336
    mural nodules on, 288
    pericoronal radiolucency, 280, 283-285
  draining, 216, 217, 219
  epidermal inclusion, 546-547

Cyst—cont'd
  eruption, 195
  follicular, 283-285, 546-547
  globulomaxillary, 300-301, 303, 304
  incisive canal, 271, 303-305
    interradicular radiolucency, 303-305
    midpalatine cyst *versus,* 328
    solitary cystlike radiolucency, 311
    solitary cystlike radiolucency not necessarily contacting teeth, 326, 327
  lymphoepithelial, 118, 227-228, 537
  maxillary sinus, 470
  median mandibular, 271, 306-307
  midpalatine
    solitary cystlike radiolucency, 311
    solitary cystlike radiolucency not necessarily contacting teeth, 326-328
  multilocular, 334-337, 353
  multiple separate, well-defined radiolucency, 381-382
  muscle overlying, 35
  nasolabial, 575
  nasopalatine, 152
  nasopalatine duct, 303-305
  nonradicular, 271-272
  odontogenic, 289-290, 291, 300, 301
  palatine papilla, 305
  periodontal, 305-306
  primordial, 271
    interradicular radiolucency, 300
    odontogenic keratocyst *versus,* 320
    solitary cystlike radiolucency, 311
    solitary cystlike radiolucency not necessarily contacting teeth, 321
  radicular, 256-259
    fluctuance of, 35
    lateral, 299, 300
    lingual mandibular bone defect *versus,* 318
    midpalatine cyst *versus,* 328
    multilocular, 336
    radiographic considerations, 256-259
    traumatic bone cyst *versus,* 270
  residual
    lingual mandibular bone defect *versus,* 318
    mixed radiolucent-radiopaque appearance, 434
    multilocular, 336
    odontogenic keratocyst *versus,* 320
    solitary cystlike radiolucency, 311
    solitary cystlike radiolucency not necessarily contacting teeth, 312-314
  sebaceous
    aspirate from, 23
    chronic draining, 219
    consistency of, 30
    mobility of, 25
    in neck, 529
  sinus draining, 38
  Stafne's, 328-329
  superficial, brownish, bluish, or black, 194-195
  thyroglossal, 24, 535, 536
  traumatic bone, 300
    interradicular radiolucency, 300
    periapical radiolucency, 270-271
    pseudomultilocular radiolucency, 334
    solitary cystlike radiolucency, 311
    solitary cystlike radiolucency not necessarily contacting teeth, 314-315, 316
Cystic hygroma, 30, 538-539
Cystic odontoma, 431
Cysticercosis, 507
Cytoid body, 76

Cytology, exfoliative, 11
Cytomegalovirus, 607, Plate F

D

Dandruff, 554
Dane particle, 613
Dapsone, 81
Darier's disease, 119, 159
ddC; *see* Zalcitabine
ddI; *see* Didanosine
Deficiency anemia, 94
Deficiency states, 92-93, 94
Delayed tooth eruption as chief complaint, 40
Delta hepatitis, 613-614
Dense bone island, 460
Dental follicle, 279
Dental laboratory studies, 9-10
Dentigerous cyst, 145, 266, 267
   interradicular radiolucency, 300
   multilocular, 336
   mural nodules on, 288
   pericoronal radiolucency, 280, 283-285
Dentin, 30, 449-450
Dentoalveolar abscess, 211-212
   chronic and acute, 259-263
   pulpoperiapical radiolucency, 259-263
   sinus draining chronic, 217, 218
Dentures
   candidiasis mucositis and, 63-64
   epulis fissuratum and, 139
   papillary hyperplasia of palate and, 140-141
   stomatitis and, 63-64
Dermatitis, seborrheic, 554
Dermatitis medicamentosa, 554-555
Dermatomyositis, 552-553
Dermoid
   aspirate from, 23
   consistency of, 30
   sebaceous cyst *versus,* 529
   submental, 535, 536
   yellow, 228
Desmoplastic ameloblastoma, 445
Desquamative gingivitis, 83
Developmental abnormalities of lip, 576-578
Developmental periodontal cyst, 305-306
Developmental submandibular gland defect of mandible, 315
Diabetes mellitus, 76
Diagnostic sequence, 39-46
   classification of lesion, 42
   development of differential diagnosis, 42-43, 44, 45, 46
   development of working diagnosis, 45-46
   formulation of final diagnosis, 46
   list of possible diagnoses, 42
   patient examination, 39-41
   two or more lesions present, 44-45
Didanosine, 607
Differential diagnosis, 1-46
   auscultation in, 38
   biopsy, 10-11
   consultation, 12
   dental laboratory studies, 9-10
   diagnostic sequence, 39-46
      classification of lesion, 42
      development of differential diagnosis, 42-43, 44, 45, 46
      development of working diagnosis, 45-46
      formulation of final diagnosis, 46
      list of possible diagnoses, 42

Differential diagnosis—cont'd
   diagnostic sequence—cont'd
      patient examination, 39-41
      two or more lesions present, 44-45
   exfoliative cytology, 11
   importance of normal anatomy and histology, 14-15, 16, 17, 18
   inspection in, 16-24
      aspirate, 23-24
      aspiration, 20-23
      color, 16-19
      contours, 16
      flat and raised entities, 20
      needle biopsy, 24
      surfaces, 19-20, 21, 22
   medical laboratory studies, 9
   palpation in, 24-38
      anatomic regions and planes involved, 25
      borders of mass, 26-27
      consistency of mass, 28, 29-31, 32-33
      consistency of surrounding tissue, 27
      extent of mass, 26
      fluctuance and emptiability, 28-33, 34, 35
      lesions demonstrating variable fluctuance, 33-34, 35, 37, 38
      mobility, 25-26
      painless, tender, or painful, 34-38
      size and shape, 27-28
      solitary or multiple lesions, 38
      sturdiness of underlying tissue, 27
      surface temperature, 24-25
      thickness of overlying tissue, 27
      unilateral or bilateral mass, 38
   percussion in, 38
   toluidine blue staining, 11-12
Differential white blood cell count, 621
Diffuse gangrenous stomatitis, 124-125
Diffuse sclerosing osteomyelitis
   fibrous dysplasia *versus,* 486
   florid cementoosseous dysplasia *versus,* 511
   solitary radiopacity not necessarily contacting teeth, 487-488, 489
Diflucan; *see* Fluconazole
Digital radiography, 6, 7
Disarticulation, 237
Discoid lupus erythematosus, 87
   facial manifestations, 551, 552
   immunofluorescence findings, 77
   leukoplakia *versus,* 102-103
Double lip, 577
Drug reaction, Plate D
   cutaneous facial lesions, 554-555
   lichenoid, 77
   predisposition to oral candidiasis, 61
Drug-induced osteoporosis, 399
Dry mouth, 41, 85
Dysosteosclerosis, 518
Dysplasia
   cleidocranial, 284, **506-507**
   fibrous
      diffuse sclerosing osteomyelitis *versus,* 488
      mixed radiolucent-radiopaque, 437-439, 447
      multiple major radiographic appearances, 620
      periapical cementoosseous dysplasia *versus,* 419-420
      polyostotic, 515
      proliferative periostitis *versus,* 492
      solitary ill-defined radiolucency, 376
      solitary radiolucency with ragged and poorly defined borders, 363-365
      solitary radiopacity not necessarily contacting teeth, 484-486
   florid cementoosseous, 509-511, 515-516

Dysplasia—cont'd
  focal cementoosseous, 269
    condensing or sclerosing osteitis *versus,* 459-460
    mature complex odontoma *versus,* 492
    mixed radiolucent-radiopaque, 437
    multiple separate radiopacities, 503-504
    periapical idiopathic osteosclerosis *versus,* 462
    periapical radiopacity, 463-465
    solitary cystlike radiolucency not necessarily contacting teeth, 326
    solitary radiopacity not necessarily contacting teeth, 483-484
  multiple radiolucent jaw lesions in, 390
  periapical cementoosseous, 266-269
    condensing or sclerosing osteitis *versus,* 459
    mature complex odontoma *versus,* 492
    mixed radiolucent-radiopaque, 418-420
    multiple separate radiopacities, 503-504
    periapical granuloma *versus,* 257
    periapical idiopathic osteosclerosis *versus,* 462
    periapical radiopacity, 463-465
    retained root tip *versus,* 417
    traumatic bone cyst *versus,* 270-271

E

Ecchymosis, 187-189
Echovirus, 531
Ectopic calcification, 470-475
Ectopic geographic tongue, 85-86, Plate D
Ectopic thyroid gland, 119
Edematous tissue, 31
Elderly
  bony or calcified lesions, 44
  soft tissue lesions, 43
Electrogalvanic and mercury contact allergy
  keratotic white lesion in, 110-111
  leukoplakia *versus,* 102
Ellsworth-Howard test, 383
Embedded tooth, 505-506
Embryonal rests, 22
Emphysema, 30
Emptiability of mass, 28-33, 34, 35
Encephalotrigeminal angiomatosis, 568
Endocrinopathies, 61
Energex-B, 617
Enostosis, 460
Enucleation
  of adenomatoid odontogenic tumor, 288
  of benign nonodontogenic tumor, 330
  bone, 236
  of dentigerous cyst, 284
  of incisive canal cyst, 305
  of midpalatine cyst, 328
  of multilocular cyst, 337
  of odontogenic keratocyst, 320
  of residual cyst, 313
Enzyme-linked immunosorbent assay, 597
Eosinophilic granuloma, 307, 331, 387
Eosinophils, normal lab values, 621
Ephelis, 20
Epidermal inclusion cyst, 546-547
Epidermal lesion, premalignant and malignant, 540-543, 544
Epidermis, 14, 15
Epidermoid
  aspirate from, 23
  consistency of, 30, 32
  facial, 546-547
  freely movable mass, 25
  of lip, 564-565

Epidermoid—cont'd
  sebaceous cyst *versus,* 529
  submental, 535, 536
  uvula, 118
  yellow, 228
Epidermolysis bullosa, 22
Epithelial mass, 26
Epithelial tissue, 15
Epstein-Barr virus, 601-602
Epstein's pearls, 195
Epulis fissuratum, 139-140, Plate A
Epulis granulomatosum, 142-143
Epulis of newborn, 157
Erosion, 163
Erosive lichen planus, Plate C
  multiple ulcerations in, 75-77, 78
  red and white lesions in, 128
Eruption cyst, 145, 195, 284
Eruption hematoma, 195
Erysipelas, 557
Erythema migrans, 90
Erythema multiforme, Plate C
  of lip, 570-571
  multiple ulcerations in, 78-80
  surface of, 22
Erythremia, 86-87
Erythrocytes, 622
Erythroleukoplakia, 128
Erythromycin, 262
Erythroplakia, Plate B, Plate H
  premalignant, 589
  solitary red lesion, 57-59
Ewing's sarcoma, 293, 373
  multiple major radiographic appearances, 620
  proliferative periostitis *versus,* 491-492
  solitary ill-defined radiolucency, 377
Excision
  of benign nonodontogenic tumor, 330
  of cementoossifying fibroma, 329
  of epulis granulomatosum, 143
  of hemangioma, 191
  of inflammatory hyperplasia lesion, 137
  of mucocele, 193
  in oral cancer, 592
  in oral melanoma, 200
  of papilloma, 146
  of peripheral fibroma with calcification, 144
  of peripheral giant cell lesion, 142
Excisional biopsy, 10, 54
Exfoliative cytology, 11
Exophytic lesion, 131-161
  anatomic structures, 132-134, 135
  central, 144-146, 147
  fibrous hyperplasia, 137-144
    acquired hemangioma, 143
    epulis fissuratum, 139-140
    epulis granulomatosum, 142-143
    hormonal therapy, 139
    papillary hyperplasia of palate, 140-141
    parulis, 140
    peripheral fibroma with calcification, 143-144
    peripheral giant cell lesion, 141-142
    pulp polyp, 142
    pyogenic granuloma, 138-139
  hemangioma, lymphangioma, and varicosity, 144
  inflammatory hyperplasia, 136-137
  minor salivary gland tumors, 149-154

Exophytic lesion—cont'd
  mucocele and ranula, 144
  nevus and melanoma, 155, 156
  in oral melanoma, 199
  peripheral benign mesenchymal tumors, 154-155
  peripheral malignant mesenchymal tumors, 156, 157
  peripheral metastatic tumors, 155-156
  rarities, 156-160
  squamous cell carcinoma, 146-149, 151
  tori and exostoses, 134-136
  traumatized tumors and, 175
  verrucous carcinoma, 149
Exophytic squamous cell carcinoma
  solitary red lesion, 59-60
  surface of, 22
Exostosis
  consistency of, 31
  exophytic, 134-136
  generalized radiopacity, 517
  multiple separate radiopacities, 500-501
  periapical radiopacity, 469
  proliferative periostitis versus, 492
  solitary radiopacities not necessarily contacting teeth, 477-478, 479
  solitary radiopacity not necessarily contacting teeth, 477-478, 479
Extent of mass, 26
External oblique ridge, 454
Exudate
  in draining mucocele and ranula, 213
  in oroantral fistula, 214

F

Facial artery calcification, 472, 475
Facial skin lesion, 540-560
  acne and acneiform dermatoses, 555-556
  amyloidosis, 559
  bacterial infections, 556-557
  benign tumors of epidermal appendages, 543-545
  connective tissue diseases, 551-553
  cutaneous reactions to actinic radiation, 554
  drug eruptions, 554-555
  melanocytic tumors, 547-548, 549
  papulosquamous dermatitides, 553-554
  premalignant and malignant, 540-543, 544
  tumorlike conditions, 546-547
  vascular tumors, 548-551
  viral infections, 557-558
  xanthelasma, 558-559
Factor analysis, 621
False periapical radiopacities, 467-475
  anatomic structures, 467, 468
  ectopic calcifications, 470-475
  foreign bodies, 469-470
  impacted teeth, supernumerary teeth, and compound odontomas, 467-469
  mucosal cyst of maxillary sinus, 470
  rarities, 475
  retained root tips, 469
  tori, exostoses, and peripheral osteomas, 469
Familial adenomatosis coli, 516
Familial gingival fibromatosis, 158
Fatty tumor, 30
Fauces, 582
FCOD; see Focal cementoosseous dysplasia
Fever blister, 570
Fibrin clot, 226
Fibrin deposits in lichen planus, 76
Fibrinogen, 621

Fibroma
  ameloblastic, 280, 290-291, 292
  with calcification, 143-144
  cementoossifying, 269, 294, 431
    curettement or excision of, 329
    exostosis versus, 479
    mixed radiolucent-radiopaque, 420-423, 440, 441, 447
    periapical cementoosseous dysplasia versus, 420
    solitary cystlike radiolucency, 311
    solitary cystlike radiolucency not necessarily contacting teeth, 328-329
  consistency of, 31
  giant cell, 138, 157
  multilocular radiolucency, 349
  odontogenic, 143, 620
  ossifying and cementifying, 352
  smooth-surfaced mass, 20
Fibromyxoma, odontogenic, 293
Fibroodontoma, ameloblastic, 428, 429
Fibroosseous lesions of periodontal ligament origin, 620
Fibrosarcoma, 31, 33
Fibrosis
  in inflammatory hyperplastic lesion, 136, 137
  submucous, 106
Fibrous dysplasia, 363-365
  diffuse sclerosing osteomyelitis versus, 488
  mixed radiolucent-radiopaque, 437-439, 447
  multiple major radiographic appearances, 620
  periapical cementoosseous dysplasia versus, 419-420
  polyostotic, 515
  proliferative periostitis versus, 492
  solitary ill-defined radiolucency, 376
  solitary radiolucency with ragged and poorly defined borders, 363-365
  solitary radiopacity not necessarily contacting teeth, 484-486
Fibrous hyperplasia, 137-144
  acquired hemangioma, 143
  epulis fissuratum, 139-140
  epulis granulomatosum, 142-143
  hormonal therapy, 139
  inflammatory, 137-138
  of lip, 572-573
  papillary hyperplasia of palate, 140-141
  parulis, 140
  peripheral fibroma with calcification, 143-144
  peripheral giant cell lesion, 141-142
  pigmented, 197
  pulp polyp, 142
  pyogenic granuloma, 138-139
Field cancerization, 589
Final diagnosis, 12, 46
Fine-needle aspiration, 10-11
Firm consistency, 28
First-echelon node, 525, 536
Fissures, 180
Fistula, 211-217
  chronic draining alveolar abscess, 211-212
  differential diagnosis, 222-223
  draining chronic osteomyelitis, 215-216
  draining cyst, 216, 217, 219
  draining mucocele and ranula, 213
  oroantral, 142, **213-214**
  orocutaneous, 221-222
  oronasal, 215
  patent nasopalatine duct, 216-217
  pustule, 217
  salivary gland, 220-221
  sinus draining chronic dentoalveolar abscess, 217, 218
  suppurative infection of parotid and submandibular glands, 212-213

Flat wart, 558
Floor of mouth
    cavernous hemangioma, 191
    epidermoid and dermoid cysts, 228
    erythematous macules, 51
    exophytic squamous cell carcinoma, 146
    intraoral lesions, 583
    ranula, 194
    recurrent aphthous ulcer, 167
    verrucous carcinoma, 113
Florid cementoosseous dysplasia, 509-511, 515-516
Flossing, 169
Fluconazole, 62, 63, 601
Fluctuance
    lesions demonstrating variable, 33-34, 35, 37, 38
    of mass, 28-33, 34, 35
    of neck mass, 525
Fluocinonide, 164
Focal cementoosseous dysplasia, 269
    condensing or sclerosing osteitis *versus,* 459-460
    mature complex odontoma *versus,* 492
    mixed radiolucent-radiopaque, 437
    multiple separate radiopacities, 503-504
    periapical idiopathic osteosclerosis *versus,* 462
    periapical radiopacity, 463-465
    solitary cystlike radiolucency not necessarily contacting teeth, 326
    solitary radiopacity not necessarily contacting teeth, 483-484
Focal epithelial hyperplasia, 159, 566
Focal osteoporotic bone marrow defect, 249, 310, 321-322
Focal sclerosing osteomyelitis, 483, 486-487
Foliate papillae, 132, 133
Follicular cyst, 283-285, 546-547
Follicular space, 279-283
Fordyce's granules, 15, 225-226
Foreign body, 465-466, 469-470, 494, 498
Fovea palatinae, 209-210
Fracture in multiple myeloma, 385
Freckle, 20
Frey's syndrome, 221
Furcation involvement, 299

G

Gangrenous stomatitis
    candidiasis *versus,* 124
    sloughing, pseudomembranous, necrotic white lesion, 124-125
Gardner's syndrome, 203, 516
Garre's osteomyelitis, 488
Gender
    development of differential diagnosis, 42, 45
    oral cancer and, 588
Generalized radiopacities, 508-518
    differential diagnosis, 515-516
    florid cementoosseous dysplasia, 509-511, 515-516
    osteopetrosis, 512-515
    Paget's disease, 511-512, 513, 515-516
    rarities, 515, 516, 517, 518
Generalized rarefactions, 392-413
    differential diagnosis, 409-412
    hereditary hemolytic anemia, 400-405
    homeostasis of bone, 392-393
    hyperparathyroidism, 393-397
    Langerhans' cell disease, 407
    leukemia, 405-406
    multiple myeloma, 408
    normal variations in bone radiodensity, 393
    osteomalacia, 399-400
    osteoporosis, 397-399

Generalized rarefactions—cont'd
    Paget's disease, 407-408
    rarities, 409, 410, 411
Genial tubercles, 132, 454, 455
Gentian violet, 62-63
Geographic tongue, 90-92
Giant cell fibroma, 138, 157
Giant cell granuloma, 195-196, 323-325
    brownish, bluish, or black, 195-196
    between central incisors, 307
    globulomaxillary radiolucency, 304
    multilocular radiolucency, 340, 341
    multiple major radiographic appearances, 620
    myxoma *versus,* 343
    periapical radiolucency, 274
Giant cell lesion, 141-142
    brown, 390
    in hyperparathyroidism, 325-326, 340, 341, 396
        multilocular radiolucencies, 353
        solitary cystlike radiolucency, 311
        solitary cystlike radiolucency not necessarily contacting teeth, 325-326
Gingiva
    amalgam tattoo, 186
    benign mucous membrane pemphigoid, 80-81
    erythroplakia, 59
    hemangioendothelioma, 205
    intraoral lesions, 581
    Kaposi's sarcoma, 605
    peripheral fibroma with calcification, 143
    recurrent intraoral herpes simplex lesion, 167, 168-169
    verrucous carcinoma, 113
Gingivitis
    acquired immunodeficiency syndrome-associated, 602-604, 605, Plate E
    acute necrotic ulcerative, 171, Plate E
        in human immunodeficiency virus infection, 602-604
        red lesions with necrotic component, 128-129
        sickle cell anemia *versus,* 122
        sloughing, pseudomembranous, necrotic white lesion, 121-122
    desquamative, 83
    erythroplakia *versus,* 59
    marginal, Plate E
    mouthbreathing, 158
    plasma cell, 85, Plate D
    during pregnancy, Plate B
Gingivostomatitis, herpetic, Plate C, Plate D
Globulomaxillary cyst, 300-301, 303, 304
Glossitis
    deficiency states and, 92
    median rhomboid, 92, 93
    migratory, 90-92
        keratotic white lesion in, 106
        red and white lesions in, 128
Glossitis areata exfoliativa, 90
Glossitis areata migrans, 90-92
Glucose, blood chemistry, 622
Goiter, 534
Granular cell lesion, 118
Granular cell myoblastoma, 21, 157
Granuloma
    central giant cell
        multilocular radiolucency, 340, 341, 353
        solitary cystlike radiolucency, 311
        solitary cystlike radiolucency not necessarily contacting teeth, 323-325
    eosinophilic, 307, 387

Granuloma—cont'd
  giant cell, 195-196
    brownish, bluish, or black, 195-196
    between central incisors, 307
    globulomaxillary radiolucency, 304
    multilocular radiolucency, 340, 341
    multiple major radiographic appearances, 620
    myxoma *versus,* 343
    periapical radiolucency, 274
  multiple separate, well-defined radiolucency, 381-382
  periapical, 255, 256
  pyogenic, 120, 121, 549-550, Plate B
    fibrous hyperplasia in, 138-139
    red lesions with necrotic component in, 129
    squamous cell carcinoma *versus,* 148
Greater palatine foramen, 247
Gumma, 179
  oronasal fistula and, 215
  syphilitic, 172-174

H

Hair follicle, 17
Hairy leukoplakia, 102
  in acquired immunodeficiency syndrome, 599, **601-602**
  keratotic white lesion in, 115
Hairy tongue
  black, 196-197
  white, 111
  yellow, 226
Halitosis, 41
Hamular process, 453
Hand-foot-and-mouth disease
  primary herpetic gingivostomatitis *versus,* 73-74
  recurrent intraoral herpes simplex lesion *versus,* 168
Hand-Schuller-Christian syndrome, 387
Hard palate
  intraoral lesions, 582
  tori, 134, 136
Hashimoto's disease, 534
Havrix, 617
Healing surgical site, 434-435
Heavy metal lines, 203-204
Heck's disease, 566
Hemangioendothelioma of gingiva, 205
Hemangioma, 144, 548-549
  acquired, 143
  amalgam tattoo *versus,* 187
  aspiration of, 24
  brownish, bluish, or black, 190-192
  capillary, Plate A
  central bone, 348-349
  congenital, 54
  consistency of, 30
  emptiability of, 37
  erythematous macule *versus,* 53
  intrabony, multilocular radiolucency and, 348-349
  of lip, 567
  multiple major radiographic appearances, 620
  red exophytic squamous cell carcinoma *versus,* 60
  red inflammatory hyperplasia lesion *versus,* 54
Hemangiosarcoma, 273
Hematocrit, 621
Hematologic blood values, 621
Hematologic disorders, 61
Hematoma, 189-190
  consistency of, 31
  eruption, 195

Hematoma—cont'd
  ossifying subperiosteal
    mixed radiolucent-radiopaque, 445, 447
    solitary radiopacity not necessarily contacting teeth, 493
  proliferative periostitis *versus,* 492
Hematopoietic bone marrow defect, 360
Hemochromatosis, 206-207, 568
Hemoglobin content, 621
Hemolysis, 229
Hemolytic anemia
  hereditary, 400-405
  sickle cell anemia and, 403-405
  thalassemia and, 401-402
Hemophilia, 294, 351
Hemorrhage
  as chief complaint, 40
  clotting abnormalities, 621
  in vascular malformations and central hemangioma of bone, 348
Hemosiderin, 323
Hepatitis, 611-619
  acute, 611-612
  delta, 613-615
  dental implications for, 618
  prophylaxis and vaccines, 616-617
Hepatitis A, 612
Hepatitis A vaccine, 617
Hepatitis B, 612-614, 615
Hepatitis B surface antigen, 613
Hepatitis B vaccine, 617
Hepatitis C, 614-615
Hepatitis D, 613-615
Hepatitis E, 616
Hepatitis F and G, 616
Heptavax-B, 617
Herald lesion of generalized stomatitis, 67
Hereditary benign intraepithelial dyskeratosis, 116
Hereditary hemolytic anemia, 400-405
Hereditary hemorrhagic telangiectasia, 568
Heroin-induced thrombocytopenic purpura, 159
Herpangina, 168
Herpes labialis, 570, 571
Herpes simplex, 163, Plate F
  candidiasis *versus,* 124
  human immunodeficiency virus-associated, 606
  in lip infection, 569-570, 571
  recurrent/intraoral, 167-169
    herpetic gingivostomatitis and, 73-75
Herpes zoster, 557-558
  human immunodeficiency virus-associated, 606
  vesicles of, 97, 119
Herpetic gingivostomatitis, Plate C, Plate D
Herpetic whitlow, 168
Herpetiform aphtha, 170
Herpetiform ulcer, 73
Hibernoma, 30
Histiocytosis X, 386-389
Histoplasmosis, 31
History; *see* Patient history
Homeostasis of bone, 392-393
Homogenous erythroplakia, 58
Homogenous leukoplakia, Plate G
Honeycomb, 334
Hormonal therapy, 139
Human immunodeficiency virus infection, 596-610
  course of disease, 598-599
  demography and epidemiology, 98, 597, 599
  gingivitis in, Plate E

Human immunodeficiency virus infection—cont'd
oral manifestations, 599-606
risk of transmission to and from dental community, 607-608
surveillance classification, 597-598
treatment and prognosis, 606-607
virus types, 596-597
Human immunodeficiency virus type 1, 596-597
Human immunodeficiency virus type 2, 596-597
Human papillomavirus, 145, 558
Hutchinson's incisors, 173
Hydroxypropyl cellulose, 166
Hydroxypropyl methylcellulose, 164
Hyoid bone, 524
Hyperbilirubinemia, 229
Hypercalcemia, 384
Hypercementosis
condensing or sclerosing osteitis *versus,* 459-460
multiple separate radiopacities, 504
periapical idiopathic osteosclerosis *versus,* 462
periapical radiopacity, 466-467
Hyperostosis, infantile cortical, 515
Hyperostotic border, 458
Hyperparathyroidism
generalized rarefactions, 393-397
giant cell lesion of, 325-326, 340, 341
serum values in, 411
Hyperplasia, 20, 131
adenoid, 153
adenomatoid, 158
benign lymphoid, 526
consistency of, 30
fibrous, 137-144
acquired hemangioma, 143
epulis fissuratum, 139-140
epulis granulomatosum, 142-143
hormonal therapy, 139
of lip, 572-573
papillary hyperplasia of palate, 140-141
parulis, 140
peripheral fibroma with calcification, 143-144
peripheral giant cell lesion, 141-142
pigmented, 197
pulp polyp, 142
pyogenic granuloma, 138-139
focal epithelial lip, 159, 566
of follicular spaces, 282, 283
inflammatory, 136-144, Plate A
exophytic, 136-137
red exophytic squamous cell carcinoma *versus,* 60
red metastatic tumor *versus,* 68
solitary red lesion, 53-54
of maxillary sinus lining, 265-266
multiple fibroepithelial, 160
nontender lymphoid, 526
papillary, Plate A
nicotine stomatitis *versus,* 104
of palate, 140-141
phenytoin, 158
sebaceous, 546
surface of, 22
verrucous, 114
Hyperplastic candidiasis
red and white lesions in, 128
white keratotic lesion in, 115
Hypertrophy, 20, 131
Hypophosphatemia
in multiple myeloma, 384-385
serum values in, 411

I
Icterus, 229
Idiopathic CD4+ T-lymphocytopenia, 598
Idiopathic osteosclerosis, 458
multiple separate radiopacities, 504
periapical radiopacity, 458-459
solitary radiopacity not necessarily contacting teeth, 480-481, 482
Idiopathic thrombocytopenic purpura, 568
Imaging, computer-assisted, 6-9, 10-11
Immunoassay for human immunodeficiency virus, 597
Immunodeficiency
predisposition to oral candidiasis, 61
recurrent intraoral herpes simplex and, 169
Immunofluorescence studies
in benign mucous membrane pemphigoid, 81
in lichen planus, 76, 77, 78
in pemphigus, 82-83
Immunoglobulin G, 83
Impacted tooth
dentigerous cyst and, 284
multiple separate radiopacities, 505-506
periapical radiopacity, 467-469
pericoronal space, 281, 282
solitary radiopacity not necessarily contacting teeth, 478-479
Impetigo, 556-557
Incisional biopsy, 10
Incisive canal, 245, 246, 451
Incisive canal cyst, 271
interradicular radiolucency, 303-305
midpalatine cyst *versus,* 328
solitary cystlike radiolucency, 311
solitary cystlike radiolucency not necessarily contacting teeth, 326, 327
Incisive foramen, 245, 246, 297, 298
Incisive fossa, 245, 246
Indinavir, 607
Infantile cortical hyperostosis, 492, 515
Infection
in condensing or sclerosing osteitis, 459
consistency of, 31
parotid and submandibular glands, 212-213
Infectious hepatitis, 612; *see also* **Hepatitis**
Infectious mononucleosis, 189
Inferior dental canal, 239-240
Inflammation
borders of, 27
consistency of, 31
in osteosclerosis, 458
pain in, 34-36
sclerosing osteitis and, 481
surface temperature in, 25
tonsillar, 526
Inflammatory hyperplasia, Plate A
exophytic, 136-137
red exophytic squamous cell carcinoma *versus,* 60
red metastatic tumor *versus,* 68
solitary red lesion, 53-54
Inflammatory periodontal cyst, 305, 306
Ingrown hairs, 557
Inspection, 16-24
aspirate, 23-24
aspiration, 20-23
color, 16-19
contours, 16
flat and raised entities, 20
needle biopsy, 24
surfaces, 19-20, 21, 22
Interleukin-1, 257
Interleukin-6, 257

Intermaxillary suture, 245
Internal oblique ridge, 454
Interradicular radiolucencies, 296-308
    anatomic, 296-298, 299
    benign nonodontogenic tumors and tumorlike conditions, 306
    furcation involvement, 299
    globulomaxillary cyst, 300-301, 303, 304
    incisive canal cyst, 303-305
    lateral periodontal cyst, 305-306
    lateral radicular cyst, 299, 300
    malignancies, 305
    median mandibular cyst, 306-307
    odontogenic tumors, 300, 301, 302
    periodontal pockets, 298, 299
    primordial cyst, 300
    rarities, 307
    traumatic bone cyst, 300
Interstitial keratitis, 173
Intrabony fibroma, 349
Intrabony neurilemoma, 352
Intraepithelial carcinoma, 100
Intramucosal nevus, 200-201
Irreversible leukoplakia, 100
Irritant contact dermatitis, 555
Isomorphic effect, 553
Itraconazole, 62
Ivy bleeding time, 621

J

Jaundice, 229, Plate B
    carotenemia *versus,* 230
    in viral hepatitis, 611
Jaw
    anatomic radiolucencies, 248-250
        developing tooth crypt, 249, 250
        marrow space, 248-249
        nutrient canal, 249, 250
        periodontal ligament space, 248
        pulp chamber and root canal, 248
    anatomic radiopacities, 449-456
        anterior nasal spine, 451, 452
        bone, 450, 451
        coronoid process, 453
        external oblique ridge, 454
        genial tubercles, 454, 455
        maxillary tuberosity, 453
        mental ridge, 454
        mineralized tissue shadows, 456
        mylohyoid ridge, 454
        nasal septum and boundaries of nasal fossae, 450-451, 452
        pterygoid plates and pterygoid hamulus, 453
        soft tissue shadows, 455, 456
        teeth, 449-450
        walls and floor of maxillary sinus, 451, 452
        zygomatic process of maxilla and zygomatic bone, 451-453
    changes in hyperparathyroidism, 394-396
    focal osteoporotic bone marrow defect, 321-322
    generalized radiopacities, 508-518
        differential diagnosis, 515-516
        florid cementoosseous dysplasia, 509-511, 515-516
        osteopetrosis, 512-515
        Paget's disease, 511-512, 513, 515-516
        rarities, 515, 516, 517, 518
    generalized rarefactions, 392-413
        differential diagnosis, 409-412
        hereditary hemolytic anemia, 400-405
        homeostasis of bone, 392-393
        hyperparathyroidism, 393-397

Jaw—cont'd
    generalized rarefactions—cont'd
        Langerhans' cell disease, 407
        leukemia, 405-406
        multiple myeloma, 408
        normal variations in bone radiodensity, 393
        osteomalacia, 399-400
        osteoporosis, 397-399
        Paget's disease, 407-408
        rarities, 409, 410, 411
    metastatic tumors to, 346-347, 365
    normal variations in radiodensity, 393
    solitary radiolucency cystlike, not necessarily contacting teeth, 309-332
        ameloblastoma, 321, 322
        anatomic patterns, 310-312
        benign nonodontogenic tumor, 329-330
        central giant cell granuloma or lesion, 323-325
        early stage of cementoossifying fibroma, 328-329
        focal cementoosseous dysplasia, 326
        focal osteoporotic bone marrow defect of jaw, 321-322
        giant cell lesion of hyperparathyroidism, 325-326
        incisive canal cyst, 326, 327
        lingual mandibular bone defect, 315-318
        midpalatine cyst, 326-328
        odontogenic keratocyst, 318-320
        postextraction socket, 312, 313
        primordial cyst, 321
        rarities, 330, 331
        residual cyst, 312-314
        surgical defect, 322-323
        traumatic bone cyst, 314-315, 316
    solitary radiolucency with ragged and poorly defined borders, 356-379
        chondrosarcoma, 368-372
        chronic osteitis, 357
        chronic osteomyelitis, 358-360
        differential diagnosis, 374-378
        fibrous dysplasia, 363-365
        hematopoietic bone marrow defect, 360
        malignant minor salivary gland tumors, 366-367
        metastatic tumors to jaw, 365
        osteogenic sarcoma-osteolytic type, 367-368, 369
        rarities, 371, 372-373
        squamous cell carcinoma, 360-363
Junctional nevus, 201, 547
Juvenile hemangioma, 549

K

Kaposi's sarcoma, 604-606, Plate F
    acquired immunodeficiency syndrome and, 604-606
    brownish, bluish, or black, 204, 205
    erythroplakia *versus,* 59
    facial, 550-551
    in human immunodeficiency virus infection, 599
    inflammatory hyperplasia *versus,* 137
    lip lesion in, 568
    red exophytic squamous cell carcinoma *versus,* 60
    red inflammatory hyperplasia lesion *versus,* 54
    red metastatic tumor *versus,* 68
    solitary red lesion, 68
Keratin
    leukoplakia and, 99
    verrucous carcinoma and, 114
Keratoacanthoma, 148
    facial, 542
    of lip, 571-572
    squamous cell carcinoma *versus,* 179
    surface of, 22

Keratocyst, odontogenic, 343, 345
   solitary cystlike radiolucency, 311
   solitary cystlike radiolucency not necessarily contacting teeth, 318-320
Keratosis
   actinic, 540-541, 564
   seborrheic, 546
   white entities and, 96-117
Keratotic white lesion, 97-117
   electrogalvanic and mercury contact allergy, 110-111
   hairy leukoplakia, 115
   hypertrophic or hyperplastic candidiasis, 115
   leukoedema, 97-98
   leukoplakia, 98-103, 108
   lichen planus, 106-110
   lichenoid drug reaction, 110
   linea alba buccalis, 98, 99
   migratory glossitis, 106
   nicotine stomatitis, 103-104
   papilloma, verruca vulgaris, and condyloma acuminatum, 111, 112
   peripheral scar tissue, 106
   rarities, 117, 118, 119
   red lesions with, 128
   skin grafts, 117, 118
   smokeless tobacco lesion, 104-105
   verrucous carcinoma, 113-115
   white exophytic squamous cell carcinoma, 111, 112, 113
   white hairy tongue, 111
   white sponge nevus, 115-117
Ketoconazole, 62, 63
Ketones, 622
Koebner's phenomenon, 553

L

Labial melanotic macule, 566, 567
Labial mucosa, 97
   intraoral lesions of, 580-581
Laboratory tests
   human immunodeficiency virus, 597
   normal values, 621-622
Lactate dehydrogenase, 622
Lamina dura
   hyperparathyroidism and, 394
   osteoporosis and, 397
   radiographic considerations, 255
   radiopacity of, 450
   thalassemia and, 402
   tooth socket sclerosis and, 502
Lamina propria, 14, 15
   erythematous macule, 51
   plasma cell gingivitis and, 85
Laminography, 6
Langerhans' cell disease, 274, 331
   basal cell nevus syndrome *versus,* 384
   chronic localized type, 372
   generalized rarefactions, 407
   multiple separate, well-defined radiolucency, 386-389
Laryngeal carcinoma, 527
Laryngocele, 30
Lateral cervical sinus, 219
Lateral fossa, 298
Lateral periodontal cyst, 305-306
Lateral pterygoid plate, 453
Lateral radicular cyst, 299, 300
Lateral region of neck, 524
   masses in, 535-539
Lee-White clotting time, 621

Leiomyoma of tongue, 154
Lentigo maligna melanoma, 198
Leser-Trélat sign, 546
Lesion
   anatomic location, 42-43, 46
   classification, 42
   detection and examination, 39
   reexamination, 41-42
   two or more present, 44-45
Letterer-Siwe disease, 387
Leucine aminopeptidase, 622
Leukemia
   generalized rarefactions, 405-406
   gingival ulcer in, 175
Leukocyte tumor necrosis factor, 165
Leukocytes
   disorders of, 61
   urinalysis, 622
Leukoedema, 97-98
   leukoplakia *versus,* 103
   white sponge nevus *versus,* 116
Leukoplakia, 98-103, 108
   hairy, 601-602
   nicotine stomatitis, 103
   premalignant, 589
   speckled, 99
Lichen planus, 106-110, Plate C
   chronic ulcerative stomatitis *versus,* 84
   leukoplakia *versus,* 103
   of lip, 563-564
   migratory glossitis *versus,* 91
   multiple ulcerations in, 75-77, 78
   white lesions and, 106-110
Lichenoid drug reaction, 77, 128
Lichenoid dysplasia, 75
Linea alba buccalis, 98, 99
Lingual foramen, 240, 241
Lingual mandibular bone defect, 311, **315-318**
   solitary cystlike radiolucency and, 315-318
Lingual thyroid gland, 157
Lingual tonsil, 132-133, 134
Lining mucosa, 17, 49-50
Lip, 561-579
   angioedema, 574
   aphthae, 568-569, 570
   brown and red lesions, 566-568, 569
   cavernous hemangioma, 191
   chancre, 173
   cheilitis glandularis, 576
   cheilitis granulomatosa and Melkersson-Rosenthal syndrome, 576
   cleft, 576-577
   contact allergy, 575
   double, 577
   erythema multiforme, 79, **570-571**
   erythematous macules, 51
   herpes simplex virus infection, 569-570, 571
   keratoacanthoma, 571-572
   lipoma, 574
   lower lip sinuses, 577, 578
   mucocele, 144, 193, 573-574
   multiple pigmentations, 567-568
   nasolabial cyst, 575
   nodular fibrous hyperplasia, 572-573
   oral melanotic macule, 192
   primary herpetic gingivostomatitis, 73
   salivary gland tumor and, 574-575
   sialolithiasis and, 575

Lip—cont'd
  superimposed radiopacity, 456
  syphilis and, 572
  traumatic ulcer, 568, 570
  white lesion, 561-566
Lipase, 622
Lipid proteinosis, 229-230
Lipochrome, 230
Lipoma, 154, **227**
  consistency of, 30
  of lip, 574
  midpalatine cyst *versus,* 326
  salivary gland tumor *versus,* 153
Liposarcoma, 30
Lobular capillary hemangioma, 549
Loose teeth as chief complaint, 40
Lower lip sinuses, 577, 578
Ludwig's angina, 54-55, 56, 526, Plate B
Lupus erythematosus, 87-88, Plate D
  leukoplakia *versus,* 102-103
  multiple ulcerations in, 87-88
  red and white lesions in, 128
Lymph nodes
  calcified, 474, 475, 496
  enlarged, 525-526
    cervical, 591
    squamous cell, 591
  lateral neck masses, 535-538
  metastasis, 591
  of neck, 522, 524-525
  oral squamous cell carcinoma and, 362
Lymphadenitis, 219, 526-527
Lymphadenopathy, 600
Lymphangioma, 144
  of alveolar ridge, 195
  brownish, bluish, or black, 197
  consistency of, 30
  pebbly surfaced mass, 22
Lymphocytes, 621
Lymphoepithelial cyst, 118, **227-228,** 537
Lymphoid hyperplasia
  benign, 526
  nontender, 526
Lymphoma, 528-529, Plate J
  bone, 438, 446
  consistency of, 31, 32
Lymphonodular pharyngitis, acute, 226-227
Lymphosarcoma, 157, 409, 620

M

Macular hemangioma
  erythroplakia *versus,* 59
  solitary red lesion, 65, 66
Macule, 20
  allergic, 65, 66
  erythema multiforme, 79
  impetigo contagiosa, 556
  labial melanotic, 566, 567
  melanotic, 192-193
  oral melanoma, 199
  red, Plate B
  traumatic erythematous, Plate A
Maffucci's syndrome, 191
Magnetic resonance imaging, 8-9
Major aphthous ulcer, 169-170
Major palatine foramen, 247
Malabsorption, osteomalacia and, 399

Malignancy
  borders of mass, 26-27
  consistency of, 31
  interradicular radiolucency, 305
  intraoral, 590
  leukoplakia and, 100
  lichen planus and, 106
  in multiple myeloma, 385
  periapical radiolucency, 272-276
  perioral, 590
  predisposition to oral candidiasis, 61
  smokeless tobacco lesion and, 105
Malignant melanoma, 548, 549
Malnutrition, osteoporosis and, 399
Mandible
  ameloblastoma, 338
  anatomic radiolucencies, 239-244
    airway shadow, 240, 242
    anterior buccal mandibular depression, 244
    cortical plate mandibular defects, 244
    lingual foramen, 240, 241
    mandibular canal, 239-240
    mandibular foramen, 239
    medial sigmoid depression, 242, 243
    mental foramen, 240, 241
    mental fossa, 242, 243
    midline symphysis, 242, 243
    pseudocyst of condyle, 244
    submandibular fossa, 240, 242
  anatomic radiopacities, 454-455
    external oblique ridge, 454
    genial tubercles, 454, 455
    mental ridge, 454
    mylohyoid ridge, 454
  aneurysmal bone cyst, 343
  cherubism, 340
  fibrous dysplasia, 364
  focal osteoporotic bone marrow defects, 321
  midline cyst of, 313
  multilocular cyst, 334
  osteoporotic, 397, 398
  phlebolith in, 497
  secondary tumors, 346
  tori, 134, 136
  traumatic bone cyst, 314
Mandibular angular cortex, 397
Mandibular canal, 239-240
Mandibular depression, anterior buccal, 244
Mandibular foramen, 239
Mandibular infected buccal cyst, 258
Marble bone disease, 512-515
Marginal gingivitis, Plate E
Marrow space, 248-249
  multilocular radiolucency, 334, 335
  multiple, 381
  solitary cystlike radiolucency, 310
Marsupialization, 194, 236
Mass
  borders of, 26-27
  extent of, 26
  fluctuance and emptiability of, 28-33, 34, 35
  inspection of, 16-24
    aspirate, 23-24
    aspiration, 20-23
    color, 16-19
    contours, 16
    flat and raised entities, 20

Mass—cont'd
  inspection of—cont'd
    needle biopsy, 24
    surfaces, 19-20, 21, 22
  mobility of, 25-26
  neck, 521-539
    general characteristics, 525
    lateral, 535-539
    median-paramedian, 534-535, 536
    parotid region, 532-534
    pathologic, 525-529
    physical examination, 522-525
    submandibular region, 529-532
  of nonspecific location, 525-529
  painless, tender, or painful, 34-38
  palpation of, 24-38
    anatomic regions and planes involved, 25
    borders, 26-27
    consistency, 28, 29-31, 32-33
    consistency of surrounding tissue, 27
    extent, 26
    fluctuance and emptiability, 28-33, 34, 35
    lesions demonstrating variable fluctuance, 33-34, 35, 37, 38
    mobility, 25-26
    painless, tender, or painful, 34-38
    size and shape, 27-28
    solitary or multiple lesions, 38
    sturdiness of underlying tissue, 27
    surface temperature, 24-25
    thickness of overlying tissue, 27
    unilateral or bilateral, 38
  size and shape, 27-28
  solitary or multiple, 38
  unilateral or bilateral, 38
Masticatory mucosa, 17, 49-50
Materia alba, 120
Maxilla
  ameloblastoma, 338
  anatomic radiolucencies, 245-248
    greater palatine foramen, 247
    incisive foramen, incisive canal, and superior foramina of incisive
      canal, 245, 246
    intermaxillary suture, 245
    maxillary sinus, 246-247, 248
    nares, 246
    nasal cavity, 245
    nasolacrimal duct or canal, 246, 247
  anatomic radiopacities, 450-453
    anterior nasal spine, 451, 452
    coronoid process, 453
    maxillary tuberosity, 453
    nasal septum and boundaries of nasal fossae, 450-451, 452
    pterygoid plates and pterygoid hamulus, 453
    walls and floor of maxillary sinus, 451, 452
    zygomatic process and zygomatic bone, 451-453
  desmoplastic ameloblastoma, 445
  fibrous dysplasia, 364
  odontoma, 424
  osteoporotic, 397
  Paget's disease and, 512
  retained roots in, 479
Maxillary canine
  adenomatoid odontogenic tumor of, 288
  normal follicular space, 281
Maxillary incisor region, 451
Maxillary ridge melanoma, 199
Maxillary sinus, 246-247, 248
  ameloblastoma, 338

Maxillary sinus—cont'd
  anatomic radiopacity, 451, 452
  antrolith in, 496
  cancer of, 362, 363, 590, Plate J
  cystlike outpouching of, 310, 312
  endodontic filling material in, 494
  hyperplasia of lining, 265-266
  interradicular radiolucency, 297, 298
  mucosal cyst of, 470
  multilocular radiolucency, 334, 335
Maxillary sinusitis, 214
Maxillary tuberosity, 453
McCune-Albright syndrome, 363
Mean corpuscular hemoglobin concentration, 621
Mean corpuscular hemoglobin content, 621
Mean corpuscular volume, 621
Medial sigmoid depression, 242, 243
Median mandibular cyst, 271, 306-307
Median rhomboid glossitis, 92, 93
Median sigmoid depression, 312
Median-paramedian region of neck, 522-524
  masses in, 534-535, 536
Medical laboratory studies, 9
Medication, predisposition to oral candidiasis, 61
Mediterranean anemia, 401-403
Melanin, 183
Melanocyte, 183
Melanocytic nevus
  facial, 547
  of lip, 566
Melanocytic tumor, 547-548, 549
Melanoma, 197-200
  consistency of, 31
  exophytic, 155, 156
  of lip, 566
  oral, 200
  superficial, Plate J
Melanoplakia, 183-184
  amalgam tattoo *versus,* 187
  melanoma *versus,* 200
  melanotic macule *versus,* 192
Melanotic macule, 192-193, 566, 567
  oral, 191-193
Melkersson-Rosenthal syndrome, 576
Membrane pemphigoid, 77
Mental foramen, 240, 241, 298
Mental fossa, 242, 243
Mental ridge, 454
Mercury contact allergy
  keratotic white lesion in, 110-111
  leukoplakia *versus,* 102
Mesenchymal tumor, 22
  exophytic, 154-155, 156, 157
  exophytic small cell carcinoma *versus,* 148
  inflammatory hyperplasia *versus,* 137
  periapical radiolucency, 274
  peripheral, 154-155
Metastatic tumor, Plate J
  basal cell nevus syndrome *versus,* 384
  bronchogenic, 330, 365
  to cervical nodes, 527-528
  consistency of, 31
  exophytic, 155-156
  jawbone, to the, 346-347
  lymph node, 591
  multilocular radiolucency, 346-347, 353
  multiple major radiographic appearances, 620
  multiple separate, well-defined radiolucency, 386

Metastatic tumor—cont'd
to oral soft tissue, 67-68
osteoblastic, 442-444, 447
red inflammatory hyperplasia lesion *versus,* 54
solitary ill-defined radiolucency, 376
solitary radiolucency with ragged and poorly defined borders, 365
solitary red lesion in, 67-68
Metronidazole, 262
Miconazole, 62
Midline cyst of mandible, 313
incisive canal cyst and, 303-305
palatal, 326-328
Midline suture, 297
Midline symphysis, 242, 243
Midpalatine cyst
solitary cystlike radiolucency, 311
solitary cystlike radiolucency not necessarily contacting teeth, 326-328
Miescher's syndrome, 576
Migratory glossitis, 90-92
keratotic white lesion in, 106
red and white lesions in, 128
Migratory mucositis, 85 86
Mikulicz' disease, 85, 533-534
Mineralized tissue shadows, 455, 456
Mixed radiolucent-radiopaque lesions
associated with teeth, 415-432
adenomatoid odontogenic tumor, 426-428
ameloblastic fibroodontoma, 428, 429
calcifying crown of developing tooth, 415-416
calcifying epithelial odontogenic tumor, 428-431
calcifying odontogenic neoplasm, 428, 429
cementoossifying fibroma, 420-423
odontoma, 423-426
periapical cementoosseous dysplasia, 418-420
rare periapical mixed lesions, 421, 422, 423
rarefying and condensing osteitis, 417-418
rarities, 431
tooth root with rarefying osteitis, 416-417
not necessarily contacting teeth, 433-448
cementoossifying fibroma, 440, 441, 447
chondroma and chondrosarcoma, 444-445, 447
chronic osteomyelitis, 434, 435-436, 447
desmoplastic ameloblastoma, 445
fibrous dysplasia, 437-439, 447
focal cementoosseous dysplasia, 437
healing surgical site, 434-435
ossifying subperiosteal hematoma, 445, 447
osteoblastic metastatic carcinoma, 442-444, 447
osteogenic sarcoma, 440-442, 447
osteoradionecrosis, 436, 447
Paget's disease, 439-440, 447
rarities, 445-447
Mobility of mass, 25-26, 525
Mole, 566
Molluscum contagiosum, Plate F
Monocytes, normal lab values, 621
Mosaic wart, 558
Mouthbreathing gingivitis, 158
Mouthrinse
carcinogenic properties, 589
oral mucosal white lesions associated with, 99
Mucobuccal fold, 227
Mucocele, 144
brownish, bluish, or black, 193-194
consistency of, 30
draining, 213
fluctuance of, 35
of lip, 573-574

Mucocele—cont'd
mucoepidermoid tumor *versus,* 202
surface of, 22
Mucoepidermoid carcinoma, 202
Mucoepidermoid tumor, 366
Mucosa
alveolar
amalgam tattoo, 186
intraoral lesions of, 581
buccal
amalgam tattoo, 186
erythematous macules, 51
exophytic intramucosal nevus on, 201
Fordyce's granules, 225
hairy leukoplakia, 602
intraoral lesions of, 580-581
leukoedema, 97
lichen planus, 107
linea alba, 98
oral lipoma, 227
recurrent intraoral herpes simplex lesion, 167, 168-169
smoker's melanosis, 185
verrucous carcinoma, 113
labial, 97, 580-581
lining, 17, 49-50
masticatory, 17, 49-50
oral
lupus erythematosus lesions of, 87
normal color, 16-17, 19, 49-50
polycythemia, 87
primary herpetic gingivostomatitis, 73
Mucosal cyst of maxillary sinus, 470
Mucositis
allergic, 129
denture, 63-64
radiation, Plate D
ulcer in, 171
Mucous glands
consistency, 29
diagram of, 15
Mucous membrane, 14
benign pemphigoid of, 80-81
melanoplakia on, 184
of palate, 582
Mucous patch, 572
Mucous retention cyst, 573
Mucous-producing salivary gland tumors, 202
Mulberry molar, 173
Multilocular cyst, 334-337, 353
Multilocular radiolucencies, 333-355
ameloblastoma, 337-340
anatomic patterns, 334, 335
aneurysmal bone cyst, 343-346
central giant cell granuloma, 340, 341
cherubism, 340-342
differential diagnosis, 353, 354
giant cell lesion of hyperparathyroidism, 340, 341
metastatic tumor to jaw, 346-347
multilocular cyst, 334-337
odontogenic keratocyst, 343, 345
odontogenic myxoma, 342-343, 344
rarities, 349-352
vascular malformations and central hemangioma of bone, 348-349
Multiple basal cell nevus syndrome, 284
Multiple fibroepithelial hyperplasia, 160
Multiple myeloma
basal cell nevus syndrome *versus,* 384
generalized rarefactions, 408

Multiple myeloma—cont'd
 multiple separate, well-defined radiolucency, 384-386
 serum values in, 411
Multiple neurofibromatosis, 202-203
Multiple separate, well-defined radiolucencies, 380-391
 anatomic variations, 380-381
 basal cell nevus syndrome, 382-384
 Langerhans' cell disease, 386-389
 metastatic carcinoma, 386
 multiple cysts or granulomas, 381-382
 multiple myeloma, 384-386
 rarities, 389-391
Multiple separate radiopacities, 500-508
 cleidocranial dysplasia, 506-507
 embedded or impacted teeth, 505-506
 hypercementosis, 504
 idiopathic osteosclerosis, 504
 mature periapical or focal cementoosseous dysplasia, 503-504
 periapical condensing osteitis, 504, 505
 rarities, 507, 508
 retained roots, 501, 502
 socket sclerosis, 501-503
 tori and exostoses, 500-501
Multiple ulcerations
 acute atrophic candidiasis, 80
 allergies, 86
 benign mucous membrane pemphigoid, 80-81
 chronic ulcerative stomatitis, 84
 desquamative gingivitis, 83
 erosive lichen planus, 75-77, 78
 erythema multiforme, 78-80
 etiology, 72
 lupus erythematosus, 87-88
 pemphigus, 81-83
 plasma cell gingivitis, 85
 polycythemia, 86-87
 primary herpetic gingivostomatitis, 73-75
 radiation and chemotherapy mucosites, 84
 rarities, 88
 recurrent aphthous stomatitis and Behçet syndrome, 72-73
 stomatitis areata migrans, 85-86
 xerostomia, 85
Mumps, 531
Munro's abscess, 86
Mural ameloblastoma, 285-288
Mural cholesteatoma, 287
Mural nodule, 288
Mycelex; *see* Clotrimazole
Mycosis fungoides, 124
Mylohyoid ridge, 454, 468
Myoblastoma
 consistency of, 31
 granular cell, 21, 157
Myoma, 31, 154
Myositis ossificans, 472
Myxoma
 consistency of, 30, 32
 cystlike, 330
 odontogenic, 320, **342-343,** 344
  multilocular radiolucency and, 342-343

N

Nare, 246
Nasal cavity, 245
 transitional cell carcinoma, Plate J
Nasal fossa, 245, 450-451, 452
Nasal septum, 450-451, 452

Nasolabial cyst, 575
Nasolacrimal canal, 246, 247
Nasolacrimal duct, 246, 247, 312
Nasopalatine cyst, 152
Nasopalatine duct, 216-217
Nasopalatine duct cyst, 303-305
Neck masses, 521-539
 anatomy and, 522-525
 general characteristics, 525
 lateral, 535-539
 median-paramedian, 534-535, 536
 parotid region, 532-534
 pathologic, 525-529
 physical examination, 522-525
 submandibular region, 529-532
Necrosis
 in gummas, 174
 sloughing, pseudomembranous, necrotic white lesion, 124
Necrotizing sialometaplasia, 177, 179
Needle biopsy, 24
Neoplasia, 131
Nerve, 15
Neurilemoma, 306, 329
Neurofibroma
 consistency of, 31
 on palate, 154
 plexiform, midpalatine cyst *versus,* 326
Neurogenic tumor, 537-538
Neuroma
 amputation, 154, 155
 consistency of, 31
Neutrophils, normal lab values, 621
Nevus
 brownish, bluish, or black, 200-202
 exophytic, 155, 156
 of lip, 566
 melanotic macule *versus,* 193
 white sponge, 115-117
Nevus araneus, 550
Nevus flammeus, 549
Nevus of Ota, 548
Nicotine stomatitis, 103-104, Plate D
 palatine papillomatosis *versus,* 141
 red and white lesions in, 128
 solitary red lesion in, 57
 white lesion in, 103-104
Nizoral; *see* Ketoconazole
Nodular fibrous hyperplasia of lip, 572-573
Nodular melanoma, 199
Nonmalignant giant cell tumor, 323
Nonpyogenic soft tissue odontogenic infection, 54-55, 56
Nonradicular cyst, 271-272
Nontender lymphoid hyperplasia, 526
Normocalcemic hyperparathyroidism, 394
Nose, 455, 468
Nutrient canal, 249, 250, 297, 298
Nutritional deficiencies, 61
Nystatin, 62

O

Occlusal problem as chief complaint, 40
Occupational acne, 555
Odontogenic cyst, 300, 301
 calcifying, 289-290, 291, 293
Odontogenic fibroma, 620
Odontogenic fibromyxoma, 293
Odontogenic infection, ulcer from, 170-171

Odontogenic keratocyst, 343, 345
   solitary cystlike radiolucency, 311
   solitary cystlike radiolucency not necessarily contacting teeth, 318-320
Odontogenic myxoma, 342-343, 344
   multilocular radiolucencies, 353
   odontogenic keratocyst *versus,* 320
   pericoronal radiolucency and, 289
Odontogenic tumor, 300, 301, 302
   adenomatoid
      mixed radiolucent-radiopaque, 426-428
      pericoronal radiolucency, 289, 290
   calcifying epithelial, 428-431
   dental follicle *versus,* 279-281
   interradicular radiolucency, 300, 301, 302
Odontoma, 423
   ameloblastic, 349, 446
   complex, 423
      periapical idiopathic osteosclerosis *versus,* 463
      periapical radiopacity, 467
      solitary radiopacity not necessarily contacting teeth, 492-493
   compound, 467-469
   compound-complex, 423
   cystic, 431
   interradicular radiolucency, 300, 301, 302
   maxillary, 424
   mixed radiolucent-radiopaque, 423-426
   multiple major radiographic appearances, 620
   solitary radiopacity not necessarily contacting teeth, 492-493
Operational diagnosis, 45-46
Oral cancer, 587-595
   detection, 590-591
   epidemiology, 587
   etiology, 587-588
   lymph node metastasis, 591
   management, 592
   premalignant lesions and predisposing conditions, 589
   prevention, 592-593
   risk factors, 587-589
   triage of lesions, 591-592
Oral mucosa
   lupus erythematosus lesions of, 87
   normal color variation in, 16-17, 19, 49-50
   polycythemia, 87
   primary herpetic gingivostomatitis, 73
Oral mucous membrane, 79, 581
Oral system
   importance of normal anatomy and histology, 14, 15-16, 17-18
   lymphatic drainage, 527
   tissues of, 15
Oral ulcer
   aphthous, Plate B, Plate F
      human immunodeficiency virus-associated, 607
      of lip, 568-569, 570
      recurrent, 165-167
      red lesions with necrotic component, 128
   defined, 163
   of lip, 568-572
   multiple
      acute atrophic candidiasis, 80
      allergies, 86
      benign mucous membrane pemphigoid, 80-81
      chronic ulcerative stomatitis, 84
      desquamative gingivitis, 83
      erosive lichen planus, 75-77, 78
      erythema multiforme, 78-80
      etiology, 72
      lupus erythematosus, 87-88

Oral ulcer—cont'd
   multiple—cont'd
      pemphigus, 81-83
      plasma cell gingivitis, 85
      polycythemia, 86-87
      primary herpetic gingivostomatitis, 73-75
      radiation and chemotherapy mucositides, 84
      rarities, 88
      recurrent aphthous stomatitis and Behçet syndrome, 72-73
      stomatitis areata migrans, 85-86
      xerostomia, 85
   in pyogenic granuloma, 138
   with red halo, 54, 55
   of salivary gland tumor, 153
   solitary, 162-181
      differential diagnosis, 176-180
      generalized mucositides and vesiculobullous diseases, 171
      minor salivary gland tumors, 176, 177
      from odontogenic infection, 170-171
      rarities, 176, 177
      secondary to systemic disease, 174-175
      sloughing, pseudomembranous, 171
      squamous cell carcinoma, 171-172
      syphilis chancre and gumma, 172-174
      traumatic, 164, 165
      traumatized tumors, 175, 176
   solitary recurrent, 165-170
      aphthous, 165-167
      atypical intraoral herpes simplex, 168-169
      Behçet syndrome, 170
      herpetiform aphtha, 170
      intraoral herpes simplex, 167-168
      major aphthous ulcer, 169-170
   tori and exostoses *versus,* 134
Organ consistency, 28
Oroantral fistula, 142, 213-214
Orocutaneous fistula, 221-222
Oronasal fistula, 215
Oropharyngeal lesion, 582
Ossifying and cementifying fibroma, 352
Ossifying subperiosteal hematoma
   mixed radiolucent-radiopaque, 445, 447
   solitary radiopacity not necessarily contacting teeth, 493
Osteitis
   condensing/sclerosing, periapical radiopacity and, 459-460
   multiple major radiographic appearances, 620
   rarefying and condensing, 417-418
   solitary ill-defined radiolucency, 376
   solitary radiolucency with ragged and poorly defined borders, 357
   solitary radiopacity not necessarily contacting teeth, 481-483
   tooth root with rarefying, 416-417
Osteitis fibrosa, 394
Osteitis fibrosa generalisata, 394
Osteoblast, 392-393
Osteoblastic metastatic carcinoma, 416
   mixed radiolucent-radiopaque, 442-444, 447
   radiolucent-radiopaque image, 438
Osteoblastoma
   multiple major radiographic appearances, 620
   periapical idiopathic osteosclerosis *versus,* 463
Osteoclast, 393
Osteogenic sarcoma, 273, Plate J
   consistency of, 31, 33
   mixed radiolucent-radiopaque, 440-442, 447
   periapical idiopathic osteosclerosis *versus,* 463
   proliferative periostitis *versus,* 492
   radiolucent-radiopaque image, 438

Osteogenic sarcoma—cont'd
  retained root tip *versus,* 416
  solitary ill-defined radiolucency, 377
  solitary radiolucency with ragged and poorly defined borders, 367-368, 369
Osteoma
  consistency of, 31
  peripheral, periapical radiopacity, 469
  proliferative periostitis *versus,* 492
  solitary radiopacities not necessarily contacting teeth, 477-478, 479
Osteomalacia
  generalized rarefactions, 399-400
  serum values in, 411
Osteomyelitis
  chronic
    diffuse sclerosing, 487-488
    draining, 215-216
    focal sclerosing, 486-487
    mixed radiolucent-radiopaque, 434, 435-436, 447
    solitary radiolucency with ragged and poorly defined borders, 358-360
  mixed radiolucent-radiopaque appearance, 439
  multiple major radiographic appearances, 620
  periapical abscess and, 263-265
  pulpoperiapical radiolucency, 263-265
  solitary ill-defined radiolucency, 376
  solitary radiopacity not necessarily contacting teeth, 486-487
  treatment, 360
Osteopetrosis, 512-515
Osteoporosis
  generalized rarefactions, 397-399
  serum values in, 411
Osteoradionecrosis
  cutaneous sinus secondary to, 216
  mixed radiolucent-radiopaque, 436, 447
  osteomyelitis *versus,* 358
Osteosarcoma, 367-368
  consistency of, 31
  multiple major radiographic appearances, 620
Osteosclerosing tumor, 458
Osteosclerosis
  idiopathic, 458
    multiple separate radiopacities, 504
    periapical radiopacity, 458-459
    solitary radiopacity not necessarily contacting teeth, 480-481, 482
  solitary radiopacity not necessarily contacting teeth, 480-481, 482
  tooth socket sclerosis, 501-503
Oxygen partial pressure, 622

P

Pachyonychia congenita, 116
Packed cell volume, 621
Paget's disease
  early stage, 407-408
  fibrous dysplasia *versus,* 484-486
  generalized radiopacities, 511-512, 513, 515-516
  generalized rarefactions, 407-408
  intermediate stage, 439-440
  mature stage, 511-512
  mixed radiolucent-radiopaque, 439-440, 447
  multiple major radiographic appearances, 620
  osteomyelitis *versus,* 265
  periapical or focal cementoosseous dysplasia *versus,* 503
  radiolucent-radiopaque image, 438-439
  serum values in, 411
Pain
  as chief complaint, 40
  in dentoalveolar abscess, 212
Pain—cont'd
  in draining cyst, 216
  in infection of submandibular gland, 213
  in mass palpation, 34-38
  in multiple myeloma, 384
  in oroantral fistula, 214
  in osteomalacia, 400
  in pulpoperiapical infection, 261
  in superficial abscess, 226
Palate, 97
  erythematous macules, 51
  exophytic squamous cell carcinoma, 146
  fovea palatinae, 210
  intraoral lesions, 582
  Kaposi's sarcoma, 605
  major recurrent aphthous ulcer, 170
  masses, 152
  melanoma, 199
  neurofibroma, 154
  normal color, 18
  papillary hyperplasia, 140-141
  petechiae and ecchymotic patches, 188
  pseudomembranous candidiasis on, 122
  psoriasis, 88
  tori, 134, 136
  verrucous carcinoma, 113
Palatine papilla cyst, 305
Palatine papillomatosis, 140-141
Palatine space abscess, 152
  from maxillary molar, 145
  midpalatine cyst *versus,* 326
Palatoglossal arch, 50, 167, Plate A
Palpation, 24-38
  anatomic regions and planes involved, 25
  borders of mass, 26-27
  consistency of mass, 28, 29-31, 32-33
  consistency of surrounding tissue, 27
  extent of mass, 26
  fluctuance and emptiability, 28-33, 34, 35
  lesions demonstrating variable fluctuance, 33-34, 35, 37, 38
  mobility, 25-26
  of neck mass, 522
  painless, tender, or painful, 34-38
  size and shape, 27-28
  solitary or multiple lesions, 38
  sturdiness of underlying tissue, 27
  surface temperature, 24-25
  of surgical defect, 323
  thickness of overlying tissue, 27
  unilateral or bilateral mass, 38
Panneck infection, 538
Panoramic radiography, 6
Papillary cyst adenoma, 35
Papillary cystadenoma lymphomatosum, 35
Papillary cystic adenoma, 30
Papillary hyperplasia, Plate A
  nicotine stomatitis *versus,* 104
  of palate, 140-141
Papilloma, 145, 146
  exophytic small cell carcinoma *versus,* 148
  keratotic white lesion in, 111, 112
  red exophytic squamous cell carcinoma *versus,* 60
  red inflammatory hyperplasia lesion *versus,* 54
  rough-surfaced mass, 21
  squamous cell, 562-563
  surface of, 22
Papillomatosis, 57
Papulosquamous dermatitides, 553-554

Paradental cyst, 284

Parathyroid hormone, calcium homeostasis and, 393

Paresthesia as chief complaint, 41

Parotid fascia, 532, 533

Parotid gland, 522
  bilateral enlargement, 533-534
  fistula, 220
  masses within, 532-533
  sialadenitis, 533
  suppurative infection of, 212-213
  tumor, Plate I

Parotid region of neck, 522, 523, 532-534

Parotitis, 220

Partial anodontia, 505

Partial thromboplastin time, 621

Parulis, 140, 262

Patent nasopalatine duct, 216-217

Patient history, 5-9, 10, 11

PCOD; *see* Periapical cementoosseous dysplasia

Pemphigoid, benign mucous membrane, 80-81, Plate C

Pemphigus, Plate C
  immunofluorescence findings, 77
  multiple ulcerations in, 81-83

Penicillin
  in dentoalveolar abscess, 262
  in syphilis, 174

Percussion, 38

Periadenitis mucosa necrotica recurrens, 169-170

Periapical cementoosseous dysplasia, 266-269
  condensing or sclerosing osteitis *versus,* 459
  mature complex odontoma *versus,* 492
  mixed radiolucent-radiopaque, 418-420
  multiple separate radiopacities, 503-504
  periapcial idiopathic osteosclerosis *versus,* 462
  periapical granuloma *versus,* 257
  periapical radiopacity, 463-465
  retained root tip *versus,* 417
  traumatic bone cyst *versus,* 270-271

Periapical condensing osteitis, 504, 505

Periapical granuloma, 255, 256

Periapical idiopathic osteosclerosis, 460-463

Periapical infection, 217

Periapical mixed lesions, 415-423
  calcifying crown of developing tooth, 415-416
  cementoossifying fibroma, 420-423
  periapical cementoosseous dysplasia, 418-420
  rare periapical mixed lesions, 421, 422, 423
  rarefying and condensing osteitis, 417-418
  tooth root with rarefying osteitis, 416-417

Periapical radiolucencies, 252-278
  anatomic patterns, 253-254
  dentigerous cyst, 266, 267
  malignant tumors, 272-276
  nonradicular cysts, 271-272
  periapical cementoosseous dysplasia, 266-269
  periodontal disease, 269-270
  pulpoperiapical, 253-265
    chronic and acute dentoalveolar abscess, 259-263
    hyperplasia of maxillary sinus lining, 265-266
    osteomyelitis, 263-265
    periapical granuloma, 256
    periapical scar, 259, 260
    radicular cyst, 256-259
    root resorption, 256
    surgical defect, 263, 264
  rarities, 274, 275, 276
  traumatic bone cyst, 270-271

Periapical radiopacities, 457-476
  false, 467-475
    anatomic structures, 467, 468
    ectopic calcifications, 470-475
    foreign bodies, 469-470
    impacted teeth, supernumerary teeth, and compound odontomas, 467-469
    mucosal cyst of maxillary sinus, 470
    rarities, 475
    retained root tips, 469
    tori, exostoses, and peripheral osteomas, 469
  sclerosing and sclerosed condition, 457-458
  sclerosing osteitis and idiopathic osteosclerosis, 458-459
  true, 459-467
    condensing or sclerosing osteitis, 459-460
    foreign bodies, 465-466
    hypercementosis, 466-467
    idiopathic osteosclerosis, 460-463
    mature periapical cementoosseous dysplasia or focal cementoosseous dysplasia, 463-465
    rarities, 467
    unerupted succedaneous teeth, 465

Periapical scar, 259, 260

Pericoronal mixed lesions, 423-431
  adenomatoid odontogenic tumor, 426-428
  ameloblastic fibroodontoma, 428, 429
  calcifying epithelial odontogenic tumor, 428-431
  odontoma, 423-426
  rarities, 431

Pericoronal radiolucencies, 279-295
  adenomatoid odontogenic tumor, 289, 290
  ameloblastic fibroma, 290-291, 292
  ameloblastoma, 289
  calcifying odontogenic cyst, 289-290, 291
  dentigerous cyst, 283-285
  differential diagnosis, 292-294
  pericoronal or follicular space, 279-283
  rarities, 291, 293, 294
  unicystic ameloblastoma, 285-288

Pericoronal space, 279-283

Periodontal abscess, 262

Periodontal cyst, 305-306

Periodontal disease
  acquired immunodeficiency syndrome-associated, 602-604, 605
  periapical radiolucency, 269-270

Periodontal ligament, 211

Periodontal ligament space, 248

Periodontal pocket, 298, 299

Periodontitis, Plate E

Perioral dermatitis, 556

Perioral system
  importance of normal anatomy and histology, 14, 15-16, 17-18
  malignancy, 590
  tissues of, 15

Periostitis ossificans, 488
  proliferative, 488-490

Peripheral fibroma with calcification, 143-144

Peripheral giant cell granuloma, 195-196

Peripheral odontogenic fibroma WHO-type, 143

Peripheral osteoma, 469

Peripheral scar tissue, 106

Persistent tuberculum impar, 157

Petechia, 187-189

Peutz-Jeghers syndrome, 203, 204, 568

pH, 622

Pharyngitis, acute lymphonodular, 226-227

Pharynx
  intraoral lesions of, 582
  lymphosarcoma in, 157

Phenotype switching, *Candida,* 60
Phenytoin hyperplasia, 158
Phlebectasia linguae, 185, 186
Phlebolith, 472, 474, 497
Phosphorus, 622
Photoallergic dermatitis, 554
Phototoxic reactions, 554
Physical examination, 5-9, 10, 11, 39-41
   of neck mass, 522-525
   in oral cancer, 589
Pigmentation
   in fibrous hyperplasia, 197
   of lip, 567-568, 569
   silver, 207
Pindborg tumor, 426, 428-431
   pericoronal mixed lesions and, 428-431
Pink as clinical feature, 16-17, 19
Pits, fistulas, and draining lesions, 209-224
Plantar wart, 558
Plaque, 120
Plasma cell, multiple myeloma and, 385
Plasma cell cheilitis, 575
Plasma cell gingivitis, 85, Plate D
Platelets, normal lab values, 621
Pleomorphic adenoma, 31, 33
Plexiform neurofibroma
   consistency of, 30, 32
   midpalatine cyst *versus,* 326
   salivary gland tumor *versus,* 153
Plunging ranula, 194
Poison ivy, 556
Polycythemia, 86-87
Polymerase chain reaction for human immunodeficiency virus, 597
Polyostotic fibrous dysplasia, 515
Port-wine stain, 549
Positron emission tomography, 8, 360
Postextraction socket
   multiple, 381
   solitary cystlike radiolucency, 311
   solitary cystlike radiolucency not necessarily contacting teeth, 312, 313
Postinfection pit, 210-211
Postmenopausal osteoporosis, 397-399
Postsurgical bone defect, 620
Postsurgical pit, 210, 211
Potassium, serum, 622
Preauricular pit, 219
Pregnancy
   chloasma gravidarum during, 205-206
   gingivitis during, Plate B
   hormonal tumor, 139
Premalignant lesion, 589
   actinic keratoses and, 540-541
   cutaneous facial, 540-543, 544
Primary herpetic gingivostomatitis
   multiple ulcerations in, 73-75
   recurrent aphthous stomatitis *versus,* 73
Primordial cyst, 271
   interradicular radiolucency, 300
   odontogenic keratocyst *versus,* 320
   solitary cystlike radiolucency, 311
   solitary cystlike radiolucency not necessarily contacting teeth, 321
Proliferative periostitis
   mixed radiolucent-radiopaque appearance, 435
   multiple major radiographic appearances, 620
   solitary radiopacity not necessarily contacting teeth, 488-492
Proliferative verrucous leukoplakia, 114, 115, Plate G
Prophylaxis for hepatitis, 616-618

Protein
   blood chemistry, 622
   urinalysis, 622
Proteinosis, lipid, 229-230
Prothrombin consumption test, 621
Prothrombin time
   in acute viral hepatitis, 612
   normal lab values, 621
Pseudocyst of condyle, 244
Pseudofolliculitis barbae, 557
Pseudofracture in osteomalacia, 400
Pseudohypha of *Candida albicans,* 61
Pseudohypoparathyroidism with osteitis fibrosa, 394
Pseudomembranous candidiasis, 128, Plate A
Pseudotumor of hemophilia, 294, 351
Psoriasis, 553-554
   on palate, 88, 177
   tongue lesion, 91
Pterygoid plates and pterygoid hamulus, 453
Puberty, hormonal tumor, 139
Pulp chamber, 248
Pulp polyp, 142
Pulpoperiapical disease, 265-266
Pulpoperiapical radiolucencies, 253-265
   chronic and acute dentoalveolar abscess, 259-263
   osteomyelitis, 263-265
   periapical granuloma, 256
   periapical scar, 259, 260
   radicular cyst, 256-259
   root resorption, 256
   surgical defect, 263, 264
Punch biopsy, 10
Purpura, 187-189
Purpuric macule
   erythroplakia *versus,* 59
   solitary red lesion, 52-53
Pus, 23
   in dentoalveolar abscess, 211
   in neck mass, 525
   in panneck infection, 538
   in sialadenitis, 532
   in submandibular abscess, 529-530
Pustule, 217, 557
Pyogenic granuloma, 120, 121, 549-550, Plate B
   fibrous hyperplasia in, 138-139
   red lesions with necrotic component in, 129
   squamous cell carcinoma *versus,* 148
Pyogenic space infection, 31
Pyostomatitis vegetans, 228-229

R

Race, development of differential diagnosis, 42
Radiation mucositis, Plate D
   multiple ulcerations in, 84
   red lesions with necrotic component in, 129
Radicular cyst, 256-259
   fluctuance of, 35
   lateral, 299, 300
   lingual mandibular bone defect *versus,* 318
   midpalatine cyst *versus,* 328
   multilocular, 336
   radiographic considerations, 256-259
   traumatic bone cyst *versus,* 270
Radiography, 5-6, 235-237
Radiolucency
   anatomic, 238-251
   interradicular, 296-298, 299

Radiolucency—cont'd
anatomic—cont'd
mandibular, 239-244
maxillary, 245-248
multilocular, 334, 335
structures common to both jaws, 248-250
generalized rarefactions in, 392-413
interradicular, 296-308
anatomic, 296-298, 299
benign nonodontogenic tumors and tumorlike conditions, 306
furcation involvement, 299
globulomaxillary cyst, 300-301, 303, 304
incisive canal cyst, 303-305
lateral periodontal cyst, 305-306
lateral radicular cyst, 299, 300
malignancies, 305
median mandibular cyst, 306-307
odontogenic tumors, 300, 301, 302
periodontal pockets, 298, 299
primordial cyst, 300
rarities, 307
traumatic bone cyst, 300
multilocular, 333-355
ameloblastoma, 337-340
anatomic patterns, 334, 335
aneurysmal bone cyst, 343-346
central giant cell granuloma, 340, 341
cherubism, 340-342
differential diagnosis, 353, 354
giant cell lesion of hyperparathyroidism, 340, 341
metastatic tumor to jaw, 346-347
multilocular cyst, 334-337
odontogenic keratocyst, 343, 345
odontogenic myxoma, 342-343, 344
rarities, 349-352
vascular malformations and central hemangioma of bone, 348-349
multiple separate, well-defined, 380-391
anatomic variations, 380-381
basal cell nevus syndrome, 382-384
Langerhans' cell disease, 386-389
metastatic carcinoma, 386
multiple cysts or granulomas, 381-382
multiple myeloma, 384-386
rarities, 389-391
periapical, 252-278
anatomic patterns, 253-254
dentigerous cyst, 266, 267
malignant tumors, 272-276
nonradicular cysts, 271-272
periapical cementoosseous dysplasia, 266-269
periodontal disease, 269-270
pulpoperiapical, 253-265; *see also* Pulpoperiapical radiolucencies
pulpoperiapical disease and hyperplasia of maxillary sinus lining, 265-266
rarities, 274, 275, 276
traumatic bone cyst, 270-271
pericoronal, 279-295
adenomatoid odontogenic tumor, 289, 290
ameloblastic fibroma, 290-291, 292
ameloblastoma, 289
calcifying odontogenic cyst, 289-290, 291
dentigerous cyst, 283-285
differential diagnosis, 292-294
pericoronal or follicular space, 279-283
rarities, 291, 293, 294
unicystic ameloblastoma, 285-288

Radiolucency—cont'd
solitary, with ragged and poorly defined borders, 356-379
chondrosarcoma, 368-372
chronic osteitis, 357
chronic osteomyelitis, 358-360
differential diagnosis, 374-378
fibrous dysplasia, 363-365
hematopoietic bone marrow defect, 360
malignant minor salivary gland tumors, 366-367
metastatic tumors to jaw, 365
osteogenic sarcoma-osteolytic type, 367-368, 369
rarities, 371, 372-373
squamous cell carcinoma, 360-363
solitary cystlike, not necessarily contacting teeth, 309-332
ameloblastoma, 321, 322
anatomic patterns, 310-312
benign nonodontogenic tumor, 329-330
central giant cell granuloma or lesion, 323-325
early stage of cementoossifying fibroma, 328-329
focal cementoosseous dysplasia, 326
focal osteoporotic bone marrow defect of jaw, 321-322
giant cell lesion of hyperparathyroidism, 325-326
incisive canal cyst, 326, 327
lingual mandibular bone defect, 315-318
midpalatine cyst, 326-328
odontogenic keratocyst, 318-320
postextraction socket, 312, 313
primordial cyst, 321
rarities, 330, 331
residual cyst, 312-314
surgical defect, 322-323
traumatic bone cyst, 314-315, 316
Radionuclide imaging, 7-8, 9, 10
Radiopacity
anatomic, 449-456
anterior nasal spine, 451, 452
bone, 450, 451
coronoid process, 453
external oblique ridge, 454
genial tubercles, 454, 455
maxillary tuberosity, 453
mental ridge, 454
mineralized tissue shadows, 456
mylohyoid ridge, 454
nasal septum and boundaries of nasal fossae, 450-451, 452
pterygoid plates and pterygoid hamulus, 453
soft tissue shadows, 455, 456
teeth, 449-450
walls and floor of maxillary sinus, 451, 452
zygomatic process of maxilla and zygomatic bone, 451-453
generalized, 508-518
differential diagnosis, 515-516
florid cementoosseous dysplasia, 509-511, 515-516
osteopetrosis, 512-515
Paget's disease, 511-512, 513, 515-516
rarities, 515, 516, 517, 518
multiple separate, 500-508
cleidocranial dysplasia, 506-507
embedded or impacted teeth, 505-506
hypercementoses, 504
idiopathic osteosclerosis, 504
mature periapical or focal cementoosseous dysplasia, 503-504
periapical condensing osteitis, 504, 505
rarities, 507, 508
retained roots, 501, 502
socket sclerosis, 501-503
tori and exostoses, 500-501

Radiopacity—cont'd
periapical, 457-476
anatomic structures, 467, 468
condensing or sclerosing osteitis, 459-460
ectopic calcifications, 470-475
foreign bodies, 465-466, 469-470
hypercementosis, 466-467
idiopathic osteosclerosis, 458-459, 460-463
impacted teeth, supernumerary teeth, and compound odontomas, 467-469
mature periapical cementoosseous dysplasia or focal cementoosseous dysplasia, 463-465
mucosal cyst of maxillary sinus, 470
rarities, 467, 475
retained root tips, 469
sclerosing and sclerosed condition, 457-458
sclerosing osteitis and idiopathic osteosclerosis, 458-459
tori, exostoses, and peripheral osteomas, 469
unerupted succedaneous teeth, 465
solitary, not necessarily contacting teeth, 477-499
condensing or sclerosing osteitis, 481-483
diffuse sclerosing osteomyelitis, 487-488, 489
fibrous dysplasia, 484-486
focal sclerosing osteomyelitis, 486-487
idiopathic osteosclerosis, 480-481, 482
mature complex odontoma, 492-493
mature focal cementoosseous dysplasia, 483-484
ossifying subperiosteal hematoma, 493
projected radiopacities, 493-498
proliferative periostitis, 488-492
retained roots, 479-480, 481
tori, exostoses, and peripheral osteomas, 477-478, 479
unerupted, impacted, and supernumerary teeth, 478-479
Ranula, 144
brownish, bluish, or black, 194
consistency of, 30, 32
draining, 213
surface of, 22
Rarefactions, generalized, 392-413
differential diagnosis, 409-412
hereditary hemolytic anemia, 400-405
homeostasis of bone, 392-393
hyperparathyroidism, 393-397
Langerhans' cell disease, 407
leukemia, 405-406
multiple myeloma, 408
normal variations in bone radiodensity, 393
osteomalacia, 399-400
osteoporosis, 397-399
Paget's disease, 407-408
rarities, 409, 410, 411
Rarefying and condensing osteitis, 417-418
Rarefying osteitis of endodontic origin, 299
Rash in systemic lupus erythematosus, 552
Raynaud's phenomenon, 553
Recombivax HB, 617
Recontouring, 237
Recurrent aphthous stomatitis, 72-73, 568-569, 570, Plate B
Recurrent oral ulcer, 165-170
aphthous, 165-167, 169-170
atypical intraoral herpes simplex, 168-169
Behçet syndrome, 170
herpetiform aphtha, 170
human immunodeficiency virus-associated, 607
intraoral herpes simplex, 167-168
Red and white lesions, 127-129
Red blood cell values, 621

Red conditions; *see also* **Red lesion**
generalized, 71-88
acute atrophic candidiasis, 80
allergies, 86
benign mucous membrane pemphigoid, 80-81
chronic ulcerative stomatitis, 84
desquamative gingivitis, 83
erosive lichen planus, 75-77, 78
erythema multiforme, 78-80
etiology, 72
lupus erythematosus, 87-88
pemphigus, 81-83
plasma cell gingivitis, 85
polycythemia, 86-87
primary herpetic gingivostomatitis, 73-75
radiation and chemotherapy mucositides, 84
rarities, 88
recurrent aphthous stomatitis and Behçet syndrome, 72-73
stomatitis areata migrans, 85-86
xerostomia, 85
of tongue, 90-95
deficiency states and, 92-93, 94
median rhomboid glossitis, 92, 93
migratory glossitis, 90-92
rarities, 93, 94
xerostomia, 93, 94
Red exophytic squamous cell carcinoma, 59-60
Red lesion
of lip, 566-568, 569
with necrotic component, 128-129
solitary, 49-70
allergic macules, 65, 66
candidiasis, 60-65
carcinoma in situ, 57-59
chemical or thermal erythematous macule, 55-57
erythroplakia, 57-59
exophytic red squamous cell carcinoma, 59-60
herald lesion of generalized stomatitis, 67
inflammatory hyperplasia lesions, 53-54
Kaposi's sarcoma, 68
macular hemangiomas and telangiectasias, 65, 66
metastatic tumors to soft tissue, 67-68
nicotine stomatitis, 57
nonpyogenic soft tissue odontogenic infection, 54-55, 56
normal variation in oral mucosa, 49-50
purpuric macules, 52-53
red macular squamous cell carcinoma, 57-59
reddish ulcers, 54, 55
traumatic erythematous macules and erosions, 50-52
vesiculobullous disease, 67
Red macular squamous cell carcinoma, 57-59
Red macule, Plate B
Red parulis, Plate A
Reddish ulcer, 54, 55
Reduced enamel epithelium, 279
Refraction phenomena, 183
Reiter's syndrome, 88, 91
Renal dysfunction
in hyperparathyroidism, 396
in multiple myeloma, 385
Rendu-Osler-Weber syndrome
lip lesion in, 568
petechial lesions and, 188
telangiectasia in, 65
Resection
of ameloblastoma, 340
of chondrosarcoma, 372

Resection—cont'd
  of odontogenic keratocyst, 320
  with or without continuity defect, 236
  of vascular malformations of bone, 349
Residual cyst
  lingual mandibular bone defect *versus,* 318
  mixed radiolucent-radiopaque appearance, 434
  multilocular, 336
  odontogenic keratocyst *versus,* 320
  solitary cystlike radiolucency, 311
  solitary cystlike radiolucency not necessarily contacting teeth,
    312-314
Retained root
  mixed radiolucent-radiopaque, 416-417
  multiple separate radiopacities, 501, 502
  periapical radiopacity, 469
  solitary radiopacity not necessarily contacting teeth, 479-480, 481
Retention phenomenon mucocele, 153
Reticular lichen planus, Plate C
Reticulum cell sarcoma
  ill-defined, ragged radiolucency, 371
  multiple major radiographic appearances, 620
  solitary ill-defined radiolucency, 377
Retinoblastoma, 411
Retrocuspid papilla, 134
Retromolar papilla, 134
Retromolar region, 582
Reversible leukoplakia, 100
Rhabdomyoma, 154
  consistency of, 32
  mobility of, 26
Rhabdomyosarcoma, 157, 273
Rhinolith, 473-474
Rhinophyma, 556
Riedel's thyroiditis, 535
Ritonavir, 607
Root canal, 248
Root resorption
  in chondrosarcoma, 445
  pulpoperiapical radiolucency, 256
  radiographic considerations, 256
Rosacea, 55-556
Rough surfaced mass, 22
Rubbery consistency, 28

S

Saddle nose, 173
Saliva as chief complaint, 41
Salivary gland
  calculus, 471-472, 473
  fistula or sinus, 220-221
  palpation of, 25
  suppurative infection of, 212-213
Salivary gland tumor
  consistency of, 31
  exophytic, 149-154
  lip manifestations, 574-575
  mucous-producing, 202
  red metastatic tumor *versus,* 68
  small cell carcinoma *versus,* 149
  **solitary radiolucency with ragged and poorly defined borders,
    366-367, 377**
  surface of, 22
  ulcerated, 176, 177
Sarcoma
  Ewing's, 293, 373
    multiple major radiographic appearances, 620

Sarcoma—cont'd
  Ewing's—cont'd
    proliferative periostitis *versus,* 491-492
    solitary ill-defined radiolucency, 377
  osteogenic, 273
    mixed radiolucent-radiopaque, 440-442, 447
    **solitary radiolucency with ragged and poorly defined borders,
      367-368, 369**
  reticulum cell, 620
Scar tissue
  keratotic white lesion, 106
  periapical radiolucency, 259, 260
Schwannoma, 31
Scintigraphy, 8
Scleroderma, 553
Sclerosing agents, 191-192
Sclerosing liposarcoma, 31
Sclerosing osteitis
  periapical radiopacity, 458-460
  solitary radiopacity not necessarily contacting teeth,
    481-483
Sclerosing osteomyelitis, 458
Sebaceous cyst
  aspirate from, 23
  chronic draining, 219
  consistency of, 30
  mobility of, 25
  in neck, 529
Sebaceous gland, 15, 17
Sebaceous hyperplasia, 546
Seborrheic dermatitis, 554
Seborrheic keratosis, 21, 22, 546
Second brachial sinus, 219
Senile hemangioma, 549
Senile osteoporosis, 397-399
Sensory nerve encroachment, 36-38
Serology
  in hepatitis A, 612
  in hepatitis B, 614, 615
  in lupus erythematosus, 87
Serous glands, 15
Serum alkaline phosphatase, 400
Serum electrolytes and blood gas, 622
Serum enzymes, 622
Serum glutamic oxaloacetic transaminase, 622
Serum glutamic pyruvic transaminase, 622
Shingles, 557
Sialadenitis, 530-532, 533
Sialolith, 471-472, 473
  of minor salivary gland, 498
  multiple separate radiopacities, 508
  in Wharton's duct, 158, 494
Sialolithiasis, 575
Sickle cell anemia
  acute necrotic ulcerative gingivitis *versus,* 122
  generalized rarefactions, 403-405
  oral ulcers in, 174, 175
Sickle cell crisis, 403
Silver pigmentation, 207
Sinuses, 218-221
  differential diagnosis, 222-223
  lower lip, 577, 578
  thyroglossal duct, 218-219
Size and shape of mass, 27-28
Sjögren's syndrome, 85
  parotid enlargement in, 534
  tongue changes in, 94

Solitary radiolucency—cont'd
  cystlike, not necessarily contacting teeth—cont'd
    benign nonodontogenic tumor, 329-330
    central giant cell granuloma or lesion, 323-325
    early stage of cementoossifying fibroma, 328-329
    focal cementoosseous dysplasia, 326
    focal osteoporotic bone marrow defect of jaw, 321-322
    giant cell lesion of hyperparathyroidism, 325-326
    incisive canal cyst, 326, 327
    lingual mandibular bone defect, 315-318
    midpalatine cyst, 326-328
    odontogenic keratocyst, 318-320
    postextraction socket, 312, 313
    primordial cyst, 321
    rarities, 330, 331
    residual cyst, 312-314
    surgical defect, 322-323
    traumatic bone cyst, 314-315, 316
  with ragged and poorly defined borders, 356-379
    chondrosarcoma, 368-372
    chronic osteitis, 357
    chronic osteomyelitis, 358-360
    differential diagnosis, 374-378
    fibrous dysplasia, 363-365
    hematopoietic bone marrow defect, 360
    malignant minor salivary gland tumors, 366-367
    metastatic tumors to jaw, 365
    osteogenic sarcoma-osteolytic type, 367-368, 369
    rarities, 371, 372-373
    squamous cell carcinoma, 360-363
Solitary radiopacities not necessarily contacting teeth, 477-499
  condensing or sclerosing osteitis, 481-483
  diffuse sclerosing osteomyelitis, 487-488, 489
  fibrous dysplasia, 484-486
  focal sclerosing osteomyelitis, 486-487
  idiopathic osteosclerosis, 480-481, 482
  mature complex odontoma, 492-493
  mature focal cementoosseous dysplasia, 483-484
  ossifying subperiosteal hematoma, 493
  projected radiopacities, 493-498
  proliferative periostitis, 488-492
  retained roots, 479-480, 481
  tori, exostoses, and peripheral osteomas, 477-478, 479
  unerupted, impacted, and supernumerary teeth, 478-479
Solitary red lesion, 49-70
  allergic macules, 65, 66
  candidiasis, 60-65
  carcinoma in situ, 57-59
  chemical or thermal erythematous macule, 55-57
  erythroplakia, 57-59
  exophytic red squamous cell carcinoma, 59-60
  herald lesion of generalized stomatitis, 67
  inflammatory hyperplasia lesions, 53-54
  Kaposi's sarcoma, 68
  macular hemangiomas and telangiectasias, 65, 66
  metastatic tumors to soft tissue, 67-68
  nicotine stomatitis, 57
  nonpyogenic soft tissue odontogenic infection, 54-55, 56
  normal variation in oral mucosa, 49-50
  purpuric macules, 52-53
  red macular squamous cell carcinoma, 57-59
  reddish ulcers, 54, 55
  traumatic erythematous macules and erosions, 50-52
  vesiculobullous disease, 67
Sonography, 9, 11
Sores as chief complaint, 40
Space abscess, 22

Specific gravity of urine, 622
Speckled erythroplakia, 59, Plate G
Speckled leukoplakia, 101, 128, Plate G
Spider angioma, 550
Splenomegaly in sickle cell anemia, 403
Squamous cell carcinoma, 179-180, Plate B, Plate G, Plate H, Plate I
  consistency of, 31, 33
  exophytic, 146-149, 151
  etiology, 587-588
  facial, 541-542
  inflammatory hyperplasia *versus,* 137
  intraoral, 588
  keratoacanthoma *versus,* 542
  laryngeal, 527
  lichen planus and, 75
  lymph node metastatis, 581
  management, 592
  orocutaneous fistula and, 221
  periapical radiolucency, 274-275
  premalignancy, 589
  prevention, 587-588
  red and white lesions in, 128
  red metastatic tumor *versus,* 68
  risk factors, 587-588
  solitary ill-defined radiolucency, 376, 377
  solitary radiolucency with ragged and poorly defined borders, 360-363
  symptoms and signs, 589-590
  tumor classification, 592
  ulcerative, 171-172
  white exophytic, 111, 112, 113
Squamous cell papilloma, 562-563
Stafne's cyst, 316-318, 328-329
Stain, toluidine blue, 11-12
Staphylococcal node abscess, 529-530
Staphylococcus aureus
  in angular cheilitis, 562
  in infection of parotid and submandibular glands, 212
Static bone cyst, 315
Sternocleidomastoid muscle mass, 536-537
Stevens-Johnson syndrome, 79, 570-571, Plate C
Stomatitis
  aphthous, 72-73, 568-569, 570
  chronic ulcerative, 84
  denture, 63-64
  diffuse gangrenous, 124-125
  herald lesion of generalized, 67
  major ulcer, 169-170
  nicotine, 57, 103-104
  red lesions with necrotic component, 128
Stomatitis areata migrans, 85-86
Strawberry hemangioma, 549
Streptococcal infection
  aspiration in, 23-24
  consistency of, 31
Striae of Wickham, 563
Sturdiness of underlying tissue, 27
Sturge-Weber syndrome
  lip lesion in, 568
  red macular hemangioma in, 65, 66
Subcutaneous tissue of neck, 522
Submandibular fossa, 240, 242
Submandibular gland, 522
  masses separate from, 529
  masses within, 530, 531
  sialadenitis, 530-531
  sialolith, 472

Submandibular gland—cont'd
  suppurative infection of, 212-213
  ultrasound image of, 11
Submandibular lymph node, 472
Submandibular region of neck, 522, 523
  masses in, 529-532
Submaxillary gland
  palpation of, 25
  sialoliths in, 495
Submental mass, 535
Submucous fibrosis, 106
Subperiosteal erosion, 394, 395
Subperiosteal hematoma, 620
Subtraction radiography, 6-7
Superficial abscess, 226
Superficial cyst, 194-195
Superficial melanoma, Plate J
Superficial nodule of tonsillar tissue, 226
Superficial spreading melanoma, 192-193, 198-199
Superimposed osteomyelitis, 447
Superimposed radiopacities, 455, 456
Superior foramina of incisive canal, 245, 246
Supernumerary tooth
  impacted, 468
  periapical radiopacity, 467-469
  solitary radiopacity not necessarily contacting teeth, 478-479
Suppurative lymphadenitis, 219
Surface as clinical feature, 19-20, 21, 22
Surface temperature, 24-25
Surgical defect, 263, 264
  pulpoperiapical radiolucency, 263, 264
  solitary cystlike radiolucency, 311, 322-323
Surgical dressing reaction, Plate D
Surgical procedures, standardized terms, 236-237
Sutton's disease, 106, 169-170
Sweat glands, 17
Swelling as chief complaint, 41
Sycosis barbae, 557
Syphilis
  candidiasis *versus,* 123
  chancre and gumma, 172-174
  lip manifestations, 572
  oronasal fistula and, 215
Syphilitic glossitis, 93, 94
Syringoma, 543-545
Systemic disease ulcer
  secondary, 174-175
  sloughing, pseudomembranous, necrotic white lesion in, 124
Systemic lupus erythematosus, 87
  discoid lesion in, 564
  facial manifestations, 551-552
  immunofluorescence findings, 77
Systemic sclerosis of lip, 564-565

T
Telangiectasia, 65, 66
Temporomandibular joint, 6
Tennis racket, 334
Tentative diagnosis, 45-46
Teratoma, 228
Tetracycline, 73, 166
Thalassemia, 401-403
Thermal erythematous macule, 55-57
Thickness of overlying tissue, 27
Third molar
  basal cell nevus syndrome and, 383
  calcifying crowns of, 416

Third molar—cont'd
  cementoossifying fibroma, 441
  developing tooth crypt, 250
  primordial cyst, 321
  unerupted, 478
Thrombin time, 621
Thrombocytopenic purpura, 188
Thyroglossal cyst, 24, 535, 536
Thyroglossal duct sinus, 218-219
Thyroid, 522-524
  cartilage of, 524
  ectopic, 119
  lingual, 157
  mass in, 534-535, 536
Thyroiditis, 534
Thyrotoxic osteoporosis, 399
Tissue
  consistency of, 28
  human immunodeficiency virus in, 596
  inspection of, 16-24
    aspirate, 23-24
    aspiration, 20-23
    color, 16-19
    contours, 16
    flat and raised entities, 20
    needle biopsy, 24
    surfaces, 19-20, 21, 22
  oral and perioral, 15
  palpation of, 24-38
    anatomic regions and planes involved, 25
    borders of mass, 26-27
    consistency of mass, 28, 29-31, 32-33
    consistency of surrounding tissue, 27
    extent of mass, 26
    fluctuance and emptiability, 28-33, 34, 35
    lesions demonstrating variable fluctuance, 33-34, 35, 37, 38
    mobility, 25-26
    painless, tender, or painful, 34-38
    size and shape, 27-28
    solitary or multiple lesions, 38
    sturdiness of underlying tissue, 27
    surface temperature, 24-25
    thickness of overlying tissue, 27
    unilateral or bilateral mass, 38
TNM system, 592
Tobacco, oral cancer and, 588
Toluidine blue staining, 11-12
Tomography, 6
Tongue
  candidiasis on, 123
  cavernous hemangioma, 191
  erythematous macules, 51
  exophytic squamous cell carcinoma, 146
  fissured, 180
  hairy
    black, 196-197
    white, 111
    yellow, 226
  hairy leukoplakia, 602
  intraoral lesions of, 582-583
  Kaposi's sarcoma, 605
  leiomyoma of, 154
  lymphatic drainage, 528
  magnetic resonance scan through, 10
  papilloma, 146
  red conditions, 90-95
    deficiency states and, 92-93, 94

Tongue—cont'd
 red conditions—cont'd
  median rhomboid glossitis, 92, 93
  migratory glossitis, 90-92
  rarities, 93, 94
  xerostomia, 93, 94
 varicosity, 185, 186
 verrucous carcinoma, 113
Tonsillar node, 526
Tonsillar tissue, 226
Tooth
 anatomic radiopacity, 449-450
 impacted
  dentigerous cyst and, 284
  multiple separate radiopacities, 505-506
  periapical radiopacity, 467-469
  pericoronal space, 281, 282
  solitary radiopacity not necessarily contacting teeth, 478-479
 multiple major radiographic appearances, 620
 root with rarefying osteitis, 416-417
 supernumerary
  impacted, 468
  periapical radiopacity, 467-469
  solitary radiopacity not necessarily contacting teeth, 478-479
Tooth crypt
 developing, 249, 250
 interradicular radiolucency, 297
 solitary cystlike radiolucency, 310-312
Tooth enamel, 449-450
Tooth eruption, dental follicle and, 279
Tooth socket sclerosis, 501-503
Torus
 consistency of, 33
 exophytic, 134-136
 generalized radiopacity, 517
 multiple separate radiopacities, 500-501
 periapical radiopacity, 469
 proliferative periostitis *versus,* 492
 solitary radiopacity not necessarily contacting teeth, 477-478, 479
Transitional cell carcinoma of nasal cavity, Plate J
Transverse processes, 524
Trauma, hematoma and, 189
Traumatic bone cyst
 interradicular radiolucency, 300
 periapical radiolucency, 270-271
 pseudomultilocular radiolucency, 334
 solitary cystlike radiolucency, 311
 solitary cystlike radiolucency not necessarily contacting teeth, 314-315, 316
Traumatic erythema, 59
Traumatic erythematous macule, 50-52, Plate A
Traumatic ulcer, 164, 165
 of lip, 568, 570
 sloughing, pseudomembranous, necrotic white lesion, 120
Traumatized tumor, ulcer in, 175, 176
Trench mouth, 121
Treponema pallidum, 172
Triamcinolone acetonide, 164
Trichoepithelioma, 543, 544
True periapical radiopacities, 459-467
 condensing or sclerosing osteitis, 459-460
 foreign bodies, 465-466
 hypercementosis, 466-467
 idiopathic osteosclerosis, 460-463
 mature periapical cementoosseous dysplasia or focal cementoosseous dysplasia, 463-465
 rarities, 467
 unerupted succedaneous teeth, 465

Tuberculous adenitis, 527
Tuberculous node, 30, 32
Tumor
 borders of mass, 26-27
 classification in oral cancer, 592
 odontogenic, 300, 301, 302
 painful, 36
Turban tumor, 545
Tylenol burn, Plate D

U

Ulcer
 aphthous, Plate B, Plate F
  human immunodeficiency virus-associated, 607
  of lip, 568-569, 570
  recurrent, 165-167
  red lesions with necrotic component, 128
 defined, 163
 of lip, 568-572
 multiple
  acute atrophic candidiasis, 80
  allergies, 86
  benign mucous membrane pemphigoid, 80-81
  chronic ulcerative stomatitis, 84
  desquamative gingivitis, 83
  erosive lichen planus, 75-77, 78
  erythema multiforme, 78-80
  etiology, 72
  lupus erythematosus, 87-88
  pemphigus, 81-83
  plasma cell gingivitis, 85
  polycythemia, 86-87
  primary herpetic gingivostomatitis, 73-75
  radiation and chemotherapy mucositides, 84
  rarities, 88
  recurrent aphthous stomatitis and Behçet syndrome, 72-73
  stomatitis areata migrans, 85-86
  xerostomia, 85
 in pyogenic granuloma, 138
 with red halo, 54, 55
 of salivary gland tumor, 153
 solitary, 162-181
  differential diagnosis, 176-180
  generalized mucositides and vesiculobullous diseases, 171
  minor salivary gland tumors, 176, 177
  from odontogenic infection, 170-171
  rarities, 176, 177
  secondary to systemic disease, 174-175
  sloughing, pseudomembranous, 171
  squamous cell carcinoma, 171-172
  syphilis chancre and gumma, 172-174
  traumatic, 164, 165
  traumatized tumors, 175, 176
 solitary recurrent, 165-170
  aphthous, 165-167
  atypical intraoral herpes simplex, 168-169
  Behçet syndrome, 170
  herpetiform aphtha, 170
  intraoral herpes simplex, 167-168
  major aphthous ulcer, 169-170
 tori and exostoses *versus,* 134
Ulcerative carcinoma, 22
Ultrasonography, 9, 11
Unerupted tooth
 periapical radiopacity, 465
 solitary radiopacity not necessarily contacting teeth, 478-479

Unicystic ameloblastoma, 285-288
Universal precautions in viral hepatitis, 618
Uremia, oral ulcers in, 174, 175
Uremic stomatitis, 88
Uric acid, 622
Urinalysis, 622
Uvula, 582

V

Vaccine
   hepatitis, 616-618
   human immunodeficiency virus, 607
Varicella, 557
Varicosity, 144, **185-186**
   consistency of, 30
   hemangioma *versus,* 191
Vascular lesion, multilocular radiolucency and, 348-349
Vascular malformation, 348-349
Vascular tumor
   consistency of, 30
   cutaneous facial, 548-551
Venereal wart, 558
Verruca vulgaris, 145, 146
   exophytic small cell carcinoma *versus,* 148
   keratotic white lesion in, 111, 112
   leukoplakia *versus,* 101-102
   of lip, 563
   red inflammatory hyperplasia lesion *versus,* 54
   surface of, 22
Verruciform xanthoma, 119
Verrucous carcinoma, 113-115, Plate G
   exophytic, 148, 149
   keratotic white lesion in, 113-115
   leukoplakia *versus,* 102
   surface of, 22
   verrucous hyperplasia *versus,* 114
Verrucous hyperplasia, 114
Verrucous leukoplakia, 100, Plate G
   proliferative, 114
Vesicle of recurrent intraoral herpes simplex lesion, 167-168
Vesiculobullous disease
   red and white lesion, 129
   solitary red lesion, 67
   ulcer in, 171
Vestibule lesion, 580-581
Vincent's infection, 121-122, 602-603
Viral hepatitis, 611-619
   acute, 611-612
   dental implications, 617, 618
   medical management, 616
   prophylaxis and vaccines, 616-618
   type A, 612
   type B, 612-614, 615
   type C, 614-615
   type E, 616
   type F and G, 616
Viral infection, cutaneous facial lesions, 557-558
Viral warts, 558
Vitamin C deficiency, 399
Vitamin D deficiency
   osteomalacia and, 399
   serum values in, 411
von Recklinghausen's disease, 202-203

W

Waldeyer's ring, 132-133, 134
Wart, 558

Warthin's tumor
   consistency of, 30
   fluctuance of, 35
Wen, 547
Western blot test, 597
Wharton's duct sialolith, 494
White as clinical feature, 17-18
White blood cell values, 621
White hairy leukoplakia, Plate E
White hairy tongue, 111
White lesion, 96-126
   keratotic, 97-117
      electrogalvanic and mercury contact allergy, 110-111
      hairy leukoplakia, 115
      hypertrophic or hyperplastic candidiasis, 115
      leukoedema, 97-98
      leukoplakia, 98-103, 108
      lichen planus, 106-110
      lichenoid drug reaction, 110
      linea alba buccalis, 98, 99
      migratory glossitis, 106
      nicotine stomatitis, 103-104
      papilloma, verruca vulgaris, and condyloma acuminatum, 111, 112
      peripheral scar tissue, 106
      rarities, 117, 118, 119
      skin grafts, 117, 118
      smokeless tobacco lesion, 104-105
      verrucous carcinoma, 113-115
      white exophytic squamous cell carcinoma, 111, 112, 113
      white hairy tongue, 111
      white sponge nevus, 115-117
   of lip, 561-566
   red lesions with, 128
   sloughing, pseudomembranous, necrotic, 117-125
      acute necrotic ulcerative gingivitis, 121-122
      candidiasis, 122-124
      chemical burns, 120-121
      diffuse gangrenous stomatitis, 124-125
      necrotic ulcers of systemic disease, 124
      plaque, 120
      pyogenic granuloma, 120, 121
      thrush, 122-124
      traumatic ulcer, 120
      trench mouth, 121-122, 602-603
      Vincent's infection, 121-122, 602-603
White sponge nevus, 101, 115-117
Working diagnosis, 45-46

X

Xanthelasma, 558-559
Xanthoma, 30
Xerostomia
   as chief complaint, 41
   multiple ulcerations in, 85
   red lesions with necrotic component, 129
   red tongue of, 93, 94

Y

Yellow as clinical feature, 18
Yellow conditions, 225-231
   acute lymphonodular pharyngitis, 226-227
   carotenemia, 230
   epidermoid and dermoid cysts, 228
   fibrin clots, 226
   Fordyce's granules, 225-226
   jaundice or icterus, 229
   lipid proteinosis, 229-230

Yellow conditions—cont'd
  lipoma, 227
  lymphoepithelial cyst, 227-228
  lymphonodular pharyngitis, 226-227
  pyostomatitis vegetans, 228-229
  rarities, 230
  superficial abscess, 226
  superficial nodules of tonsillar tissue, 226
  yellow hairy tongue, 226
Yellow hairy tongue, 226

Z

Zalcitabine, 607
Zidovudine, 607
Zygomatic bone, 451-453
Zygomatic process, 451-453